AF722259

Respiratory Physiology and Therapeutics

Respiratory Physiology and Therapeutics

Editor: Briana Johnson

AMERICAN
MEDICAL PUBLISHERS
www.americanmedicalpublishers.com

AMERICAN
MEDICAL PUBLISHERS
www.americanmedicalpublishers.com

Cataloging-in-Publication Data

Respiratory physiology and therapeutics / edited by Briana Johnson.
p. cm.
Includes bibliographical references and index.
ISBN 979-8-88740-575-9
1. Respiratory organs. 2. Respiratory organs--Diseases. 3. Respiratory organs--Diseases--Treatment.
4. Respiration. I. Johnson, Briana.
RC731 .R47 2023
616.2--dc23

© American Medical Publishers, 2023

American Medical Publishers,
41 Flatbush Avenue,
1st Floor, New York,
NY 11217, USA

ISBN 979-8-88740-575-9 (Hardback)

This book contains information obtained from authentic and highly regarded sources. Copyright for all individual chapters remain with the respective authors as indicated. All chapters are published with permission under the Creative Commons Attribution License or equivalent. A wide variety of references are listed. Permission and sources are indicated; for detailed attributions, please refer to the permissions page and list of contributors. Reasonable efforts have been made to publish reliable data and information, but the authors, editors and publisher cannot assume any responsibility for the validity of all materials or the consequences of their use.

Trademark Notice: Registered trademark of products or corporate names are used only for explanation and identification without intent to infringe.

Contents

Preface

Human respiratory system is composed of oropharynx, nose, trachea, larynx, bronchi, bronchioles and lungs. The basic function of the respiratory system is to perform gas exchange between the environment and the bloodstream. There are various conditions that affect the respiratory system, including asthma, infection, aging, allergies, and respiratory diseases, such as chronic obstructive pulmonary disease (COPD) and lung cancer. The treatments for respiratory diseases include medications, lung transplant and interventional bronchoscopy. Some preventive measures such as regular exercise, eating a healthy diet, and quitting smoking play a crucial role in the management of these diseases. This book includes some of the vital pieces of work being conducted across the world, on various topics related to the physiology and therapeutics of respiratory diseases. From theories to research to practical applications, case studies related to all contemporary topics of relevance to this field of study have been included herein. This book will provide comprehensive knowledge to the readers.

All of the data presented henceforth, was collaborated in the wake of recent advancements in the field. The aim of this book is to present the diversified developments from across the globe in a comprehensible manner. The opinions expressed in each chapter belong solely to the contributing authors. Their interpretations of the topics are the integral part of this book, which I have carefully compiled for a better understanding of the readers.

At the end, I would like to thank all those who dedicated their time and efforts for the successful completion of this book. I also wish to convey my gratitude towards my friends and family who supported me at every step.

Editor

1

Where we Stand: Lung Organotypic Living Systems that Emulate Human-Relevant Host–Environment/Pathogen Interactions

*Rocio J. Jimenez-Valdes[1], Uryan I. Can[1], Brian F. Niemeyer[1] and Kambez H. Benam[1,2,3]**

[1] Division of Pulmonary Sciences and Critical Care Medicine, Department of Medicine, University of Colorado Anschutz Medical Campus, Aurora, CO, United States, [2] Department of Bioengineering, University of Colorado Denver, Aurora, CO, United States, [3] Linda Crnic Institute for Down Syndrome, University of Colorado Anschutz Medical Campus, Aurora, CO, United States

***Correspondence:**
Kambez H. Benam
kambez.benam@cuanschutz.edu

Lung disorders such as chronic obstructive pulmonary disease (COPD) and lower respiratory tract infections (LRTIs) are leading causes of death in humans globally. Cigarette smoking is the principal risk factor for the development of COPD, and LRTIs are caused by inhaling respiratory pathogens. Thus, a thorough understanding of host–environment/pathogen interactions is crucial to developing effective preventive and therapeutic modalities against these disorders. While animal models of human pulmonary conditions have been widely utilized, they suffer major drawbacks due to inter-species differences, hindering clinical translation. Here we summarize recent advances in generating complex 3D culture systems that emulate the microarchitecture and pathophysiology of the human lung, and how these platforms have been implemented for studying exposure to environmental factors, airborne pathogens, and therapeutic agents.

Keywords: spheroids, organoids, bio-scaffolds, precision cut lung slices, bronchial biopsies, 3D bioprinting, lung-on-a-chip, inhalation models

INTRODUCTION

Lung disorders represent a great socioeconomic challenge and a major burden on health care systems worldwide; chronic obstructive pulmonary disease (COPD) and lower respiratory tract infections (LRTIs) are the third and fourth leading causes of death globally, respectively (World Health Organization [WHO], 2018). Cigarette smoke exposure is the principal risk factor for COPD development and exacerbation, and LRTIs are consequent to inhalation of airborne pathogens. Therefore, a better understanding of the pulmonary system at health and disease and recreation of respiratory host–environment/pathogen interactions are crucial if we are to prevent and treat lung disorders. While animal models of human respiratory conditions have been instrumental in advancing our knowledge, they suffer major drawbacks due to inter-species (e.g., genetic, homeostatic physiology, pathology, and respiratory tree anatomy, airway histology, etc.) differences hindering clinical translation. Rodent animal models, for instance, which have widely been applied to shed light on signaling networks and lung development, are fundamentally different from humans in terms of lung cellular composition, airway branching, and immune system function (Rackley and Stripp, 2012). Besides, rodents are obligate nose breathers with intricate and highly developed nasal turbinates that lead to different particulate deposition patterns compared to humans during breathing (Hecht, 2005). Due to these factors, rodents at best are passive inhalers and, unlike humans, are unable to actively inhale therapeutic candidates or cigarette smoke.

To circumvent some of these shortcomings with animal models, simple two-dimensional (2D) cell culture models that emulate naturally present lung air–liquid interface (ALI) have been developed to study human lung pathophysiology *in vitro* (Prunieras et al., 1983). Recently, these systems have been used in combination with cell exposure systems that mimic the natural route of exposure of lung epithelium to environmental factors in order to measure the risks of potentially damaging inhaled nanoparticles (Lenz et al., 2009) or cigarette smoke (Thorne and Adamson, 2013). However, despite their use of primary human lung airway epithelial cells (hAECs) and recapitulation of mucociliated histology, they have several limitations in recreating organ-level functionalities of the human lung. For example, they do not enable (1) real-time analysis of dynamic intercellular (e.g., leukocyte-endothelial cell) interactions under physiological flow, (2) study of inhalation exposure to whole cigarette smoke, as a representative inhaled material, under physiological breathing airflow without disturbing ALI, (3) recreation of blood-like vascular perfusion to continually supply nutrients and growth factors, (4) introduction and perturbation of vascular and airflow shear stress to simulate different pathophysiological conditions, and (5) high-resolution kinetic analysis of biological responses (e.g., the time-course release of secreted factors, like cytokines/chemokines, in response to pathogenic challenge) (Fang and Eglen, 2017; Ainslie et al., 2019). In addition, these platforms are commonly used in the absence of sub-epithelial extracellular matrix (ECM; Yamaya et al., 1992; Gray et al., 1996).

Recent advances in tissue engineering and microfabrication have led to the development and application of more complex 3D culture systems and biomimetic microfluidic platforms to capture the structural and functional complexity of the human lung (Miller and Spence, 2017). In this review, we assess these state-of-the-art complex *in vitro* lung models, and the efforts made to expose these models to environmental factors, pathogens, and therapeutic agents. Finally, we discuss future directions on tackling the challenges of *in vitro* lung models that were observed over the past decade and share our vision on how to further enhance these models for more accurate and better clinical translation.

RECENT ADVANCES IN CREATING COMPLEX 3D *IN VITRO* MODELS OF HUMAN LUNG

Spheroids and Organoids

Among the simplest of the 3D lung models are spheroids. Spheroids are multicellular sphere-like culture systems that enable recapitulation of cell–cell interactions; they are either utilized as freely floating cell aggregates or get seeded onto 3D bio-scaffolds (Ainslie et al., 2019). Spheroids utilize tumor-derived cells, patient-derived xenograft cells, and immortalized cell lines, and have been applied to study intercellular interactions and response to therapies in the context of cancer (Ekert et al., 2014; Meenach et al., 2016; Klameth et al., 2017; Lewis et al., 2018), lung progenitor cells differentiation (Chimenti et al., 2017), and pulmonary fibrosis (Surolia et al., 2017). However, spheroid culture systems still suffer deficiencies such as a lack of vasculature and ALI, hard to control cell ratios and aggregate size, as well as a failure to mimic organ function (Fang and Eglen, 2017); therefore, spheroids do not represent good *in vitro* lung models to study host–environment/pathogen interactions. Another similar yet distinct preclinical system is organoids; these are cultured organ-specific cell types, which are derived from a population of stem cells (adult or pluripotent), and are capable of maintaining stem cells during *in vitro* culture. During formation, organoids develop into 3D tissues that recreate *in vivo*-observed microanatomy through self-organization (Fang and Eglen, 2017; Ainslie et al., 2019). Compared to spheroids, organoids exhibit long-term viability and rely on internal developmental processes (rather than cell–cell adhesions) to drive tissue/organ-like microarchitecture formation. Human lung organoids have been generated to replicate bronchi/bronchioles (Konishi et al., 2016; Mccauley et al., 2017; Miller et al., 2018), alveoli (Zacharias et al., 2018), and even multi-lineage structures (Dye et al., 2016). While helpful in advancing our understanding of the respiratory system, particularly from a developmental perspective, this models lack several of key organ features such as vascularization, and mechanical forces associated with breathing, and it is difficult to obtain fully differentiated lung cell types (Barkauskas et al., 2017). Lung organoids have been sparsely used for host–environment/pathogen exposure studies, since the organoid lumen, which represents the apical surface of the lungs through which a natural exposure would occur *in vivo*, is difficult to access, thus treatments or stimuli are applied in the environment in which the organoids are embedded. In this scenario, murine organoids have been infected with influenza virus (Quantius et al., 2016), and human organoids have been infected with respiratory syncytial virus (RSV; Sachs et al., 2019). Some attempts have been made to microinject pathogens or their by-products into organoids using custom made tools, primarily in gastrointestinal organoids (Williamson et al., 2018); however, in lung organoids, this technique has only been applied to propagate Cryptosporidium, a protozoan parasite (Heo et al., 2018).

Precision Cut Lung Slices

To address the disconnection that often exists in spheroids and organoids in including both cellular and organ-level complexities *in vitro*, some groups have turned to an *ex vivo* system called precision cut lung slices (PCLS), which maintain the cellular structure and the biological processes of the lung (Ainslie et al., 2019). Importantly, PCLS generation from healthy explants and diseased tissue can reveal differences in the cellular and molecular interactions within the microenvironment of the lung. Disease modeling of healthy tissue can be achieved *ex vivo* through mimicking disease characteristics and used for exploring therapeutic treatments (Alsafadi et al., 2020). Precision cut lung slices have been applied for cytotoxicity assessment to low-molecular-weight (LMW) chemicals (Lauenstein et al., 2014), evaluation of biological responses to inflammatory stimuli such as lipopolysaccharide endotoxin (LPS), macrophage-activating lipopeptide-2 (MALP-2), interferon gamma (IFNgamma) (Henjakovic et al., 2008), and recreation of pathologies such as pulmonary fibrosis, through the use of a combination of profibrotic growth factors and signaling molecules (Alsafadi et al., 2017) and COPD models induced with 1-(3-Hydroxy-5-(thiophen-2-yl)phenyl)-3-(naphthalen-2-yl)urea (FzM1) (Skronska-Wasek et al., 2017). However, PCLS are often cultivated only for short periods of time (they are very challenging to maintain viable and functional for weeks), their use is impacted by the limited availability of whole/resected organ for slicing, and they only represent a brief snapshot of the cell populations in the tissue. Besides, the PCLS cannot fully recapitulate all attributes seen *in vivo*; for instance, there are major challenges with preserving arteriole morphology and localization of lung airway smooth muscle cells (Sanderson, 2011). Precision cut lung slices can reproduce the initial interactions and inflammatory responses to industrial chemicals (Lauenstein et al., 2014) and pathogens [e.g., influenza viruses (Liu et al., 2015), rhinovirus (Beale et al., 2014), *Yersinia pestis* (Banerjee et al., 2019), and *Coxiella burnetiid* (Graham et al., 2016)] in the human respiratory system; however, the extent to which the immune response can replicate the *in vivo* situation is limited, as demonstrated by Neuhaus et al. (2017), who observed that LPS-induced tumor necrosis factor-alpha (TNF-α) secretion decreased significantly over a period of 15 days, and it is not possible to recruit non-resident immune cells. Moreover, while murine-derived PCLS models have been adapted to study the effects of cigarette smoke (Donovan et al., 2016), the PCLS per se have not been utilized for inhalation exposure studies *in vitro*, principally because the route of administration represents a challenge (e.g., physiological ALI cannot be established in this model system), and often the entire slice is bathed in the compound or stimulant of interest (Liu et al., 2019). Changing from ALI conditions to liquid-submerged conditions represents a drawback, as it impacts epithelial cells' glycoprotein secretion profile, tight junction integrity, and permeability (Grainger et al., 2006). In addition, the physio-chemical properties of pulmonary stimuli such as airborne pollutants, gaseous substances, novel medications, and therapeutic agents can alter when in liquid suspension (Upadhyay and Palmberg, 2018). In addition to this, PCLS become static systems, lacking the shear flows associated with air and blood flow in the ALI and vascular endothelium, respectively, which could impact cell–cell/ECM responses and interactions in tissues.

Bronchial Biopses

Bronchial biopsies are samples of airway tissue obtained from the carinae of large and small cartilaginous airways. These samples are often fixed and used to measure airway remodeling by morphometric analyses of airway epithelial mucin stores, measurements of reticular basement membrane thickness, quantification of the number and size of globlet cells, the analysis of the content and density of the smooth muscle of the airways, as well as quantification and characterization of inflammatory cells (Woodruff and Innes, 2006). In addition, some effort have been made to culture the bronchial biopsies for short-term exposure studies *in vitro*. For instance, this culture model has been used to study the effects of chemotherapeutic treatments on non-small cell lung cancer (Lang et al., 2007), to evaluate cellular responses by exposing asthmatic lung tissue to allergen *Dermatophagoides pteronyssinus* (Jaffar et al., 1999; Lordan et al., 2001; Vijayanand et al., 2010), and to test the antiviral efficacy of therapeutic drugs against influenza virus infection (Nicholas et al., 2015). The advantages of bronchial biopsies include retaining the three-dimensional structure of the lungs if the extraction procedure is successful, which requires a trained bronchoscopist, allowing sampling from healthy subjects as well as patients with lung diseases, and the minimally invasive nature of the sampling procedure. However, this system has similar drawbacks as the PCLS, and is impacted by scarcity of donor tissue availability, small sample size (usually 1–3 mm) and number of biopses that can be obtained at any given time (~4–10). In addition the *in vitro* viability in often low, therefore exposure studies on bronchial biopsies usually do not last more than a single day.

Cellularized Bio-Scaffolds

Extracellular matrix is the 3D network of extracellular macromolecules that provide structural integrity and biochemical support to tissue-resident cells. Extracellular matrix both serves as a scaffold and modulates cellular responses such as self-renewal, quiescence, migration, proliferation, phenotype maintenance, differentiation, and apoptosis (Akhmanova et al., 2015). Hydrogels can mimic ECM *in vitro* using natural products (like collagen, hyaluronic acid, chitosan, alginate, or Matrigel) or synthetic polymers [such as polyethylene glycol (PEG) or polyacrylamide (PAA)] (Zhou et al., 2018). Natural hydrogels have been predominantly used to culture lung cells and organoids (Sato et al., 2017; Zacharias et al., 2018); however, artificial matrices have been demonstrated as a viable alternative (Miller et al., 2019), since their components are biologically inert, and can be functionalized by the addition of proteins, peptides, and/or polysaccharides (Akhmanova et al., 2015).

Besides hydrogels, lung ECM can be generated via decellularization of the whole/resected lung through perfusion with detergents, which allows considerable preservation of the micro- and macro-architecture of the organ, and the ECM composition (Gilpin and Wagner, 2018). Extracellular matrix has been recognized as a bioactive medium that modulates cellular responses in its surroundings. By using cellularized bio-scaffolds it will therefore be possible to mimic some pathological alterations, and the consequent functional changes that occur in lung diseases, especially those with a chronic nature (Burgess et al., 2016). Decellularized lung scaffolds have enabled studying cell–ECM interactions in tissues of healthy people and patients with chronic lung diseases, such as lung cancer (Stratmann et al., 2014), idiopathic pulmonary fibrosis

(IPF; Van Der Velden et al., 2018), and scleroderma (Sun et al., 2016). These matrices are instrumental in evaluating lung repair and regeneration and have been recellularized with different types of human cells, including fibroblasts, endothelial cells, epithelial cells, stem cells from multiple organ sources, and organoids (Porzionato et al., 2018; Giobbe et al., 2019). However, it has not been possible to completely recellularize these matrices to allow recreation of lung physiology and function, their application has been partly hindered due to the limited number of whole/resected human lungs, and to our knowledge, their utilization [beyond regenerative medicine and orthotopic transplantation (Guenthart et al., 2019)] for studying host–environment/pathogen interactions has not been demonstrated.

3D Bioprinting

To more faithfully replicate tissue microarchitectures of the human lung, 3D bioprinting has emerged as a great technological platform ideally positioned to create finely defined and controlled biological structures and living systems by utilizing a wide array of materials (natural, synthetic, or even hybrid hydrogels) and cell types. This technology can achieve a high degree of precision in cell positioning and can be scalable for automation (Gungor-Ozkerim et al., 2018). However, 3D bioprinting has been predominantly applied for the development of vascularized tissues (Kolesky et al., 2014), rather than generating functional whole organ or organ-like mimicries. To our knowledge, only a few studies have focused on the lungs. Horvath et al. (2015) biofabricated a three-part mimetic (composed of an endothelial cell layer, basement membrane, and an epithelial cell layer) of air–blood barrier analog of the human lung alveoli within a transwell insert. While a great initiative, the study utilized cell lines, rather than primary human-derived cells, and the authors only focused on model validation (viability, cellular proliferation, and barrier function) and no data were presented on the application of the platform for the analysis of host-environment/pathogen interactions. More recently, a new method for 3D bioprinting of tissues by stereolithography was reported, whereby it was possible to make a model inspired by alveolar morphology, capable of withstanding mechanical strain for cyclical ventilation and oxygen transport (Grigoryan et al., 2019). While successful in creating entangled vascular networks of the lung alveoli, the bioprinted tissue lacked alveolar epithelial cells, and the platform was applied neither for toxicological studies nor for inhaled exposure to a respiratory pathogen or therapeutic agents. Altogether, 3D bioprinting offers the possibility of developing biologically inspired lung organotypic models; however, despite the advantages of 3D bioprinting, wide spread utilization of these techniques has been limited by the requirement of expensive and complex technologies as well as a steep learning curve.

Lung-on-a-Chip Models

Organ-on-a-Chips are biomimetic, microfluidic, cell culture devices created with microchip manufacturing methods that contain continuously perfused hollow microchannels inhabited by living tissue cells arranged to simulate organ-level physiology (Bhatia and Ingber, 2014; Benam et al., 2015). By recapitulating the multicellular architectures, tissue–tissue interfaces, chemical gradients, mechanical cues, and vascular perfusion of the body, these devices produce levels of tissue and organ functionality with well-defined structures and highly controlled microenvironments that would not be possible with conventional 2D or 3D culture systems. They also enable high-resolution, real-time imaging and *in vitro* analysis of biochemical, genetic and metabolic activities of living human cells in a functional human tissue and organ context. Adaptation of Organ-on-a-Chip technology by pulmonary scientists has led to the development of model systems that emulate human lung pathophysiology *in vitro*.

Lung-on-a-Chip devices have been developed to model different regions of the respiratory system and recapitulate *in vivo*-observed multicellular architecture and physicochemical environment of the lung (airway and alveoli). The use of this technology (Alveolus-on-a-Chip) has enabled a better understanding of different aspects of human alveolar pathologies; such as evaluating the influence of breathing-associated mechanical cues on the growth and migration pattern of Non-Small Cell Lung Cancer tumor cells (NSCLC; Hassell et al., 2017), reproducing interleukin-2 (IL-2) induced alveolar edema observed in human cancer patients at similar doses and over the same time frame, and its pharmacological inhibition (Huh et al., 2012), mimicking pulmonary thrombosis by treatment with inflammatory stimuli (TNF-α) and bacterial products (LPS) corroborated in murine models (Jain et al., 2018), studying inhaled exposure of the alveolar epithelium to aerosolized LPS and its immune-modulatory impact (Artzy-Schnirman et al., 2019), and recreating recruitment of circulating leukocytes and inflammation induction after treatment of epithelial cells with TNF-a, *Escherichia coli*, and silica nanoparticles (Huh et al., 2010). In these microphysiological systems primary, cancerous or immortalized cell line of human alveolar epithelial origin have been co-cultured with human lung microvascular endothelial cells (Huh et al., 2010, 2012; Hassell et al., 2017) or human umbilical vascular endothelial cells (HUVECs; Jain et al., 2018).

In the context of conducting airways, we have developed and applied Lung-on-a-Chip devices (Airway-on-a-Chip) for culture and differentiation of primary human epithelial cells in co-culture with primary human lung microvascular endothelial cells, to model small airways, reproduce the mechanical forces associated with inhalation-exhalation respiration cycles (airflow shear), mimic the shear forces across endothelial cell layers (via vascular flow), and recreate the ALI barrier of human airways (Benam et al., 2015, 2016a,b, 2017, 2018, 2019, 2015; Benam and Ingber, 2016; Niemeyer et al., 2018). This technology has been adapted to allow first-in-kind studies that reproduce and characterize tissue–tissue crosstalk between pulmonary epithelium and airway smooth muscle (Humayun et al., 2018) and enable better understanding infectious disease biogenesis processes through analysis of the production of inflammatory cytokines and immune cell recruitment (neutrophils) following exposure to respiratory fungi (e.g., *Aspergillus fumigatus*) and the bacteria (e.g., *Pseudomonas aeruginosa*) (Barkal et al.,

2017) by other investigators. Similay utilizing Airway-on-a-Chip we have been able to dissect inflammatory processes involved in the pathobiology of chronic lung conditions such as asthma induced by the exposure of ephitelium to IL-13 and COPD by recreating terminally differentiated mucociliated airway epithelia on-chip, and exposing cells to the viral mimic polyinosinic–polycytidylic acid (poly(I:C)) or to LPS (Benam et al., 2016b), and identify novel biomarkers of human lung diseases and test efficacy of lead therapeutic compounds (Benam et al., 2016b).

We developed a Breathing-Smoking Lung-on-a-Chip platform that recreates smoke-induced pathologies in humans (Benam et al., 2016b). The system consisted of a Lung Small Airway-on-a-Chip (Benam et al., 2016b) that reproduces the living bronchiolar tissue for exposure to inhaled whole cigarette smoke (WCS), a "microrespirator" that emulates diaphragm and rib cage function and reproduces inhalation-exhalation airflow at physiological rhythms and patterns, a "biomimetic smoking robot" (Benam et al., 2020) that mimics human mouth and generates fresh WCS

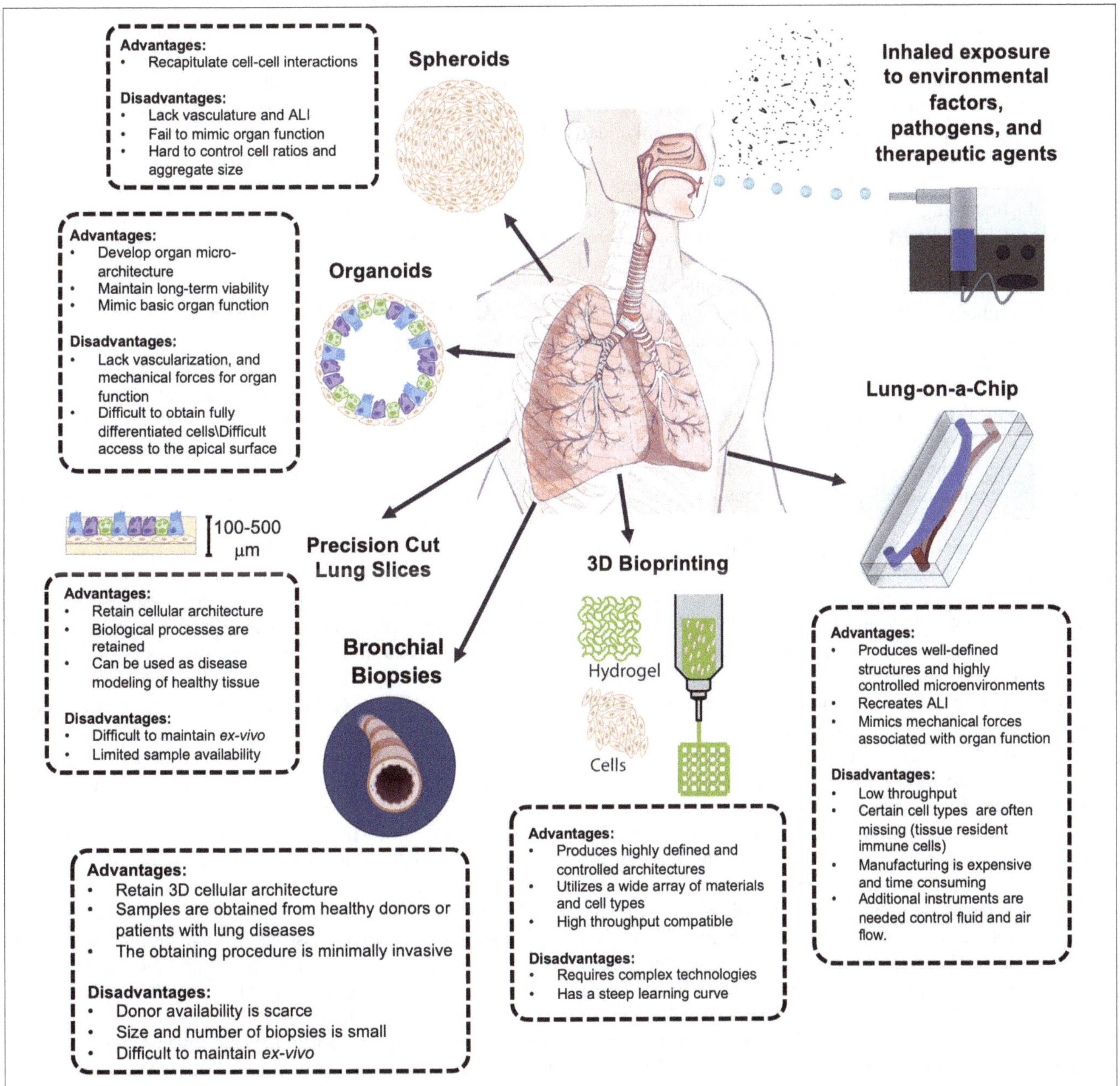

FIGURE 1 | Advantages and disadvantages of complex 3D *in vitro* culture models of the human lung for inhalation exposure studies. Each model presented has unique benefits and challenges. Improved airway modeling can be achieved through incorporating inhalation exposure systems. The digital images of human lung at the center and bronchus near the bottom left were acquired from Shutterstock and Biorender, respectively.

and regulates the passage of inhale/exhale air/smoke, and software that represents the brain of human smoker and controls "smoking topography" and "breathing" behavior. Using this platform, we flowed WCS horizontally across the apical surface of differentiated human bronchiolar epithelia (as occurs in the lungs of human smokers), from normal subjects and COPD patients, at representative smoking topography parameters for puff time, puff volume and inter-puff interval under clinically relevant breathing conditions. We found that inhaled smoke exposure transformed ciliary beat frequency (CBF) pattern, range, and variability and induced oxidative stress. Importantly, it was observed that submerging the ciliated airway epithelia with cell culture medium alone was sufficient to mask the impact of inhaled WCS on ciliary micro-pathologies. In addition, we discovered new smoke-mounted biological markers that distinguish COPD epithelia from those from healthy individuals (Benam et al., 2016a).

Recently, Elias-Kirma et al. (2020) developed an interesting model of branching Airway-on-a-Chip for toxicological evaluation of inhaled particulate matter. The authors utilized primary human bronchial epithelial cells for culture, and exposed the epithelium on-chip to anti-vanilloid receptor 1 (VR1) antibody-coated polystyrene microparticles. The microparticles were generated using a commercial aerosolizing machine and brought into contact with the cells through a pinch valve-controlled antistatic tube. While the device design in this study was unique, the exposure did not mimic what naturally occurs during rhythmic breathing cycles and the authors did not study biological impact of exposure to environmental pollutants, tobacco products or therapeutic agents.

These study implies that Lung-on-a-Chip platforms have the potential for recreation of *in vivo*-like inhaled exposure to pathogens, environmental threats, and drug treatments. However, for such platforms to be more applicable and physiologically relevant, it is important to enhance their multicellularity and complexity, for instance by the addition of parenchymal cells, such as fibroblasts, tissue-resident and circulating immune cells, muscle cells, and/or ECM. One of the drawbacks of microfluidics is that manufacturing is often expensive and time consuming; in addition, instruments such as syringe pumps or air pressure systems are required to control fluid flow within the chips. Furthermore, the devices need to become more user friendly (particularly for biologists with little/no engineering expertise) and be amenable for increased throughput. On the other hand, although microphysiological systems have great flexibility with respect to the experimental design, there are important challenges due to miniaturization, such as reduced media volumes, different media exchange rates and methods, and lower number of cells tested; finally, and an additional challenge in conducting host-pathogen/environment studies is the stimulus dose. Therefore, it is necessary to carefully evaluate these differences when comparing cell behavior and viability in microfluidic devices versus macroscopic cultures, and especially when comparing against *in vivo* results to validate the systems. Moreover, from a high-level perspective investigators utilizing Organ-on-Chip devices must consider as accurate and as feaible as possible validating and qualifying these models against tissues that they are aiming to replicate – i.e., human samples and clinical data. Lastly, we would like to mention that multiple factors have contributed to popularity and quick and widespread adaptation of PDMS for fabrication of Lung-on-a-Chip microfluidic devices. These include ability for rapid prototyping and multilayer device fabrication, optical transparency from 240 to 1100 nm (enabling utilization by various optical detection schemes), flexibility (allowing axial stretch), gas-permeablity (so that oxygen can feasibly penetrate the device and reach the cells embedded within the chip), being non-toxic, inexpensive and not breaking (like glass). However, a drawback of PDMS has been its absorption of small, hydrophobic molecules from flowing solution (Toepke and Beebe, 2006). To mitigate this, we apply either of these two approaches: (1) correcting for absorption of small hydrophobic molecules by quantifying the loss (e.g., via mass spectrometry) and (2) saturating the chips prior to cell culture or experimentation to minimize loss.

CONCLUSION AND FUTURE DIRECTIONS

In this article, we reviewed the most recent advances in creating preclinical 3D model systems that reproduce human lung pathophysiology *in vitro* and discussed their respective merits and drawbacks in the context of host-environment/pathogen interactions (**Figure 1**). It has been a long road for the transition from 2D to 3D cell culture systems; however, 3D models are gaining popularity in use and adaptation due to their critical advantages over static cell cultures. Spheroids, organoids, and PCLS have proven to be invaluable tools for studying lung development and pathologies, but they lack natural ALI and are unable to reproduce breathing-associated airflow, thus it is not possible to perform inhalation exposure studies using these platforms. Cellularized scaffolds have been widely used to study cell–ECM interactions at health and disease, and for regenerative purposes; however, these have not yet been used to assess host–environment/pathogen interactions. Recently, 3D bioprinting has emerged as a promising technique for developing more intricate lung living systems with great potential for high throughput yield; but numerous technical challenges need to be tackled and complex-system building to integrate multiple organ-specific cells and tissue (beyond generating vascularized constructs) must become a priority. In contrast, microfluidic Lung-on-a-Chip microdevices have emerged as an attractive alternative to mimic lung function and biology as seen *in vivo*. In the particular case of lung models, and more specifically in the study of the host–environment/pathogen interaction, it is important how the treatments and/or stimuli are delivered, in this sense, the microfluidic platforms have demonstrated to be very robust and physiologically relevant *in vitro* tools that can incorporate biochemical, physical and mechanical cues. We envision considerable improvement and adaption of Lung-on-a-Chip platforms for the study of host-environment/pathogen interactions. The improvements include allowing higher throughput analysis, and integration of ECM and additional cellular complexity. These microdevices will be utilized for the study of nebulized and dry powder treatments and recreation of clinically relevant exposure to airborne respiratory pathogens (instead of lung cells being exposed submerged to the infective agents). We also anticipate the *in vitro* cell culture of cellularized matrices and potentially PCLS within the Lung-on-a-Chip system to provide dynamism and enhanced viability *ex vivo*. In line with this, 3D bioprinting techniques could revolutionize the way microfluidic devices are currently manufactured, allowing for increased production and reproducibility.

AUTHOR CONTRIBUTIONS

KB conceptualized and critically revised the manuscript. RJ-V, UC, and BN drafted the manuscript. All authors contributed to the article and approved the submitted version.

REFERENCES

Ainslie, G. R., Davis, M., Ewart, L., Lieberman, L. A., Rowlands, D. J., Thorley, A. J., et al. (2019). Microphysiological lung models to evaluate the safety of new pharmaceutical modalities: a biopharmaceutical perspective. *Lab Chip* 19, 3152–3161.

Akhmanova, M., Osidak, E., Domogatsky, S., Rodin, S., and Domogatskaya, A. (2015). Physical, spatial, and molecular aspects of extracellular matrix of *in vivo* niches and artificial scaffolds relevant to stem cells research. *Stem Cells Int.* 2015:167025.

Alsafadi, H. N., Staab-Weijnitz, C. A., Lehmann, M., Lindner, M., Peschel, B., Konigshoff, M., et al. (2017). An *ex vivo* model to induce early fibrosis-like changes in human precision-cut lung slices. *Am. J. Physiol. Lung Cell. Mol. Physiol.* 312, L896–L902.

Alsafadi, H. N., Uhl, F. E., Pineda, R. H., Bailey, K. E., Rojas, M., Wagner, D. E., et al. (2020). Applications and approaches for three-dimensional precision-cut lung slices. Disease modeling and drug discovery. *Am. J. Respir. Cell Mol. Biol.* 62, 681–691. doi: 10.1165/rcmb.2019-0276tr

Artzy-Schnirman, A., Zidan, H., Elias-Kirma, S., Ben-Porat, L., Tenenbaum-Katan, J., Carius, P., et al. (2019). Capturing the onset of bacterial pulmonary infection in acini-on-chips. *Advan. Biosys.* 3:e1900026.

Banerjee, S. K., Huckuntod, S. D., Mills, S. D., Kurten, R. C., and Pechous, R. D. (2019). Modeling pneumonic plague in human precision-cut lung slices highlights a role for the plasminogen activator protease in facilitating type 3 secretion. *Infect. Immun.* 87:e00175-19.

Barkal, L. J., Procknow, C. L., Alvarez-Garcia, Y. R., Niu, M., Jimenez-Torres, J. A., Brockman-Schneider, R. A., et al. (2017). Microbial volatile communication in human organotypic lung models. *Nat. Commun.* 8:1770.

Barkauskas, C. E., Chung, M. I., Fioret, B., Gao, X., Katsura, H., and Hogan, B. L. (2017). Lung organoids: current uses and future promise. *Development* 144, 986–997. doi: 10.1242/dev.140103

Beale, J., Jayaraman, A., Jackson, D. J., Macintyre, J. D. R., Edwards, M. R., and Walton, R. P. (2014). Rhinovirus-induced IL-25 in asthma exacerbation drives type 2 immunity and allergic pulmonary inflammation. *Sci. Transl. Med.* 6:256ra134. doi: 10.1126/scitranslmed.3009124

Benam, K. H., Dauth, S., Hassell, B., Herland, A., Jain, A., and Jang, K. J. (2015). Engineered in vitro disease models. *Annu. Rev. Pathol.* 10, 195–262.

Benam, K. H., Gilchrist, S., Kleensang, A., Satz, A. B., Willett, C., and Zhang, Q. (2019). Exploring new technologies in biomedical research. *Drug Discov. Today* 24, 1242–1247. doi: 10.1016/j.drudis.2019.04.001

Benam, K. H., and Ingber, D. E. (2016). Commendation for exposing key advantage of organ chip approach. *Cell Syst.* 3:411. doi: 10.1016/j.cels.2016.11.009

Benam, K. H., Konigshoff, M., and Eickelberg, O. (2018). Breaking the in vitro barrier in respiratory medicine. engineered microphysiological systems for chronic obstructive pulmonary disease and beyond. *Am. J. Respir. Crit. Care Med.* 197, 869–875. doi: 10.1164/rccm.201709-1795pp

Benam, K. H., Mazur, M., Choe, Y., Ferrante, T. C., Novak, R., and Ingber, D. E. (2017). Human lung small airway-on-a-chip protocol. *Methods Mol. Biol.* 1612, 345–365. doi: 10.1007/978-1-4939-7021-6_25

Benam, K. H., Novak, R., Ferrante, T. C., Choe, Y., and Ingber, D. E. (2020). Biomimetic smoking robot for in vitro inhalation exposure compatible with microfluidic organ chips. *Nat. Protoc.* 15, 183–206. doi: 10.1038/s41596-019-0230-y

Benam, K. H., Novak, R., Nawroth, J., Hirano-Kobayashi, M., Ferrante, T. C., Choe, Y., et al. (2016a). Matched-comparative modeling of normal and diseased human airway responses using a microengineered breathing lung chip. *Cell Syst.* 3, 456–466.e4. doi: 10.1016/j.cels.2016.10.003

Benam, K. H., Villenave, R., Lucchesi, C., Varone, A., Hubeau, C., Lee, H. H., et al. (2016b). Small airway-on-a-chip enables analysis of human lung inflammation and drug responses *in vitro*. *Nat. Methods* 13, 151–157. doi: 10.1038/nmeth.3697

Bhatia, S. N., and Ingber, D. E. (2014). Microfluidic organs-on-chips. *Nat. Biotechnol.* 32, 760–772. doi: 10.1038/nbt.2989

Burgess, J. K., Mauad, T., Tjin, G., Karlsson, J. C., and Westergren-Thorsson, G. (2016). The extracellular matrix - the under-recognized element in lung disease? *J. Pathol.* 240, 397–409. doi: 10.1002/path.4808

Chimenti, I., Pagano, F., Angelini, F., Siciliano, C., Mangino, G., Picchio, V., et al. (2017). Human lung spheroids as *in vitro* niches of lung progenitor cells with distinctive paracrine and plasticity properties. *Stem Cells Transl. Med.* 6, 767–777. doi: 10.5966/sctm.2015-0374

Donovan, C., Seow, H. J., Bourke, J. E., and Vlahos, R. (2016). Influenza A virus infection and cigarette smoke impair bronchodilator responsiveness to beta-adrenoceptor agonists in mouse lung. *Clin. Sci.* 130, 829–837. doi: 10.1042/cs20160093

Dye, B. R., Dedhia, P. H., Miller, A. J., Nagy, M. S., White, E. S., Shea, L. D., et al. (2016). A bioengineered niche promotes *in vivo* engraftment and maturation of pluripotent stem cell derived human lung organoids. *eLife* 5:e19732.

Ekert, J. E., Johnson, K., Strake, B., Pardinas, J., Jarantow, S., Perkinson, R., et al. (2014). Three-dimensional lung tumor microenvironment modulates therapeutic compound responsiveness *in vitro*–implication for drug development. *PLoS One* 9:e92248. doi: 10.1371/journal.pone.0092248

Elias-Kirma, S., Artzy-Schnirman, A., Das, P., Heller-Algazi, M., Korin, N., and Sznitman, J. (2020). *In situ*-like aerosol inhalation exposure for cytotoxicity assessment using airway-on-chips platforms. *Front. Bioeng. Biotechnol.* 8:91. doi: 10.3389/fbioe.2020.00091

Fang, Y., and Eglen, R. M. (2017). Three-dimensional cell cultures in drug discovery and development. *SLAS Discov.* 22, 456–472. doi: 10.1177/1087057117696795

Gilpin, S. E., and Wagner, D. E. (2018). Acellular human lung scaffolds to model lung disease and tissue regeneration. *Eur. Respir. Rev.* 27:180021. doi: 10.1183/16000617.0021-2018

Giobbe, G. G., Crowley, C., Luni, C., Campinoti, S., Khedr, M., Kretzschmar, K., et al. (2019). Extracellular matrix hydrogel derived from decellularized tissues enables endodermal organoid culture. *Nat. Commun.* 10:5658.

Graham, J. G., Winchell, C. G., Kurten, R. C., and Voth, D. E. (2016). Development of an *ex vivo* tissue platform to study the human lung response to *Coxiella burnetii*. *Infect. Immun.* 84, 1438–1445. doi: 10.1128/iai.00012-16

Grainger, C. I., Greenwell, L. L., Lockley, D. J., Martin, G. P., and Forbes, B. (2006). Culture of Calu-3 cells at the air interface provides a representative model of the airway epithelial barrier. *Pharm. Res.* 23, 1482–1490. doi: 10.1007/s11095-006-0255-0

Gray, T. E., Guzman, K., Davis, C. W., Abdullah, L. H., and Nettesheim, P. (1996). Mucociliary differentiation of serially passaged normal human tracheobronchial epithelial cells. *Am. J. Respir. Cell Mol. Biol.* 14, 104–112. doi: 10.1165/ajrcmb.14.1.8534481

Grigoryan, B., Paulsen, S. J., Corbett, D. C., Sazer, D. W., Fortin, C. L., Zaita, A. J., et al. (2019). Multivascular networks and functional intravascular topologies within biocompatible hydrogels. *Science* 364, 458–464. doi: 10.1126/science.aav9750

Guenthart, B. A., O'neill, J. D., Kim, J., Fung, K., Vunjak-Novakovic, G., and Bacchetta, M. (2019). Cell replacement in human lung bioengineering. *J. Heart Lung Transplant.* 38, 215–224. doi: 10.1016/j.healun.2018.11.007

Gungor-Ozkerim, P. S., Inci, I., Zhang, Y. S., Khademhosseini, A., and Dokmeci, M. R. (2018). Bioinks for 3D bioprinting: an overview. *Biomater. Sci.* 6, 915–946.

Hassell, B. A., Goyal, G., Lee, E., Sontheimer-Phelps, A., Levy, O., Chen, C. S., et al. (2017). Human organ chip models recapitulate orthotopic lung cancer growth, therapeutic responses, and tumor dormancy *in vitro*. *Cell Rep.* 21, 508–516. doi: 10.1016/j.celrep.2017.09.043

Hecht, S. S. (2005). Carcinogenicity studies of inhaled cigarette smoke in laboratory animals: old and new. *Carcinogenesis* 26, 1488–1492. doi: 10.1093/carcin/bgi148

Henjakovic, M., Sewald, K., Switalla, S., Kaiser, D., Muller, M., Veres, T. Z., et al. (2008). *Ex vivo* testing of immune responses in precision-cut lung slices. *Toxicol. Appl. Pharmacol.* 231, 68–76. doi: 10.1016/j.taap.2008.04.003

Heo, I., Dutta, D., Schaefer, D. A., Iakobachvili, N., Artegiani, B., Sachs, N., et al. (2018). Modelling cryptosporidium infection in human small intestinal and lung organoids. *Nat. Microbiol.* 3, 814–823. doi: 10.1038/s41564-018-0177-8

Horvath, L., Umehara, Y., Jud, C., Blank, F., Petri-Fink, A., and Rothen-Rutishauser, B. (2015). Engineering an in vitro air-blood barrier by 3D bioprinting. *Sci. Rep.* 5:7974.

Huh, D., Leslie, D. C., Matthews, B. D., Fraser, J. P., Jurek, S., Hamilton, G. A., et al. (2012). A human disease model of drug toxicity-induced pulmonary edema in a lung-on-a-chip microdevice. *Sci. Transl. Med.* 4:159ra147. doi: 10.1126/scitranslmed.3004249

Huh, D., Matthews, B. D., Mammoto, A., Montoya-Zavala, M., Hsin, H. Y., and Ingber, D. E. (2010). Reconstituting organ-level lung functions on a chip. *Science* 328, 1662–1668. doi: 10.1126/science.1188302

Humayun, M., Chow, C. W., and Young, E. W. K. (2018). Microfluidic lung airway-on-a-chip with arrayable suspended gels for studying epithelial and smooth muscle cell interactions. *Lab Chip* 18, 1298–1309. doi: 10.1039/c7lc01357d

Jaffar, Z., Roberts, K., Pandit, A., Linsley, P., Djukanovic, R., and Holgate, S. (1999). B7 costimulation is required for IL-5 and IL-13 secretion by bronchial biopsy tissue of atopic asthmatic subjects in response to allergen stimulation. *Am. J. Respir. Cell Mol. Biol.* 20, 153–162. doi: 10.1165/ajrcmb.20.1.3255

Jain, A., Barrile, R., Van Der Meer, A. D., Mammoto, A., Mammoto, T., De Ceunynck, K., et al. (2018). Primary human lung alveolus-on-a-chip model of intravascular thrombosis for assessment of therapeutics. *Clin. Pharmacol. Ther.* 103, 332–340. doi: 10.1002/cpt.742

Klameth, L., Rath, B., Hochmaier, M., Moser, D., Redl, M., Mungenast, F., et al. (2017). Small cell lung cancer: model of circulating tumor cell tumorospheres in chemoresistance. *Sci. Rep.* 7:5337.

Kolesky, D. B., Truby, R. L., Gladman, A. S., Busbee, T. A., Homan, K. A., and Lewis, J. A. (2014). 3D bioprinting of vascularized, heterogeneous cell-laden tissue constructs. *Adv. Mater.* 26, 3124–3130. doi: 10.1002/adma.201305506

Konishi, S., Gotoh, S., Tateishi, K., Yamamoto, Y., Korogi, Y., Nagasaki, T., et al. (2016). Directed induction of functional multi-ciliated cells in proximal airway epithelial spheroids from human pluripotent stem cells. *Stem Cell Rep.* 6, 18–25. doi: 10.1016/j.stemcr.2015.11.010

Lang, D. S., Droemann, D., Schultz, H., Branscheid, D., Martin, C., Ressmeyer, A. R., et al. (2007). A novel human ex vivo model for the analysis of molecular events during lung cancer chemotherapy. *Respir. Res.* 8:43.

Lauenstein, L., Switalla, S., Prenzler, F., Seehase, S., Pfennig, O., Forster, C., et al. (2014). Assessment of immunotoxicity induced by chemicals in human precision-cut lung slices (PCLS). *Toxicol. In Vitro* 28, 588–599. doi: 10.1016/j.tiv.2013.12.016

Lenz, A. G., Karg, E., Lentner, B., Dittrich, V., Brandenberger, C., Rothen-Rutishauser, B., et al. (2009). A dose-controlled system for air-liquid interface cell exposure and application to zinc oxide nanoparticles. *Part. Fibre Toxicol.* 6:32. doi: 10.1186/1743-8977-6-32

Lewis, K. J. R., Hall, J. K., Kiyotake, E. A., Christensen, T., Balasubramaniam, V., and Anseth, K. S. (2018). Epithelial-mesenchymal crosstalk influences cellular behavior in a 3D alveolus-fibroblast model system. *Biomaterials* 155, 124–134. doi: 10.1016/j.biomaterials.2017.11.008

Liu, G., Betts, C., Cunoosamy, D. M., Aberg, P. M., Hornberg, J. J., Sivars, K. B., et al. (2019). Use of precision cut lung slices as a translational model for the study of lung biology. *Respir. Res.* 20:162.

Liu, R., An, L., Liu, G., Li, X., Tang, W., and Chen, X. (2015). Mouse lung slices: an *ex vivo* model for the evaluation of antiviral and anti-inflammatory agents against influenza viruses. *Antiviral Res.* 120, 101–111. doi: 10.1016/j.antiviral.2015.05.008

Lordan, J. L., Davies, D. E., Wilson, S. J., Dent, G., Corkhill, A., Jaffar, Z., et al. (2001). The role of CD28-B7 costimulation in allergen-induced cytokine release by bronchial mucosa from patients with moderately severe asthma. *J. Allergy Clin. Immunol.* 108, 976–981. doi: 10.1067/mai.2001.119740

Mccauley, K. B., Hawkins, F., Serra, M., Thomas, D. C., Jacob, A., and Kotton, D. N. (2017). Efficient derivation of functional human airway epithelium from pluripotent stem cells via temporal regulation of Wnt signaling. *Cell Stem Cell* 20, 844–857.e6. doi: 10.1016/j.stem.2017.03.001

Meenach, S. A., Tsoras, A. N., Mcgarry, R. C., Mansour, H. M., Hilt, J. Z., and Anderson, K. W. (2016). Development of three-dimensional lung multicellular spheroids in air- and liquid-interface culture for the evaluation of anticancer therapeutics. *Int. J. Oncol.* 48, 1701–1709. doi: 10.3892/ijo.2016.3376

Miller, A. J., Dye, B. R., Ferrer-Torres, D., Hill, D. R., Overeem, A. W., Shea, L. D., et al. (2019). Generation of lung organoids from human pluripotent stem cells *in vitro*. *Nat. Protoc.* 14, 518–540.

Miller, A. J., Hill, D. R., Nagy, M. S., Aoki, Y., Dye, B. R., Chin, A. M., et al. (2018). *In vitro* induction and *in vivo* engraftment of lung bud tip progenitor cells derived from human pluripotent stem cells. *Stem Cell Rep.* 10, 101–119. doi: 10.1016/j.stemcr.2017.11.012

Miller, A. J., and Spence, J. R. (2017). *In vitro* models to study human lung development, disease and homeostasis. *Physiology* 32, 246–260. doi: 10.1152/physiol.00041.2016

Neuhaus, V., Schaudien, D., Golovina, T., Temann, U. A., Thompson, C., Lippmann, T., et al. (2017). Assessment of long-term cultivated human precision-cut lung slices as an ex vivo system for evaluation of chronic cytotoxicity and functionality. *J. Occup. Med. Toxicol.* 12:13.

Nicholas, B., Staples, K. J., Moese, S., Meldrum, E., Ward, J., Dennison, P., et al. (2015). A novel lung explant model for the ex vivo study of efficacy and mechanisms of anti-influenza drugs. *J. Immunol.* 194, 6144–6154. doi: 10.4049/jimmunol.1402283

Niemeyer, B. F., Zhao, P., Tuder, R. M., and Benam, K. H. (2018). Advanced microengineered lung models for translational drug discovery. *SLAS Discov.* 23, 777–789. doi: 10.1177/2472555218760217

Porzionato, A., Stocco, E., Barbon, S., Grandi, F., Macchi, V., and De Caro, R. (2018). Tissue-engineered grafts from human decellularized extracellular matrices: a systematic review and future perspectives. *Int. J. Mol. Sci.* 19:4117. doi: 10.3390/ijms19124117

Prunieras, M., Regnier, M., and Woodley, D. (1983). Methods for cultivation of keratinocytes with an air-liquid interface. *J. Invest. Dermatol.* 81, 28s–33s.

Quantius, J., Schmoldt, C., Vazquez-Armendariz, A. I., Becker, C., El Agha, E., Wilhelm, J., et al. (2016). Influenza virus infects epithelial stem/progenitor cells of the distal lung: impact on fgfr2b-driven epithelial repair. *PLoS Pathog.* 12:e1005544. doi: 10.1371/journal.ppat.1005544

Rackley, C. R., and Stripp, B. R. (2012). Building and maintaining the epithelium of the lung. *J. Clin. Invest.* 122, 2724–2730. doi: 10.1172/jci60519

Sachs, N., Papaspyropoulos, A., Zomer-Van Ommen, D. D., Heo, I., Bottinger, L., Klay, D., et al. (2019). Long-term expanding human airway organoids for disease modeling. *EMBO J.* 38:e100300.

Sanderson, M. J. (2011). Exploring lung physiology in health and disease with lung slices. *Pulm. Pharmacol. Ther.* 24, 452–465. doi: 10.1016/j.pupt.2011.05.001

Sato, T., Morita, M., Tanaka, R., Inoue, Y., Nomura, M., Sakamoto, Y., et al. (2017). Ex vivo model of non-small cell lung cancer using mouse lung epithelial cells. *Oncol. Lett.* 63–6868.

Skronska-Wasek, W., Mutze, K., Baarsma, H. A., Bracke, K. R., Alsafadi, H. N., Lehmann, M., et al. (2017). Reduced frizzled receptor 4 expression prevents WNT/beta-catenin-driven alveolar lung repair in chronic obstructive pulmonary disease. *Am. J. Respir. Crit. Care Med.* 1.96, 172–185. doi: 10.1164/rccm.201605-0904oc

Stratmann, A. T., Fecher, D., Wangorsch, G., Gottlich, C., Walles, T., Walles, H., et al. (2014). Establishment of a human 3D lung cancer model based on a biological tissue matrix combined with a Boolean in silico model. *Mol. Oncol.* 8, 351–365. doi: 10.1016/j.molonc.2013.11.009

Sun, H., Zhu, Y., Pan, H., Chen, X., Balestrini, J. L., Lam, T. T., et al. (2016). Netrin-1 regulates fibrocyte accumulation in the decellularized fibrotic sclerodermatous lung microenvironment and in bleomycin-induced pulmonary fibrosis. *Arthritis Rheumatol.* 68, 1251–1261.

Surolia, R., Li, F. J., Wang, Z., Li, H., Liu, G., Zhou, Y., et al. (2017). 3D pulmospheres serve as a personalized and predictive multicellular model for assessment of antifibrotic drugs. *JCI Insight* 2:e91377.

Thorne, D., and Adamson, J. (2013). A review of *in vitro* cigarette smoke exposure systems. *Exp. Toxicol. Pathol.* 65, 1183–1193. doi: 10.1016/j.etp.2013.06.001

Toepke, M. W., and Beebe, D. J. (2006). PDMS absorption of small molecules and consequences in microfluidic applications. *Lab Chip* 6, 1484–1486.

Upadhyay, S., and Palmberg, L. (2018). Air-liquid interface: relevant in vitro models for investigating air pollutant-induced pulmonary toxicity. *Toxicol. Sci.* 164, 21–30. doi: 10.1093/toxsci/kfy053

Van Der Velden, J. L., Wagner, D. E., Lahue, K. G., Abdalla, S. T., Lam, Y. W., Weiss, D. J., et al. (2018). TGF-beta1-induced deposition of provisional extracellular matrix by tracheal basal cells promotes epithelial-to-mesenchymal transition in a c-Jun NH2-terminal kinase-1-dependent manner. *Am. J. Physiol. Lung Cell. Mol. Physiol.* 314, L984–L997.

Vijayanand, P., Durkin, K., Hartmann, G., Morjaria, J., Seumois, G., Staples, K. J., et al. (2010). Chemokine receptor 4 plays a key role in T cell recruitment into the airways of asthmatic patients. *J. Immunol.* 184, 4568–4574. doi: 10.4049/jimmunol.0901342

Williamson, I. A., Arnold, J. W., Samsa, L. A., Gaynor, L., Disalvo, M., Cocchiaro, J. L., et al. (2018). A high-throughput organoid microinjection platform to study gastrointestinal microbiota and luminal physiology. *Cell. Mol. Gastroenterol. Hepatol.* 6, 301–319. doi: 10.1016/j.jcmgh.2018.05.004

Woodruff, P. G., and Innes, A. L. (2006). Quantitative morphology using bronchial biopsies. *Eur. Respir. Rev.* 15, 157–161. doi: 10.1183/09059180.00010106

World Health Organization [WHO] (2018). *The Top 10 Causes of Death.* Available online at: https://www.who.int/news-room/fact-sheets/detail/the-top-10-causes-of-death (accessed March 31, 2020).

Yamaya, M., Finkbeiner, W., Chun, S., and Widdicombe, J. (1992). Differentiated structure and function of cultures from human tracheal epithelium. *Am. J. Physiol. Lung Cell. Mol. Physiol.* 262, L713–L724.

Zacharias, W. J., Frank, D. B., Zepp, J. A., Morley, M. P., Alkhaleel, F. A., Kong, J., et al. (2018). Regeneration of the lung alveolus by an evolutionarily conserved epithelial progenitor. *Nature* 555, 251–255. doi: 10.1038/nature25786

Zhou, Y., Horowitz, J. C., Naba, A., Ambalavanan, N., Atabai, K., Balestrini, J., et al. (2018). Extracellular matrix in lung development, homeostasis and disease. *Matrix Biol.* 73, 77–104.

2

Use of the Reversible Myogenic to Lipogenic Transdifferentiation Switch for the Design of Pre-Clinical Drug Screening in Idiopathic Pulmonary Fibrosis

Arun Lingampally[1,2], Matthew R. Jones[1,2], Shirisha Bagari[1,2], Chengshui Chen[1], Stefano Rivetti[1,2] and Saverio Bellusci[1,2]**

[1] Key Laboratory of Interventional Pulmonology of Zhejiang Province, Department of Pulmonary and Critical Care Medicine, First Affiliated Hospital of Wenzhou Medical University, Wenzhou, China, [2] Department of Pulmonary and Critical Care Medicine and Infectious Diseases, Universities of Giessen and Marburg Lung Center (UGMLC), Member of the German Center for Lung Research (DZL), Cardio-Pulmonary Institute, Justus-Liebig University Giessen, Giessen, Germany

***Correspondence:**
Stefano Rivetti
stefano.rivetti@innere.med.uni-giessen.de
Saverio Bellusci
saverio.bellusci@innere.med.uni-giessen.de

Idiopathic Pulmonary Fibrosis (IPF) is an end-stage lung disease characterized by excessive extracellular matrix (ECM) deposition from activated myofibroblasts (MYFs) and tissue scarring. Eventually leading to stiffening of the lung, capable of assuming only limited gas exchange function. So far two drugs, pirfenidone [acting via TGF-β (transforming growth factor beta) inhibition] and nintedanib (a pan-tyrosine kinase receptor inhibitor) have been approved for IPF patients. They both act on the activated MYF by reducing the expression of fibrotic markers. Unfortunately, these drugs are only slowing down fibrosis formation and as such do not represent a cure for this lethal, devastating disease. We previously reported that activated MYF originate, at least in part, from lung fibroblast resident cells called lipofibroblasts (LIF). During resolution, these activated MYF can transdifferentiate into LIF. We propose that this reversible myogenic/lipogenic transdifferentiation switch paradigm can be used to screen for drugs capable of triggering the lipogenic differentiation of activated MYFs. Ideally, these drugs should also induce the reduction of pro-fibrotic markers alpha smooth muscle actin2 (ACTA2) and collagen 1A1 (COL1A1) in activated MYF and as such would represent important alternatives to the approved drugs. The goal of this review is to summarize the current knowledge and limitations of the current strategies aiming to carry out methodical pre-clinical drug screening in pertinent *in vitro*, *ex vivo*, and *in vivo* models of IPF. These models include (1) *in vitro* culture of primary fibroblasts from IPF patients, (2) *ex vivo* culture of precision cut lung slices from end-stage IPF lungs obtained from transplant patients, and (3) bleomycin-induced fibrosis mouse models in the context of lineage tracing of activated MYF during resolution. For all these assays, we propose the innovative use of lipogenic read outs for the LIFs.

Keywords: idiopathic pulmonary fibrosis, aging, *in vitro* models, alveolar type 2 cells, activated myofibroblast, lipofibroblast

IDIOPATHIC PULMONARY FIBROSIS (IPF)

IPF is a fatal lung disease with unknown ethology. It is a pathological condition characterized by excessive extracellular matrix (ECM) deposition and tissue scarring, progressively leading to stiffening of the lung, respiratory paralysis, and death. IPF patients are often diagnosed at end stage, and the mean survival rate post-diagnosis is 3 years. The average annual incidence of pulmonary fibrosis is 17.4 per 100,000 persons worldwide (El Agha et al., 2017a; Zhao et al., 2020). It is widely postulated that IPF starts with repetitive injury and chronic inflammation of the alveolar epithelium. Injured epithelial cells regulate secretion of profibrotic and inflammatory mediators like matrix metalloproteins (MMP), growth factors, cytokines and chemokines (Selman and Pardo, 2006; Mora et al., 2017), which consequently results in the recruitment and chemo-attraction of activated myofibroblasts (MYFs) in the fibrotic precursor region known as fibrotic foci. Fibrotic foci are enriched with the profibrotic mediator transforming growth factor beta (TGF-β), which induces the transition of resident lung fibroblasts to MYFs. During homeostasis, TGF-β is in an inactive form bound to the ECM. However, during fibrosis, TGF-β becomes activated in the ECM and is also secreted by the alveolar epithelium (Wipff et al., 2007; Fernandez and Eickelberg, 2012; Zhao et al., 2020).

Activated MYFs are the core drivers for IPF progression and ECM deposition. Activated MYFs express alpha smooth muscle actin2 (ACTA2), and are characterized by apoptotic resistance and excessive ECM production. Activated MYFs have been proposed to arise through transdifferentiation from different precursors during fibrosis. Recent studies have shown that the activated MYFs arise from pericytes (Marriott et al., 2014), from $CD45^+$ $COL1^+$ $CXCR4^+$ bone marrow-derived circulating fibrocytes (Phillips et al., 2004) and from lipofibroblasts (LIFs) (El Agha et al., 2017b). In addition, it has been proposed that alveolar epithelial type 2 (AT2) cells could also be a source of activated MYF through a process of epithelial-to-mesenchymal transition (EMT) (Kim et al., 2006). However, this is controversial as lineage tracing of AT2 cells in mice in the context of bleomycin-induced pulmonary fibrosis does not show any contribution of AT2 cells to the newly formed myofibroblasts foci (Rock et al., 2011). Given all these potential sources of activated MYFs, it is likely that these cells constitute a quite heterogeneous population which so far has not been well-characterized. It is also likely that subpopulations in this heterogenous activated MYF population may respond differently to drugs (Kheirollahi et al., 2019).

It is therefore important to clearly define the types of read outs that will be implemented in the context of pre-clinical drug screening models in idiopathic pulmonary fibrosis. Our proposed models focus on the transdifferentiation of the MYFs into an important mesenchymal cell type, the LIFs. LIFs are proposed to be critical for the maintenance of AT2 stem cells and as such, are critical for lung repair after injury. The AT2-LIF interaction will be further developed in the next chapter.

INTERACTION BETWEEN ALVEOLAR EPITHELIAL TYPE 2 (AT2) STEM CELLS AND LIPOFIBROBLASTS (LIFS)

The alveolar epithelium consists of alveolar type 1 (AT1) and AT2 cells. AT1 cells are instrumental for gas exchange and AT2 cells secrete surfactant. At birth, pulmonary surfactant is crucial for reducing the surface tension in the alveoli thereby allowing gases exchange and for adapting to the transition from 3 to 21% oxygen (Torday, 2003; Torday et al., 2003). Recent discoveries suggest that a subpopulation of AT2 has a higher capacity for self-renewal, and the ability to differentiate to AT1 cells during homeostasis and injury (Barkauskas et al., 2013; Zacharias et al., 2018). Recent studies from Nan Tang et al. have shown that mechanical forces contribute to differentiation of the AT2 to AT1 cells during lung development and pneumonectomy (PNX)-induced alveolar regeneration. They also observed that Cdc-42 (Cell division cycle 42), a member of the RhoGTPase family, is required for differentiation of AT2 cells to AT1 cells. Ablation of *Cdc-42* in AT2 cells exhibited impaired regeneration and elevated mechanical stress, which led to the activation of latent Tgf-β. Activated Tgf-β signaling in turn led to the initiation and progression of fibrosis from the periphery to the center of the lung (Liu et al., 2016; Li et al., 2018; Wu et al., 2020). Interestingly, AT2 senescence, by activating senescence-associated secretory phenotype (SASP), and loss of AT2 cells due to persistent injury as well as altered AT2 self-renewal capacity are observed in IPF patients. AT2 cells are therefore active regulators of fibrosis. As they collaterally get damaged, this leads to the induction of the fibrotic phenotype, which includes the activation of resident fibroblast by profibrotic factors such as TGF-β (Yao et al., 2019; Parimon et al., 2020).

LIFS SIGNIFICANTLY CONTRIBUTE TO THE POOL OF ACTIVATED MYFS DURING FIBROSIS

As of today, the characteristics of the different types of resident fibroblasts in the adult lung are still unclear. During the early 1970s, two distinct types of interstitial cells were observed in neonatal rat lungs, namely, the lipid interstitial cell (aka LIF) and the non-lipid interstitial cell (O'Hare and Sheridan, 1970; Vaccaro and Brody, 1978). Lipofibroblasts are lipid droplet containing fibroblasts, anatomically located in close proximity to AT2 cells. These cells are Acta2-negative and also express Adipose differentiation related protein (*Adrp*)/Perilipin2 (*Plin2*). LIFs emerge during the late pseudoglandular stage of mouse lung development. Studies involving genetic tracing using the Fibroblast growth factor 10 ($Fgf10^{icre}$) mouse model as well as mouse mutants displaying impaired Fgf10/Fibroblast growth factor receptor 2b (Fgfr2b) signaling demonstrated the embryonic origin of LIFs and the role of Fgf10 in LIF differentiation during lung development (El Agha et al., 2014; Al Alam et al., 2015). Ablating a single allele of *Fgf10*, or its receptor *Fgfr2b*, in the mesenchyme of lungs exhibited significant decrease in LIF formation at birth. Adipocytes and LIFs share similarities in development. Fgf10 is the principal regulator of adipogenesis, Fgf10 signaling activates peroxisome proliferator activated receptor gamma (*Pparg*) expression via retinoblastoma protein and CCAAT-enhancer-binding protein alpha (pRb and C/EBPα) complex. *Fgf10* deficient mice exhibited impaired differentiation of the white adipose tissue (Sakaue et al., 2002). In addition, Fgf10 appears to also control the proliferation of the white adipose tissue (Konishi et al., 2006).

LIF synthesizes and secretes Fgf10, which acts in both a paracrine manner on the epithelium for branching morphogenesis and differentiation, and in an autocrine fashion to control the differentiation of LIF progenitors toward the lipogenic lineage (Bellusci et al., 1997; Al Alam et al., 2015; Jones et al., 2019). In the adult lung, during homeostasis and repair, LIFs contribute to the AT2 stem cell niche; LIFs and AT2 co-cultured in Matrigel formed the so-called "alveolospheres" in a 3D organoid model (Barkauskas et al., 2013). These alveolospheres are the consequence of the self-renewal of the AT2 stem cell as well as their differentiation toward AT1 cells. Interestingly, to date, surface markers specific for LIFs have not yet been discovered. Several dyes for Lipid droplets have been described such as Sudan III stains red to yellowish-red, Oil Red O stains red to reddish-orange and Sudan Black B stains black. However, LipidTOX dye appeared to be dye of choice for the assays described within this review. LipidTOX dye stains neutral lipid droplets with a remarkably high affinity and can be used to follow the formation and differentiation of cells within the lipogenic lineage. The detection of the dye via fluorescence allows the use of flow cytometry to quantify and isolate live LIFs during development and repair.

Recent studies in mice demonstrated that LIFs significantly contribute to the pool of activated MYFs during fibrosis. Using *Adrp*$^{Cre-ERT2}$ mice, a LIF genetic tracing model, it was shown that LIFs transition to an activated MYF phenotype in bleomycin-challenged mice. Surprisingly, during fibrosis resolution, a beneficial process which is happening in young mice (but unfortunately not in humans), lineage-labeled activated MYFs, labeled using the *Tg(Acta2-CreERT2); tomato*^{flox} mice, do not undergo apoptotic clearance, but instead acquire a lipogenic program to transdifferentiate back to LIFs (El Agha et al., 2017b). This reversible transdifferentiation switch from LIF to activated MYF opens the way for the testing of drugs capable of stimulating the transition of the activated MYF toward the LIF phenotype (**Figure 1**).

METABOLIC REPROGRAMING DURING FIBROSIS

The survival of a living organism is tightly associated with energy metabolism. ATP, the product of metabolism, is vital for survival and used in various cellular pathways. Metabolic dysregulation contributes to organ fibrosis through a decrease in mitochondrial biogenesis (Bueno et al., 2020). Mitochondrial biogenesis is crucial for cell survival and energy production by cellular respiration. AT2 cells in bleomycin-induced fibrosis display swollen mitochondria, a phenomenon which leads to apoptosis of the AT2 cells. A recent study indicated that thyroid hormone T3 and T4 (metabolic regulators) attenuated bleomycin-induced fibrosis in a mouse model. This antifibrotic effect was due to normalization of the mitochondrial structure and mitochondrial function, thereby inhibiting AT2 apoptosis (Yu et al., 2018). Recent studies have shown that 5' adenosine monophosphate-activated protein kinase (AMPK) activity is essential for mitochondrial biogenesis and fibrosis resolution. Reduced AMPK activation is observed in MYFs during fibrosis, leading to the accumulation of apoptotic resistant proliferative MYFs. This pathological fibrotic state is attenuated by AMPK activators, like 5-aminoimidazole-4-carboxamide ribonucleotide (AICAR) and metformin, by sensitizing MYFs to apoptosis and inhibiting their proliferation (Rangarajan et al., 2018). In brief, altered metabolism is associated with increased prevalence and incidents of fibrosis. AT2 cell regeneration and apoptotic clearance of profibrotic MYFs are essential for IPF therapy.

During homeostatic conditions, resident fibroblasts express ECM at physiological rates. The ECM regulates tissue function, maintains the 3D-structure, as well as orchestrates the repair process. During pathological states, resident fibroblasts, and the recruited fibrocytes, increase ECM deposition in the fibrotic regions. ECM is composed of fibronectin, laminin, collagens, proteoglycans, and glycosaminoglycans. Collagen is the major protein of the ECM and collagen type 1 is predominantly deposited during fibrosis. Collagen is synthesized in the endoplasmic reticulum as pre-pro-collagen and pro-collagen, then packed and secreted into the extracellular space by the Golgi apparatus. Pro-collagen is cleaved and cross-linked to form insoluble collagen fibers (Zhao et al., 2020). Collagen is mostly composed of the amino acids proline, lysine and glycine. Glycine which contributes to one third of collagen, is synthesized *de novo* by the serine-glycine one carbon pathway, a pathway that is catalyzed by the Phosphoglycerate Dehydrogenase (PHGDH) enzyme. PHGDH expression is elevated in the fibrotic foci regions and Inhibition of the PHGDH attenuated TGF-β-mediated collagen synthesis in fibrosis (Nigdelioglu et al., 2016; Hamanaka et al., 2018). In another study, Endo et al. (2003) demonstrated an increase in arginase, an enzyme which catalyzes arginine to ornithine, the precursor for proline and hydroxyproline, which contributes to ECM remodeling in bleomycin-challenged mice. Lysyl oxidases (LOX) catalyze and facilitate crosslinking of collagen and elastin by aldehyde groups, thereby inhibiting ECM degradation. Interestingly, hypoxia-inducible transcription factor (HIF) regulates LOX during hypoxia. LOX represses *E-cadherin* expression, causing EMT (Schietke et al., 2010). Inhibition or knock-down of LOX showed decreased recruitment of MYFs in bleomycin-challenged mice (Cheng et al., 2014). Glycolysis and ATP are upregulated in MYFs during fibrosis, which contributes to collagen synthesis. Fatty acid oxidation contributes to collagen degradation. Both collagen synthesis and degradation should be at physiological rates during homeostasis (Rabinowitz and Mutlu, 2019). ECM collagen unwinds and is cleaved by MMPs in the extracellular space. The cleaved collagen fibers, via fatty acid translocase

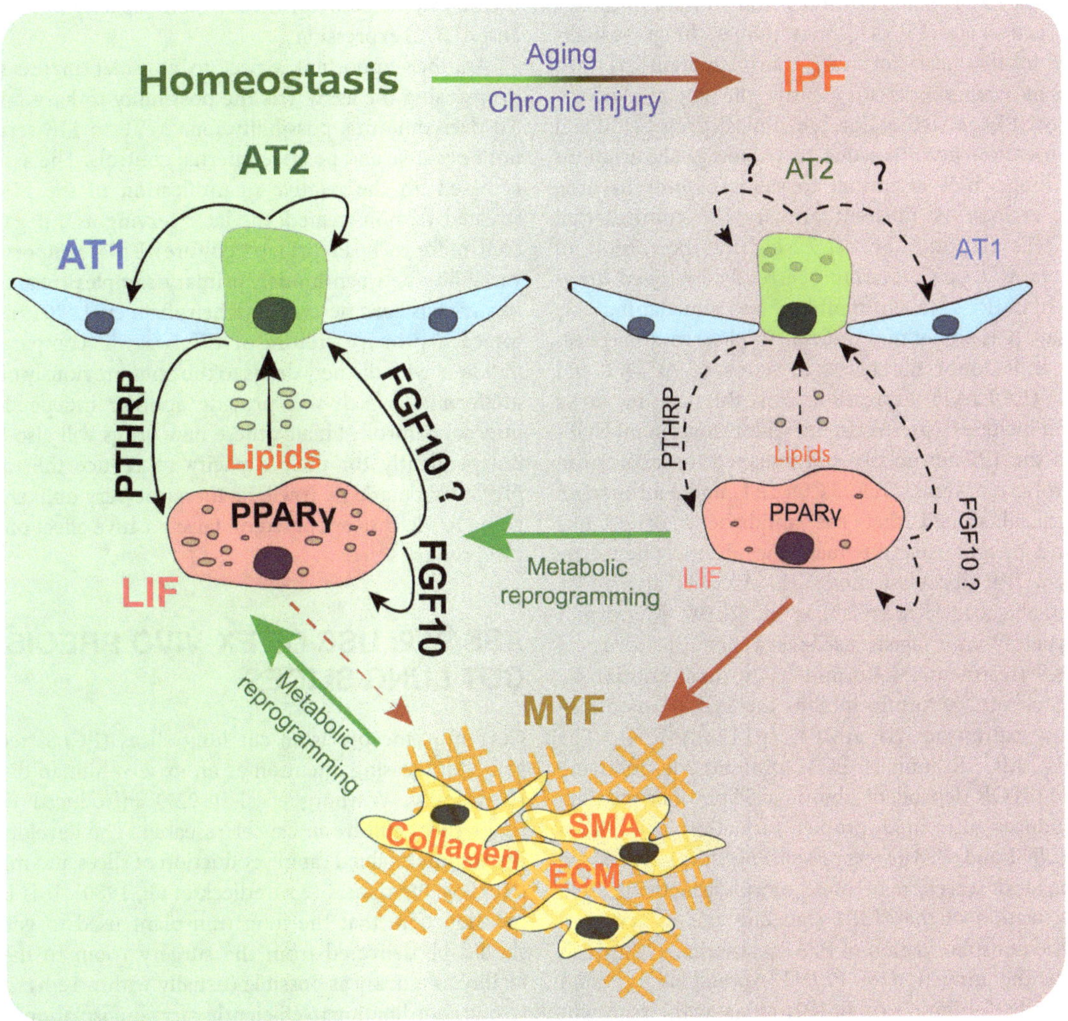

FIGURE 1 | Alveolar type 2 (AT2) and lipofibroblast (LIF) interaction during homeostasis and IPF. During homeostasis, a subset of AT2 cells helps in the renewal and maintenance of the AT2 and alveolar type 1 (AT1) pools. The PTHRP/PPARγ axis is vital for lipid trafficking and surfactant production. FGF10 signaling maintains LIFs and acts as s stem cell niche for AT2. During IPF, AT2 cells senesce. Disruption of the PTHRP/PPARγ axis and FGF10 leads to loss of LIFs. LIFs differentiate to smooth muscle actin (SMA) positive Myofibroblasts (MYF), with excessive extracellular matrix (ECM) deposition. Metabolic reprograming promotes the dedifferentiation of MYFs to LIFs, and helps retain the LIF population.

CD36 (aka platelet glycoprotein 4), translocate into fibroblasts for lysosomal degradation (Rabinowitz and Mutlu, 2019; Zhao et al., 2020). CD36 activates PPARγ, the master regulator of lipogenesis (Febbraio et al., 2001). Tgf-β upregulation during fibrosis inhibits CD36, leading to dysregulating in collagen degradation. Therefore the extensive screening of drugs capable of correcting different types of metabolic dysregulations is likely to be a very promising venue for fibrosis therapy (Zhao et al., 2020).

In a recent study, it was reported that the first line antidiabetic and metabolic drug metformin, acting as a AMPK-activator, was capable to enhance the activated MYF to LIF transition both (1) *in vitro* in primary fibroblasts from IPF patients, (2) *ex vivo* in precision cut lung slices from end-stage IPF lungs obtained from transplant patients, and (3) *in vivo* using bleomycin-induced fibrosis mouse models in the context of lineage tracing of activated MYF during resolution (Kheirollahi et al., 2019). These three types of assay constitute the base for the pre-clinical drug screening in idiopathic pulmonary fibrosis.

ASSAY 1: USE OF PRIMARY FIBROBLASTS FROM HUMAN LUNGS

Due to their ability to replicate human physiology, *in vitro* human cell-based models have been extensively used in drug testing during toxicological and pharmacological studies. Human lung fibroblast cultures were established during the early 1960s in the Wistar Institute (Hayflick and Moorhead, 1961). Later, the fibroblasts were immortalized by simian virus 40 (SV40). However, cell immortalization resulted in permanent phenotypic changes and may no longer reflect *in vitro* their normal counterpart (Jensen et al., 1963).

To circumvent this problem, primary human lung fibroblast culture from end stage IPF or Donor human lungs (usually obtained due to the need for lung transplantation) is now the standard *in vitro* model to identify the key underlying mechanisms of IPF, as well as for pre-clinical drug testing. It is critical to mention here that due to pathological variations between IPF lungs, it is important to validate, prior to drug screening, on at least 10 different primary IPF cultures that the selected cells respond (by decreasing the expression of fibrotic markers *ACTA2, COL1A1*) to currently approved drugs commonly used in IPF such as pirfenidone and nintedanib.

In this assay, it is sometimes difficult to observe differences between IPF and Donor fibroblasts in terms of ACTA2 and collagen 1A1 (COL1A1) expression. For this reason, drug screening often includes a pre-treatment with recombinant TGF-β to activates the IPF fibroblasts and enhance the expression of the profibrotic markers ACTA2, COL1A1, and Fibronectin. Recent studies illustrated that the antidiabetic drugs like metformin and rosiglitazone attenuate the fibrotic phenotype in this *in vitro* IPF fibroblast model (El Agha et al., 2017b; Rangarajan et al., 2018; Kheirollahi et al., 2019). Metformin is an anti-hyperglycemic agent used as a first line drug in type 2 diabetes treatment. Metformin has a dual, antifibrotic and lipogenic, effect. Metformin inhibits the TGF-β1 mediated ECM proteins expression via AMPK (pT172-AMPK). The AMPK agonist AICAR inhibits ECM proteins via inducing autophagy and mTOR-dependent ribosomal S6 phosphorylation. Metformin induces also lipid droplet formation as well as increase in *PLIN2* and *PPARg* expression. Metformin induced the expression and secretion of bone morphogenetic protein 2 (BMP2). Activation of the BMP2 signaling axis in activated MYFs led to the phosphorylation of PPARγ at serine-112, which in turn led to the induction of *PLIN2* expression and lipid droplet formation. Inhibition of BMP2, along with treatment with metformin, abolishes lipid droplet formation and *PLIN2* expression. However, AMPK-dependent COL1A1 inhibition was not altered in these studies.

Interestingly, compared to metformin, pirfenidone and nintedanib displayed quite a modest effect on reduction of the expression of fibrotic markers in primary IPF culture (Kheirollahi et al., 2019). This could be due to drug resistance in IPF patients upon long-term treatment and justifies the efforts for fast-tracking the discovery of new drugs.

Rosiglitazone, a PPARγ agonist and antidiabetic drug, antagonizes the TGF-β-mediated fibrotic phenotype. Time-lapse imaging of primary human lung fibroblasts with antifibrotic drugs (metformin/rosiglitazone) and LipidTOX dye is a novel model to visualize in real-time the transition from a profibrotic to an antifibrotic phenotype. This assay can be amenable to high throughput screening by adapting the culture of IPF fibroblasts to 96 or 384 wells plates and incorporating fluorescent imaging techniques or fluorescence quantification of each well through automated systems allowing the quantification of LipidTOX staining (**Figure 2**) or the total fluorescence signal through a proper cell lysis. However, in this later case, it is important to use a lysis method that will not degrade the lipids. In addition, drugs capable of inducing the lipogenic differentiation should then be validated by qPCR for their capacity to reduce *COL1A1* and *ACTA2* expression.

Another important aspect to consider in the screening of drugs using the assay 1 is the possibility to have false positives. To overcome this possibility, our MYF to LIF screen includes both negative and positive internal controls. The assay described is based on the relative quantification of the LIF phenotype (treated vs. non-treated, the later serving as a negative internal control for each IPF primary culture). This is important as a high variability between human primary samples treated with drugs *in vitro* has been described (Kheirollahi et al., 2019). In addition, for each primary culture of IPF, we will compare the results obtained with the new drugs to the ones previously obtained with metformin (which will provide another independent positive internal control). Finally, these new drugs will also be evaluated independently for their capacity to reduce the expression of profibrotic markers. It will be therefore very unlikely that we are going to select drugs based on false positive effect on the MYF to LIF primary screen.

ASSAY 2: USE OF EX-VIVO PRECISION CUT LUNG SLICES

Currently, the precision-cut lung slices (PCLS) technique has gained increasing attention as an *ex vivo* human disease model. Historically, Warburg et al. (1927) introduced the usage of tissue slices culture in cancer research. The development of the microtome enabled rapid production of slices and minimized the stress on the tissues (Krumdieck et al., 1980). It is important to mention here that the lung transplant used to generate PCLS should be delivered from the surgery room to the processing facility as quickly as possible (usually within 12 h). This requires strong coordination to efficiently carry out isolation of fibroblasts, vibratome sectioning for PCLS as well as isolation of epithelial, mesenchymal, endothelial and immune cells by flow cytometry. In addition, while it is possible to cryopreserve live cells such as primary fibroblasts, this technique is not efficient to preserve the integrity of PCLS, which therefore require fresh lungs. Initially, PCLS were used to study proximal airways in toxicological studies, and were later optimized for the distal lung tissues (Placke, 1987; Kheirollahi et al., 2019). Human lung tissues enable a more sophisticated analysis of fibrosis mechanisms and provide material for pre-clinical drug testing. PCLS are thought to preserve human physiology and lung functionality, by which interactions between cells can be maintained during fibrosis and drug testing. Use of PCLS as a secondary assay for the validation of drugs capable of inducing lipogenic differentiation (see Assay 1) is a natural and optimal follow up in the overall pre-clinical validation strategy. Due to the use of pertinent human material, PCLS reduces the challenges in the interpretation and limitations which are commonly observed in animal fibrosis models (see assay 3).

It was recently shown that metformin has antifibrotic properties in the PCLS model. In this study, 200 μm PCLS display preserved tissue architecture for up to 5 days in culture. Human IPF PCLS treated with metformin for 5 days exhibited

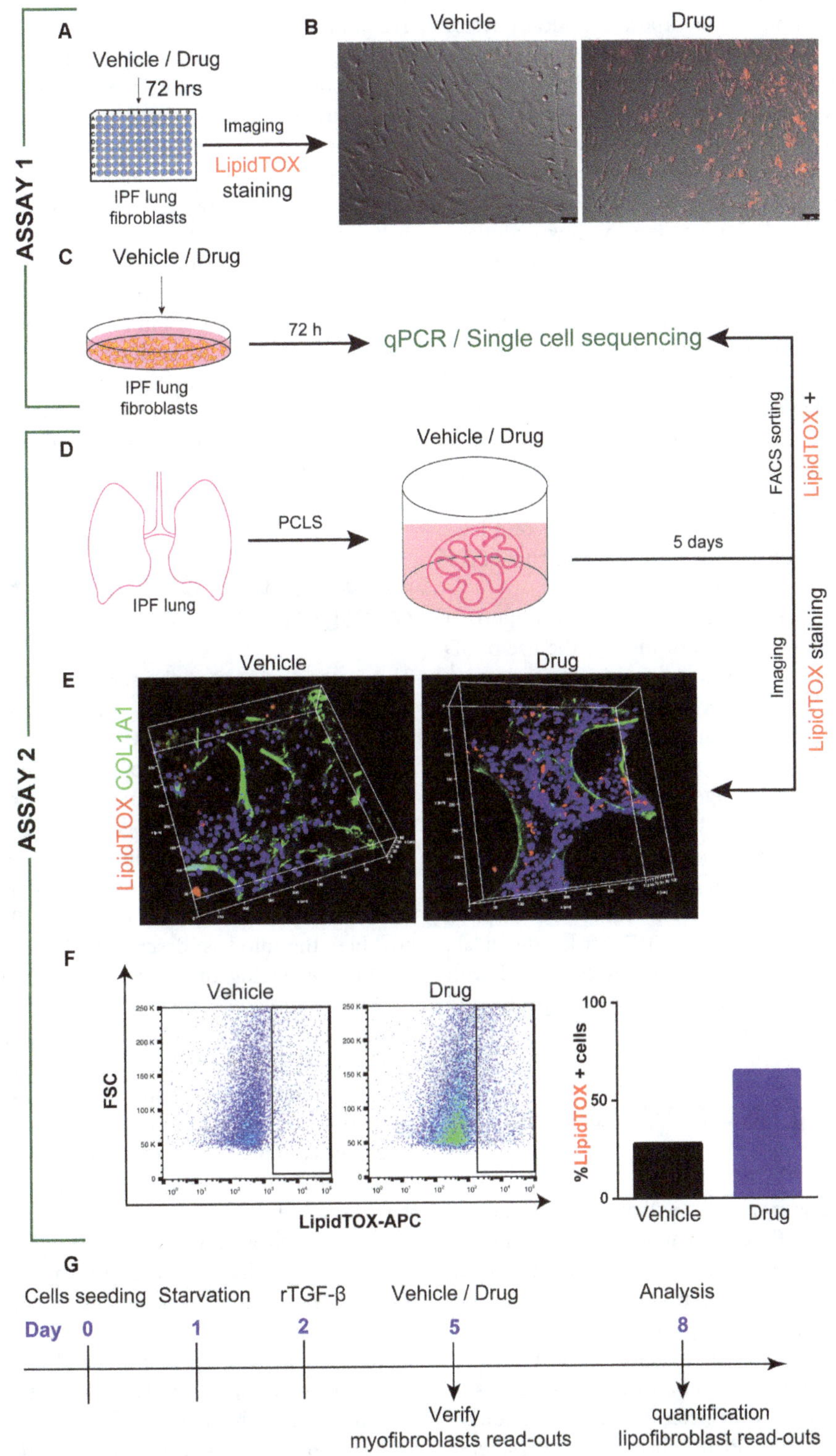

FIGURE 2 | *In vitro* drug screening models in idiopathic pulmonary fibrosis. **(A)** Experimental set-up, where primary IPF lung fibroblasts are treated with drugs or vehicle in a 96 well plate. **(B)** Time-lapse imaging with presence of LipidTOX dye to visualize lipid drops for 72 h. **(C)** Treatment of primary IPF lung fibroblasts with drugs or vehicle for 72 h and gene analysis by qPCR or single-cell sequencing. **(D)** PCLS preparation from fresh IPF lung explants and treatment of PCLS with drugs or vehicle for 5 days, FACS-sorting of LipidTOX positive cells, and analysis of genes by qPCR or single-cell sequencing. **(E)** Confocal images of PCLS after 5 days treatment and staining with LipidTOX dye and anti-Collagen1 antibody. **(F)** FACS-based analysis and quantification for vehicle and drug treated PCLS or IPF lung fibroblasts. **(G)** Timeline for assay 1 (Figure 2 adapted from Kheirollahi et al., 2019). Scale bars: **(B)** 5 μm; **(E)** 400 μm, 400 μm, 100 μm (XYZ-axis).

macroscopically a relaxed structure with open spaces. In the future, it would be important to incorporate optical/physical techniques allowing to quantify this relaxed state. Metformin treatment increased the number of LipidTOX stained cells with a corresponding decrease in collagen deposition. Such a decrease in collagen, together with other fibrotic specific proteins, as well as the induction of lipofibroblast characteristic markers (e.g., PLIN2 and PPARγ), could also be validated by western blot using the whole PCLS. Quantification by flow cytometry indicated increase in LipidTOX positive cells in the PCLS treated with metformin vs. vehicle suggesting a transition from a MYF to LIF phenotype in IPF lungs. Analysis of histological images supported that metformin attenuated fibrosis, and tissue sections confirmed the relaxed structure and open airspaces associated with decreased collagen deposition. Time-lapse imaging of PCLS with antifibrotic drugs and LipidTOX dye was a novel model used to visualize in real-time the transition from a profibrotic to an antifibrotic phenotype. As IPF lungs may not be easily available in every institution, this assay should be kept as a second level validation of the drugs identified using the primary culture of IPF fibroblasts and LipidTOX staining as a main read out.

Due to the limitation in obtaining fresh lungs, it is important to consider alternative approach. One of them is the use of 3D Matrigel-based lung organoids developed *in vitro* from human pluripotent stem cells (hPSCs). Recently, Snoeck et al. have developed a model to generate lung bud organoids (LBOs) form hPSCs. These LBOs contain pulmonary endoderm and mesoderm. LBOs cultured in Matrigel displayed the formation of branching airways and alveolar structures. This model was carried out to study the lung fibrosis associated with Hermansky–Pudlak syndrome (HPS). Deletion in hPSCs of *HPS1*, *HPS2* and *HPS4* followed by the generation of corresponding LBOs showed elevated fibrotic markers (Chen et al., 2017; Strikoudis et al., 2019). New experimental models using LBOs combined with CRISPR/Cas9 gene editing could be used as a therapeutic and drug screening model in the coming future.

HOW ARE ASSAY 1 AND 2 ADVANCING IPF RESEARCH?

The first advantage of these two assays is that human materials coming from patients with IPF are being used. This allows testing of new drugs directly on primary human cells relevant for the disease. The drawback of Assay 1 is that it is lacking the *in vivo* environment. In addition, the phenotype of the cells may change due to *in vitro* culture and in our experience, there is quite a lot of variability in the response to drugs between different sets of primary IPF fibroblast (reflecting the heterogeneity of the human population). In addition, as these IPF fibroblasts are from patients who have been treated with Pirfenidone and/or Nintedanib, the response of the IPF cells from these patients is somehow limited due likely to resistance to these drugs (Kheirollahi et al., 2019). As aforementioned, to overcome the variability between IPF fibroblasts, a pre-treatment with recombinant TGF-β is required to activate the IPF fibroblasts and enhance the expression of the profibrotic markers ACTA2, COL1A1, and Fibronectin. Furthermore, to have statistical reliable results, it is recommended to use around 10 independent primary IPF cell fibroblasts. Assay 1 is mostly testing the efficacy of new drugs in the context of resistance to the currently available drugs. It may therefore be important to treat the cells with a combination of the old drugs with the new ones under investigation to find a potential synergistic effect. The same limitations are also applicable for the assay 2, even though PCLSs represent a much better model due to the preservation of the complex cellular environment. As aforementioned, LIFs and AT2 cells interactions are crucial for the maintenance of the AT2 stem cells during homeostasis. Loss of LIFs in IPF correlates with AT2 cells injury and loss. Therefore, the analysis of new drugs using PCLS (Assay 2) should allow monitoring and quantifying the increase in LIF formation and the collateral impact on AT2 cells proliferation and differentiation. In addition, it will be important to quantify the effect of these new drugs on the restoration of the native lung structure by the clearance of the deposited collagen.

ASSAY 3: USE OF MURINE FIBROSIS MODELS

This is the last arm of the screening strategy that we propose for drugs first identified in primary culture of IPF (assay 1) and then validated using PCLS (assay 2). Murine models are widely accepted and used to study pulmonary fibrosis, due to their ability to represent the native complex biological system for understanding disease pathogenesis. Currently, various murine fibrosis models exist, including bleomycin, amiodarone, silica, asbestosis, cytokine overexpression, fluorescent isothiocyanate, and radiation-induced (Tashiro et al., 2017). Ideally and when possible, the models described above should also integrate the lineage tracing of the activated MYF [using the *Tg(Acta-CreERT2); Tomato*^{flox} mice] (El Agha et al., 2017b). This would allow an easy monitoring of the activated MYF during resolution.

However, murine models have limitations. One limitation is that young mice, capable of fibrosis resolution are often used. IPF occurs usually in old men and is unfortunately not reversible (Garcia, 2011). It would therefore be more appropriate to use older mice (around 12–18 months of age) instead of the 2–3 months old mice used in most of the studies. Aging is associated with a natural decline in physiological and cellular processes. The hallmarks of the aging process are cellular senescence, epigenetic changes, stem cell depletion, genomic mutations, mitochondrial dysfunction, metabolic changes, and altered cellular communications and interactions (Sgalla et al., 2018; Bueno et al., 2020). Aging leads to significant prevalence of chronic lung diseases like COPD and IPF. An age and sex dimorphism study revealed aged male mice are more susceptible to fibrosis than young males, and, interestingly, young and old female mice showed less fibrosis than male mice (Redente et al., 2011). In addition, most of these model do not integrate the progressive nature of the disease, which in humans takes decades to develop. Interestingly, such models mimicking the progressive injury to AT2 cells with mutation in *surfactant protein C (Sftpc)* leading to endoplasmic reticulum stress (Lawson et al., 2011) or the recently described mice displaying *Cdc-42* deletion in AT2 cells (Wu et al., 2020) are now available. If drugs can work in the context of these mouse models, then there is a higher chance that these drugs will be more efficient in humans. Prior to the initiation of clinical trials, these mouse models should definitively be included for the final selection of drugs potentially efficient in IPF.

CONCLUSION

The reversible myogenic/lipogenic switch was used as an example to illustrate different pre-clinical models. We have detailed a three arms strategy for the high flow throughput selection and subsequent validation of new drugs potentially used for the treatment of IPF patients. These drugs are selected based on their lipogenic differentiation potential as well as on their antifibrotic potential. The reversible myogenic/lipogenic switch between LIF and activated MYF is a new paradigm that has not been used so far in the context of drug screening. Finding drugs displaying this dual lipogenic/antifibrotic activity will allow restoring the functionality of the LIFs, an essential component of the AT2 stem cell niche, thereby promoting enhanced lung repair.

AUTHOR CONTRIBUTIONS

AL wrote the manuscript. MJ edited the manuscript. SBa made the illustrations. CC, SR, and SBe proposed the concept for the manuscript, guided the writing process, and made the final corrections. All authors contributed to the article and approved the submitted version.

ACKNOWLEDGMENTS

We apologize to those colleagues whose references have been omitted from this discussion due to space restrictions and our focus, we were unable to include all articles on this interesting and diverse subject matter.

REFERENCES

Al Alam, D., El Agha, E., Sakurai, R., Kheirollahi, V., Moiseenko, A., Danopoulos, S., et al. (2015). Evidence for the involvement of fibroblast growth factor 10 in lipofibroblast formation during embryonic lung development. *Development* 142, 4139–4150. doi: 10.1242/dev.109173

Barkauskas, C. E., Cronce, M. J., Rackley, C. R., Bowie, E. J., Keene, D. R., Stripp, B. R., et al. (2013). Type 2 alveolar cells are stem cells in adult lung. *J. Clin. Invest.* 123, 3025–3036. doi: 10.1172/jci68782

Bellusci, S., Grindley, J., Emoto, H., Itoh, N., and Hogan, B. L. (1997). Fibroblast growth factor 10 (FGF10) and branching morphogenesis in the embryonic mouse lung. *Development* 124, 4867–4878.

Bueno, M., Calyeca, J., Rojas, M., and Mora, A. L. (2020). Mitochondria dysfunction and metabolic reprogramming as drivers of idiopathic pulmonary fibrosis. *Redox Biol.* 33:101509. doi: 10.1016/j.redox.2020.101509

Chen, Y. W., Huang, S. X., de Carvalho, A., Ho, S. H., Islam, M. N., Volpi, S., et al. (2017). A three-dimensional model of human lung development and disease from pluripotent stem cells. *Nat. Cell Biol.* 19, 542–549. doi: 10.1038/ncb3510

Cheng, T., Liu, Q., Zhang, R., Zhang, Y., Chen, J., Yu, R., et al. (2014). Lysyl oxidase promotes bleomycin-induced lung fibrosis through modulating inflammation. *J. Mol. Cell Biol.* 6, 506–515. doi: 10.1093/jmcb/mju039

El Agha, E., Herold, S., Al Alam, D., Quantius, J., MacKenzie, B., Carraro, G., et al. (2014). Fgf10-positive cells represent a progenitor cell population during lung development and postnatally. *Development* 141, 296–306. doi: 10.1242/dev.099747

El Agha, E., Kramann, R., Schneider, R. K., Li, X., Seeger, W., Humphreys, B. D., et al. (2017a). Mesenchymal stem cells in fibrotic disease. *Cell Stem Cell* 21, 166–177. doi: 10.1016/j.stem.2017.07.011

El Agha, E., Moiseenko, A., Kheirollahi, V., De Langhe, S., Crnkovic, S., Kwapiszewska, G., et al. (2017b). Two-way conversion between lipogenic and myogenic fibroblastic phenotypes marks the progression and resolution of lung fibrosis. *Cell Stem Cell* 20, 261–273.e263. doi: 10.1016/j.stem.2016.10.004

Endo, M., Oyadomari, S., Terasaki, Y., Takeya, M., Suga, M., Mori, M., et al. (2003). Induction of arginase I and II in bleomycin-induced fibrosis of mouse lung. *Am. J. Physiol. Lung Cell Mol. Physiol.* 285, L313–L321. doi: 10.1152/ajplung.00434.2002

Febbraio, M., Hajjar, D. P., and Silverstein, R. L. (2001). CD36: a class B scavenger receptor involved in angiogenesis, atherosclerosis, inflammation, and lipid metabolism. *J. Clin. Invest.* 108, 785–791. doi: 10.1172/JCI14006

Fernandez, I. E., and Eickelberg, O. (2012). The impact of TGF-beta on lung fibrosis: from targeting to biomarkers. *Proc. Am. Thorac. Soc.* 9, 111–116. doi: 10.1513/pats.201203-023AW

Garcia, C. K. (2011). Idiopathic pulmonary fibrosis: update on genetic discoveries. *Proc. Am. Thorac. Soc.* 8, 158–162. doi: 10.1513/pats.201008-056MS

Hamanaka, R. B., Nigdelioglu, R., Meliton, A. Y., Tian, Y., Witt, L. J., O'Leary, E., et al. (2018). Inhibition of phosphoglycerate dehydrogenase attenuates bleomycin-induced pulmonary fibrosis. *Am. J. Respir. Cell Mol. Biol.* 58, 585–593. doi: 10.1165/rcmb.2017-0186OC

Hayflick, L., and Moorhead, P. S. (1961). The serial cultivation of human diploid cell strains. *Exper. Cell Res.* 25, 585–621. doi: 10.1016/0014-4827(61)90192-6

Jensen, F., Koprowski, H., and Ponten, J. A. (1963). Rapid transformation of human fibroblast cultures by simian virus. *Proc. Natl. Acad. Sci. U.S.A.* 50, 343–348. doi: 10.1073/pnas.50.2.343

Jones, M. R., Lingampally, A., Dilai, S., Shrestha, A., Stripp, B., Helmbacher, F., et al. (2019). Characterization of Tg(Etv4-GFP) and Etv5 (RFP) reporter lines in the context of fibroblast growth factor 10 signaling during mouse embryonic lung development. *Front. Genet.* 10:178. doi: 10.3389/fgene.2019.00178

Kheirollahi, V., Wasnick, R. M., Biasin, V., Vazquez-Armendariz, A. I., Chu, X., Moiseenko, A., et al. (2019). Metformin induces lipogenic differentiation in myofibroblasts to reverse lung fibrosis. *Nat. Commun.* 10:2987. doi: 10.1038/s41467-019-10839-0

Kim, K. K., Kugler, M. C., Wolters, P. J., Robillard, L., Galvez, M. G., Brumwell, A. N., et al. (2006). Alveolar epithelial cell mesenchymal transition develops in vivo during pulmonary fibrosis and is regulated by the extracellular matrix. *Proc. Natl. Acad. Sci. U.S.A.* 103, 13180–13185. doi: 10.1073/pnas.0605669103

Konishi, M., Asaki, T., Koike, N., Miwa, H., Miyake, A., and Itoh, N. (2006). Role of Fgf10 in cell proliferation in white adipose tissue. *Mol. Cell Endocrinol.* 249, 71–77. doi: 10.1016/j.mce.2006.01.010

Krumdieck, C. L., dos Santos, J., and Ho, K.-J. (1980). A new instrument for the rapid preparation of tissue slices. *Analyt. Biochem.* 104, 118–123. doi: 10.1016/0003-2697(80)90284-5

Lawson, W. E., Cheng, D. S., Degryse, A. L., Tanjore, H., Polosukhin, V. V., Xu, X. C., et al. (2011). Endoplasmic reticulum stress enhances fibrotic remodeling in the lungs. *Proc. Natl. Acad. Sci. U.S.A.* 108, 10562–10567. doi: 10.1073/pnas.1107559108

Li, J., Wang, Z., Chu, Q., Jiang, K., Li, J., and Tang, N. (2018). The strength of mechanical forces determines the differentiation of alveolar epithelial cells. *Dev. Cell* 44, 297–312.e295. doi: 10.1016/j.devcel.2018.01.008

Liu, Z., Wu, H., Jiang, K., Wang, Y., Zhang, W., Chu, Q., et al. (2016). MAPK-mediated YAP activation controls mechanical-tension-induced pulmonary alveolar regeneration. *Cell Rep.* 16, 1810–1819. doi: 10.1016/j.celrep.2016.07.020

Marriott, S., Baskir, R. S., Gaskill, C., Menon, S., Carrier, E. J., Williams, J., et al. (2014). ABCG2pos lung mesenchymal stem cells are a novel pericyte subpopulation that contributes to fibrotic remodeling. *Am. J. Physiol. Cell Physiol.* 307, C684–C698. doi: 10.1152/ajpcell.00114.2014

Mora, A. L., Rojas, M., Pardo, A., and Selman, M. (2017). Emerging therapies for idiopathic pulmonary fibrosis, a progressive age-related disease. *Nat. Rev. Drug Discov.* 16, 755–772. doi: 10.1038/nrd.2017.170

Nigdelioglu, R., Hamanaka, R. B., Meliton, A. Y., O'Leary, E., Witt, L. J., Cho, T., et al. (2016). Transforming growth factor (TGF)-beta promotes de novo serine synthesis for collagen production. *J. Biol. Chem.* 291, 27239–27251. doi: 10.1074/jbc.M116.756247

O'Hare, K. H., and Sheridan, M. N. (1970). Electron microscopic observations on the morphogenesis of the albino rat lung, with special reference to pulmonary epithelial cells. *Am. J. Anat.* 127, 181–205. doi: 10.1002/aja.1001270205

Parimon, T., Yao, C., Stripp, B. R., Noble, P. W., and Chen, P. (2020). Alveolar epithelial Type II cells as drivers of lung fibrosis in idiopathic pulmonary fibrosis. *Int. J. Mol. Sci.* 21:269. doi: 10.3390/ijms21072269

Phillips, R. J., Burdick, M. D., Hong, K., Lutz, M. A., Murray, L. A., Xue, Y. Y., et al. (2004). Circulating fibrocytes traffic to the lungs in response to CXCL12 and mediate fibrosis. *J. Clin. Invest.* 114, 438–446. doi: 10.1172/JCI20997

Placke, M. (1987). Adult peripheral lung organ culture? A model for respiratory tract toxicology. *Toxicol. Appl. Pharmacol.* 90, 284–298. doi: 10.1016/0041-008x(87)90336-x

Rabinowitz, J. D., and Mutlu, G. M. (2019). A metabolic strategy to reverse fibrosis? *Nat. Metab.* 1, 12–13. doi: 10.1038/s42255-018-0013-8

Rangarajan, S., Bone, N. B., Zmijewska, A. A., Jiang, S., Park, D. W., Bernard, K., et al. (2018). Metformin reverses established lung fibrosis in a bleomycin model. *Nat. Med.* 24, 1121–1127. doi: 10.1038/s41591-018-0087-6

Redente, E. F., Jacobsen, K. M., Solomon, J. J., Lara, A. R., Faubel, S., Keith, R. C., et al. (2011). Age and sex dimorphisms contribute to the severity of bleomycin-induced lung injury and fibrosis. *Am. J. Physiol. Lung Cell Mol. Physiol.* 301, L510–L518. doi: 10.1152/ajplung.00122.2011

Rock, J. R., Barkauskas, C. E., Cronce, M. J., Xue, Y., Harris, J. R., Liang, J., et al. (2011). Multiple stromal populations contribute to pulmonary fibrosis without evidence for epithelial to mesenchymal transition. *Proc. Natl. Acad. Sci. U.S.A.* 108, E1475–E1483. doi: 10.1073/pnas.1117988108

Sakaue, H., Konishi, M., Ogawa, W., Asaki, T., Mori, T., Yamasaki, M., et al. (2002). Requirement of fibroblast growth factor 10 in development of white adipose tissue. *Genes Dev.* 16, 908–912. doi: 10.1101/gad.983202

Schietke, R., Warnecke, C., Wacker, I., Schodel, J., Mole, D. R., Campean, V., et al. (2010). The lysyl oxidases LOX and LOXL2 are necessary and sufficient to repress E-cadherin in hypoxia: insights into cellular transformation processes mediated by HIF-1. *J. Biol. Chem.* 285, 6658–6669. doi: 10.1074/jbc.M109.042424

Selman, M., and Pardo, A. (2006). Role of epithelial cells in idiopathic pulmonary fibrosis: from innocent targets to serial killers. *Proc. Am. Thorac. Soc.* 3, 364–372. doi: 10.1513/pats.200601-003TK

Sgalla, G., Iovene, B., Calvello, M., Ori, M., Varone, F., and Richeldi, L. (2018). Idiopathic pulmonary fibrosis: pathogenesis and management. *Respir. Res.* 19:32. doi: 10.1186/s12931-018-0730-2

Strikoudis, A., Cieslak, A., Loffredo, L., Chen, Y. W., Patel, N., Saqi, A., et al. (2019). Modeling of fibrotic lung disease using 3D organoids derived from human pluripotent stem cells. *Cell Rep.* 27, 3709–3723.e3705. doi: 10.1016/j.celrep.2019.05.077

Tashiro, J., Rubio, G. A., Limper, A. H., Williams, K., Elliot, S. J., Ninou, I., et al. (2017). Exploring animal models that resemble idiopathic pulmonary fibrosis. *Front. Med.* 4:118. doi: 10.3389/fmed.2017.00118

Torday, J. S. (2003). Parathyroid hormone-related protein is a gravisensor in lung and bone cell biology. *Adv. Space Res.* 32, 1569–1576. doi: 10.1016/s0273-1177(03)90397-8

Torday, J. S., Torres, E., and Rehan, V. K. (2003). The role of fibroblast transdifferentiation in lung epithelial cell proliferation, differentiation, and repair in vitro. *Pediatr. Pathol. Mol. Med.* 22, 189–207. doi: 10.1080/pdp.22.3.189.207

Vaccaro, C., and Brody, J. S. (1978). Ultrastructure of developing alveoli. I. The role of the interstitial fibroblast. *Anat. Rec.* 192, 467–479. doi: 10.1002/ar.1091920402

Warburg, O., Wind, F., and Negelein, E. (1927). The metabolism of tumors in the body. *J. Gen. Physiol.* 8, 519–530. doi: 10.1085/jgp.8.6.519

Wipff, P. J., Rifkin, D. B., Meister, J. J., and Hinz, B. (2007). Myofibroblast contraction activates latent TGF-beta1 from the extracellular matrix. *J. Cell Biol.* 179, 1311–1323. doi: 10.1083/jcb.200704042

Wu, H., Yu, Y., Huang, H., Hu, Y., Fu, S., Wang, Z., et al. (2020). Progressive pulmonary fibrosis is caused by elevated mechanical tension on alveolar stem Cells. *Cell* 180, 107–121.e117. doi: 10.1016/j.cell.2019.11.027

Yao, C., Guan, X., Carraro, G., Parimon, T., Liu, X., Huang, G., et al. (2019). Senescence ofalveolar stem cells drives progressive pulmonary fibrosis. *bioRxiv* [Preprint], doi: 10.1101/820175

Yu, G., Tzouvelekis, A., Wang, R., Herazo-Maya, J. D., Ibarra, G. H., Srivastava, A., et al. (2018). Thyroid hormone inhibits lung fibrosis in mice by improving epithelial mitochondrial function. *Nat. Med.* 24, 39–49. doi: 10.1038/nm.4447

Zacharias, W. J., Frank, D. B., Zepp, J. A., Morley, M. P., Alkhaleel, F. A., Kong, J., et al. (2018). Regeneration of the lung alveolus by an evolutionarily conserved epithelial progenitor. *Nature* 555, 251–255. doi: 10.1038/nature25786

Zhao, X., Kwan, J. Y. Y., Yip, K., Liu, P. P., and Liu, F. F. (2020). Targeting metabolic dysregulation for fibrosis therapy. *Nat. Rev. Drug Discov.* 19, 57–75. doi: 10.1038/s41573-019-0040-5

3

Modifying and Integrating *in vitro* and *ex vivo* Respiratory Models for Inhalation Drug Screening

Aylin Cidem [1†]***, Peta Bradbury*** [1,2†]***, Daniela Traini*** [1,2] ***and Hui Xin Ong*** [1,2*]

[1] *Respiratory Technology, Woolcock Institute of Medical Research, Sydney, NSW, Australia,* [2] *Faculty of Medicine and Health, University of Sydney, Sydney, NSW, Australia*

***Correspondence:**
Hui Xin Ong
ong.hui@sydney.edu.au

† *These authors have contributed equally to this work*

For the past 50 years, the route of inhalation has been utilized to administer therapies to treat a variety of respiratory and pulmonary diseases. When compared with other drug administration routes, inhalation offers a targeted, non-invasive approach to deliver rapid onset of drug action to the lung, minimizing systemic drug exposure and subsequent side effects. However, despite advances in inhaled therapies, there is still a need to improve the preclinical screening and the efficacy of inhaled therapeutics. Innovative *in vitro* models of respiratory physiology to determine therapeutic efficacy of inhaled compounds have included the use of organoids, micro-engineered lung-on-chip systems and sophisticated bench-top platforms to enable a better understanding of pulmonary mechanisms at the molecular level, rapidly progressing inhaled therapeutic candidates to the clinic. Furthermore, the integration of complementary *ex vivo* models, such as precision-cut lung slices (PCLS) and isolated perfused lung platforms have further advanced preclinical drug screening approaches by providing *in vivo* relevance. In this review, we address the challenges and advances of *in vitro* models and discuss the implementation of *ex vivo* inhaled drug screening models. Specifically, we address the importance of understanding human *in vivo* pulmonary mechanisms in assessing strategies of the preclinical screening of drug efficacy, toxicity and delivery of inhaled therapeutics.

Keywords: drug efficacy, drug delivery, drug toxicity, inhalation therapy, isolated perfused lung, lung-on-chip, organoid, precision-cut lung slices

INTRODUCTION

Respiratory diseases are among the leading causes of mortality worldwide, with chronic obstructive pulmonary disease (COPD), lung infections (viral and bacterial), lung cancer and tuberculosis all listed in the top 10 causes of death (World Health Organisation [WHO], 2019a,b). Respiratory diseases impose an immense global health burden, with an estimated 1 billion people suffering from either acute or chronic conditions that result in upwards of 4 million deaths annually (World Health Organisation [WHO], 2014). Treatment of respiratory diseases relies on a variety of drug administration routes, however, not all routes are effective for disease or symptomatic relief. For example, when treating lung cancer, anti-cancer therapeutics are commonly administered systemically, resulting in low drug concentrations at the tumor site, reduced efficacy and multiple negative systemic side effects (Palumbo et al., 2013). Thus, a more targeted approach to the delivery and administration of anti-cancer drugs for lung cancer patients may increase therapeutic benefit and also quality of life. Whereas, oral and intravenous drug administration of high dose antibiotics and anti-inflammatory agents are commonly used to treat COPD, cystic fibrosis, pulmonary oedemas, and respiratory infections. However, both of these administration routes require the drug to be pre-processed by either liver or kidney and as a result, sustained long-term treatment strategies often cause liver/kidney toxicity and failure (Ditchfield et al., 2018). As such, a targeted delivery approach that deposits drugs directly within the lung (via inhalation) will distribute optimal and effective drug concentrations to the diseased site, minimize systemic drug exposure by negating any negative side effects, and thereby improve therapeutic efficacy, patient outcomes and patient quality of life (Borghardt et al., 2018).

The complex anatomical structure and branching of the lung present a unique challenge when attempting a targeted drug delivery approach. The airways also contain several biological barriers and properties that can limit drug uptake (transport, absorption) and subsequent efficacy (Ruge et al., 2013). Following inhalation, drugs deposited in the lung are subject to removal by the natural clearance mechanisms of the epithelium; goblet cells secrete a mucous layer to line the airways, and ciliated cells rapidly beat in a coordinated, metachronous fashion to move the mucous-trapped drug particle up, and out of the airway (Eliezer et al., 1970). While, drugs deposited in lower lung regions, for example in the alveolar space, are engulfed and removed by resident alveolar macrophages (Wanner et al., 1996; Ruge et al., 2013). However, once a drug is successfully deposited within an airway, a new challenge arises, as the epithelial cells that line the bronchial tree form tight junctions and it is these tight junctions that limit drug uptake and therefore therapeutic efficacy (Ghadiri et al., 2019). Importantly, however, it is not just the structural, physiological and biological properties of the lung that present challenges for inhaled therapies, the physiochemical and pharmacokinetic characteristics of the drug also need to be taken into account.

The physiochemical attributes of an inhaled drug interact with the biological properties of a lung to determine the deposition site, mechanism of action and therapeutic efficacy. The size of an aerosolized drug particle plays a pivotal role in determining the exact deposition site within the lung with particles of an aerodynamic diameter of 5–10 μm depositing in the larger airways, while particles less than 2 μm in diameter can be targeted to the bronchoalveolar and deep lung alveolar regions (Davies and Muir, 1966; Yeh et al., 1976; Lippmann et al., 1980). Particles with an aerodynamic diameter smaller than 0.5 μm can theoretically be delivered to the alveolar space, however, the majority of particles are immediately exhaled following inhalation due to their small size (Davies and Muir, 1966; Yeh et al., 1976; Lippmann et al., 1980). In order to evade the aforementioned clearance mechanisms of the airways, inhaled therapeutics are engineered with the appropriate surface chemistry to avoid adhesion to the mucosal layer and yet small enough for deposition beyond the large airways (Lippmann et al., 1980).

To appropriately determine key parameters of inhaled therapies (aerodynamic performance, pharmacodynamics and pharmacokinetics), *in vitro* lung models have been developed, validated and characterized to be used as preclinical screening tools. One of the key objectives for these *in vitro* research models is to mimic the structural and biological properties of the *in vivo* human lung environment to better replicate therapeutic exposure, deposition and efficacies. It is important to note that the translation of results from human *in vitro* models to *in vivo* animal (namely, rodent and pig) experimental results have proved limited and is hypothesized to be due to the anatomical, physiological and pathophysiological differences of human and animal lungs (Ware, 2008; Aun et al., 2017). In this review, we address the challenges and advances in *in vitro* and *ex vivo* respiratory research models when evaluating therapeutic efficacy of inhaled therapeutics in a preclinical setting to ensure successful translation to the clinic. Specifically, we discuss the implementation of progressive lung models (respiratory organoids, lung-on-chip platforms) and sophisticated bench-top approaches to evaluate inhaled drug delivery, efficacy and potential cytotoxicity.

CONVENTIONAL RESPIRATORY *in vitro* CELL MODELS

Mimicking the Heterogeneity of the Respiratory Microenvironment

The respiratory epithelium lines the airways and provides the principal physical barrier to transport and absorption of foreign particles, including inhaled therapies. The bronchial epithelium is composed of a heterogeneous mix of cells that stem from distinctive lung progenitor cells and can self-renew and differentiate into goblet, ciliated, or basal cells (Eliezer et al., 1970; Wanner et al., 1996; Ruge et al., 2013; Li et al., 2015). As mentioned previously, these differentiated epithelia cells protect the respiratory tract from foreign irritants such as smoke and dust, but also drug particles (Wanner et al., 1996). Epithelial cells form tight junctions between the neighboring epithelial cells to seal off the paracellular space between cells, regulating the influx and efflux of xenobiotics, but also the release of inflammatory mediators following inhalation of foreign agents, irritants and particulates to activate and recruit immune cells (Madara, 1998). Thus, mimicking these important biological barriers and properties *in vitro* has become an important tool when validating the appropriateness of a cell-based model. Numerous human bronchial epithelial cell lines have been used to recapitulate both healthy and diseased respiratory environments *in vitro to specifically evaluate drug transport in response to the biological barriers of the epithelium* (16HBE16o-, NuLi-1, and BEAS-2B (healthy human bronchial epithelial cells; Forbes et al., 2003; Garcia-Canton et al., 2013; Monnappa et al., 2016), Calu-3 and NCI-H441 (lung adenocarcinoma; Ong et al., 2011; Salomon et al., 2014); and CuFi-1 and CuFi-5 (cystic fibrosis; Molina et al., 2015; Sheikh et al., 2020).

Progress and Limitations of *in vitro* Air-Liquid Interface Models

To recapitulate luminal airflow of the respiratory system *in vitro*, an air-liquid interface (ALI) culture system has been implemented. Briefly, cells are first seeded onto the semi-permeable membrane of a Transwell support and both the apical (upper; cell) and basolateral (bottom; media) chambers are submerged in culture medium. When cell confluency is reached, media from the apical chamber removed, exposing the cultured cells to air and therefore establishing the ALI. Importantly, exposing cells to the air forces the cells to differentiate, secrete mucus and establish tight junctions, mimicking the *in vivo* respiratory environment. Furthermore, ALI respiratory models allow *in vivo* inhaled drug exposure conditions to be replicated by subjecting drug particles to the differentiated cell layer of the model. As such, ALI culture models provide a unique *in vitro* platform to mimic drug deposition onto the respiratory epithelial surface allowing downstream drug transport, efficacy and cytotoxicity studies to be performed (Grainger et al., 2006; Ong et al., 2011; Salomon et al., 2014).

Formation of the key biological parameters, namely tight junctions and differentiation is required for a successful ALI culture model to appropriately assess drug uptake, solute permeability and transport mechanisms. Various immortalized respiratory cell lines, including Calu-3, A549, 16HBE, NuLi-1, CuFi-1, and NCI-H441, have all been shown to form tight junctions and/or produce mucous under specific and appropriate ALI culture conditions (Grainger et al., 2006; Ong et al., 2011; Salomon et al., 2014; Faura Tellez et al., 2016; Latvala et al., 2016; Sheikh et al., 2020). However, many cell lines are limited in their ability to functionally recapitulate the *in vivo* respiratory epithelium. For example, the A549 cell line is unable to form functional tight junctions as A549 cells show reduced expression of the seal-forming proteins, claudin-3, -4, and -5 (Ren et al., 2016), while the Calu-3 cell line is unable to produce functional ciliary activity (Kreft et al., 2015). As a result, ALI culture systems have progressed to use primary human respiratory epithelial cells as primary cells can generate ciliated cells, mucus secretions and form tight junctions to better represent the *in vivo* respiratory epithelium (Pezzulo et al., 2011; Wang et al., 2018). However, there are several caveats to the use of primary epithelial cells as these cells have a finite population doubling and obtaining primary human respiratory epithelial cells from commercial sources is often expensive. As an alternative, primary bronchial epithelial cells can be harvested and expanded from deceased or transplanted human lungs, but this requires ethics approval and is a labor- and skill-intensive protocol. Despite these limitations, primary respiratory epithelial ALI culture models have been used to recapitulate *in vivo* airway epithelia as a biologically relevant *in vitro* drug screening platform (Ong et al., 2016). ALI culture systems have been heavily reviewed in the literature and have delivered highly impactful research outcomes (Movia et al., 2018; Upadhyay and Palmberg, 2018) however, the use of *in vitro* ALI models to determine toxicity, delivery and efficacy of inhaled therapeutics requires greater physiological and anatomical relevance. Specifically, *in vitro* respiratory models that implement breathing mechanics, aerosol deposition, and the co-culture of different cell types allow greater mechanistic and efficacious insights of novel inhalable therapeutic compounds. Thus, *in vitro* models that consider the biological and physiological diversity of the respiratory system provide an appropriate preclinical screening tool to determine how the respiratory microenvironment dictates the therapeutic response of inhaled agents (**Table 1**).

in vitro EXPERIMENTAL MODELS THAT PHYSIOLOGICALLY MIMIC THE RESPIRATORY SYSTEM TO SCREEN INHALED THERAPIES

To accurately investigate drug delivery, efficacy, and toxicity of inhaled therapies, *in vitro* experimental models that accurately resemble the *in vivo* physiology are crucial research tools. As such, *in vitro* experimental models have advanced beyond standard ALI monoculture methods to now include the mechanical and physiological parameters of breathing (the cyclic tissue stretch that occurs during inhalation and exhalation) that regulate airflow and pressure, the role of the extracellular matrix (ECM), and multiple cell types (alveolar, endothelial or smooth muscle cells etc.). To determine the preclinical success of an inhaled therapy, therapeutic dosage, efficacy and toxicity must be evaluated in a model(s) that aptly replicate the physiological parameters that influence *in vivo* drug transport mechanisms. Importantly, drug deposition in a specific lung region must first be inhaled via the mouth (oral pharyngeal) and then delivered to the airways (mouth-to-airway transit) and therefore is an important characteristic to replicate and include in preclinical screening models for inhaled therapies. Thus, the use of sophisticated 3-dimensional (3D) experimental models [organoids (**Figure 1**) and chip-based platforms (**Figure 2**)] and devices that model mouth-to-airway transit [Andersen Cascade impactor (ACI) (**Figure 3**), next-generation impactor (NGI) (**Figure 4**), and twin stage impinger (TSI) (**Figure 5**)] have advanced the preclinical screening capabilities of novel inhaled therapies.

Respiratory Organoids Recreate the 3-Dimensional Microenvironment of Airways to Evaluate Drug Efficacy and Toxicity

Respiratory organoids are 3D tissue-engineered culture systems capable of mimicking essential structural aspects of airways to screen drug pharmaceutical safety and efficacy (Jung et al., 2019; Liu et al., 2020). Unlike ALI monoculture models, respiratory organoids physiologically represent the 3D respiratory airway lumen microenvironment by promoting the growth and differentiation of multiple cell types to mimic the diverse structural branching present in airways (Barkauskas et al., 2017; van der Vaart and Clevers, 2020). Respiratory organoids are generated from primary lung and/or pluripotent stem cells that self-aggregate to form spheroids and then embedded within a complex mixture of extracellular matrix (ECM) proteins (collagens, laminin, and fibronectin) (Barkauskas et al., 2017; Chen et al., 2017; Leeman et al., 2019). Exposure to the ECM proteins provides the architectural and physiological support for sustained cell growth, differentiation,

TABLE 1 | Overview of the advantages and disadvantages of *in vitro* models used for respiratory inhalation drug screening.

In vitro model	Applications	Respiratory disease model	Advantages	Disadvantages	References
Air-liquid interface	Drug efficacy, toxicity and transport/delivery studies	COPD, cystic fibrosis, lung cancer	Mimics respiratory tract of the lung when exposed to toxic and therapeutic agents. Dose of inhalation agents highly controllable. Can be implemented in drug transport/delivery studies using impactor technologies.	Restricted to a select range of respiratory cell lines to functionally recapitulate the *in vivo* airway epithelium. Use of primary cells may possess ethical and cell-culturing limitations.	Grainger et al., 2006, 2012; Ong et al., 2011, 2014; Haghi et al., 2012; Kumar et al., 2020
OrganoidS	Drug efficacy and toxicity studies	Lung cancer, fibrosis, cystic fibrosis, viral and bacterial infections	Capacity to mimic cellular heterogeneity of lung microenvironment. Recapitulates structural architecture and cellular interactions of lung microenvironment. Ability to be implemented in personalized medicine studies through the use of patient-derived organoids	Do not possess breathing mechanics essential in airflow. Do not possess anatomical structures essential for addressing mouth-to-airway transit of inhaled therapies.	Tan et al., 2017; Jung et al., 2019; Miller et al., 2019
Lung-on-chip	Drug toxicity and efficacy studies	Severe asthma, COPD, lung cancer	Able to reproduce key morphological and biological processes of lung airway barriers through emulating cellular stretching of the alveolar microenvironment. Ability to recapitulate mechanical and shear stresses that result from cyclical breathing. Possess cellular heterogeneity and vascular flow rates to simulate the lung *in vivo* microenvironment.	Inability to evaluate aerosolized bio-pharmacokinetics observed during the mouth-to-airway transit of inhaled particles.	Huh et al., 2010, 2012; Benam et al., 2016; Konar et al., 2016

cell-cell and cell-matrix signaling pathways that encourages the correct spatially organization of heterogenous cell populations (epithelial, alveolar, mesenchymal cells) to generate luminal growth within the organoid (**Figure 1A**; Jacob et al., 2017; Tan et al., 2017; Miller et al., 2019). Therapeutic compounds are microinjected directly into the lumen of the organoid (Hill et al., 2017), organoids are integrated within microfluidic devices (via drug diffusion in solution) (Jung et al., 2019) or implanted within *in vivo* models (patient-derived xenografts) (**Figure 1B**; Tan et al., 2017; Berkers et al., 2019; Kim et al., 2019; Takahashi et al., 2019) to provide a physiologically relevant *in vitro* drug screening platform.

Respiratory organoids have been used to model the specific characteristics and physiological properties numerous respiratory diseases including to cystic fibrosis (Berkers et al., 2019; Dekkers et al., 2013; Liu et al., 2020), fibrosis (Strikoudis et al., 2019), viral and bacterial infections (Chen et al., 2017; Hill et al., 2017; Paolicelli et al., 2019), and lung cancer (Jung et al., 2019; Kim et al., 2019; Takahashi et al., 2019). The delivery of novel preclinical drug compounds to organoid models of respiratory diseases to determine therapeutic efficacy and cytotoxicity has been achieved in a variety of experimentally diverse setups. Hill et al. (2017) delivered drugs directly to the lumen by microinjection (using thin wall glass capillaries) to determine patient-specific drug transport, permeation across an epithelial barrier, efficacy, and toxicity, while preventing luminal contamination of the external growth media. Organoid integration within microfluidic devices has achieved drug delivery under flow conditions, mimicking the pulmonary system (Jung et al., 2019). By implementing flow conditions, a stable supply of nutrients and oxygen is delivered to the organoid but also allowed drug-containing medium to be delivered to the organoid thus, mimicking the diffusion uptake process of systemically delivered drugs. The study by Jung et al. (2019) developed patient-derived lung cancer organoids loaded within a microfluidic chip device to allow clinically relevant chemotherapeutic sensitivity under physiologically relevant flow conditions and determining safe therapeutic concentrations at the preclinical level.

Respiratory organoid models have also been developed to advance personalized medicine, especially for those diseases with high phenotypic and genetic variability including cystic fibrosis (Dekkers et al., 2013; Berkers et al., 2019) and lung cancer (Kim et al., 2019; Kondo and Inoue, 2019). Kim et al. (2019) derived lung cancer organoids from 36 patient tumor tissues of five different histological subtypes to determine individualized patient sensitivities, and in some cases previously unknown resistance to specific chemotherapeutics was found. The direct implantation of organoids *in vivo*, typically mice (known as PDX models), recapitulate the structural hallmarks of cancer tissue and maintain both genetic and histological characteristics of cancer. While drug delivery directly to the luminal space of the organoid is currently unavailable in these PDX models, drugs can be administered via intraperitoneal injection and the organoid then harvested for further pharmacodynamic and bio-pharmacokinetic analyses. Cystic fibrosis organoids been derived from patients with diverse genetic mutations and treatment

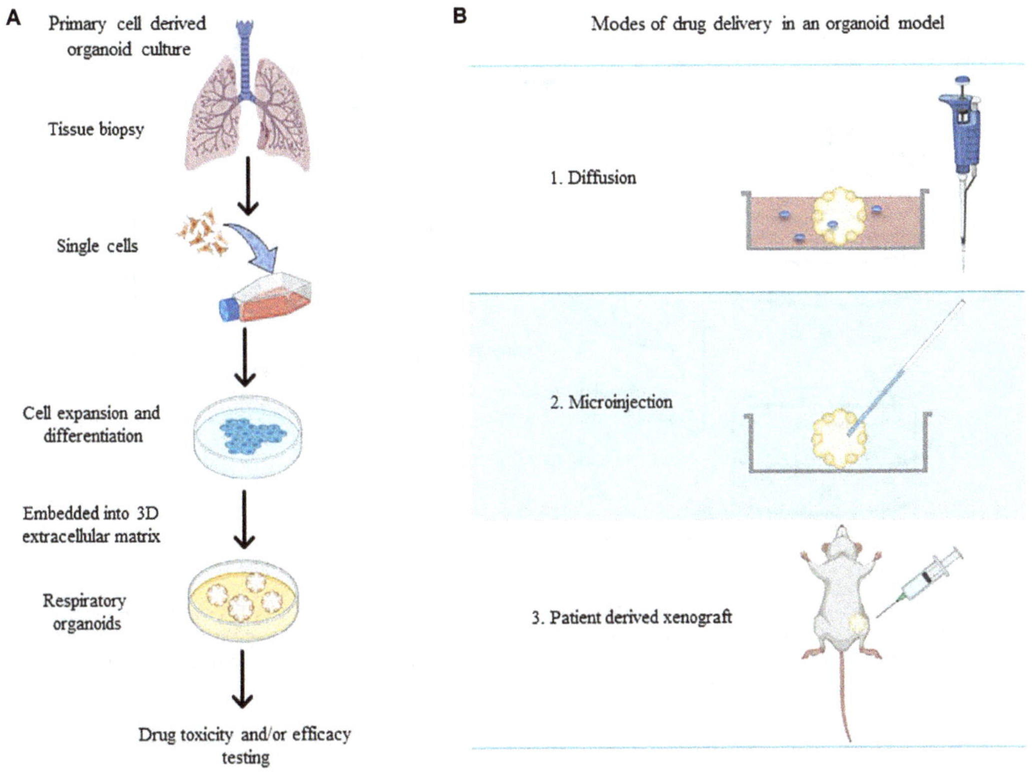

FIGURE 1 | (A) Schematic overview of methods for the generation of respiratory organoid cultures derived from primary lung cells. **(B)** The varying modes of drug treatment delivery in an organoid model (made in ©BioRender - biorender.com).

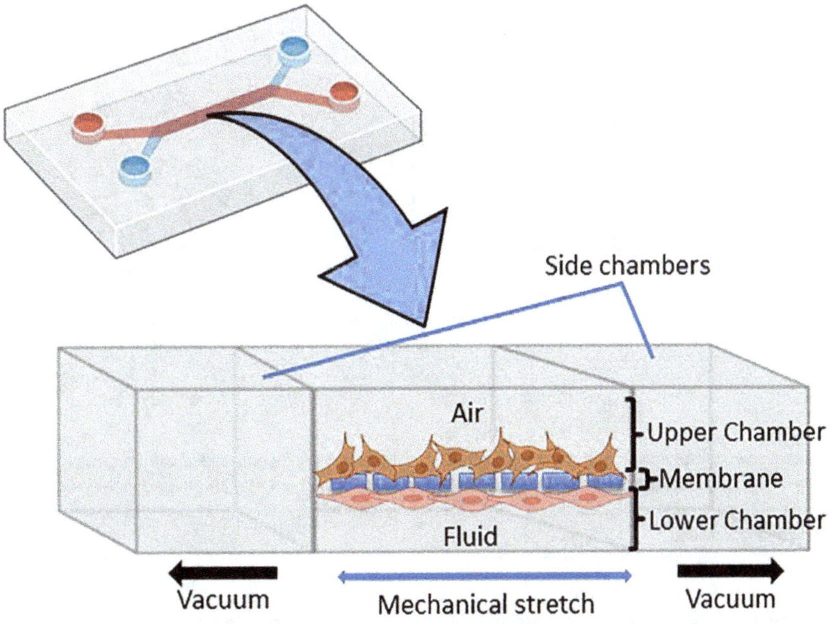

FIGURE 2 | Schematic representation of the microfluidic lung-on-chip (LOC) system. Cross-section through the LOC model displaying the upper chamber consisting of human lung epithelial cells and the lower chamber consisting of pulmonary endothelial cells divided by a thin porous membrane. Side vacuum channels stretch out the membrane and mimic *in vivo* breathing-like forces (adapted from Huh et al., 2010 and made in ©BioRender - biorender.com).

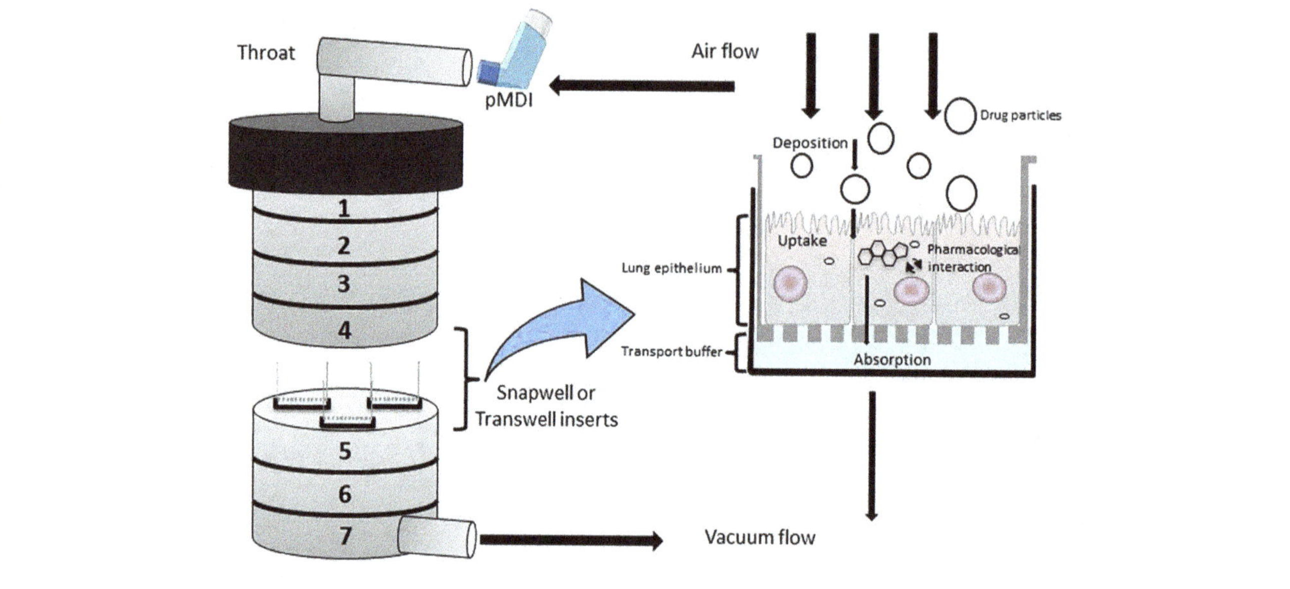

FIGURE 3 | Diagrammatic rrepresentation of a modified Anderson Cascade Impactor (mACI) with the incorporation of Snapwell or Transwell inserts embedded with respiratory cell lines at the air-liquid interface (ALI). Airflow is maintained at a controlled flow rate and generated via vacuum flow on the opposite end of the mACI to simulate airflow and allow for the assessment of mouth-to-airway transit of drug particles. Evaluation of aerosolized drug particle deposition, transport and absorption across the cell epithelia is determined through assessing inserted Transwells.

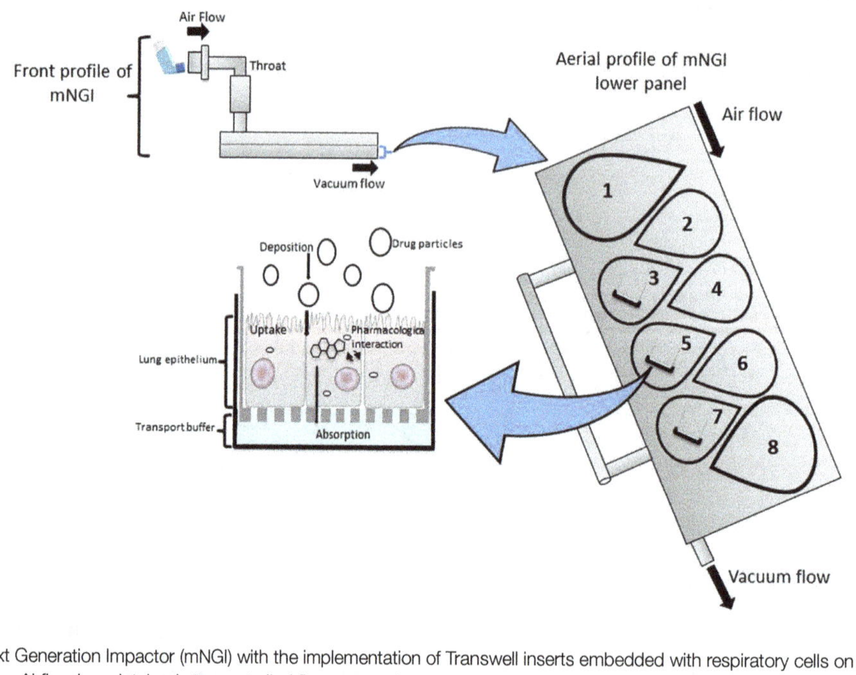

FIGURE 4 | A modified Next Generation Impactor (mNGI) with the implementation of Transwell inserts embedded with respiratory cells on stages 3, 5, and 7 at the lower panel of the apparatus. Airflow is maintained at a controlled flow rate and generated via vacuum flow on the opposite end of the mNGI allowing for the assessment of mouth-to-airway transit of drug particles. Evaluation of aerosolized drug particle deposition, transport and absorption across the cell epithelia is determined through assessing inserted Transwells.

regimens have been developed to better predict therapeutic outcomes of individual patients (Dekkers et al., 2013; Berkers et al., 2019). Drugs administrated to the culture media of patient-derived cystic fibrosis organoids showed that this was a powerful predictor of therapeutic outcomes and patient responses to single and combination drug treatment regimens for a personalized medicine approach (Dekkers et al., 2013). Thus, patient-derived organoids offer a unique *in vitro* approach to developing personalized, targeted inhalable therapies as they take into account patient-specific phenotypic differences (i.e., mucous

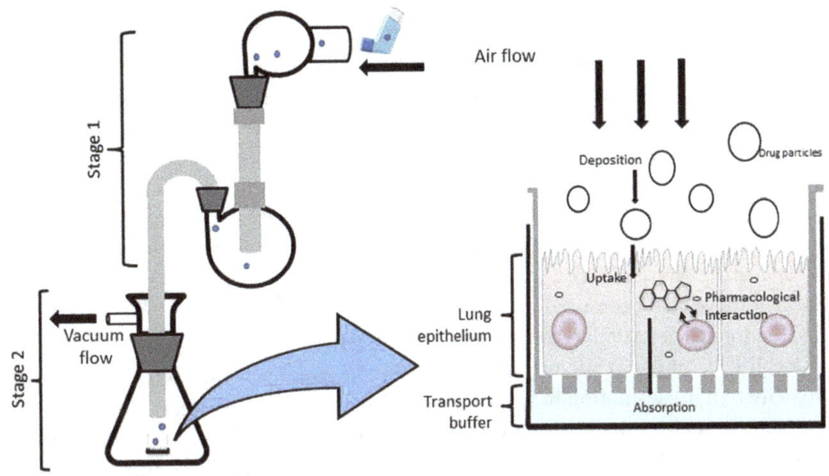

FIGURE 5 | Schematic representation of a modified Twin Stage Impinger (mTSI) with the integration of ALI cell culture insert at the base of stage 2 enabling aerosolized drugs to be deposited directly at the respiratory epithelia to better mimic *in vivo* biopharmaceutical processes of particle deposition and absorption.

production in cystic fibrosis patients or genetic mutations in lung cancer patients) known to impact drug uptake.

Respiratory organoid models serve as a tool to study disease-relevant and physiologically relevant cell-cell interactions when testing the therapeutic efficacy and toxicity of novel drug compounds. However, respiratory organoids lack not only the breathing mechanics that regulate airflow and pressure but also the anatomical structure that gives rise to the mouth-to-airway transit, both vital in determining the aerodynamic performance, pharmacodynamics and deposition of an inhaled therapy. Thus, while organoids are a novel and advantageous *in vitro* tool, they may not be the ideal research tool for screening therapeutic efficacy and toxicity of inhaled compounds as breathing mechanics and lung anatomy are vital to properly assessing the therapeutic efficacy of inhaled compounds.

Chip-Based Devices Mimic the Physiological and Mechanical Properties of a Lung to Better Predict Therapeutic Outcome of Inhaled Therapies

Organ-on-a-chip-based devices have been engineered to appropriately mimic the physiological and mechanical parameters that regulate and influence, organ homeostasis and function. In terms of the respiratory system, lung-on-chip (LOC) devices simulate the diverse physiological and mechanical parameters of an *in vivo* respiratory environment by replicating the *in vivo* breathing mechanics (the cyclic stretch of inhalation and exhalation), airflow and air pressure dynamics, cellular heterogeneity and vascular flow rates. At the cellular level, it is known that exposure to mechanical stressors, including stretch and/or changes to airflow and fluid shear stress induce proliferation (Gudipaty et al., 2017), differentiation (Edwards, 2001) and cell function (Ke et al., 2019), highlighting the importance of integrating mechanical stress when mimicking an *in vivo* environment. Thus, LOC devices have permitted *in vitro* investigations to determine the behavior of inhaled therapies (aerodynamic performance, bio-pharmacokinetics, therapeutic efficacy and toxicity) and how physiological and mechanical *in vivo* parameters impact drug uptake.

LOC devices are 3D, micro-fabricated, microfluidic devices that feature two separate chambers [an apical (top) and a basal (bottom) chamber] separated by a thin porous membrane that supports the growth, maturation and/or differentiation of distinct cell types on each side of the membrane (**Figure 2**). Importantly, each chamber can be subjected to independent dynamic flow conditions (i.e., airflow and liquid flow conditions), to better replicate the *in vivo* interplay between cell-cell, cell-matrix and cell-mechanical forces *in vitro* (Huh et al., 2010; Benam et al., 2016). The first LOC device was published by Huh et al. (2010) and reproduced key physiological and mechanical parameters of the human alveolar-capillary interface with alveolar cells seeded on the apical surface of the membrane and exposed to air with variable flow and pressure rates to simulate breathing. Pulmonary endothelial cells were applied to the basal surface of the membrane and subjected to the liquid-filled chamber under dynamic perfusion to mimic blood flow (Huh et al., 2010). The LOC device is uniquely fitted with a vacuum chamber at either side of the apical and basolateral chambers (**Figure 2**) to simulate the mechanical stretch that occurs during breathing. Taken together, LOC devices provide a more sophisticated ALI model that allows researchers to mimic the *in vivo* pulmonary interactions of the alveolar air space and blood vessels while integrating mechanical stimuli to better model drug deposition and therapeutic studies.

LOC devices model the biological, physiological and pathophysiological characteristics of the human respiratory system and therefore, have been used to assess cellular response(s) following exposure to therapeutic stimuli under dynamic flow conditions. COPD LOC devices have been engineered to measure cellular inflammatory responses to novel anti-inflammatory compounds delivered via the vascular channel (basal chamber), replicating systemic drug delivery (Benam et al., 2016). LOC devices have also been used to model cellular responses to inhaled nanoparticles (delivered apically, in solution) revealing that alveoli cells under cyclic mechanical strain show enhanced cytotoxicity and inflammation in response to nanoparticles in comparison to conventional 2D culture systems that do not possess mechanical force regimens (Huh et al., 2010). Interestingly Huh et al. (2010) also identified that cyclic strain enhanced epithelial and endothelial uptake and therapeutic efficacy of nanoparticles, confirming the importance of integrating mechanical parameters in *in vitro* models.

Chip-based devices have diversified from the single organ on a chip (i.e., LOC) to now include body-on-a-chip (BOC) [sometimes referred to as multi-organ-on-a-chip (MOC)] technologies that can be used to predict the complex organ cross-talk that occurs during drug delivery, metabolism and toxicity (both local and systemic). Concerning the respiratory system, exposure to inhaled therapies and/or toxicants enhances the complexity and physiological relevance of multiple tissue responses, including liver and kidney. The co-culture of 3D respiratory organoids with liver spheroid cultures integrated within a single chip device saw the arrival of the lung/liver-on-a-chip BOC device (Bovard et al., 2018). By incorporating the liver model, Bovard et al. (2018) were able to test both the toxicity of inhaled compounds and metabolites and further monitor the toxicity profile of the administered compounds in both organs *in vitro* (Bovard et al., 2018). Similarly, Miller et al. (2020) engineered a multi-organ breast cancer BOC device to compare the efficacy and toxicity of inhaled and/or intravenously delivered anticancer drug, curcumin. For physiological relevance, the breast cancer BOC device integrated both the liver (complete with recirculating flow), and the lung (including ALI and breathing mechanics to replicate gas exchange, and contraction and expansion) (Miller et al., 2020). Interestingly, curcumin was only found to significantly induce lung toxicity when the device was under static conditions but when breathing mechanics were added to the device, lung cell viability was not affected. Taken together, both the Bovard et al. (2018) and Miller et al. (2020) studies have highlighted the importance of appropriately mimicking the *in vivo* physiological environment to determine therapeutic efficacy and cytotoxicity but also determine the involvement and cross-talk of multiple organs.

LOCs and BOCs offer tremendous potential to be utilized as a dynamic inhaled drug screening platform, with future opportunities to integrate clinically relevant aerosolized inhalation therapy exposure systems as the current mode of drug treatment relies on the direct delivery of solubilized drug into the apical chamber. While LOCs and BOCs mimic the mechanical strain of breathing and the respiratory air-liquid microenvironment, these platforms are not optimized to study "real" aerosol characteristics and interactions during mouth-to-airway transit of drug particles. Importantly, the anatomical and physiological elements of the human respiratory system (including the upper airways: mouth, pharynx and larynx and the lower airways: bronchial branching, mucosal lining, and humidity) need be integrated within *in vitro* models to allow for greater clinical relevance when assessing inhalation therapies.

In vitro Mouth-to-Airway Transit Delivery Models

The anatomical and physiological elements of the human respiratory system (including bronchial branching, mucosal lining, and humidity) need be integrated within *in vitro* models to allow for greater clinical relevance. Both the upper and lower airways contribute to the challenges that govern targeted delivery and disposition of inhaled particles of therapeutic concentration at a specific region of the lung (bronchial epithelium, alveolar space, smooth muscle) can be problematic as significant concentrations of the drug is lost in the upper airways, i.e., during mouth-to-airway transit (Ong et al., 2015). Furthermore, mouth-to-airway transit of inhaled compounds dictates the aerosol deposition at specific anatomical lung regions, an important characteristic to model *in vitro* for *in vivo* relevance. To model aerosol behavior in a physiological and anatomical realistic environment, various impactor technologies (Anderson Cascade impactor, next-generation impactor, twin stage impinger) have been developed and then modified to couple with cell culture models, allowing greater *in vivo* relevance of drug deposition and therapeutic efficacy *in vitro*. While previous reviews have extensively described the use of impactor technologies as inhalation therapy models for drug delivery (Marple et al., 2003a,b, 2004; Haghi et al., 2014a), this section of our review will focus on the advances in these technologies. Conventional *in vitro* impactor studies have utilized ALI culture models to measure the permeability of a drug solution once pipetted onto the cell layer but overlook the important physiochemical characteristics of aerosolized particles (size, surface chemistry and morphology) that affect *in vivo* drug deposition, therapeutic efficacy and therefore clinical relevance. Thus, attempts have been made to modify conventional impactors to study deposition and permeability of aerosolized drugs on respiratory cell culture models.

Cascade Impactors

Cascade impactors are multi-staged *in vitro* tools used to characterize aerosol performance at different regions of the lung. Both the Anderson Cascaded Impactor (ACI; **Figure 3**) and the Next Generation Impactor (NGI; **Figure 4**) designed to measure the size distribution and concentration of an aerosolized sample under flow conditions. Each stage of a cascade impactor corresponds to a specific region of the lung and therefore the size of the particle dictates the region that the particle can be deposited. For example, Stage 0 corresponds to the mouth and typically allows only those particles with a diameter of less than 10 μm to pass through (cascade) to the following stage. Stage 7 represents the alveolar space and will only allow particles with a diameter of 0.4 μm to enter the stage. Importantly, drug concentration can also be determined at each stage thus, predicting the concentration of drug deposited at specific lung regions.

The ACI is a vertical cascade apparatus and is the primary method for characterizing aerosolized particle deposition of inhaled compounds (**Figure 3**). Haghi et al. (2014b) developed a modified ACI (mACI) that incorporated ALI models of Calu-3 cells inserted within the mACI at stages 4–7 that represented the deep lung region (the base of the trachea to the alveolar space). By integrating the ALI culture models within the ACI, deposition and subsequent permeability of inhalable Ventolin (salbutamol sulfate) and Qvar (beclomethasone dipropionate) formulations were conducted with drug formulations delivered via an inhaler device [known as a pressurized metered dose inhaler (pMDI)] to provide for clinically relevant administration of inhaled therapies (Haghi et al., 2014b). The mACI model presented in the Haghi et al. (2014b) study demonstrated reproducible and similar patterns of particle deposition when compared to an unmodified ACI, confirming the mACI model as a reliable *in vitro* tool to evaluate micro-particle deposition, permeability and therapeutic efficacy on respiratory epithelia using a delivery system that modeled mouth-to-airway drug transit.

The NGI is a horizontal cascade apparatus used to predict *in vivo* drug behavior that has also been modified to include an ALI cell culture model (mNGIs) able to determine aerosol deposition and transport across cell epithelia (Shur and Price, 2016; van Rensburg et al., 2018; Kumar et al., 2020). mNGIs have been engineered to deliver aerosolized particles under controlled vacuum flow to ALI cultured Calu-3 cells at stages 2, 3, and 4 (van Rensburg et al., 2018) and stages 3, 5, and 7 (Kumar et al., 2020), highlighting the versatility and adaptability of an mNGI depending on a researchers needs. The mNGI has been utilized to examine the uptake of a pMDI administrated aerosolized glucocorticoid (anti-inflammatory) of various particle sizes to determine how particle size influenced not only aerodynamic performance, but also anti-inflammatory efficacy *in vitro* (Kumar et al., 2020). Thus, modified cascade impactors are important and valid *in vitro* drug screening tools, as the integration of cell-based platforms (ALI cultured cells) permit investigations that evaluate *in vivo* deposition of aerosol particles, cellular response and therapeutic efficacy of novel inhaled compounds.

Twin Stage Impingers

The modern-day glass twin stage impinger (TSI) apparatus allows aerosolized compounds to be delivered at a simulated oropharynx (mid pharynx) and particles are then separated by size throughout the two stages of the device (**Figure 5**). The first stage of the TSI replicates the upper airways, while the second stage resembles the lower airways. It is important to note that the TSI does not fully simulate the mouth-to-airway transit as the drug is delivered at the mid pharynx rather than a simulated oral pharyngeal orifice however, the aerosolized fraction that is delivered and collected in the first stage of the TSI has been shown to positively correlate with drug amounts collected in the mouth and throat (Hallworth and Westmoreland, 1987). Regardless, the TSI remains an important and widely used *in vitro* tool to determine the aerodynamic performance of an inhaled therapeutic as particle trajectories can be determined to identify the site-specific deposition of an aerosolized drug (Mendes et al., 2009). Similar to the mNGI and mACI, a modified version of the TSI (mTSI) has integrated an ALI cell culture model at the base of stage 2 (**Figure 5**) enabling aerosolized drugs (delivered via a pMDI) to be deposited directly at the respiratory epithelia to better mimic *in vivo* biopharmaceutical processes (**Figure 5**; Grainger et al., 2012; Haghi et al., 2012; Ong et al., 2014). The integration of a microfluidic device as a nebulization platform for pulmonary drug delivery alongside a TSI has been implemented in a study by Qi et al. (2009), demonstrating the use of microfluidics as an efficient means to generate appropriate aerosolized drug particles. A TSI was utilized to confirm the mean aerosol diameter produced by the device, demonstrating the high efficiency of drug particle delivery and the overall viability of the microfluidic platform for inhalation therapy (Qi et al., 2009). It would be of great interest to further enhance and modify TSI models by incorporating alternative *in vitro* cell culture systems (organoids, LOC/BOC devices etc.) to better mimic the respiratory microenvironment for evaluating inhaled drug particle transport, absorption and bio-pharmacokinetics.

The use of *in vitro* cellular models alone, or in combination with microfluidic devices or mouth-to-airway transit models, has increased in our knowledge of cellular behavior following exposure to inhaled compounds. However, cell-based approaches alone or integrated, are unable to holistically mimic the structural and mechanical diversity of a human lung that determine the biological and physiological characteristics of respiration. While the obvious solution is to go directly to *in vivo* rodent and pig models, the translational data acquired from animal respiratory disease models are limited in providing mechanistic insight into human pathologies (Ware, 2008), highlighting the demand for alternative research platforms that better recapitulate the dynamic architecture and complex cellularity of a human lung. Thus, inhaled drug delivery investigations conducted on whole lung tissue (*ex vivo*) models permit a thorough understanding drug behavior *in vivo*, as *ex vivo* lung tissue samples retain *in vivo* airway structure, architecture, cellular heterogeneity and importantly, the microenvironment.

ADVANCES IN *ex vivo* RESEARCH MODELS OFFER TRANSLATIONAL PRECLINICAL, THERAPEUTIC RELEVANCE WHEN SCREENING NOVEL INHALED THERAPIES

Ex vivo lung models provide opportunities to study the performance and therapeutic efficacy of inhaled drugs in either healthy or diseased lungs. As *ex vivo* lung models retain the 3-dimensional lung structure and native microenvironment (cell-cell, cell-matrix interactions), *ex vivo* drug studies can specifically investigate the role the *in vivo* lung environment plays in determining drug transport kinetics, cytotoxicity and therapeutic efficacy. This next section of the review will focus on two *ex vivo* models, precision-cut lung slices (PCLS) and isolated perfused lungs (IPL) (summarized in **Table 2**).

Precision-Cut Lung Slices Maintain Complex Multi-Dimensional and Multi-Cellular Interactions to Appropriately Determine *in vivo* Therapeutic Efficacy

Precision-cut lung slices are sections harvested from lung tissue immediately following *post mortem*, sliced (100–300 μm) and submerged in culture media to retain functional physiological and cellular interactions while maintaining anatomical and structural diversity of a lung (Placke and Fisher, 1987; Liu et al., 2019). This preservation of lung architecture provides for a clinically relevant *ex vivo* respiratory platform to study therapeutic efficacy and cytotoxicity. Thus, PCLS have emerged as a powerful research tool and offer a more complex mechanistic understanding of drug interactions with the multicellular and multidimensional properties of a lung (Hess et al., 2016; Hansen et al., 2016; Cedilak et al., 2019; Liu et al., 2019). In addition, PCLS provide opportunities to assess preclinical, translational studies that determine therapeutic concentrations and efficacies of drugs delivered to different lung regions and have also allowed for cross-species comparisons—with PCLS reportedly prepared from a variety of species including rodent, sheep and human lung tissue (Danov et al., 2018; Lehmann et al., 2018; Yilmaz et al., 2019).

PCLS have been utilized in studies as pre-validation platforms to screen compound toxicity and drug efficacy (Hess et al., 2016; Danov et al., 2018; Cedilak et al., 2019). Drug delivery to *ex vivo* PCLS is often via submersion in drug-containing medium (Nassimi et al., 2009; Neuhaus et al., 2013, 2014; Paranjpe et al., 2013) or direct liquid infusion (via culture medium) to the airway (Hess et al., 2016) as the ventilated delivery of compounds (to mimic inhaled delivery) to PCLS models is currently unattainable. To work around this limitation of PCLS models, Nassimi et al. (2010) administered aerosolized nanoparticles to live BALB/c mice using a jet-driven aerosol generator in a closed Plexiglas box system, mice were then sacrificed and PCLS were generated (Nassimi et al., 2010). Cytotoxicity of PCLS models, regardless of the route of drug delivery, can be assessed by measuring changes to mitochondrial activity, metabolic activity, cytokine release, or imaging of Live/Dead staining of the whole lung section (Nassimi et al., 2010; Neuhaus et al., 2013, 2014; Paranjpe et al., 2013; Hess et al., 2016). PCLS models have further been developed to mimic the complex structure and function relationship of the pulmonary system with connected heart and lung harvested from mice and then sliced (Paranjpe et al., 2013). Paranjpe et al. (2013) determined the therapeutic efficacy of nanoparticles with loaded with Sildenafil (Viagra) as a novel inhalable treatment of pulmonary hypertension. Exposure of the formulated Sildenafil-loaded SLN solutions to the heart and lung slices showed that the IC_{50} value for lung slices was higher than that of heart slices, suggesting that directly targeting the lungs with higher drug concentrations would achieve maximal therapeutic

TABLE 2 | Overview of the advantages and disadvantages of *ex vivo* models used for respiratory inhalation drug screening.

Ex vivo model	Applications	Respiratory disease model	Advantages	Disadvantages	References
Precision cut lung slices	Drug toxicity and efficacy studies	Pulmonary hypertension	High reproducibility of the platform. Preservation of the lung architecture allowing for a true representation of lung structural response to experimental stimuli. Retain functional cellular interactions for a multicellular response.	Lack of translation of treatment to clinical inhalation applications and dosing evaluation. Inability to mimic ventilation, mechanical stretch, or perfusion observed in human lung.	Paranjpe et al., 2013; Hansen et al., 2016; Hess et al., 2016; Liu et al., 2019
Isolated perfused lungS	Drug delivery/transport and efficacy studies	Severe asthma	Maintains functioning of lung tissue. Intact lung provides for a multicellular response to drug stimuli. Suitable for the direct administration of inhalation drug therapies using inhalable delivery systems. Ability for controlled dosing of drug stimuli.	Typically derived of rodent or rabbit origin which differs in tracheobronchial anatomical and structural composition when compared to human lungs.	Hochhaus et al., 1997; Beck-Broichsitter et al., 2009; Eriksson et al., 2018

efficacy in the heart and relieve pulmonary hypertension (Paranjpe et al., 2013).

The use of *ex vivo* PCLS models to determine *in vivo* toxicities and therapeutic efficacies are a clinically relevant, pre-validation research platform. As PLCS models consist of whole lung tissue and maintain the complex multi-dimensional and multi-cellular interactions of respiratory, immune and neuronal cells, PCLS models are better placed to properly mimic a therapeutic response to a delivered drug. While PCLS have obvious limitations, namely the inability to mimic ventilation, mechanical stretch or perfusion, this model has been successfully used to determine the preclinical pharmacotoxicology and therapeutic efficacy of novel compounds within an *in vivo* environment (Liu et al., 2019). However, to study the region-specific deposition of inhaled drugs and subsequent transport analysis, an alternative model(s) is required to obtain greater clinical relevance.

Isolated Perfused Lungs Are a Unique Platform to Determine Inhaled Drug Aerodynamic Performance and Bio-Pharmacokinetics

Isolated perfused lungs are prepared by encasing the whole lung of a rodent or rabbit within an artificial thoracic chamber at physiologically relevant conditions (37°C, 5% CO_2) and supplying a perfusion buffer (termed perfusate) to mimic pulmonary circulation and ensure the sustained tissue survival and function. In IPL *ex vivo* models, drug agents can be administered directly into the lungs using inhalable delivery systems such as nebulizers, modified nebulizers (AeroProbe), aerosolizers (DustGun) or syringe insufflator (MicroSprayer, PennCentury) (Tronde et al., 2002; Gerde et al., 2004; Ewing et al., 2008; Beck-Broichsitter et al., 2010; Selg et al., 2013) to replicate trachea-to-airway drug transit. However, when replicating mouth-to-airway drug transit in IPL models, delivery devices are limited due to the differences in the oral pharyngeal anatomy between humans and animals. Furthermore, the device selected for inhaled drug delivery or aerosolization are as equally important as the physiochemical properties of the formulation when determining aerosol performance, deposition and efficacy. Nevertheless, *ex vivo* IPL offers a unique opportunity to test inhaled drug delivery in a platform that is physiologically and biologically similar to a human lung allowing drug aerodynamic and bio-pharmacokinetic parameters to be studied.

IPL models are used to determine the uptake of inhaled agents across the pulmonary epithelium, the subsequent rate of drug absorption and therapeutic efficacy (Hochhaus et al., 1997; Bosquillon et al., 2017; Eriksson et al., 2018). IPL has been used to explore the drug transport profiles of inhaled (ventilated)/nebulized compounds, or nanoparticles, that have been formulated to achieve deposition in the tracheal, bronchial or alveolar lung regions with high drug permeability, absorption and retention (Tronde et al., 2002; Ewing et al., 2006; Beck-Broichsitter et al., 2009; Selg et al., 2013; Eriksson et al., 2020). IPL platforms have also integrated sophisticated imaging techniques (photon correlation spectroscopy, laser Doppler anemometry, atomic force microscopy and fluorescence spectroscopy) to allow real-time analysis of drug stability during nebulization, distribution profiles after nebulization (Beck-Broichsitter et al., 2009), further validating IPL as a useful preclinical model for screening novel inhaled drugs.

IPL models are typical of rodent or rabbit origin and it is important that users are aware of the differences in tracheobronchial anatomical and structural composition between animal and human lungs. Not only do the airway diameters of rodent lungs differ to that of human lungs, but rodent lungs are monopodial with asymmetrical branching, while human lungs are dichotomous with symmetrical branching (Phalen et al., 1978; Yeh et al., 1979). While these differences in airway structure have obvious implications for modeling the delivery and deposition of inhaled compounds (Hofmann et al., 1989), IPL offer a generalized understanding of inhaled drug behavior within branched luminal space. It is important to note that IPL models are unable to replicate the initial drug transit mechanisms specifically, inhalation via the oral pharyngeal orifice thus, IPL offers a physiologically relevant platform of the tracheal, bronchial and alveolar regions to screen novel inhaled therapies.

Research platforms used to screen novel inhaled therapeutic compounds, inherently suggests that the research is focused toward finding a treatment for a specific disease or disease phenotype. Yet interestingly, the vast majority of research conducted that utilize IPL as a research tool are conducted on healthy animal lungs. It has long been established that the structural and mechanical properties of diseased lungs alter not only the biological and physiological environment but also the lung capacity (the volume of air able to be inspired and expired) of individuals (Bates et al., 2007). For example, emphysema patients have a significantly reduced lung capacity as a result of the progressive destruction of alveolar spaces and structural properties of the lungs. Therefore, is it important that the relevant mechanical, structural and physiological characteristics of the disease are appropriately modeled to obtain appropriate aerodynamic and bio-pharmacokinetic information when screening preclinical, inhaled therapies.

CONCLUSION

There is currently no single faultless universal model for evaluating the delivery, efficacy and toxicity of inhaled therapies thus, a single preclinical model cannot be advocated. The use of multiple, relevant experimental approaches to screen inhaled therapies is essential for the translation of preclinical inhaled drug candidates to clinical practice. The ideal scientific strategy is influenced by numerous factors including the physicochemical properties of the drug, the disease of interest, and the available laboratory resources. Furthermore, when selecting an appropriate model, researchers must understand the limitations and capabilities of *in vitro* and/or *ex vivo* platforms to be implemented in their study. It is therefore critical to understand both the benefits and drawbacks of each scientific platform to appropriately answer the specific research question and to maximize the relevance of the results obtained. Thus, the implementation of multiple experimental platforms provides for greater relevance and validation of models for clinical relevance.

The predictive power of *in vitro* and *ex vivo* correlations for preclinical inhaled therapies has been extensively reviewed in the literature (Sakagami, 2006, 2020; Nahar et al., 2013; Nickel et al., 2016; Ehrmann et al., 2020) and comparisons of *in vitro* and *ex vivo* data have been used to establish, validate and compare experimental models with known *in vivo* responses (Sakagami, 2006, 2020; Nahar et al., 2013; Nickel et al., 2016; Ehrmann et al., 2020). The most common *in vivo* tool used for comparative inhaled therapy studies to date is the ALI culture model, while the most common complementary *ex vivo* model is the IPL platform, with studies demonstrating results that are comparable to *in vivo* data (Nassimi et al., 2010; Ong et al., 2014; Bosquillon et al., 2017). The *in vivo* predictive capabilities of *in vitro* and *ex vivo* methodologies when performed side-by-side have the potential to enhance novel drug screening platforms and bridge the translation from preclinical testing to the patient population. Innovative drug screening platforms can accelerate and facilitate preclinical therapeutic studies to allow for more informed decisions on potential inhalation drug candidates for future use in clinical trials. Thus, the rapidly evolving and innovative research space of 3D *in vitro* and *ex vivo* platforms to model respiratory diseases and evaluate the therapeutic potential of inhalation drug candidates provides promising avenue for screening preclinical inhaled therapies.

AUTHOR CONTRIBUTIONS

AC and PB prepared the manuscript. AC and HO prepared tables and figures. HO, PB, and DT provided critical feedback as all authors contributed equally towards conceptualization of the finalized manuscript.

REFERENCES

Aun, M. V., Bonamichi-Santos, R., Arantes-Costa, F. M., Kalil, J., and Giavina-Bianchi, P. (2017). Animal models of asthma: utility and limitations. *J. Asthma Allergy* 10, 293–301. doi: 10.2147/jaa.S121092

Barkauskas, C. E., Chung, M. I., Fioret, B., Gao, X., Katsura, H., and Hogan, B. L. (2017). Lung organoids: current uses and future promise. *Development* 144, 986–997. doi: 10.1242/dev.140103

Bates, J. H., Davis, G. S., Majumdar, A., Butnor, K. J., and Suki, B. (2007). Linking parenchymal disease progression to changes in lung mechanical function by percolation. *Am. J. Respir. Crit. Care Med.* 176, 617–623. doi: 10.1164/rccm.200611-1739OC

Beck-Broichsitter, M., Gauss, J., Gessler, T., Seeger, W., Kissel, T., and Schmehl, T. (2010). Pulmonary targeting with biodegradable salbutamol-loaded nanoparticles. *J. Aerosol. Med. Pulm. Drug Deliv.* 23, 47–57. doi: 10.1089/jamp.2009.0759

Beck-Broichsitter, M., Gauss, J., Packhaeuser, C. B., Lahnstein, K., Schmehl, T., Seeger, W., et al. (2009). Pulmonary drug delivery with aerosolizable nanoparticles in an ex vivo lung model. *Int. J. Pharm.* 367, 169–178. doi: 10.1016/j.ijpharm.2008.09.017

Benam, K. H., Villenave, R., Lucchesi, C., Varone, A., Hubeau, C., Lee, H. H., et al. (2016). Small airway-on-a-chip enables analysis of human lung inflammation and drug responses in vitro. *Nat. Methods* 13, 151–157. doi: 10.1038/nmeth.3697

Berkers, G., van Mourik, P., Vonk, A. M., Kruisselbrink, E., Dekkers, J. F., de Winter-de Groot, K. M., et al. (2019). Rectal organoids enable personalized treatment of cystic fibrosis. *Cell. Rep.* 26, 1701.e3–1708.e3. doi: 10.1016/j.celrep.2019.01.068

Borghardt, J. M., Kloft, C., and Sharma, A. (2018). Inhaled therapy in respiratory disease: the complex interplay of pulmonary kinetic processes. *Can. Respir. J.* 2018:2732017. doi: 10.1155/2018/2732017

Bosquillon, C., Madlova, M., Patel, N., Clear, N., and Forbes, B. (2017). A comparison of drug transport in pulmonary absorption models: isolated perfused rat lungs, respiratory epithelial cell lines and primary cell culture. *Pharm. Res.* 34, 2532–2540. doi: 10.1007/s11095-017-2251-y

Bovard, D., Sandoz, A., Luettich, K., Frentzel, S., Iskandar, A., Marescotti, D., et al. (2018). A lung/liver-on-a-chip platform for acute and chronic toxicity studies. *Lab. Chip.* 18, 3814–3829. doi: 10.1039/c8lc01029c

Cedilak, M., Banjanac, M., Belamarić, D., Paravić Radičević, A., Faraho, I., Ilić, K., et al. (2019). Precision-cut lung slices from bleomycin treated animals as a model for testing potential therapies for idiopathic pulmonary fibrosis. *Pulm. Pharmacol. Ther.* 55, 75–83. doi: 10.1016/j.pupt.2019.02.005

Chen, Y. W., Huang, S. X., de Carvalho, A., Ho, S. H., Islam, M. N., Volpi, S., et al. (2017). A three-dimensional model of human lung development and disease from pluripotent stem cells. *Nat. Cell. Biol.* 19, 542–549. doi: 10.1038/ncb3510

Danov, O., Jiménez Delgado, S. M., Obernolte, H., Seehase, S., Dehmel, S., Braubach, P., et al. (2018). Human lung tissue provides highly relevant data about efficacy of new anti-asthmatic drugs. *PLoS One* 13:e0207767. doi: 10.1371/journal.pone.0207767

Davies, C. N., and Muir, D. C. (1966). Deposition of inhaled particles in human lungs. *Nature* 211, 90–91. doi: 10.1038/211090a0

Dekkers, J. F., Wiegerinck, C. L., de Jonge, H. R., Bronsveld, I., Janssens, H. M., de Winter-de Groot, K. M., et al. (2013). A functional CFTR assay using primary cystic fibrosis intestinal organoids. *Nat. Med.* 19, 939–945. doi: 10.1038/nm.3201

Ditchfield, N., Gilchrist, F. J., Davies, S. J., and Carroll, W. (2018). Strategies to prevent kidney injury from antibiotics in people with cystic fibrosis. *Cochrane Database Syst. Rev.* 2018:CD013032. doi: 10.1002/14651858.CD013032

Edwards, Y. S. (2001). Stretch stimulation: its effects on alveolar type II cell function in the lung. *Comp. Biochem. Physiol. A Mol. Integr. Physiol.* 129, 245–260. doi: 10.1016/s1095-6433(01)00321-x

Ehrmann, S., Schmid, O., Darquenne, C., Rothen-Rutishauser, B., Sznitman, J., Yang, L., et al. (2020). Innovative preclinical models for pulmonary drug delivery research. *Expert Opin. Drug Deliv.* 17, 463–478. doi: 10.1080/17425247.2020.1730807

Eliezer, N., Sadé, J., Silberberg, A., and Nevo, A. C. (1970). The role of mucus in transport by cilia. *Am. Rev. Respir. Dis.* 102, 48–52. doi: 10.1164/arrd.1970.102.1.48

Eriksson, J., Sjögren, E., Lennernäs, H., and Thörn, H. (2020). Drug absorption parameters obtained using the isolated perfused rat lung model are predictive of rat in vivo lung absorption. *AAPS J.* 22:71. doi: 10.1208/s12248-020-00456-x

Eriksson, J., Sjögren, E., Thörn, H., Rubin, K., Bäckman, P., and Lennernäs, H. (2018). Pulmonary absorption - estimation of effective pulmonary permeability and tissue retention of ten drugs using an ex vivo rat model and computational analysis. *Eur. J. Pharm. Biopharm.* 124, 1–12. doi: 10.1016/j.ejpb.2017.11.013

Ewing, P., Blomgren, B., Ryrfeldt, A., and Gerde, P. (2006). Increasing exposure levels cause an abrupt change in the absorption and metabolism of acutely inhaled benzo(a)pyrene in the isolated, ventilated, and perfused lung of the rat. *Toxicol. Sci.* 91, 332–340. doi: 10.1093/toxsci/kfj104

Ewing, P., Eirefelt, S. J., Andersson, P., Blomgren, A., Ryrfeldt, A., and Gerde, P. (2008). Short inhalation exposures of the isolated and perfused rat lung to respirable dry particle aerosols; the detailed pharmacokinetics of budesonide, formoterol, and terbutaline. *J. Aerosol. Med. Pulm. Drug Deliv.* 21, 169–180. doi: 10.1089/jamp.2007.0654

Faura Tellez, G., Willemse, B. W., Brouwer, U., Nijboer-Brinksma, S., Vandepoele, K., Noordhoek, J. A., et al. (2016). Protocadherin-1 localization and cell-adhesion function in airway epithelial cells in asthma. *PLoS One* 11:e0163967. doi: 10.1371/journal.pone.0163967

Forbes, B., Shah, A., Martin, G. P., and Lansley, A. B. (2003). The human bronchial epithelial cell line 16HBE14o- as a model system of the airways for studying drug transport. *Int. J. Pharm.* 257, 161–167. doi: 10.1016/s0378-5173(03)00129-7

Garcia-Canton, C., Minet, E., Anadon, A., and Meredith, C. (2013). Metabolic characterization of cell systems used in in vitro toxicology testing: lung cell system BEAS-2B as a working example. *Toxicol. In Vitro* 27, 1719–1727. doi: 10.1016/j.tiv.2013.05.001

Gerde, P., Ewing, P., Låstbom, L., Ryrfeldt, A., Waher, J., and Lidén, G. (2004). A novel method to aerosolize powder for short inhalation exposures at high concentrations: isolated rat lungs exposed to respirable diesel soot. *Inhal. Toxicol.* 16, 45–52. doi: 10.1080/08958370490258381

Ghadiri, M., Young, P. M., and Traini, D. (2019). Strategies to enhance drug absorption via nasal and pulmonary routes. *Pharmaceutics* 11:113. doi: 10.3390/pharmaceutics11030113

Grainger, C. I., Greenwell, L. L., Lockley, D. J., Martin, G. P., and Forbes, B. (2006). Culture of Calu-3 cells at the air interface provides a representative model of the airway epithelial barrier. *Pharm. Res.* 23, 1482–1490. doi: 10.1007/s11095-006-0255-0

Grainger, C. I., Saunders, M., Buttini, F., Telford, R., Merolla, L. L., Martin, G. P., et al. (2012). Critical characteristics for corticosteroid solution metered dose inhaler bioequivalence. *Mol. Pharm.* 9, 563–569. doi: 10.1021/mp200415g

Gudipaty, S. A., Lindblom, J., Loftus, P. D., Redd, M. J., Edes, K., Davey, C. F., et al. (2017). Mechanical stretch triggers rapid epithelial cell division through Piezo1. *Nature* 543, 118–121. doi: 10.1038/nature21407

Haghi, M., Ong, H. X., Traini, D., and Young, P. (2014a). Across the pulmonary epithelial barrier: integration of physicochemical properties and human cell models to study pulmonary drug formulations. *Pharmacol. Ther.* 144, 235–252. doi: 10.1016/j.pharmthera.2014.05.003

Haghi, M., Traini, D., Bebawy, M., and Young, P. M. (2012). Deposition, diffusion and transport mechanism of dry powder microparticulate salbutamol, at the respiratory epithelia. *Mol. Pharm.* 9, 1717–1726. doi: 10.1021/mp200620m

Haghi, M., Traini, D., and Young, P. (2014b). In vitro cell integrated impactor deposition methodology for the study of aerodynamically relevant size fractions from commercial pressurised metered dose inhalers. *Pharm. Res.* 31, 1779–1787. doi: 10.1007/s11095-013-1282-2

Hallworth, G. W., and Westmoreland, D. G. (1987). The twin impinger: a simple device for assessing the delivery of drugs from metered dose pressurized aerosol inhalers. *J. Pharm. Pharmacol.* 39, 966–972. doi: 10.1111/j.2042-7158.1987.tb03142.x

Hansen, N. U., Karsdal, M. A., Brockbank, S., Cruwys, S., Rønnow, S., and Leeming, D. J. (2016). Tissue turnover of collagen type I, III and elastin is elevated in the PCLS model of IPF and can be restored back to vehicle levels using a phosphodiesterase inhibitor. *Respir. Res.* 17:76. doi: 10.1186/s12931-016-0394-8

Hess, A., Wang-Lauenstein, L., Braun, A., Kolle, S. N., Landsiedel, R., Liebsch, M., et al. (2016). Prevalidation of the ex-vivo model PCLS for prediction of respiratory toxicity. *Toxicol. In Vitro* 32, 347–361. doi: 10.1016/j.tiv.2016.01.006

Hill, D. R., Huang, S., Nagy, M. S., Yadagiri, V. K., Fields, C., Mukherjee, D., et al. (2017). Bacterial colonization stimulates a complex physiological response in the immature human intestinal epithelium. *eLife* 6:e29132. doi: 10.7554/eLife.29132

Hochhaus, G., Möllmann, H., Derendorf, H., and Gonzalez-Rothi, R. J. (1997). Pharmacokinetic/pharmacodynamic aspects of aerosol therapy using glucocorticoids as a model. *J. Clin. Pharmacol.* 37, 881–892. doi: 10.1002/j.1552-4604.1997.tb04262.x

Hofmann, W., Koblinger, L., and Martonen, T. B. (1989). Structural differences between human and rat lungs: implications for Monte Carlo modeling of aerosol deposition. *Health Phys.* 57(Suppl. 1), 41–46. doi: 10.1097/00004032-198907001-00005

Huh, D., Leslie, D. C., Matthews, B. D., Fraser, J. P., Jurek, S., Hamilton, G. A., et al. (2012). A human disease model of drug toxicity-induced pulmonary edema in a lung-on-a-chip microdevice. *Sci. Transl. Med.* 4:159ra147. doi: 10.1126/scitranslmed.3004249

Huh, D., Matthews, B. D., Mammoto, A., Montoya-Zavala, M., Hsin, H. Y., and Ingber, D. E. (2010). Reconstituting organ-level lung functions on a chip. *Science* 328, 1662–1668. doi: 10.1126/science.1188302

Jacob, A., Morley, M., Hawkins, F., McCauley, K. B., Jean, J. C., Heins, H., et al. (2017). Differentiation of human pluripotent stem cells into functional lung alveolar epithelial cells. *Cell Stem Cell* 21, 472.e10–488.e10. doi: 10.1016/j.stem.2017.08.014

Jung, D. J., Shin, T. H., Kim, M., Sung, C. O., Jang, S. J., and Jeong, G. S. (2019). A one-stop microfluidic-based lung cancer organoid culture platform for testing drug sensitivity. *Lab. Chip.* 19, 2854–2865. doi: 10.1039/c9lc00496c

Ke, Y., Karki, P., Zhang, C., Li, Y., Nguyen, T., Birukov, K. G., et al. (2019). Mechanosensitive Rap1 activation promotes barrier function of lung vascular endothelium under cyclic stretch. *Mol. Biol. Cell.* 30, 959–974. doi: 10.1091/mbc.E18-07-0422

Kim, M., Mun, H., Sung, C. O., Cho, E. J., Jeon, H. J., Chun, S. M., et al. (2019). Patient-derived lung cancer organoids as in vitro cancer models for therapeutic screening. *Nat. Commun.* 10:3991. doi: 10.1038/s41467-019-11867-6

Konar, D., Devarasetty, M., Yildiz, D. V., Atala, A., and Murphy, S. V. (2016). Lung-on-a-chip technologies for disease modeling and drug development. *Biomed. Eng. Comput. Biol.* 7(Suppl. 1), 17–27. doi: 10.4137/becb.S34252

Kondo, J., and Inoue, M. (2019). Application of cancer organoid model for drug screening and personalized therapy. *Cells* 8:470. doi: 10.3390/cells8050470

Kreft, M. E., Jerman, U. D., Lasič, E., Hevir-Kene, N., Rižner, T. L., Peternel, L., et al. (2015). The characterization of the human cell line Calu-3 under different culture conditions and its use as an optimized in vitro model to investigate bronchial epithelial function. *Eur. J. Pharm. Sci.* 69, 1–9. doi: 10.1016/j.ejps.2014.12.017

Kumar, V., Bariwal, J., Narang, A. S., Tso, J., Cheong, J., and Mahato, R. I. (2020). Functional similarity of modified cascade impactor to deposit drug particles on cells. *Int. J. Pharm.* 583:119404. doi: 10.1016/j.ijpharm.2020.119404

Latvala, S., Hedberg, J., Möller, L., Odnevall Wallinder, I., Karlsson, H. L., and Elihn, K. (2016). Optimization of an air-liquid interface exposure system for assessing toxicity of airborne nanoparticles. *J. Appl. Toxicol.* 36, 1294–1301. doi: 10.1002/jat.3304

Leeman, K. T., Pessina, P., Lee, J. H., and Kim, C. F. (2019). Mesenchymal stem cells increase alveolar differentiation in lung progenitor organoid cultures. *Sci. Rep.* 9:6479. doi: 10.1038/s41598-019-42819-1

Lehmann, M., Buhl, L., Alsafadi, H. N., Klee, S., Hermann, S., Mutze, K., et al. (2018). Differential effects of Nintedanib and Pirfenidone on lung alveolar epithelial cell function in ex vivo murine and human lung tissue cultures of pulmonary fibrosis. *Respir. Res.* 19:175. doi: 10.1186/s12931-018-0876-y

Li, F., He, J., Wei, J., Cho, W. C., and Liu, X. (2015). Diversity of epithelial stem cell types in adult lung. *Stem Cells Int.* 2015:728307. doi: 10.1155/2015/728307

Lippmann, M., Yeates, D. B., and Albert, R. E. (1980). Deposition, retention, and clearance of inhaled particles. *Br. J. Ind. Med.* 37, 337–362. doi: 10.1136/oem.37.4.337

Liu, G., Betts, C., Cunoosamy, D. M., Åberg, P. M., Hornberg, J. J., Sivars, K. B., et al. (2019). Use of precision cut lung slices as a translational model for the study of lung biology. *Respir. Res.* 20:162. doi: 10.1186/s12931-019-1131-x

Liu, Z., Anderson, J. D., Deng, L., Mackay, S., Bailey, J., Kersh, L., et al. (2020). Human nasal epithelial organoids for therapeutic development in cystic fibrosis. *Genes* 11:603. doi: 10.3390/genes11060603

Madara, J. L. (1998). Regulation of the movement of solutes across tight junctions. *Annu. Rev. Physiol.* 60, 143–159. doi: 10.1146/annurev.physiol.60.1.143

Marple, V. A., Olson, B. A., Santhanakrishnan, K., Mitchell, J. P., Murray, S. C., and Hudson-Curtis, B. L. (2003a). Next generation pharmaceutical impactor (a new impactor for pharmaceutical inhaler testing). Part II: archival calibration. *J. Aerosol. Med.* 16, 301–324. doi: 10.1089/089426803769017668

Marple, V. A., Olson, B. A., Santhanakrishnan, K., Roberts, D. L., Mitchell, J. P., and Hudson-Curtis, B. L. (2004). Next generation pharmaceutical impactor: a new impactor for pharmaceutical inhaler testing. Part III. extension of archival calibration to 15 L/min. *J. Aerosol. Med.* 17, 335–343. doi: 10.1089/jam.2004.17.335

Marple, V. A., Roberts, D. L., Romay, F. J., Miller, N. C., Truman, K. G., Van Oort, M., et al. (2003b). Next generation pharmaceutical impactor (a new impactor for pharmaceutical inhaler testing). part I: design. *J. Aerosol. Med.* 16, 283–299. doi: 10.1089/089426803769017659

Mendes, P. J., Sousa, J. M., and Pinto, J. F. (2009). Prediction of the deposition of dry powder aerosols. *AAPS J.* 11, 186–194. doi: 10.1208/s12248-009-9095-2

Miller, A. J., Dye, B. R., Ferrer-Torres, D., Hill, D. R., Overeem, A. W., Shea, L. D., et al. (2019). Generation of lung organoids from human pluripotent stem cells in vitro. *Nat. Protoc.* 14, 518–540. doi: 10.1038/s41596-018-0104-8

Miller, P. G., Chen, C. Y., Wang, Y. I., Gao, E., and Shuler, M. L. (2020). Multiorgan microfluidic platform with breathable lung chamber for inhalation or intravenous drug screening and development. *Biotechnol. Bioeng.* 117, 486–497. doi: 10.1002/bit.27188

Molina, S. A., Stauffer, B., Moriarty, H. K., Kim, A. H., McCarty, N. A., and Koval, M. (2015). Junctional abnormalities in human airway epithelial cells expressing F508del CFTR. *Am. J. Physiol. Lung Cell. Mol. Physiol.* 309, L475–L487. doi: 10.1152/ajplung.00060.2015

Monnappa, A. K., Bari, W., Choi, S. Y., and Mitchell, R. J. (2016). Investigating the responses of human epithelial cells to predatory bacteria. *Sci. Rep.* 6:33485. doi: 10.1038/srep33485

Movia, D., Bazou, D., Volkov, Y., and Prina-Mello, A. (2018). Multilayered Cultures of NSCLC cells grown at the Air-Liquid Interface allow the efficacy testing of inhaled anti-cancer drugs. *Sci. Rep.* 8:12920. doi: 10.1038/s41598-018-31332-6

Nahar, K., Gupta, N., Gauvin, R., Absar, S., Patel, B., Gupta, V., et al. (2013). In vitro, in vivo and ex vivo models for studying particle deposition and drug absorption of inhaled pharmaceuticals. *Eur. J. Pharm. Sci.* 49, 805–818. doi: 10.1016/j.ejps.2013.06.004

Nassimi, M., Schleh, C., Lauenstein, H. D., Hussein, R., Hoymann, H. G., Koch, W., et al. (2010). A toxicological evaluation of inhaled solid lipid nanoparticles used as a potential drug delivery system for the lung. *Eur. J. Pharm. Biopharm.* 75, 107–116. doi: 10.1016/j.ejpb.2010.02.014

Nassimi, M., Schleh, C., Lauenstein, H. D., Hussein, R., Lübbers, K., Pohlmann, G., et al. (2009). Low cytotoxicity of solid lipid nanoparticles in in vitro and ex vivo lung models. *Inhal. Toxicol.* 21(Suppl. 1), 104–109. doi: 10.1080/08958370903005769

Neuhaus, V., Chichester, J. A., Ebensen, T., Schwarz, K., Hartman, C. E., Shoji, Y., et al. (2014). A new adjuvanted nanoparticle-based H1N1 influenza vaccine induced antigen-specific local mucosal and systemic immune responses after administration into the lung. *Vaccine* 32, 3216–3222. doi: 10.1016/j.vaccine.2014.04.011

Neuhaus, V., Schwarz, K., Klee, A., Seehase, S., Förster, C., Pfennig, O., et al. (2013). Functional testing of an inhalable nanoparticle based influenza vaccine using a human precision cut lung slice technique. *PLoS One* 8:e71728. doi: 10.1371/journal.pone.0071728

Nickel, S., Clerkin, C. G., Selo, M. A., and Ehrhardt, C. (2016). Transport mechanisms at the pulmonary mucosa: implications for drug delivery. *Expert Opin. Drug Deliv.* 13, 667–690. doi: 10.1517/17425247.2016.1140144

Ong, H. X., Benaouda, F., Traini, D., Cipolla, D., Gonda, I., Bebawy, M., et al. (2014). In vitro and ex vivo methods predict the enhanced lung residence time of liposomal ciprofloxacin formulations for nebulisation. *Eur. J. Pharm. Biopharm.* 86, 83–89. doi: 10.1016/j.ejpb.2013.06.024

Ong, H. X., Jackson, C. L., Cole, J. L., Lackie, P. M., Traini, D., Young, P. M., et al. (2016). Primary air-liquid interface culture of nasal epithelium for nasal drug delivery. *Mol. Pharm.* 13, 2242–2252. doi: 10.1021/acs.molpharmaceut.5b00852

Ong, H. X., Traini, D., Bebawy, M., and Young, P. M. (2011). Epithelial profiling of antibiotic controlled release respiratory formulations. *Pharm. Res.* 28, 2327–2338. doi: 10.1007/s11095-011-0462-1

Ong, H. X., Traini, D., Loo, C. Y., Sarkissian, L., Lauretani, G., Scalia, S., et al. (2015). Is the cellular uptake of respiratory aerosols delivered from different devices equivalent? *Eur. J. Pharm. Biopharm.* 93, 320–327. doi: 10.1016/j.ejpb.2015.04.012

Palumbo, M. O., Kavan, P., Miller, W. H. Jr., Panasci, L., Assouline, S., Johnson, N., et al. (2013). Systemic cancer therapy: achievements and challenges that lie ahead. *Front. Pharmacol.* 4:57. doi: 10.3389/fphar.2013.00057

Paolicelli, G., Luca, A., Jose, S. S., Antonini, M., Teloni, I., Fric, J., et al. (2019). Using lung organoids to investigate epithelial barrier complexity and IL-17 signaling during respiratory infection. *Front. Immunol.* 10:323. doi: 10.3389/fimmu.2019.00323

Paranjpe, M., Neuhaus, V., Finke, J. H., Richter, C., Gothsch, T., Kwade, A., et al. (2013). In vitro and ex vivo toxicological testing of sildenafil-loaded solid lipid nanoparticles. *Inhal. Toxicol.* 25, 536–543. doi: 10.3109/08958378.2013.810315

Pezzulo, A. A., Starner, T. D., Scheetz, T. E., Traver, G. L., Tilley, A. E., Harvey, B. G., et al. (2011). The air-liquid interface and use of primary cell cultures are important to recapitulate the transcriptional profile of in vivo airway epithelia. *Am. J. Physiol. Lung Cell. Mol. Physiol.* 300, L25–L31. doi: 10.1152/ajplung.00256.2010

Phalen, R. F., Yeh, H. C., Schum, G. M., and Raabe, O. G. (1978). Application of an idealized model to morphometry of the mammalian tracheobronchial tree. *Anat. Rec.* 190, 167–176. doi: 10.1002/ar.1091900202

Placke, M. E., and Fisher, G. L. (1987). Adult peripheral lung organ culture–a model for respiratory tract toxicology. *Toxicol. Appl. Pharmacol.* 90, 284–298. doi: 10.1016/0041-008x(87)90336-x

Qi, A., Friend, J. R., Yeo, L. Y., Morton, D. A., McIntosh, M. P., and Spiccia, L. (2009). Miniature inhalation therapy platform using surface acoustic wave microfluidic atomization. *Lab. Chip* 9, 2184–2193. doi: 10.1039/b903575c

Ren, H., Birch, N. P., and Suresh, V. (2016). An optimised human cell culture model for alveolar epithelial transport. *PLoS One* 11:e0165225. doi: 10.1371/journal.pone.0165225

Ruge, C. A., Kirch, J., and Lehr, C. M. (2013). Pulmonary drug delivery: from generating aerosols to overcoming biological barriers-therapeutic possibilities and technological challenges. *Lancet Respir. Med.* 1, 402–413. doi: 10.1016/s2213-2600(13)70072-9

Sakagami, M. (2006). In vivo, in vitro and ex vivo models to assess pulmonary absorption and disposition of inhaled therapeutics for systemic delivery. *Adv. Drug Deliv. Rev.* 58, 1030–1060. doi: 10.1016/j.addr.2006.07.012

Sakagami, M. (2020). In vitro, ex vivo and in vivo methods of lung absorption for inhaled drugs. *Adv. Drug Deliv. Rev.* 58, 9–10. doi: 10.1016/j.addr.2020.07.025

Salomon, J. J., Muchitsch, V. E., Gausterer, J. C., Schwagerus, E., Huwer, H., Daum, N., et al. (2014). The cell line NCl-H441 is a useful in vitro model for transport studies of human distal lung epithelial barrier. *Mol. Pharm.* 11, 995–1006. doi: 10.1021/mp4006535

Selg, E., Ewing, P., Acevedo, F., Sjöberg, C. O., Ryrfeldt, A., and Gerde, P. (2013). Dry powder inhalation exposures of the endotracheally intubated rat lung, ex vivo and in vivo: the pulmonary pharmacokinetics of fluticasone furoate. *J. Aerosol. Med. Pulm. Drug Deliv.* 26, 181–189. doi: 10.1089/jamp.2012.0971

Sheikh, Z., Bradbury, P., Pozzoli, M., Young, P. M., Xin Ong, H., and Traini, D. (2020). An in vitro model for assessing drug transport in cystic fibrosis treatment: characterisation of the CuFi-1 cell line. *Eur. J. Pharm. Biopharm.* 156, 121–130. doi: 10.1016/j.ejpb.2020.09.002

Shur, J., and Price, R. (2016). Predictive in vitro dissolution methods for orally inhaled drug products. *Respir. Drug Deliv.* 1121–130.

Strikoudis, A., Cieślak, A., Loffredo, L., Chen, Y. W., Patel, N., Saqi, A., et al. (2019). Modeling of fibrotic lung disease using 3D organoids derived from human pluripotent stem cells. *Cell. Rep.* 27, 3709.e5–3723.e5. doi: 10.1016/j.celrep.2019.05.077

Takahashi, N., Hoshi, H., Higa, A., Hiyama, G., Tamura, H., Ogawa, M., et al. (2019). An in vitro system for evaluating molecular targeted drugs using lung patient-derived tumor organoids. *Cells* 8:481. doi: 10.3390/cells8050481

Tan, Q., Choi, K. M., Sicard, D., and Tschumperlin, D. J. (2017). Human airway organoid engineering as a step toward lung regeneration and disease modeling. *Biomaterials* 113, 118–132. doi: 10.1016/j.biomaterials.2016.10.046

Tronde, A., Baran, G., Eirefelt, S., Lennernäs, H., and Bengtsson, U. H. (2002). Miniaturized nebulization catheters: a new approach for delivery of defined aerosol doses to the rat lung. *J. Aerosol. Med.* 15, 283–296. doi: 10.1089/089426802760292627

Upadhyay, S., and Palmberg, L. (2018). Air-liquid interface: relevant in vitro models for investigating air pollutant-induced pulmonary toxicity. *Toxicol. Sci.* 164, 21–30. doi: 10.1093/toxsci/kfy053

van der Vaart, J., and Clevers, H. (2020). Airway organoids as models of human disease. *J. Intern. Med.* doi: 10.1111/joim.13075

van Rensburg, L., van Zyl, J. M., and Smith, J. (2018). Deposition and transport of linezolid mediated by a synthetic surfactant Synsurf(®) within a pressurized metered dose inhaler: a Calu-3 model. *Drug Des. Devel. Ther.* 12, 1107–1118. doi: 10.2147/dddt.S147035

Wang, H., He, L., Liu, B., Feng, Y., Zhou, H., Zhang, Z., et al. (2018). Establishment and comparison of air-liquid interface culture systems for primary and immortalized swine tracheal epithelial cells. *BMC Cell. Biol.* 19:10. doi: 10.1186/s12860-018-0162-3

Wanner, A., Salathé, M., and O'Riordan, T. G. (1996). Mucociliary clearance in the airways. *Am. J. Respir. Crit. Care Med.* 154(6 Pt 1), 1868–1902. doi: 10.1164/ajrccm.154.6.8970383

Ware, L. B. (2008). Modeling human lung disease in animals. *Am. J. Physiol. Lung Cell. Mol. Physiol.* 294, L149–L150. doi: 10.1152/ajplung.00472.2007

World Health Organisation [WHO] (2014). *Global Status Report on Noncommunicable Diseases 2014.* Geneva: World Health Organisation.

World Health Organisation [WHO] (2019a). *Burden of COPD.* Geneva: World Health Organisation.

World Health Organisation [WHO] (2019b). *The Top 10 Causes of Death.* Geneva: World Health Organization.

Yeh, H. C., Phalen, R. F., and Raabe, O. G. (1976). Factors influencing the deposition of inhaled particles. *Environ. Health Perspect.* 15, 147–156. doi: 10.1289/ehp.7615147

Yeh, H. C., Schum, G. M., and Duggan, M. T. (1979). Anatomic models of the tracheobronchial and pulmonary regions of the rat. *Anat. Rec.* 195, 483–492. doi: 10.1002/ar.1091950308

Yilmaz, Y., Williams, G., Walles, M., Manevski, N., Krähenbühl, S., and Camenisch, G. (2019). Comparison of rat and human pulmonary metabolism using precision-cut lung slices (PCLS). *Drug Metab. Lett.* 13, 53–63. doi: 10.2174/1872312812666181022114622

4

Pulmonary Surfactant and Drug Delivery: An Interface-Assisted Carrier to Deliver Surfactant Protein SP-D into the Airways

*Cristina García-Mouton†, Alberto Hidalgo†‡, Raquel Arroyo‡, Mercedes Echaide, Antonio Cruz and Jesús Pérez-Gil**

Department of Biochemistry and Molecular Biology, Faculty of Biology, Research Institute "Hospital 12 de Octubre (imas12)," Complutense University, Madrid, Spain

***Correspondence:** Jesús Pérez-Gil jperezgil@bio.ucm.es*

† These authors have contributed equally to this work

***‡Present address:** Alberto Hidalgo, Helmholtz Institute for Pharmaceutical Research Saarland, Helmholtz Center for Infection Research, Saarbrücken, Germany Raquel Arroyo, Division of Neonatology and Pulmonary Biology, Perinatal Institute, Cincinnati Children's Hospital Medical Center, Cincinnati, OH, United States*

This work is focused on the potential use of pulmonary surfactant to deliver full-length recombinant human surfactant protein SP-D (rhSP-D) using the respiratory air-liquid interface as a shuttle. Surfactant protein D (SP-D) is a collectin protein present in the pulmonary surfactant (PS) system, involved in innate immune defense and surfactant homeostasis. It has been recently suggested as a potential therapeutic to alleviate inflammatory responses and lung diseases in preterm infants suffering from respiratory distress syndrome (RDS) or bronchopulmonary dysplasia (BPD). However, none of the current clinical surfactants used for surfactant replacement therapy (SRT) to treat RDS contain SP-D. The interaction of SP-D with surfactant components, the potential of PS as a respiratory drug delivery system and the possibility to produce recombinant versions of human SP-D, brings the possibility of delivering clinical surfactants supplemented with SP-D. Here, we used an *in vitro* setup that somehow emulates the respiratory air-liquid interface to explore this novel approach. It consists in two different compartments connected with a hydrated paper bridge forming a continuous interface. We firstly analyzed the adsorption and spreading of rhSP-D alone from one compartment to another over the air-liquid interface, observing low interfacial activity. Then, we studied the interfacial spreading of the protein co-administered with PS, both at different time periods or as a mixed formulation, and which oligomeric forms of rhSP-D better traveled associated with PS. The results presented here demonstrated that PS may transport rhSP-D long distances over air-liquid interfaces, either as a mixed formulation or separately in a close window time, opening the doors to empower the current clinical surfactants and SRT.

Keywords: pulmonary surfactant, interfacial delivery, respiratory drug delivery, air-liquid interface, lipid-protein interaction

INTRODUCTION

Surfactant protein D (SP-D) is a C-type calcium-dependent lectin that belongs to the collectin family. It is involved in the innate immune properties of pulmonary surfactant (PS) (Crouch et al., 1994; Crouch, 2000) and contributes to alveolar and surfactant homeostasis (Korfhagen et al., 1998). PS is a lipid-protein material essential for the process of breathing that has been proposed as potent drug delivery system (Van't Veen et al., 1996; De Backer et al., 2013; Banaschewski et al., 2015; Hidalgo et al., 2015, 2017). PS is mainly composed by lipids (90% by mass), mainly phospholipids, and four different proteins (6–8% by mass): two hydrophobic (SP-B and SP-C) and two hydrophilic (SP-A and SP-D) (Pérez-Gil, 2008; Parra and Pérez-Gil, 2015). SP-B and SP-C are essential for the maintenance and organization of PS at the air-liquid interface, while SP-A and SP-D are mostly involved in innate immune defense (Perez-Gil and Weaver, 2010). PS enables the process of breathing by lowering the surface tension of the layer of water covering the whole respiratory surface, minimizing the work of breathing and avoiding the alveolar collapse. Apart from the interfacial and immune defense functions, its composition and interfacial properties confers PS the possibility to spread efficiently over air-liquid interfaces and transport therapeutic molecules by surfing the respiratory surface, what has been called an interfacial delivery (Hidalgo et al., 2020).

As the rest of collectins, SP-D monomers (43 kDa) contain four different structural domains: a short N-terminal region enriched in cysteines, a collagen-like domain of Gly-X-Y repetitions, a neck region with α-helical structure and a C-terminal carbohydrate recognition domain (CRD), which constitutes the key structure for most of the protein functions and interactions (Orgeig et al., 2011; Casals et al., 2018). Monomers may associate into trimers (130 kDa), constituting the minimal functional unit to allow the recognition of specific molecules through the CRD. Trimers can also associate forming hexamers, dodecamers (520 kDa) and the so-called "fuzzy balls," which have been recently considered as the most potent oligomeric form of SP-D in bacterial aggregation (Arroyo et al., 2018, 2020). By recognizing a wide range of pathogens and foreign particles mostly through the CRD, SP-D promotes opsonization and aggregation and further clearance by phagocytic alveolar cells (Orgeig et al., 2011; Watson et al., 2019). Additionally, it also modulates the release of pro- and anti-inflammatory mediators via toll-like receptors and calreticulin/CD91 (Kingma and Whitsett, 2006; Sorensen, 2018).

Due to the immuno-modulatory and anti-inflammatory potential of SP-D, its delivery through the airways has been proposed in recent years as a potential therapeutic approach to alleviate inflammatory processes in the lungs. Since Clark and Reid highlighted in 2003 the potential benefits of delivering recombinant fragments of human SP-D (rfhSP-D) as a potential therapy to reduce inflammation in neonatal chronic lung disease, cystic fibrosis and emphysema (Clark and Reid, 2003), few works have explored this anti-inflammatory strategy and how this protein can be delivered through the airways. The instillation of rfhSP-D alone showed a reduction of inflammation derived from allergy in mice (Strong et al., 2003; Liu et al., 2005) or LPS in lambs (Ikegami et al., 2006) using recombinant fragments or full length recombinant human SP-D (rhSP-D), respectively. A recent study demonstrated the benefits of encapsulating SP-D in PLGA nanoparticles as a sustained release approach during several days from the administration (Cohen et al., 2020). In spite of the therapeutic effects of SP-D, the current commercially available clinical surfactants are all still lacking SP-D. However, since SP-D interacts with pulmonary surfactant components (Korfhagen et al., 1998), preferentially with phosphatidylinositol (PI) (Ogasawara et al., 1992), the possibility of delivering clinical surfactants supplemented with rhSP-D has also been explored showing enhanced anti-inflammatory effects of PS/SP-D formulations on ventilation- (Sato et al., 2010) and LPS-derived (Ikegami et al., 2007) inflammation in lambs and mice, respectively. However, to the best of our knowledge, the capability of PS to transport SP-D interfacially to optimize PS/SP-D formulations and delivery has not been studied.

Therefore, in the present study we have evaluated for the first time (1) the possibility of SP-D to adsorb into and spread over air-liquid interfaces, (2) whether PS enhances this process, and (3) the influence of PS structures to interact with the different oligomeric forms of SP-D (i.e., trimers, hexamers and "fuzzy balls"). To do so, we used self-designed vehiculization setups consisting in two aqueous compartments connected by an interfacial bridge, and different PS/SP-D preparations and modes of administration were tested.

MATERIALS AND METHODS

Unless otherwise indicated, all chemicals and reagents were purchased from commercial suppliers (i.e., Sigma-Aldrich®, Merck KGaA or Macron Fine Chemicals™). Water was filtered and treated with a Merck-Millipore Direct-Q3 purification system and further distilled for the surface balance experiments.

Pulmonary Surfactant Preparations

Native Surfactant

Native pulmonary surfactant (NS) was isolated from bronchoalveolar lavage (BAL) of fresh slaughtered porcine lungs as previously described (Taeusch et al., 2005). Briefly, BAL was centrifuged at 1,000 g for 5 min to eliminate cells and tissue debris. Then, it was subsequently ultracentrifuged for 1 h at 100,000 g and 4°C. Pellets, containing the surfactant complexes, were resuspended in 16% NaBr 0.9% NaCl to perform a discontinuous NaBr density gradient at 120,000 g for 2 h at 4°C to purify the surfactant complexes from other cell membranes. After the gradient, pulmonary surfactant complexes, concentrated between the lighter (0.9% NaCl) and the medium dense solution (13% NaBr 0.9% NaCl), were homogenized with 0.9% NaCl and stored at −80°C until used.

Surfactant Organic Extract

Surfactant organic extract (OE), containing all the lipids plus the hydrophobic proteins SP-B and SP-C, was obtained following the organic extraction protocol established by Blight and Dyer (Bligh and Dyer, 1959). A mixture of chloroform/methanol/water (1:2:1 v/v/v) was added to the NS and incubated during 30 min at 37°C to allow protein flocculation. An additional volume of water and chloroform were added to the mixture and centrifuged 5 min at 3,000 g and 4°C. The fraction at the bottom containing the hydrophobic components of NS (organic phase) was collected. The upper fraction (aqueous phase) was subjected to two successive lavages by adding two volumes of chloroform and centrifuged 5 min at 3,000 g and 4°C. Finally, the material recovered was stored at −20°C until used.

To prepare aqueous suspensions from OE, proper amounts of the material were dried under a nitrogen stream and further vacuum for 2 h to form a dry film without organic solvent traces. The dried films were reconstituted by hydration with a buffer solution (5 mM Tris, 150 mM NaCl, pH 7.4) during 1 h at 45°C, shacking vigorously every 10 min. When needed, the aqueous solution was sonicated in ice during 2 min (burst for 0.6, and 0.4 s between bursts) at 65% amplitude for 7 cycles in a UP 200S sonifier, with a 2 mm microtip.

Poractant α

Poractant α, commercially available as Curosurf®, was obtained from Chiesi Farmaceutici S.p.A. (Parma, Italy) at a concentration of 80 mg/mL.

Recombinant Human SP-D (rhSP-D)

rhSP-D was provided by Airway Therapeutics Inc. It has been produced and purified as previously described by Arroyo et al. (2018). All the different clones used have been previously analyzed by atomic force microscopy (AFM) to qualitatively and quantitatively characterize the oligomeric forms of the protein.

Fluorescent Labeling of rhSP-D

rhSP-D was conjugated with the amine-reactive fluorescent dye Alexa Fluor 488. First, the protein was exchanged to Hepes buffer (10 mM Hepes, 200 mM NaCl, 1 mM EDTA, pH 7.4) by dialysis at 4°C, in which the labeling reaction would take place. The proper amount of the probe, dissolved in methanol, to get a 1:20 (mol/mol) protein/probe ratio was dried under a nitrogen stream and under vacuum for 30 min and further dissolved in water. To shift the pH to values near 9 and activate amines, $NaHCO_3$ was added to the solution. Then, the labeling reaction was performed for 1 h at room temperature with continuous stirring. Finally, to separate fluorescently labeled protein (F-rhSP-D) from the free probe, the solution was dialyzed against Histidine buffer (5 mM His, 200 mM NaCl, 1 mM EDTA, pH 6).

Interfacial Assays

In the present study, the adsorption and spreading properties of rhSP-D by itself and the delivery capabilities of PS were characterized in Wilhelmy and vehiculization troughs.

Adsorption Tests

To evaluate the interfacial adsorption of the protein, experiments were performed using a single Wilhelmy trough (NIMA technologies, Coventry, UK). To do so, 1.8 mL of a buffered solution (5 mM Tris, 150 mM NaCl, pH 7.4) was placed in the Wilhelmy trough and an aqueous aliquot of 10 μL at 0.34 mg/mL (3.4 μg) of rhSP-D was injected into the subphase close to the surface, before monitoring the changes in surface pressure during 100 min with a pressure sensor (NIMA technologies, Coventry, UK). The subphase was constantly stirred to reduce diffusion limitation and thermostated at 25 ± 1°C.

Spreading and Vehiculization Assays

In order to explore the interfacial spreading capabilities of SP-D and its potential interface-assisted vehiculization by PS, an *in vitro* vehiculization setup was used (Yu and Possmayer, 2003; Hidalgo et al., 2017). Briefly, it consists in two different troughs containing a buffered solution (5 mM Tris, 150 mM NaCl, pH 7.4) connected by an interfacial bridge. One of the troughs is used as a donor (surface area: 315 mm^2; subphase volume: 1.8 mL), somehow mimicking delivery at the upper airways, and the other as the recipient, which emulates the target surfaces at the distal airways and may vary depending on the experiment. Both troughs are connected by an interfacial bridge (6 cm length × 1 cm width), made of a hydrated filter paper (No. 1 Whatman filter paper), which creates a continuous air-liquid interface between both compartments, somehow recreating the conductive airways (**Supplementary Figure 1**). The filter paper was hydrated by submersion into the same buffer solution during 5 min before connecting both compartments. The samples were added directly onto the donor interface by drop deposition. This should simulate the arrival of surfactant or surfactant/drug drops, either upon nebulization or direct bolus deposition, into the upper airways. Changes in surface pressure were simultaneously monitored in both donor and recipient compartments (pressure sensors from NIMA technologies, Coventry, UK). An increase of surface pressure at the donor trough indicates that the sample adsorbs into the air-liquid interface. The increase of surface pressure at the recipient trough is a signal indicating that the sample can interfacially spread over the air-liquid interface. This interfacial spreading of material is likely governed by Marangoni convection. The surface tension gradient between both connected compartments leads to the spread of material from the donor, where the surface tension is lower (higher surface pressure) and near the equilibrium, to the recipient trough, where the surface tension is initially high (low surface pressure) (Borgas and Grotberg, 1988; Grotberg and Gaver III, 1996; Halpern et al., 1998). To determine whether PS can transport SP-D, the recipient interface was measured by fluorescence or visualized under transmission electron microscopy (TEM) or atomic force microscopy (AFM) as detailed in the next sections. The experimental temperature was maintained constant at 25 ± 1°C. Different vehiculization setups and samples were used for each assay:

Spreading Properties of rhSP-D Alone

An aliquot of 20 μL at 0.6 mg/mL (12 μg) of rhSP-D, an amount enough to have an excess of protein, was added by drop deposition onto the donor interface connected to a recipient trough with a surface area of 25 cm^2 and 25 mL subphase volume. To determine the fluorescence of F-shSP-D, a smaller version of the recipient trough (surface area: 315 mm^2; subphase volume: 1.8 mL) was used in order to collect the whole volume.

Interfacial Vehiculization of a Combined PS/rhSP-D Formulation

An aqueous suspension of OE was incubated with rhSP-D (1% by mass with respect to lipids) at 37°C for 30 min. In these experiments, a rhSP-D clone enriched with higher amounts of fuzzy ball oligomers (82% by weight of total protein mass) compared with the average quantity [29% weight (Arroyo et al., 2018)] was used to facilitate its detection and recognition under the microscopes. Then, an aqueous aliquot of 15 μL at 50 mg/mL (750 μg) of OE was added by drop deposition onto the donor interface connected to the recipient trough (surface area: 25 cm^2; subphase volume: 25 mL). To visualize the protein under TEM and AFM, the interfacial films were transferred to carbon-coated cupper grids and mica plates, respectively, as explained in the next sections. In addition, to evaluate the differential vehiculization of the oligomeric forms of rhSP-D, the aqueous suspension of OE was sonicated or not prior incubation with 1% rhSP-D by mass. In this case, a Langmuir-Blodgett trough (surface area: 60–184 cm^2; subphase volume: 350 mL) was used as recipient to transfer the interfacial film onto mica plates.

Co-administration of PS and rhSP-D

In an attempt to strategize a sequential co-administration of PS and rhSP-D and understand the mechanisms of the interaction and interfacial spreading of PS and rhSP-D, we added both materials sequentially instead of as a combined formulation to the donor compartment connected to the recipient trough (surface area: 25 cm^2; subphase volume: 25 mL). The clinical surfactant Curosurf (50 μL at 80 mg/mL; 4 mg) and the fluorescent derivative of rhSP-D (15 μL at 1 mg/mL; 15 μg) were used for these experiments. In a first scenario, Curosurf was firstly added by drop deposition onto the donor interface and F-rhSP-D 70 s later. This favors the interaction of the protein with a previously-formed surfactant interfacial film at the donor compartment and allows to analyze whether, in the case of interactions with Curosurf, the interfacial spreading driving forces promote the interfacial vehiculization of F-rhSP-D. In a second scenario, F-rhSP-D was first added onto the donor interface by drop deposition and Curosurf 70 s later to evaluate whether the surfactant can somehow take the SP-D that potentially diffuses through the aqueous subphase and transport it interfacially. The interface from the recipient trough was collected after 30 min to measure the fluorescence spectra. Additionally, experiments applying OE in organic solvent (Chloroform/Methanol 2:1 v/v) were performed to avoid the formation of surface-associated structures. To do so, 20 μL of OE at 18 μg/μL (360 μg) were added by drop deposition onto the donor interface and, 10 min later for letting the organic solvents evaporate, 2.5% (9 μg; data not shown) and 5% (18 μg) of rhSP-D by mass with respect to lipids was also added on top of the donor surfactant-occupied interface by drop deposition. A Langmuir-Blodgett trough (surface area: 60–184 cm^2; subphase volume: 350 mL) was used as recipient to transfer the interfacial film onto mica plates for AFM analysis.

Fluorescence Spectroscopy

The vehiculization of the fluorescently-labeled F-rhSP-D by PS was detected by collecting the interface of the recipient trough and measuring the fluorescence of the covalently attached Alexa Fluor 488 ($\lambda_{excitation} = 490$ nm; $\lambda_{emission} = 525$ nm) in an Aminco Browman Series 2 spectrofluorometer. The emission spectra were measured at 25°C.

Atomic Force Microscopy (AFM)

This technique was used to visualize the oligomers of rhSP-D that were transported by PS over the air-liquid interface. The transference of the interfacial film at the target recipient surface to mica supports was performed following two different methods: (1) by direct deposition of the mica plate on top of the interface of the recipient trough, or (2) by forming Blodgett films using a Langmuir-Blodgett trough as the recipient compartment. In the latter method, the mica plate was cleaved and submerged into the buffered subphase prior sample addition. At the end of each experiment, the mica plate was progressively raised maintaining the surface pressure constant at 20 mN/m (barrier speed: 25 cm^2/min; dipper speed: 5 mm/min). We selected that transfer pressure in order to avoid the potential exclusion of some components and the formation of three-dimensional structures that would hinder the acquisition of images under AFM. Images were acquired using an AFM from Nanotec (Nanotec Electrónica, Madrid, Spain) with PointProbePlus tips (Nanosensors, Neuchâtel, Switzerland), or a NanoScope IIIa scanning probe microscope (Bruker, Billerica, USA) with TESP-SS tips (Bruker, Billerica, USA), in the Centro Nacional de Biotecnología (CNB, CSIC) and ICTS Centro Nacional de Microscopía Electrónica (Universidad Complutense de Madrid). Samples were imaged in tapping mode in air, at room temperature and low humidity. The images were processed using the WSxM freeware and the NanoScope Analysis software.

Transmission Electron Microscopy

To observe the surfactant structures and confirm that PS can transport rhSP-D over air-liquid interfaces, carbon-coated cupper grids (EMS400-Cu, Gilder grids) were deposited on the interface of the recipient troughs and incubated for 30 s. Then, the grids were directly incubated for 1 min with 2% uranyl acetate (w/v) to perform negative staining. Samples were observed under a JEOL JEM-1010 transmission electron microscope (ICTS Centro Nacional de Microscopía Electrónica, Universidad Complutense de Madrid) at a magnification of 40,000x and 120,000x.

Dynamic Light Scattering (DLS)

In order to characterize the OE samples after sonication, the hydrodynamic radius (R_H) of aqueous suspensions in the presence or the absence of 1% rhSP-D by mass were determined using a DynaPro MS/X DLS detector equipped with a 824.7 nm-laser (Wyatt Inc). R_H was calculated by the Stokes-Einstein equation (Equation 1):

$$D = \frac{k_B \cdot T}{6\pi \eta R_H} \tag{1}$$

where D is the translational diffusion coefficient, k_B the Boltzman constant, T the temperature, and η the viscosity. Water used to dilute the samples was 10 times filtered using filters of 0.22 μm (Q-Pod, Merck). Polydispersity values smaller than 15% were considered to correspond to monodisperse samples.

RESULTS

Interfacial Properties and Spreading of rhSP-D Alone

As shown in **Figure 1A**, the surface pressure does not increase during the first 40 min. Then, it raises to values around 5 mN/m. It indicates that the protein slowly adsorbs into the air-liquid interface, but long periods of time are required to have enough amount of protein at the interface to cause a slight increase of surface pressure.

Figure 1B shows the interfacial spreading of rhSP-D by means of changes in surface pressure during 40 min both in donor and recipient compartments. Surface pressure at donor compartment increases until stabilizing at a limited surface pressure of ~3 mN/m. Then, it slightly decreases as the surface pressure at the recipient compartment increases. The stabilization of the pressure at the donor trough and its subsequent decrease could indicate a transient adsorption of the protein into the interface and further diffusion to the recipient trough. However, once the surface pressure at the recipient equals the pressure at the donor compartment, the latter increases as well, indicating a continuous adsorption of rhSP-D at the donor interface until the interface stabilizes. To confirm the presence of the protein in the recipient trough, interfacial films were transferred to carbon-coated cupper grids and observed by TEM (**Supplementary Figure 2**), but no traces of SP-D were observed. Therefore, we also performed the vehiculization assays using the fluorescent derivative of rhSP-D. In this case, the smallest recipient trough was used to collect the whole volume (1.8 mL) and also measure the F-rhSP-D that might diffuse and dilute away from the interface into the subphase. As observed in **Figure 1C**, fluorescence was detected in the recipient compartment, suggesting that rhSP-D may actually cross the bridge alone from the donor to the recipient trough. However, the fluorescent signal was very low and maximal sensitivity in the fluorometer was required to detect it.

Interfacial Delivery of rhSP-D in the Presence of Pulmonary Surfactant

Once analyzed the adsorption and spreading properties of the rhSP-D alone confirming low interfacial adsorption and spreading capabilities, the next step was to analyze how the presence of PS influences the interface-assisted vehiculization process. To do so, different strategies were followed including a PS/rhSP-D combined formulation and the addition of PS and rhSP-D separately.

Interfacial Vehiculization of a Combined PS/rhSP-D Formulation

Figure 2A shows that right after addition of OE/rhSP-D mixture, the surface pressure at the donor compartment increases sharply above 30 mN/m, indicating a proper interfacial adsorption of the formulation. After 10 min, the surface pressure in the recipient trough starts increasing as well, though this increase seems to be lower than the one observed in the donor compartment. This, together with the high error bars could indicate that rhSP-D could somehow affect or modulate the adsorption and spreading capabilities of pulmonary surfactant, something that needs further exploration to elucidate the relevant factors involved in this potential effect. In spite of the donor-to-recipient diffusion of OE/rhSP-D, the surface pressure at the donor trough always remained stable, indicating a rapid and continuous adsorption and spreading of new material from the surface-associated reservoirs at the donor compartment.

To confirm the potential of OE to transport rhSP-D over the air-liquid interface, the material placed at the recipient interface was transferred onto carbon-coated cupper grids and mica plates for TEM and AFM visualization, respectively. The micrographs obtained by TEM (**Figure 2B**) shows accumulation at the interface of fuzzy-ball-like structures, recognizable by the higher electron density of the central N-terminal collagenous stem. These structures are similar to the ones observed somewhere else (Holmskov, 2000). The AFM phase images (**Figure 2C**) demonstrated the presence of rhSP-D fuzzy balls at the air-liquid interface, appearing both grouped and isolated.

Understanding the Mechanisms Behind the Interaction and Interfacial Spreading of PS and rhSP-D

Figures 3A,B show Π-time isotherms adding first Curosurf or F-rhSP-D, respectively. In both scenarios, Curosurf reaches the equilibrium surface pressure (around 40 mN/m) in the donor compartment right after injection, and subsequently the surface pressure in the recipient trough also increased. The injection of F-rhSP-D after 70 s in the presence of the preformed surfactant film does not induce further changes in surface pressure either in the donor neither in the recipient. This indicates that the protein does not affect the interfacial and spreading properties of Curosurf. After 30 min, the recipient interface was collected to measure the fluorescence of F-rhSP-D. As shown in **Figure 3C**, F-rhSP-D was detected at the recipient trough in both scenarios. Although no statistically significant differences were observed ($p = 0.078$), the injection of Curosurf prior to the protein seems to show a tendency to enhance the vehiculization, which could indicate a more extensive interaction with rhSP-D at the air-liquid interface when surfactant structures are already adsorbed at the interface.

To avoid formation of surface-associated reservoirs and to have both donor and recipient interfaces saturated with surfactant and stable prior to the addition of rhSP-D, OE in organic solvent was firstly applied onto the donor air-liquid interface. **Figure 4A** shows that OE rapidly spreads over the interface, reaching and stabilizing at the equilibrium surface pressure. Then, to allow organic solvent to evaporate, rhSP-D was applied at the donor interface 10 min later. At the end of the experiment, the recipient interface was transferred onto a mica plate for detecting the presence of rhSP-D by AFM analysis. As observed in the images shown in **Figure 4B**, rhSP-D was not detectable at the recipient interface.

Differential Vehiculization of Oligomeric Forms of rhSP-D by Pulmonary Surfactant

In an attempt to elucidate whether the different oligomers are transported differently and whether surfactant structure

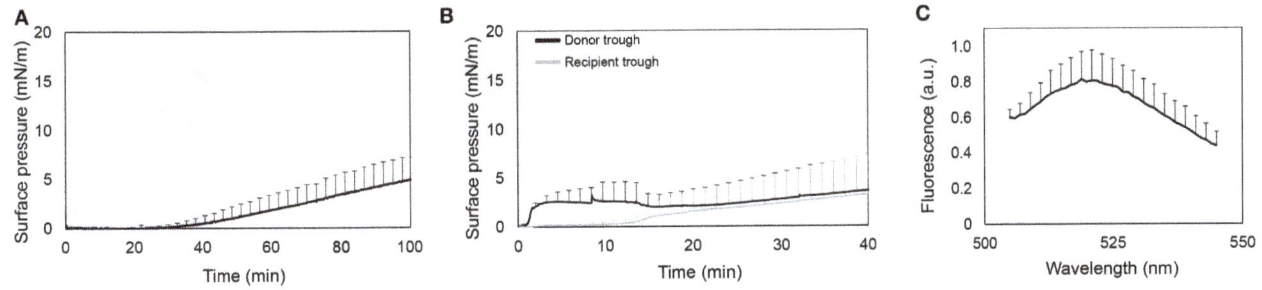

FIGURE 1 | Interfacial activity of rhSP-D. **(A)** Recording of surface pressure as a function of time for the adsorption of an aliquot of 10 μL at 0.34 mg/mL (3.4 μg) of rhSP-D injected into the subphase of a Wilhelmy balance. **(B)** Adsorption and spreading isotherms of rhSP-D upon injection of an aliquot of 20 μL at 0.6 mg/mL (12 μg) of the protein at the air-liquid interface in a double-Wilhelmy balance. Surface pressure measured in the donor (black line) and recipient troughs (gray line). **(C)** Fluorescence emission spectra of the F-rhSP-D detected in the whole volume taken from the recipient trough at the end of the experiments. Data represented by the mean and standard deviations of three different replicates.

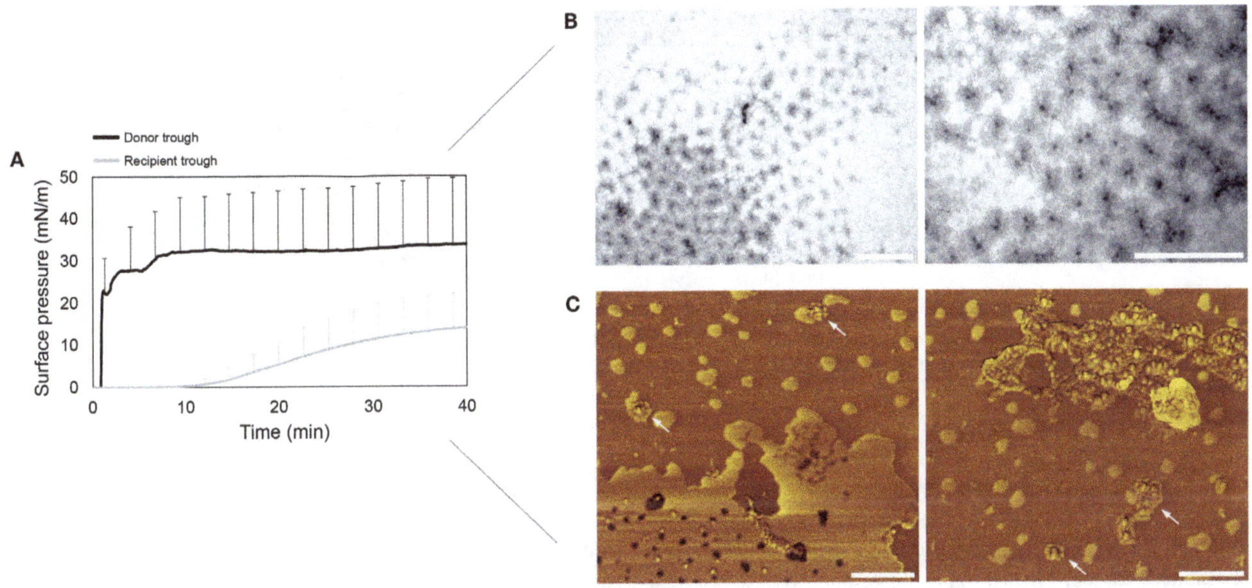

FIGURE 2 | Pulmonary surfactant vehiculization of rhSP-D over the air-liquid interface. **(A)** Adsorption and spreading isotherm of a suspension of the organic extract from native surfactant (OE) reconstituted and mixed with rhSP-D at 1% protein/lipid (w/w) ratio. An aqueous aliquot of 15 μL (50 mg/mL; 750 μg) of the material were deposited dropwise at the donor interface in the double-Wilhelmy balance and changes in surface pressure were measured in both troughs. Mean and standard deviations were obtained from three replicates. **(B)** Transmission electron microscopy (TEM) micrographs of the rhSP-D fuzzy balls detected at the recipient air-liquid interface upon surfactant-promoted interfacial vehiculization. **(C)** rhSP-D vehiculized by surfactant detected at the recipient air-liquid interface by atomic force microscopy (AFM) phase images. Some examples of fuzzy balls are pointed with white arrows. Scale bar: 400 nm.

could influence this process, vehiculization of the OE/rhSP-D combination was assessed with sonicated and non-sonicated OE suspensions. The sonication process favors the formation of smaller surfactant vesiculated structures with higher curvature (García-Fojeda et al., 2019), which has been proposed to promote interaction of amphiphilic proteins. As observed in **Supplementary Figure 3**, sonication induced fragmentation of OE vesicles observable by means of more monodispersed population of smaller vesicles. The presence of rhSP-D caused a shift in the peak to larger sizes in both sonicated and non-sonicated surfactant, indicating an interaction of rhSP-D with surfactant membranes.

Figure 5A compares the Π-time isotherms of both donor and recipient compartments upon application of sonicated or non-sonicated samples. After 30 min, the interfacial film at the recipient trough was transferred onto a mica plate at a constant surface pressure of 20 mN/m to avoid the formation of multilayered structures and the exclusion of material from the interface once higher pressures are reached. The surfactant vehiculization of rhSP-D by both approaches was demonstrated by observing the presence of rhSP-D oligomers under the AFM (see **Figure 5B**). Coexistence of liquid-condensed (L_c) and liquid-expanded (L_e) lipid phases are differentiable in **Figure 5B**, where L_c domains exhibit round-shaped areas with an average

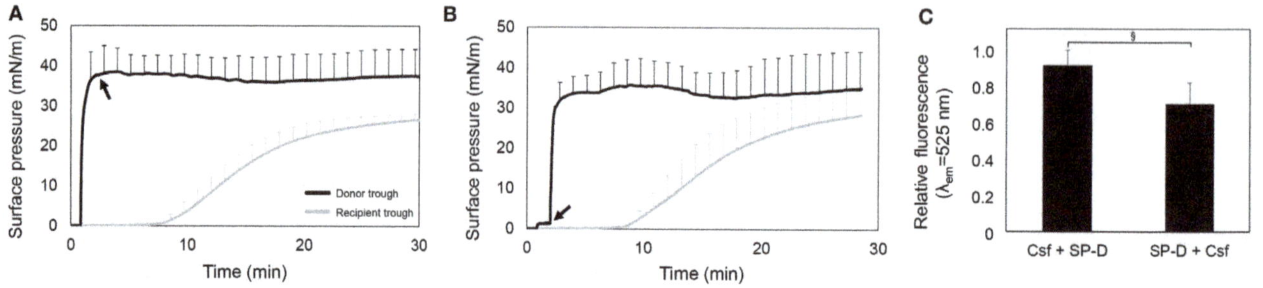

FIGURE 3 | rhSP-D conjugated with Alexa Fluor 488 transported over the interface by the association with Curosurf (Csf). **(A)** Adsorption and spreading isotherm obtained from the interfacial injection of 50 μL (80 mg/mL; 4 mg) of Curosurf and, 70 s after, 15 μL (1 mg/mL; 15 μg) of F-rhSP-D (black arrow), measured in the double-Langmuir balance. **(B)** Pressure-time isotherm upon injection of, first, F-rhSP-D and, 70 s after, Curosurf (black arrow), in a double-Langmuir balance. **(C)** Relative fluorescence emission at λ_{em} = 525 nm of the material collected from the recipient interface by aspiration at the end of each experiment. Data represent mean and standard deviation calculated from three different experiments. Pair *t*-test: (§) $p = 0.078$.

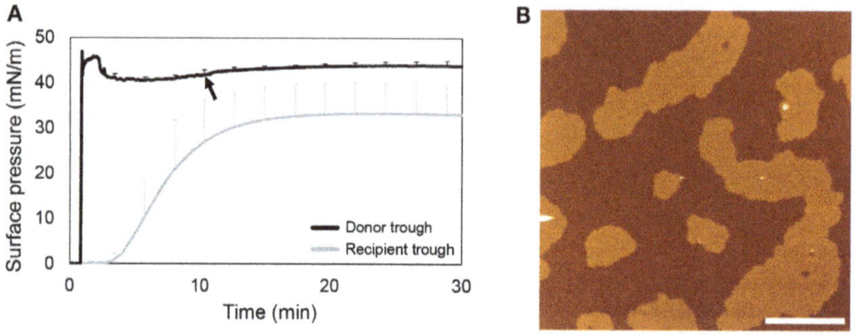

FIGURE 4 | rhSP-D association to the interface in the absence of surfactant-associated reservoirs. **(A)** Spreading isotherm of OE in organic solvent in a double-Langmuir balance and **(B)** AFM height image obtained from the transference of the recipient interfacial film after the spreading of 360 μg of OE in organic solvent and the injection of 5% w/w rhSP-D 10 min after (black arrow in **A**). Three replicates were performed to obtain mean and standard deviation data.

difference in height of 5.5 ± 0.89 Å (mean ± SD) surrounded by more extended L_e phases (see **Supplementary Figure 4A**), consistent with previous observations (Yuan and Johnston, 2002; Blanco et al., 2012). The percentage of area that occupied big (>200 nm) or small (<200 nm) L_c domains was also analyzed, but no differences were observed between the films formed by sonicated or non-sonicated samples (**Supplementary Figure 4B**). SP-D molecules are predominately distributed associated with the L_e phase compared with the fraction of the protein seen associated with L_c-L_e boundaries (**Figure 5C**). Interestingly, the protein seems to present a closed configuration of their collagenic arms, and seems to be at least partly buried into the lipid film, observed as protein molecules with similar height but shorter in length than previously described (Arroyo et al., 2018) (**Supplementary Figure 4C**). This particular configuration makes difficult to identify the number of trimers taking part of each oligomer. To assess whether smaller or larger oligomeric forms were preferentially transported by interfacial films assembled from smaller or larger surfactant vesicles, we quantified the oligomers including trimers or hexamers on one group and higher ordered dodecamers and fuzzy balls on the other (see **Figures 5D,E**). In both cases, when using sonicated or non-sonicated surfactant suspensions, an apparently larger number of trimers/hexamers were transported from the donor to the recipient trough in comparison with the proportion of dodecamers and fuzzy balls vehiculized and with the proportion of smaller and larger oligomers in this preparation when examined on plain mica (roughly 50% of each). No significant differences were observed when comparing sonicated and non-sonicated samples, although the intrinsic variability of the few replicas examined prevents a clear conclusion at this stage. The proportion of SP-D trimers and hexamers observed as associated with the interfacial film seems to be higher when smaller surfactant vesicles were accessible to the protein, possibly indicating a trend of the smaller oligomers to interact better with highly curved membranes.

DISCUSSION

Pulmonary surfactant protein SP-D plays essential roles in alveolar immunity and surfactant metabolism (Clark and Reid, 2003). However, the current clinical surfactants used for surfactant replacement therapy (SRT) to treat infant respiratory distress syndrome (RDS), a common cause of morbidity and mortality in preterm neonates characterized by pulmonary immaturity and lack of PS, lack the hydrophilic collectins SP-A and SP-D (Johansson and Curstedt, 2019; Hentschel et al., 2020). Therefore, in this study we have investigated the possibility that

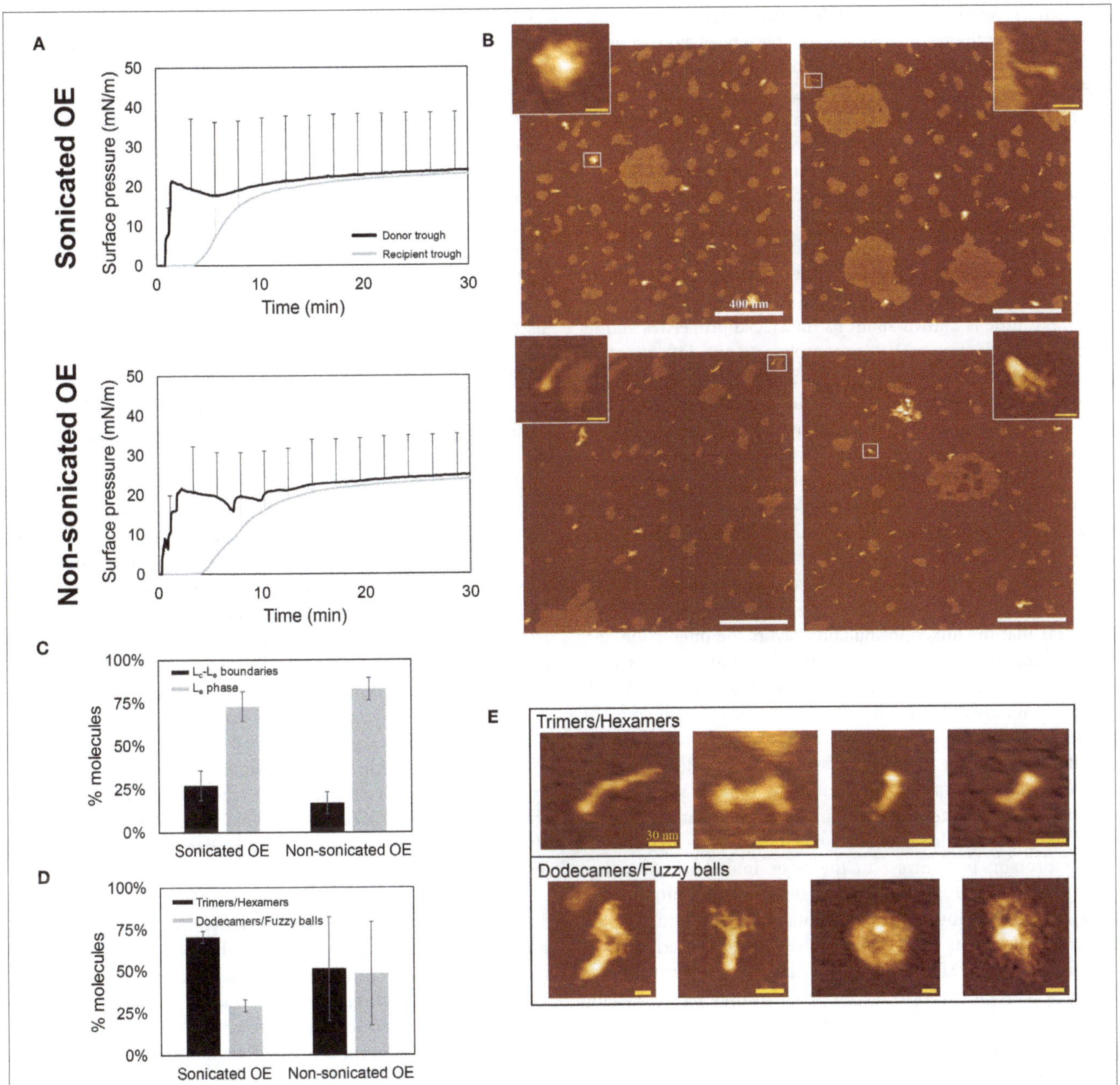

FIGURE 5 | Analysis of rhSP-D oligomers transported over the air-liquid interface associated to surfactant complexes. An aqueous aliquot of OE/rhSP-D at 50 mg/mL (750 µg) and 1% rhSP-D by mass (7.5 µg) was applied at the donor interface. **(A)** Adsorption and spreading isotherms performed in the double-Langmuir balance. **(B)** AFM height images taken after transference onto mica surface of the recipient interfacial film. Data obtained by the vehiculization of sonicated (top) or non-sonicated (bottom) OE before mixing with 1% w/w rhSP-D. Scale bar: 400 nm. Zoom regions show examples of rhSP-D oligomers corresponding to the areas highlighted with white rectangles. Scale bar: 30 nm. **(C)** Percentage of rhSP-D oligomers found at the L_c-L_e boundaries (black) or distributed into the L_e phase (gray) upon vehiculization by sonicated or non-sonicated surfactant. **(D)** Quantitative distribution of smaller and larger rhSP-D oligomers observed in surfactant films, upon association of the protein with sonicated or non-sonicated surfactant structures. **(E)** Representative AFM images of the different SP-D oligomers grouped into trimers/hexamers and dodecamers/fuzzy balls. Scale bar: 30 nm.

protein SP-D could interact with interfacial surfactant films and, through the interface, diffuse over the whole respiratory surface, which could facilitate its function to encounter, interact and label for clearance potential harmful entities impinging the surfactant film, the first barrier exposed to the outer environment in the lungs. In the study, we have used a recombinant form of human SP-D. Our experiments are therefore also useful to show how the combination of the protein with PS could be a useful strategy to facilitate an efficient delivery of the protein through the airways as a therapeutic option, using PS as a shuttle. The use of PS as a drug delivery system to carry and distribute different therapeutic molecules over the respiratory surfaces have been studied in the recent years both *in vitro* and *in vivo* (Van't Veen et al., 1996; Hidalgo et al., 2017, 2020; Baer et al., 2018). The combination of exogenous PS with rhSP-D could have the potential to serve as a preventive or therapeutic approach to treat inflammatory responses and lung diseases in preterm infants such as RDS or bronchopulmonary dysplasia (BPD) (Ikegami et al., 2007; Sato et al., 2010).

The research about SP-D has been focused around its immune roles and anti-inflammatory properties (Crouch et al., 1995; Cai et al., 1999; Liu et al., 2005; Ikegami et al., 2006; Cohen et al., 2020), but little is known about its interfacial properties and its potential combination with PS to complement anti-inflammatory actions, or to define novel therapeutic approaches through the airways. In this work, we report a low interfacial adsorption and spreading properties of rhSP-D by itself on clean air-water interfaces. However, in the presence of pulmonary surfactant, either delivered as a PS/rhSP-D combined formulation or co-administered one right after the other, rhSP-D efficiently traveled associated to air-liquid interfaces. Although the combination of rhSP-D with PS seems to slightly affect the interfacial performance of PS revealed by lower surfaces pressures reached at the recipient compartment and larger experimental variability, it is clear that the mixed formulation favors the interaction and permanence of the protein at the interface and, consequently, its spreading over it (**Figure 2**). When rhSP-D was applied with the donor interface already occupied by PS, it was also detected in the recipient compartment, indicating that the protein is able to interact with pre-existing surfactant films at the interface and used them as a sort of shuttle to rapidly spread long distances via the interface. Similarly, the fact that adding PS right after rhSP-D also promoted the interfacial vehiculization of the protein, in contrast to the poor interfacial spreading of rhSP-D alone (**Figures 1**, **3**), suggests that the protein can shift from a free form in the aqueous bulk phase to a lipid-associated state that is competent to diffuse over the interface. We propose that SP-D/lipid complexes, or alternatively, the interaction of SP-D with any of the hydrophobic surfactant proteins present in the film, converts SP-D into a form that is stably associated with the interface and facilitates its "surfing" capabilities. The injection of rhSP-D on top of a pre-formed surfactant film that had reached surface pressure values of around 15 mN/m, produced an instantaneous and visible increase in surface pressure, confirming the rapid adsorption of the protein into the interface and its insertion into the surfactant film (data not shown). These observations are consistent with the effect on the initial surface pressure as a consequence of SP-D adsorption that was described by Taneva et al. (1997). At surface pressures above ~30 mN/m, SP-D, as occurring with other hydrophilic proteins, cannot penetrate into the lipid films. Thus, rhSP-D may somehow attach to either PS at the interface or the PS reservoirs at the subphase, most likely through the interaction of its CRD with PS phospholipids (Ogasawara et al., 1992; Persson et al., 1992), and leverage the interfacial spreading forces even without their previous combination. This opens the possibility to deliver rhSP-D as a mixed formulation together with PS or administered in a close time window but separately one after the other, without the necessity to develop *de-novo* PS/rhSP-D combined formulations, which could reduce time and costs associated with the design and implementation of clinical trials *ad hoc*.

Nonetheless, when rhSP-D was applied with both donor and recipient interfaces completely saturated with PS to emulate the physiological conditions, the protein was not detected in the recipient compartment (**Figure 4**). This could indicate that SP-D could be able to interact and spread mainly in physiological contexts where surfactant has been depleted from the interface for some reason. However, the absence of breathing-like interfacial compression/expansion dynamics in the current experiments could limit the behavior of SP-D compared with the potential action of the protein *in vivo*. We have recently demonstrated that breathing dynamics could be essential to understand the interfacial behavior of surfactant, particularly with respect to potential interface-assisted spreading capabilities and release processes (Hidalgo et al., 2020), as a consequence of surface tension-driven interfacial flows and the potential progressive exclusion of material from the interface (Borgas and Grotberg, 1988; Pastrana-Rios et al., 1994; Grotberg and Gaver III, 1996; Halpern et al., 1998; Keating et al., 2012; Hidalgo et al., 2020). These effects could be important to promote the spreading of new material coming from upstream reservoirs and better distribute the therapeutics over the respiratory surface (Hidalgo et al., 2020). Thus, further experiments are needed to explore the interfacial delivery of rhSP-D in saturated interfaces subjected to breathing-like dynamic conditions.

The structures of SP-D identified in the images taken by TEM and AFM (**Figures 2**, **5**) are consistent with those obtained in previous studies (Holmskov, 2000; Arroyo et al., 2018), though the association/vehiculization with PS seem to modulate their conformation slightly. All the oligomers analyzed presented a closed conformation, with the collagen domains and the CRD heads less defined. This is likely a consequence of their association with phospholipid surfaces, as it occurs with other hydrophilic proteins (Maget-Dana and Ptak, 1995), something that should be investigated in more detail. We also found a differential vehiculization of the different rhSP-D oligomers over the air-liquid interface. Trimers and hexamers are apparently better transported associated to pulmonary surfactant than dodecamers and fuzzy balls (**Figure 5**). This can be related with their smaller size and a facilitated diffusion associated with the interfacial film. This effect could have some consequences on the role of SP-D in PS homeostasis. SP-D seems to be involved in the regulation of surfactant lipid pool sizes, contributing somehow to the transformation of surfactant large aggregates into small aggregates, preferentially taken up by alveolar type II pneumocytes but not macrophages (Horowitz et al., 1997; Ikegami et al., 2000). Still, when higher order oligomers-enriched batches, the most active oligomers in bacterial aggregation (Arroyo et al., 2020), were used (**Figure 2**), PS was also able to transport them efficiently.

Although our data suggests that PS improves the travel of SP-D across air-liquid interfaces, the Wilhelmy balance results may not be identical to the properties of the alveolar air-liquid interface. In addition, it is uncertain how much PS is needed to facilitate SP-D movement. It is possible that PS levels may be sufficient to achieve maximum SP-D distribution even in surfactant depleted conditions such as RDS.

The above limitations notwithstanding, altogether, this work points out the potential synergistic effect that PS/rhSP-D formulations could have to empower surfactant replacement therapy (SRT) to treat infants with RDS or BPD. It could also offer new possibilities to use SRT in acute lung injuries such as acute respiratory distress syndrome (ARDS) or lung infections in both children and adults. The administration of exogenous surfactants either animal-derived (Kesecioglu et al., 2009) or synthetic (Spragg et al., 2004) has failed so far for treating ARDS, possibly, at least in part, due to the presence in the airways of surfactant inhibitors such as serum components or phospholipases (Autilio et al., 2020) derived from severe inflammation processes and the damage of alveolar epithelium. The incorporation of recombinant forms of human SP-D could contribute to mitigate the inflammation process at the distal airways and enhance the efficacy of SRT. Interestingly, SP-D has also demonstrated different anti-infective activities including antifungal actions (Madan et al., 2001; Ordonez et al., 2019), abilities to recognize and promote virus and bacterial killing and clearance (Crouch, 2000; Hillaire et al., 2013) and specifically binding to the highly glycosylated S-protein of coronavirus inhibiting their replication (Leth-Larsen et al., 2007). Thus, an efficient administration of SP-D could also be beneficial for the treatment of diseases associated with lung infection such as the current COVID-19 pandemic caused by the SARS-CoV-2 virus. The administration of SP-D combined with PS to patients suffering from severe ARDS could help to mitigate lung inflammation and counteract the secondary bacterial and viral infection. In summary, the optimization of PS/rhSP-D formulations could be interesting to empower the current clinical surfactants increasing their potential to replace the lack or damaged endogenous surfactant, to open damaged and poorly-aerated areas in the lungs and to act as a carrier distributing rhSP-D over the respiratory surface. A similar principle could be explored to optimize surfactant-promoted vehiculization of other therapeutic proteins along the interface, including versions of the proteins that could be modified to facilitate their association with surfactant and a efficient interface-driven vehiculization through the airways.

AUTHOR CONTRIBUTIONS

CG-M and AH designed the study, acquired data by performing most of laboratory experiments, interpreted data, and drafted the manuscript. RA acquired data by performing some experiments. ME and AC supervised some data analyses. JP-G conceptualized the study, supervised the whole work, and interpreted all the data. All authors critically revised the paper for important intellectual content and finally approved the paper in the present form. All authors agreed to be accountable for all aspects of the work in ensuring that questions related to the accuracy or integrity of any part of the work were appropriately investigated and resolved.

ACKNOWLEDGMENTS

Authors are indebted to Dr. Fernando Moreno-Herrero and his team, at the National Center of Biotechnology (CNB-CSIC) for their technical assistance with the AFM experiments.

REFERENCES

Arroyo, R., Echaide, M., Moreno-Herrero, F., Perez-Gil, J., and Kingma, P. S. (2020). Functional characterization of the different oligomeric forms of human surfactant protein SP-D. *Biochim. Biophys. Acta Prot. Proteom.* 1868:140436. doi: 10.1016/j.bbapap.2020.140436

Arroyo, R., Martin-Gonzalez, A., Echaide, M., Jain, A., Brondyk, W., Rosenbaum, J., et al. (2018). Supramolecular assembly of human pulmonary surfactant protein SP-D. *J. Mol. Biol.* 430, 1495–1509. doi: 10.1016/j.jmb.2018.03.027

Autilio, C., Echaide, M., Shankar-Aguilera, S., Bragado, R., Amidani, D., Salomone, F., et al. (2020). Surfactant injury in the early phase of severe meconium aspiration syndrome. *Am. J. Respir. Cell Mol. Biol.* 63, 327–337. doi: 10.1165/rcmb.2019-0413OC

Baer, B., Veldhuizen, E. J., Possmayer, F., Yamashita, C., and Veldhuizen, R. (2018). The wet bridge transfer system: a novel tool to assess exogenous surfactant as a vehicle for intrapulmonary drug delivery. *Discov. Med.* 26, 207–218. Available online at: https://www.discoverymedicine.com/Brandon-Baer/2018/11/wet-bridge-transfer-exogenous-surfactant-intrapulmonary-drug-delivery/

Banaschewski, B. J. H., Veldhuizen, E. J. A., Keating, E., Haagsman, H. P., Zuo, Y. Y., Yamashita, C. M., et al. (2015). Antimicrobial and biophysical properties of surfactant supplemented with an antimicrobial peptide for treatment of bacterial pneumonia. *Antimicrob. Agents Chemother.* 59, 3075–3083. doi: 10.1128/AAC.04937-14

Blanco, O., Cruz, A., Ospina, O. L., López-Rodriguez, E., Vázquez, L., and Pérez-Gil, J. (2012). Interfacial behavior and structural properties of a clinical lung surfactant from porcine source. *Biochim. Biophys. Acta* 1818, 2756–2766. doi: 10.1016/j.bbamem.2012.06.023

Bligh, E., and Dyer, W. (1959). A rapid method of lipid extraction and purification. *Can. J. Biochem. Physiol.* 37, 911–917. doi: 10.1139/y59-099

Borgas, M. S., and Grotberg, J. B. (1988). Monolayer flow on a thin film. *J. Fluid Mech.* 193, 151–170. doi: 10.1017/S0022112088002095

Cai, G.-Z., Griffin, G. L., Senior, R. M., Longmore, W. J., and Moxley, M. A. (1999). Recombinant SP-D carbohydrate recognition domain is a chemoattractant for human neutrophils. *Am. J. Physiol. Lung Cell. Mol. Physiol.* 276, L131–L136. doi: 10.1152/ajplung.1999.276.1.L131

Casals, C., Campanero-Rhodes, M. A., García-Fojeda, B., and Solís, D. (2018). The role of collectins and galectins in lung innate immune defense. *Front. Immunol.* 9:1998. doi: 10.3389/fimmu.2018.01998

Clark, H., and Reid, K. (2003). The potential of recombinant surfactant protein D therapy to reduce inflammation in neonatal chronic lung disease, cystic fibrosis, and emphysema. *Arch. Dis. Child* 88, 981–984. doi: 10.1136/adc.88.11.981

Cohen, S. A., Kingma, P. S., Whitsett, J., Goldbart, R., Traitel, T., and Kost, J. (2020). SP-D loaded PLGA nanoparticles as drug delivery system for prevention and treatment of premature infant's lung diseases. *Int. J. Pharm.* 585:119387.

doi: 10.1016/j.ijpharm.2020.119387

Crouch, E., Persson, A., Chang, D., and Heuser, J. (1994). Molecular structure of pulmonary surfactant protein D (SP-D). *J. Biol. Chem.* 269, 17311–17319.

Crouch, E. C. (2000). Surfactant protein-D and pulmonary host defense. *Respir. Res.* 1:6. doi: 10.1186/rr19

Crouch, E. C., Persson, A., Griffin, G. L., Chang, D., and Senior, R. M. (1995). Interactions of pulmonary surfactant protein D (SP-D) with human blood leukocytes. *Am. J. Respir. Cell Mol. Biol.* 12, 410–415. doi: 10.1165/ajrcmb.12.4.7695920

De Backer, L., Braeckmans, K., Demeester, J., De Smedt, S. C., and Raemdonck, K. (2013). The influence of natural pulmonary surfactant on the efficacy of siRNA-loaded dextran nanogels. *Nanomedicine* 8, 1625–1638. doi: 10.2217/nnm.12.203

García-Fojeda, B., González-Carnicero, Z., De Lorenzo, A., Minutti, C. M., De Tapia, L., Euba, B., et al. (2019). Lung surfactant lipids provide immune protection against Haemophilus influenzae respiratory infection. *Front. Immunol.* 10:458. doi: 10.3389/fimmu.2019.00458

Grotberg, J. B., and Gaver III, D. P. (1996). A synopsis of surfactant spreading research. *J. Coll. Interf. Sci.* 178, 377–378. doi: 10.1006/jcis.1996.0130

Halpern, D., Jensen, O., and Grotberg, J. (1998). A theoretical study of surfactant and liquid delivery into the lung. *J. Appl. Physiol.* 85, 333–352. doi: 10.1152/jappl.1998.85.1.333

Hentschel, R., Bohlin, K., Van Kaam, A., Fuchs, H., and Danhaive, O. (2020). Surfactant replacement therapy: from biological basis to current clinical practice. *Pediatr. Res.* 88, 176–183. doi: 10.1038/s41390-020-0750-8

Hidalgo, A., Cruz, A., and Pérez-Gil, J. (2015). Barrier or carrier? Pulmonary surfactant and drug delivery. *Eur. J. Pharm Biopharm.* 95, 117–127. doi: 10.1016/j.ejpb.2015.02.014

Hidalgo, A., Garcia-Mouton, C., Autilio, C., Carravilla, P., Orellana, G., Islam, M. N., et al. (2020). Pulmonary surfactant and drug delivery: vehiculization, release and targeting of surfactant/tacrolimus formulations. *J. Control. Release* 329, 205–222. doi: 10.1016/j.jconrel.2020.11.042

Hidalgo, A., Salomone, F., Fresno, N., Orellana, G., Cruz, A., and Perez-Gil, J. (2017). Efficient interfacially driven vehiculization of corticosteroids by pulmonary surfactant. *Langmuir* 33, 7929–7939. doi: 10.1021/acs.langmuir.7b01177

Hillaire, M. L., Haagsman, H. P., Osterhaus, A. D., Rimmelzwaan, G. F., and Van Eijk, M. (2013). Pulmonary surfactant protein D in first-line innate defence against influenza A virus infections. *J. Innate Immun.* 5, 197–208. doi: 10.1159/000346374

Holmskov, U. (2000). Collectins and collectin receptors in innate immunity [based on 9 publications]. *APMIS Suppl.* 100, 1–59. doi: 10.1111/j.1600-0463.2000.tb05694.x

Horowitz, A., Kurak, K., Moussavian, B., Whitsett, J., Wert, S., Hull, W., et al. (1997). Preferential uptake of small-aggregate fraction of pulmonary surfactant *in vitro*. *Am. J. Physiol. Lung Cell. Mol. Physiol.* 273, L468–L477. doi: 10.1152/ajplung.1997.273.2.L468

Ikegami, M., Carter, K., Bishop, K., Yadav, A., Masterjohn, E., Brondyk, W., et al. (2006). Intratracheal recombinant surfactant protein D prevents endotoxin shock in the newborn preterm lamb. *Am. J. Respir. Crit. Care Med.* 173, 1342–1347. doi: 10.1164/rccm.200509-1485OC

Ikegami, M., Scoville, E. A., Grant, S., Korfhagen, T., Brondyk, W., Scheule, R. K., et al. (2007). Surfactant protein-D and surfactant inhibit endotoxin-induced pulmonary inflammation. *Chest* 132, 1447–1454. doi: 10.1378/chest.07-0864

Ikegami, M., Whitsett, J. A., Jobe, A., Ross, G., Fisher, J., and Korfhagen, T. (2000). Surfactant metabolism in SP-D gene-targeted mice. *Am. J. Physiol. Lung Cell. Mol. Physiol.* 279, L468–L476. doi: 10.1152/ajplung.2000.279.3.L468

Johansson, J., and Curstedt, T. (2019). Synthetic surfactants with SP-B and SP-C analogues to enable worldwide treatment of neonatal respiratory distress syndrome and other lung diseases. *J. Intern. Med.* 285, 165–186. doi: 10.1111/joim.12845

Keating, E., Zuo, Y. Y., Tadayyon, S. M., Petersen, N. O., Possmayer, F., and Veldhuizen, R. A. (2012). A modified squeeze-out mechanism for generating high surface pressures with pulmonary surfactant. *Biochim. Biophys. Acta* 1818, 1225–1234. doi: 10.1016/j.bbamem.2011.12.007

Kesecioglu, J., Beale, R., Stewart, T. E., Findlay, G. P., Rouby, J.-J., Holzapfel, L., et al. (2009). Exogenous natural surfactant for treatment of acute lung injury and the acute respiratory distress syndrome. *Am. J. Respir. Crit. Care Med.* 180, 989–994. doi: 10.1164/rccm.200812-1955OC

Kingma, P. S., and Whitsett, J. A. (2006). In defense of the lung: surfactant protein A and surfactant protein D. *Curr. Opin. Pharmacol.* 6, 277–283. doi: 10.1016/j.coph.2006.02.003

Korfhagen, T. R., Sheftelyevich, V., Burhans, M. S., Bruno, M. D., Ross, G. F., Wert, S. E., et al. (1998). Surfactant protein-D regulates surfactant phospholipid homeostasis *in vivo*. *J. Biol. Chem.* 273, 28438–28443. doi: 10.1074/jbc.273.43.28438

Leth-Larsen, R., Zhong, F., Chow, V. T., Holmskov, U., and Lu, J. (2007). The SARS coronavirus spike glycoprotein is selectively recognized by lung surfactant protein D and activates macrophages. *Immunobiology* 212, 201–211. doi: 10.1016/j.imbio.2006.12.001

Liu, C. F., Chen, Y. L., Shieh, C. C., Yu, C. K., Reid, K., and Wang, J. Y. (2005). Therapeutic effect of surfactant protein D in allergic inflammation of mite-sensitized mice. *Clin. Exp. Allergy* 35, 515–521. doi: 10.1111/j.1365-2222.2005.02205.x

Madan, T., Kishore, U., Singh, M., Strong, P., Clark, H., Hussain, E. M., et al. (2001). Surfactant proteins A and D protect mice against pulmonary hypersensitivity induced by Aspergillus fumigatus antigens and allergens. *J. Clin. Invest.* 107, 467–475. doi: 10.1172/JCI10124

Maget-Dana, R., and Ptak, M. (1995). Interactions of surfactin with membrane models. *Biophys. J.* 68, 1937–1943. doi: 10.1016/S0006-3495(95)80370-X

Ogasawara, Y., Kuroki, Y., and Akino, T. (1992). Pulmonary surfactant protein D specifically binds to phosphatidylinositol. *J. Biol. Chem.* 267, 21244–21249.

Ordonez, S. R., Van Eijk, M., Salazar, N. E., De Cock, H., Veldhuizen, E. J., and Haagsman, H. P. (2019). Antifungal activities of surfactant protein D in an environment closely mimicking the lung lining. *Mol. Immunol.* 105, 260–269. doi: 10.1016/j.molimm.2018.12.003

Orgeig, S., Morrison, J. L., and Daniels, C. B. (2011). Evolution, development, and function of the pulmonary surfactant system in normal and perturbed environments. *Compr. Physiol.* 6, 363–422. doi: 10.1002/cphy.c150003

Parra, E., and Pérez-Gil, J. (2015). Composition, structure and mechanical properties define performance of pulmonary surfactant membranes and films. *Chem. Phys. Lipids* 185, 153–175. doi: 10.1016/j.chemphyslip.2014.09.002

Pastrana-Rios, B., Flach, C. R., Brauner, J. W., Mautone, A. J., and Mendelsohn, R. (1994). A direct test of the "Squeeze-Out" hypothesis of lung surfactant function. external reflection FT-IR at the air/wave interface. *Biochemistry* 33, 5121–5127. doi: 10.1021/bi00183a016

Pérez-Gil, J. (2008). Structure of pulmonary surfactant membranes and films: the role of proteins and lipid–protein interactions. *Biochim. Biophys. Acta* 1778, 1676–1695. doi: 10.1016/j.bbamem.2008.05.003

Perez-Gil, J., and Weaver, T. E. (2010). Pulmonary surfactant pathophysiology: current models and open questions. *Physiology* 25, 132–141. doi: 10.1152/physiol.00006.2010

Persson, A. V., Gibbons, B. J., Shoemaker, J. D., Moxley, M. A., and Longmore, W. J. (1992). The major glycolipid recognized by SP-D in surfactant is phosphatidylinositol. *Biochemistry* 31, 12183–12189. doi: 10.1021/bi00163a030

Sato, A., Whitsett, J. A., Scheule, R. K., and Ikegami, M. (2010). Surfactant protein-d inhibits lung inflammation caused by ventilation in premature newborn lambs. *Am. J. Respir. Crit. Care Med.* 181, 1098–1105. doi: 10.1164/rccm.200912-1818OC

Sorensen, G. L. (2018). Surfactant protein D in respiratory and non-respiratory diseases. *Front. Med.* 5:18. doi: 10.3389/fmed.2018.00018

Spragg, R. G., Lewis, J. F., Walmrath, H.-D., Johannigman, J., Bellingan, G., Laterre, P.-F., et al. (2004). Effect of recombinant surfactant protein C–based surfactant on the acute respiratory distress syndrome. *New Eng. J. Med.* 351, 884–892. doi: 10.1056/NEJMoa033181

Strong, P., Townsend, P., Mackay, R., Reid, K., and Clark, H. (2003). A recombinant fragment of human SP-D reduces allergic responses in mice sensitized to house dust mite allergens. *Clin. Exp. Immunol.* 134, 181–187. doi: 10.1046/j.1365-2249.2003.02281.x

Taeusch, H. W., De La Serna, J. B., Perez-Gil, J., Alonso, C., and Zasadzinski, J. A. (2005). Inactivation of pulmonary surfactant due to serum-inhibited adsorption and reversal by hydrophilic polymers: experimental. *Biophys. J.* 89, 1769–1779. doi: 10.1529/biophysj.105.062620

Taneva, S., Voelker, D. R., and Keough, K. M. (1997). Adsorption of pulmonary surfactant protein D to phospholipid monolayers at the air- water interface. *Biochemistry* 36, 8173–8179. doi: 10.1021/bi963040h

Van't Veen, A., Mouton, J. W., Gommers, D., and Lachmann, B. (1996). Pulmonary surfactant as vehicle for intratracheally instilled tobramycin in mice infected with Klebsiella pneumoniae. *Br. J. Pharmacol.* 119, 1145–1148. doi: 10.1111/j.1476-5381.1996.tb16016.x

Watson, A., Phipps, M. J., Clark, H. W., Skylaris, C.-K., and Madsen, J. (2019). Surfactant proteins A and D: trimerized innate immunity proteins with an affinity for viral fusion proteins. *J. Innate Immun.* 11, 13–28. doi: 10.1159/000492974

Yu, S.-H., and Possmayer, F. (2003). Lipid compositional analysis of pulmonary surfactant monolayers and monolayer-associated reservoirs. *J. Lipid Res.* 44, 621–629. doi: 10.1194/jlr.M200380-JLR200

Yuan, C., and Johnston, L. (2002). Phase evolution in cholesterol/DPPC monolayers: atomic force microscopy and near field scanning optical microscopy studies. *J. Microsc.* 205, 136–146. doi: 10.1046/j.0022-2720.2001.00982.x

5

A Custom-Made Device for Reproducibly Depositing Pre-Metered Doses of Nebulized Drugs on Pulmonary Cells *in vitro*

Justus C. Horstmann[1,2], Chelsea R. Thorn[3], Patrick Carius[1,2], Florian Graef[1†], Xabier Murgia[1†], Cristiane de Souza Carvalho-Wodarz[1*] and Claus-Michael Lehr[1,2]*

[1] Helmholtz Institute for Pharmaceutical Research Saarland (HIPS), Saarbrücken, Germany, [2] Department of Pharmacy, Saarland University, Saarbrücken, Germany, [3] Clinical and Health Science, University of South Australia, Adelaide, SA, Australia

***Correspondence:**
Xabier Murgia
xabi_murgia@hotmail.com
Cristiane de Souza Carvalho-Wodarz
cristiane.carvalho@helmholtz-hips.de

† Present address:
Florian Graef,
Bayer AG, Leverkusen, Germany
Xabier Murgia,
Gaiker Technology Centre, Bizkaia, Spain

The deposition of pre-metered doses (i.e., defined before and not after exposition) at the air–liquid interface of viable pulmonary epithelial cells remains an important but challenging task for developing aerosol medicines. While some devices allow quantification of the deposited dose after or during the experiment, e.g., gravimetrically, there is still no generally accepted way to deposit small pre-metered doses of aerosolized drugs or pharmaceutical formulations, e.g., nanomedicines. Here, we describe a straightforward custom-made device, allowing connection to commercially available nebulizers with standard cell culture plates. Designed to tightly fit into the approximately 12-mm opening of either a 12-well Transwell® insert or a single 24-well plate, a defined dose of an aerosolized liquid can be directly deposited precisely and reproducibly (4.8% deviation) at the air–liquid interface (ALI) of pulmonary cell cultures. The deposited dose can be controlled by the volume of the nebulized solution, which may vary in a range from 20 to 200 μl. The entire nebulization-deposition maneuver is completed after 30 s and is spatially homogenous. After phosphate-buffered saline (PBS) deposition, the viability and barrier properties transepithelial electrical resistance (TEER) of human bronchial epithelial Calu-3 cells were not negatively affected. Straightforward in manufacture and use, the device enables reproducible deposition of metered doses of aerosolized drugs to study the interactions with pulmonary cell cultures grown at ALI conditions.

Keywords: inhalation, aerosol, pulmonary drug delivery, epithelial cells, air–liquid interface

INTRODUCTION

The development of drugs against pulmonary diseases requires testing of both safety and efficacy. In this context there recently has been a growing interest in using *in vitro* cell culture models to replace, reduce, and refine animal experiments (Tannenbaum and Bennett, 2015; Ehrmann et al., 2020). Initially, such tests were and still are performed with submerged cell culture models (Pulskamp et al., 2007; Rothen-Rutishauser et al., 2007; Metz et al., 2020). However, as patients inhale drugs as an aerosol, air–liquid interface

(ALI) models are more physiologically relevant (Lacroix et al., 2018). It has been shown that testing of aerosolized excipients under ALI conditions is, in many ways, different from testing under liquid-covered conditions (LCCs) (Brandenberger et al., 2010; Paur et al., 2011; Upadhyay and Palmberg, 2018). For instance, drug transport rates across *in vitro* cell culture inserts depend on the donor compartment concentrations and are, therefore, dramatically increased when drugs are applied as dry particles without any additional liquid at the ALI (Bur et al., 2010). Vice versa, adverse effects could be shown at lower doses in ALI conditions compared with LCC, albeit only the nominal—not the cell-delivered dose—would be obtained for submerged culture conditions (Loret et al., 2016). On the contrary, there is also evidence that the culture conditions do not affect the dose-specific efficacy of certain drugs (e.g., bortezomib) in A549 lung epithelial cells (Lenz et al., 2014). Once inhaled *in vivo*, particles tend to land on a layer of mucus or thin lining fluid (e.g., pulmonary surfactant) that is only 1/10 of the particles' size (Bastacky et al., 1995). Modeling physiological situations when developing models and protocols for meaningful *in vitro* tests is, therefore, pivotal (Bastacky et al., 1995; Hiemstra et al., 2018).

To date, several laboratory methods have already been described to deposit aerosolized drugs on epithelial cells, such as modified impactors or impingers (Cooney et al., 2004; Bur et al., 2009), using electrostatic attraction forces (Jeannet et al., 2016; Frijns et al., 2017) or insufflator devices developed initially for animals (Blank et al., 2006; Bur et al., 2010). Vibrating mesh nebulizers (i.e., Omron NE-U22) have been used to deposit pH-sensitive archeosomes onto macrophages covered with pulmonary surfactant in classic 24-well plates (Altube et al., 2017). While depositing a fine mist onto cell cultures seems trivial, ALI conditions are hardly used, adding complexity to the application. There has also been considerable interest in the pharmaceutical application of dry powders. To study the deposition of metered aerosols from commercially available dry powder inhaler (DPI) devices, systems such as the Pharmaceutical Aerosol Deposition Device on Cell Cultures (PADDOCC) (Hein et al., 2010, 2011) or the Vitrocell® Dry Powder Chamber (Hittinger et al., 2017) have been developed. Other commercially available devices, including the Cultex Devices (Cultex® Technology, 2020), the PreciseInhale®, and XposeALI® (Inhalation Sciences, 2020), and the PRIT® System (Fraunhofer P.R.I.T® Systems, 2020), have emerged; and more details are described in recent review articles (Schneider-Daum et al., 2019; Ehrmann et al., 2020). However, the Vitrocell® Cloud systems—originally called Air-liquid Interface Cell Exposure-Cloud (ALICE-Cloud) (Lenz et al., 2014), have become quite popular, as seen in the number of recent publications in both the field of (nano-)particle toxicity (Chortarea et al., 2017; He et al., 2020) and preclinical drug testing (Röhm et al., 2017; D'Angelo et al., 2018). The available standard device consists of a polycarbonate chamber connected to a vibrating mesh nebulizer (Aeroneb® Lab nebulizer unit), generating a cloud of liquid aerosol settling down on multiple Transwell® inserts at the same time. These wells sit in a base module that controls the temperature of the cell medium, and the cell-delivered dose can be determined with a quartz crystal microbalance (Lenz et al., 2009, 2014). Only recently, the Vitrocell® Cloud MAX has been introduced (Vitrocell® Cloud Systems, 2020), which was designed for metered-dose delivery to one Transwell® insert at a time (Cei et al., 2020).

Nevertheless, experimental setups enabling the controlled deposition of predetermined aerosol doses onto one Transwell® insert at a time for exposure of pulmonary epithelial cells under ALI conditions are seldomly available. To close this gap, we here present an easy-to-make and easy-to-use device, consisting of a machined polyoxymethylene (POM) cylinder, which directs a single aerosol dose generated by a vibrating mesh nebulizer (Aeroneb® Lab nebulizer unit) to the bottom of individual wells or inserts of standard multi-well plates. The data presented here demonstrate its suitability to reproducibly deposit pre-metered doses by nebulizing between 20 and 200 µl of an aqueous drug solution and a nanoparticle pharmaceutical drug formulation. Apart from cleaning the device after use, no further maintenance is needed, making it easy to handle under sterile conditions. A proof-of-concept experiment with Transwell® insert-grown Calu-3 cells revealed no signs of cytotoxicity, and the epithelial barrier function as measured by the transepithelial electrical resistance (TEER) was the same as for untreated cells. The system has already been successfully employed earlier by our group for other tasks (Graef et al., 2018) but was so far not further described in detail concerning its construction or application to deposit single doses of drugs on cells.

MATERIALS AND METHODS

Manufacturing of the Chamber and Setup of the System

The deposition device is made of POM and was produced at the workshop of Saarland University (Saarbrücken, Germany). With a standard (computerized numerical control)-milling machine, the cylinder is made from a rod following the dimensions shown in **Figure 1A**. The cylindrical device has a wider opening to fit on the nebulizer and a smaller opening to fit in a 12-well Transwell® insert, Cat. No. 3460, with a pore size of 0.4 µm (Corning™ Costar™, Lowell, MA, United States, **Figure 1B**). An Aeroneb® Lab nebulizer unit (standard VMAD, 4.0–6.0 µm droplet diameter) plugged into the deposition device was used and is connected to an Aerogen® USB controller (both Aerogen®, Galway, Ireland). The device's wider opening contains a rim to fit the nebulizer, which stops at the edge of the rim after an 8-mm distance from the entrance (**Figure 1A**). The rim contains a circular cavity to fit a rubber ring to connect the device in the nebulizing process and prevent aerosol loss. The cylinder itself tapers conically to the opening leading outside to the smaller protruding outlet. This part at the bottom opening is designed precisely to fit the dimensions of a 12-well Transwell® insert (**Figure 1B**). It does not touch the Transwell® membrane or the well's walls and leads the aerosol exactly on the apical side of the membrane and not to the basolateral side. Alternatively, the system can also be placed on 24-well plates instead of Transwell® inserts.

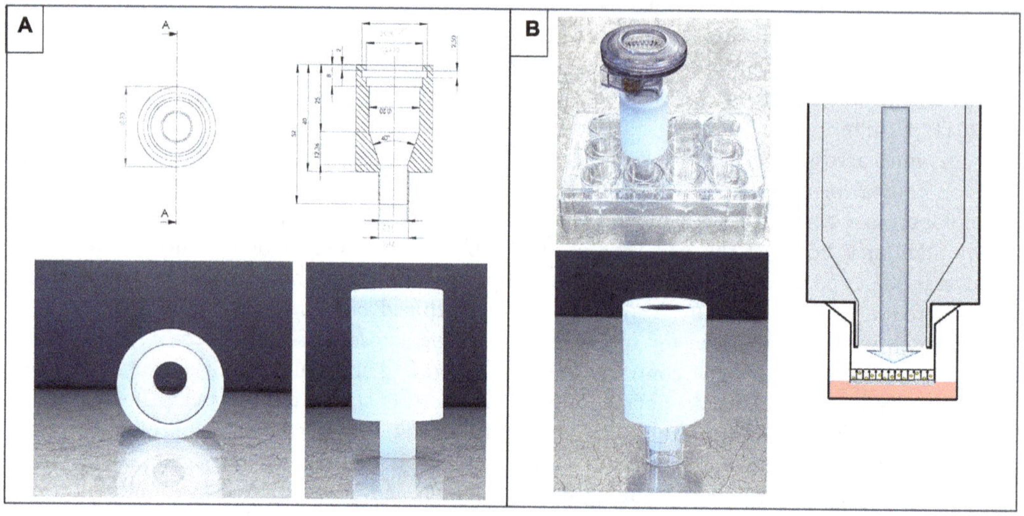

FIGURE 1 | Design and dimensions of the deposition system. **(A)** Technical drawing and images of the device alone. **(B)** Nebulizer connected to deposition device on top of Transwell® inserts ready for nebulization on cells (top image) and details of placement in an insert (bottom). On the right side, schematic view of the process of nebulization in a Transwell® insert.

Aerosol Generation and Deposition Protocol

In aerosol deposition studies, sodium fluorescein salt (Sigma-Aldrich) was used at various concentrations (as indicated, 2.5, 25, 100, or 250 μg/ml) diluted in phosphate-buffered saline (PBS; without calcium and magnesium, Sigma-Aldrich, D8537) or loaded into lipid liquid crystalline nanoparticles (LCNPs) as a model pharmaceutical formulation described below. To deposit aerosols, the system is assembled as described. To initialize the nebulization process, 100 μl of PBS was aerosolized three times in the whole system (nebulizer + device). The system is then placed on the respective wells. A volume of 20–200 μl from the desired liquid (or particle suspension) is added to the nebulizer mesh. Once the nebulization process is finished (shown by a small puff of a cloud above the mesh), the nebulizer is kept over the well for another 30 s (or as indicated) to allow the cloud to settle. The nebulizer and the device are separated again, and the remaining solution drops are removed from the downstream side of the mesh membrane by gently wiping with a (sterile) tissue. After the experiments were finished, the nebulizer and device are cleaned with (sterile) deionized water.

To contrast the solution, lipid nanoparticles (LCNPs) loaded with sodium fluorescein (3.5 mg/ml) or tobramycin (5 mg/ml, free base, Sigma-Aldrich) were formed with monoolein (MO; Myverol 18-99K; part number: 5D01253, Kerry Ingredients, and Flavors), as previously described (Thorn et al., 2020). The sodium fluorescein-LCNPs (250 μg/ml) were aerosolized onto Transwell® inserts at volumes of 20–200 μl, to compare with the sodium fluorescein solution. These studies were obtained in another lab as the studies done with free sodium fluorescein to compare the reproducibility of the method. For tobramycin, the aerosolization of a solution was compared with the tobramycin-LCNPs with 200 μl of varying concentrations (0.1, 0.2, 1, and 2 mg/ml) into 24-well plates.

Drug Deposition Studies in 24-Well Plates

Nebulization with sodium fluorescein (as a surrogate drug) was done as described above. First, parameters affecting drug deposition were changed in order to characterize the system. Two hundred microliters of PBS was filled into 24-well plates, and sodium fluorescein was deposited. Different invested volumes were tested under constant concentration and settling time (20, 50, 100, and 200 μl; 100 μg/ml, 30 s). Different concentrations were tested under constant volume and settling time (2.5, 25, and 250 μg/ml; 20 and 200 μl, 30 s); and different settling times were analyzed under constant volume and concentration (0, 30, and 60 s; 20 μl, 100 μg/ml, and 200 μl with 25 μg/ml). Multiple dosing of the drug was analyzed by nebulizing either 200 μl of 25 μg/ml or 20 μl of 100 μg/ml with 30-s settling time. The deposition was done two and three times in one well.

Analysis of the Deposited Amounts and Total Recovery of Aerosolized Material

The deposition system was set up as described and placed on Transwell® inserts. Two hundred microliters of PBS was filled on the apical and basolateral sides of the Transwell® inserts to analyze the deposited substance. Basolateral liquid did not touch the bottom side of the Transwell® membrane to prevent free diffusion. Sodium fluorescein or LCNPs in PBS were deposited as described (with 30-s settling time). Afterward, the nebulizer and the device were separated carefully and placed on Petri dishes. Each part was rinsed with 3 ml of PBS in the Petri dishes. One hundred microliters of the apical and basolateral sides and from either the nebulizer or device rinse fluid was withdrawn to analyze deposited mass. The drug deposition efficiency percentage was calculated by the mass of substance in the acceptor well divided by the mass invested in nebulizer times 100.

The fluorescence intensity of sodium fluorescein determined the aerosol-deposited dose measured in 96-well plates at 485-nm excitation and 550-nm emission wavelength with a plate reader (Tecan Trading AG, Infinite M200 Pro). Sodium fluorescein-LCNPs were detected via solubilizing the LCNPs with 0.05% Triton-X and quantifying sodium fluorescein via fluorescent spectroscopy plate reader (Inspire Multimode Plate reader, Perkin Elmer). Similarly, tobramycin was quantified after solubilizing the LCNPs in 0.05% Triton-X in 0.9% sodium chloride and filtration with 4-mm Millex® syringe filters. Liquid chromatography–tandem mass spectrometry (LC-MS) with a Dionex UltiMate 3000 Binary Rapid Separation LC System (Thermo Scientific) coupled with a TSQ Quantum Access Max (QQQ, Thermo Scientific) and a modified ion-pairing method was used for quantification. Trifluoroacetic acid (0.1%), heptafluorobutyric acid (0.1%), and pentafluoropropionic acid (0.1%) were added to eluent A (acetonitrile) and eluent B (water), as a mobile phase. A Zorbax Eclipse xdb C-18 column (5 μm, 50 * 4.6 mm, Agilent, Santa Clara, CA, United States) with C18 guard column was used as the analytical column. At a flow of 0.7 ml/min, samples were run with a gradient of eluents A and B, beginning at 20:80 (first minute), changing to 70:30 (1–3.5 min), and restored to 20:80 (3.5–4.5 min). Three microliters of the samples was injected and quantified by positive electrospray ionization (ESI+) and selected reaction monitoring (SRM) of the ion 468.184 → 323.960. A total of nine replicates were analyzed per concentration.

Viability Testing and Transepithelial Electrical Resistance Measurement After Aerosol Deposition on Calu-3 Cells

The Calu-3 HTB-55 cell line was received from American Type Culture Collection (ATCC®) and cultivated in minimum essential medium supplemented with Earle's salts, L-glutamine, 1% non-essential amino acids (NEAAs), 1 mM of sodium pyruvate, and 10% fetal calf serum (FCS) (all Gibco™, Thermo Fisher Scientific Inc. Waltham, MA, United States). The medium was changed every 2–3 days while using passages between 35 and 55. For experiments, cells were detached using trypsin/EDTA, and 1×10^5 cells were seeded per Transwell® insert. After 3 days, cells were switched to ALI conditions and grown for a total of 11–13 days until being used in the experiments.

Before PBS is aerosolized, the basolateral medium was changed. The controls included wells not exposed to nebulization and inserts with 1% Triton-X 100 (Sigma-Aldrich) in the basolateral medium (control consisting of dead cells). The deposition on cells was done under sterile conditions. Transwell® inserts in a 12-well plate were placed on a heating plate at 37°C. Then, one insert was transferred into a new, empty, 12-well plate with a sterile tweezer, and the aerosolization-deposition maneuver of PBS was performed, as previously described. Permeable supports were placed back to the original well plate filled with 500 μl of medium on the basolateral side. Inserts were incubated at 37°C and 5% CO_2 for 24 h. Lactate dehydrogenase (LDH) release was assessed with a kit based on color reaction (Roche, Cytotoxicity Detection Kit) from the basolateral medium according to the manufacturer's advice. The color change was detected with a spectrophotometer (ThermoFisher™, Multiskan™ GO) and calculated in % viability of the respective controls. To measure TEER, cells were incubated for another hour at submerged conditions (500/1,500 μl) with the medium. Then, TEER was assessed via electrical Volt-Ohm-meter (EVOM2, World Precision Instruments) with STX2 chopstick electrodes. Values were corrected to the Transwell® insert (1.12 cm^2) area and the respective value of a blank insert (between 90 and 120 $\Omega \cdot cm^2$). After that, cells were put back to ALI conditions by replacing the medium with 500 μl of fresh medium on the basolateral side and stored in an incubator.

Nanoparticle Aerosol Deposition Evaluation With the Spatial Distribution

The deposition in the Transwell® inserts was also assessed for spatial distribution using the described method with sodium fluorescein-LCNPs. To ensure no intentional manipulation, directly after sodium fluorescein-LCNP deposition, the membranes were left to equilibrate at room temperature for 1 h. The bottom of the Transwell® insert was then attached to coverslips (#1.5) with Dako Mounting medium (Agilent Technologies). An inverted fluorescent microscope (Olympus IX53) connected to CoolLed pE-300 illuminator system was used with a 2 × objective to visualize the deposition of sodium fluorescein-LCNPs on the membranes, from the bottom side up. Sodium fluorescein was illuminated with the blue-green LED filter and adjusted according to an untreated Transwell® membrane. Three replicates at each volume tested were imaged. ImageJ extracted the fluorescent intensities per pixel across the midline of the membrane's diameter. For each membrane, four lines were systematically drawn horizontally, vertically, and diagonally in each direction, splitting the membranes into eight parts to obtain an average fluorescent intensity profile. The pixel distances were equated to a numerical distance of the membrane. The pixels' intensities were converted to a heat map, where the highest intensities were represented by a red color and the lowest intensities by blue. For quantitative analysis, the average fluorescent intensities were correlated to the mean intensity. The intensities were normalized for each volume invested with the highest value in each data equated to an arbitrary value of one and the lowest to zero and plotted against the membrane's diameter.

Statistical Analysis

Differences were tested for statistical significance by one-way ANOVA, followed by Tukey's multiple comparisons test for all solution deposition analyses. The statistical comparison between solution-LCNP formulation and Transwell®-well plate inserts were performed by a two-way ANOVA, followed by a Sidak's multiple comparisons test. $P < 0.05$ were considered statistically significant as described in the respective figure legends. Error bars indicate standard deviation (SD). All statistical tests were performed with GraphPad Prism® 8.

RESULTS

Effects of Concentration, Settling Time, and Repeated Deposition

The entire setup consisted of (1) a commercially available nebulizer (e.g., Aeroneb® Lab nebulizer and Aerogen® USB controller) plugged on the (2) custom-made deposition device (as described in the section "Materials and Methods"), which is then (3) placed on either the well of a standard 24-well plate or a 12-well Transwell® insert. The deposition system itself (**Figure 1A**) is designed not to touch the bottom of the well/Transwell® insert and forms a closed chamber together with the well/Transwell® insert, leaving 5.5-mm distance to the insert or 5.7 mm to the well plate bottom (**Figure 1B**).

To explore the reproducibility and identify critical factors for aerosol deposition with this device, we investigated the effect of different concentrations, settling times, and multiple depositions (**Figure 2**). Apart from those factors, the invested volume is the most critical factor, as the generated aerosol deposits directly in a single well. Preliminary trials revealed that invested volumes lower than 20 μl show very high SDs, discouraging the application of smaller volumes (data not shown). This is probably related to the characteristics of the nebulizer's vibrating mesh, which also propels substance to the apical side of the vibrating mesh. Beginning with 20 μl, the SD of the measured dose for repeated experiments was acceptable in our experiments (22%). At the higher end, 200 μl turned out to be the largest volume to be reproducibly deposited (4.8% SD), since higher volumes lead to condensing drops on the inside wall of the device that dropped out on the well. Notably, these volumes are much smaller than in clinical settings, where volumes of up to 5 ml are used with similar nebulizers (Dolovich and Dhand, 2011; Aerogen® , 2020). On account of this, both 20 and 200 μl of invested volumes were further analyzed. A 10-fold change in invested substance concentration did not lead to higher deposition efficiencies at either 20 or 200 μl ($p \leq 0.6$, **Figures 2A,B**, respectively).

Regardless of the nebulized volume, longer settling times (time after complete nebulization of invested liquid) had a positive influence on the deposition efficiency, in line with the observation that the generated aerosol cloud is still settling after the end of the nebulization itself. When nebulizing 200 μl, a 30-s settling time was found to be necessary, but further increasing it to 60 s did not significantly improve deposition efficiency (**Figures 2A,B**). In the case of 20 μl, which takes only about 3 s for nebulization, the benefit of a 30-s waiting time became still more prominent and was therefore adopted as routine for the protocol.

To show that a distinct dose is precisely deposited and can even be enlarged linearly by its increment, multiple repeated depositions were performed for both small and high volumes (**Figure 2**). After each respective nebulization step, the nebulized dose was added up and reproducibly deposited multiple times to achieve the desired dose. Even so, R^2-values show a more precise deposition with 200 μl of volume than with 20 μl (0.9420 vs. 0.8482).

The Deposited Mass Linearly Depends on the Invested Volume

After identifying the range of possible volumes between 20 and 200 μl and the necessary settling time of 30 s, we asked if the volume of the nebulized solution could control the deposited amount of a dissolved compound. Hence, the system was tested with increasing volumes of sodium fluorescein (100 μg/ml)

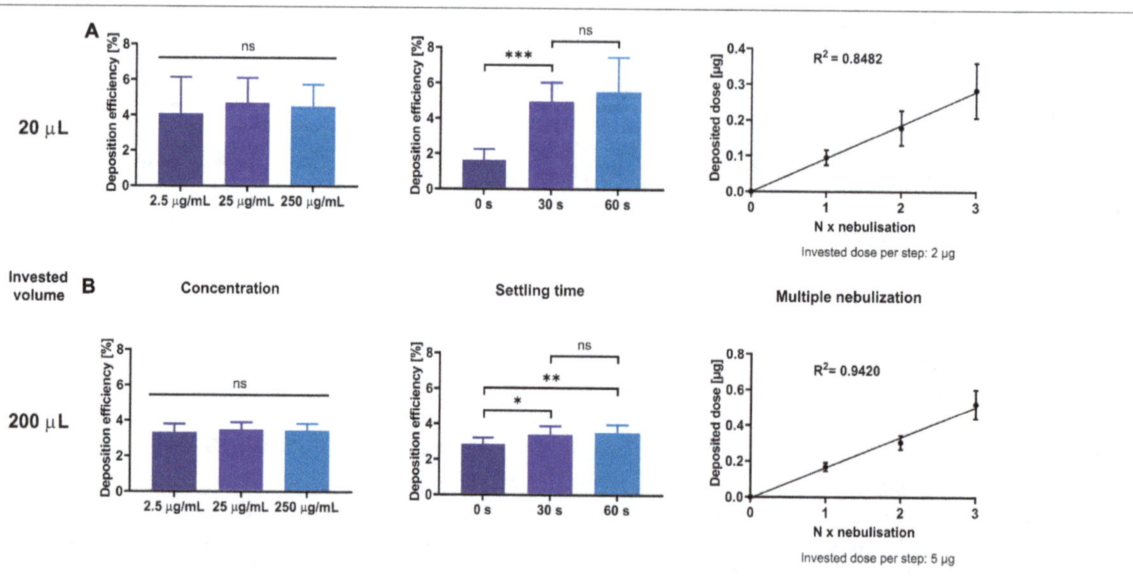

FIGURE 2 | Deposition characteristics at different concentrations, settling time, and multiple nebulization steps. Sodium fluorescein solution is deposited as described in the section "Materials and Methods." Either 20 μl **(A)** or 200 μl **(B)** was used for nebulization. From left to right, 10-fold increasing concentrations were nebulized, the efficiency of different settling times after the end of nebulization processes was assessed, and respective doses nebulized one or more times into one well at 30-s settling time were analyzed, as indicated. Error bars show standard deviation. One-way ANOVA, Tukey's multiple comparisons test, ns $p > 0.12$; *$p < 0.033$; **$p < 0.002$; ***$p < 0.001$. $N = 9$ of three experiments.

to confirm this hypothesis. Six repetitions were performed and analyzed in triplicate for each volume tested, yielding 18 observations for each data point. As shown in **Figure 3A**, the deposited dose increased linearly and thus can be controlled by the invested volume (R^2: 0.9706). Not surprisingly, calculating and plotting the deposition efficiency of the same dataset show that the smaller the invested volume, the higher the SD (1.44 for 20 μl and 0.18 for 200 μl) (**Figure 3B**). Nevertheless, the system allows to deposit a finite pre-metered dose with reasonable reproducibility, and the invested volume may control this dose.

Mass Balance Reveals the Distribution of the Deposited Substance in the System

Consistently, about 4% of the nebulized dose was deposited in the well. Therefore, the question arises where the rest of the nebulized substance goes. Besides the mass deposited on the apical side of a Transwell® insert, we also quantified the amounts deposited in the device itself and remaining in the nebulizer after loading it with 20, 100, and 200 μl of a 25 μg/ml sodium fluorescein solution (**Table 1**). With increasing volume, the relative amount of deposited mass in the device increased from 46 to 63%, as did the relative amount remaining in the nebulizer (from 21 to 27%). The respective amounts of mass deposited on the inserts remained around 4%. As calculated by the sum of the amounts collected in all three compartments (=total recovery), the total recovery was 80% after nebulization with 20 μl but increased to 93 and 94% after nebulization of 100 and 200 μl, respectively. After deposition on the apical side of the Transwell® insert, no substance was found on the basolateral side, confirming that the tapered cylinder structure restricts the deposition to the apical side (data not shown). As described, this is tested in Transwell® inserts with a pore size of 0.4 μm and without contact to basolateral medium to avoid free diffusion.

Analysis of Reproducibility of Deposition Between Free Drug and Particles and Well Plates

The deposition of sodium fluorescein as an aerosolized solution or in a pharmaceutical formulation (i.e., LCNPs) was compared

TABLE 1 | Total recovery of substance in the system after nebulization and deposition on the apical side of permeable supports.

	20 μl	100 μl	200 μl
Nebulizer	20.5 ± 12.2	34.2 ± 2.83	27.2 ± 3.64
Device	45.8 ± 9.37	55.4 ± 3.32	63.0 ± 8.77
Transwell	5.52 ± 0.84	3.31 ± 0.54	3.43 ± 0.23
Total recovery	79.7 ± 9.02	92.9 ± 2.02	93.5 ± 8.51

20, 100, and 200 μl of sodium fluorescein solution are nebulized at 25 μg/ml as described in the section "Materials and Methods." The relative abundance of deposited substance in each part of the system is displayed for each nebulized volume. "Total recovery" is the sum of the relative abundance of each invested volume. Error represents standard deviation. N = 9 of three experiments; 100 μl, N = 6 of three experiments.

to evaluate the robustness of using the device for other applications in a wider pharmaceutical field. Deposition of sodium fluorescein was performed in another lab than the deposition of sodium fluorescein formulation (Lab 1: Helmholtz Institute for Pharmaceutical Research Saarland; Lab 2: University of South Australia). When investing 20, 100, or 200 μl, sodium fluorescein's deposition efficiency as a free solution or in LCNPs was comparable (**Figure 4A**). While only the 20 μl of free sodium fluorescein showed a slight, statistically significant increase, all other groups showed a deposition efficiency that was well comparable. The same trend was observed by comparing the deposition of free sodium fluorescein into a 24-well plate and Transwell® inserts, which was essentially the same, except for the 20 μl deposition into Transwell® (**Figure 4B**). The variation in the accuracy of pipetted micro-volumes increases toward lower volumes, which may further explain the variation observed at 20 μl of invested volume. Compared with a different compound (i.e., tobramycin), the deposition efficiency remained consistent at ~4% ($p > 0.05$, **Figure 5**) across 0.1–2 mg/ml invested concentrations at 200 μl of invested volume, in both conditions of a solution and LCNPs. This is the same as sodium fluorescein deposition efficiency, proving the usability of this surrogate substance. Generally, the deposition of different formulations and drugs on different well plates demonstrates the high versatility of using this device.

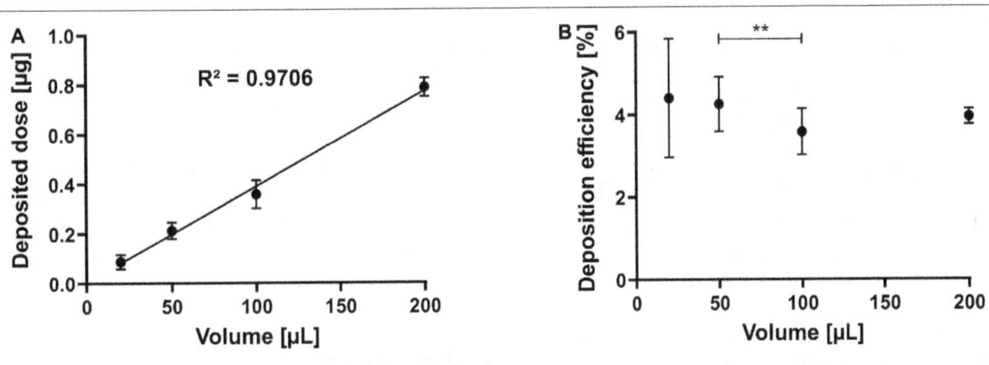

FIGURE 3 | Linearity by dose and efficiency. Sodium fluorescein solution is nebulized as described in the section "Materials and Methods." **(A)** Deposited dose of a 100 μg/ml solution at different invested volumes. **(B)** Deposition efficiency at different invested volumes. Error bars indicate standard deviation. *N* = 18 of six experiments (for 20 and 200 μl) and *N* = 21 of seven experiments (for 50 and 100 μl). One-way ANOVA, Tukey's multiple comparisons test; $^{**}p = 0.002$.

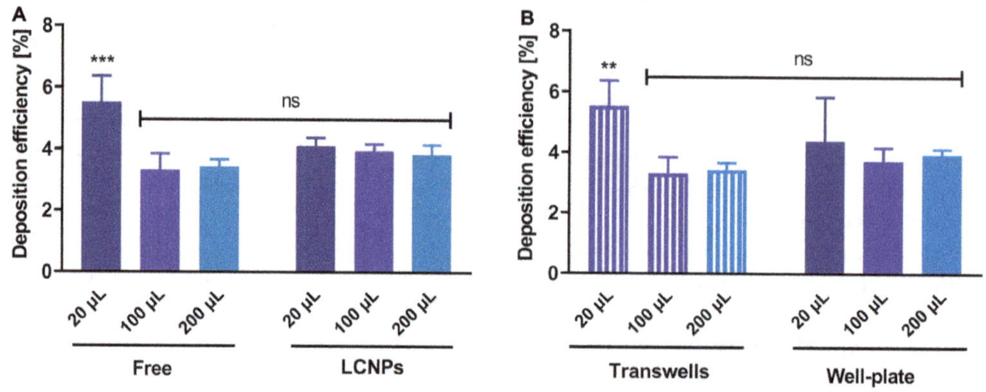

FIGURE 4 | Comparison of deposition efficiency of different volumes, substances, and wells. **(A)** Deposition efficiencies of free sodium fluorescein and LCNPs loaded with sodium fluorescein. Substance deposited on the apical side of permeable supports was analyzed (the section "Materials and Methods"), $N = 9$ of two experiments (for 20 µl of free and LCNP, 100 and 200 µl of LCNP); $N = 6$ of two experiments (for 100 µl of free); $N = 8$ of three experiments (for 200 µl of free). **(B)** Comparison of deposition efficiency on 24-well plates and Transwell® inserts. Sodium fluorescein was nebulized using the device as described. Either the device deposited on Transwell® inserts or 24-well plate inserts. Data show mean and standard deviation. $N = 9$ of three experiments; 100 µl, $N = 6$ of two experiments. Two-way ANOVA, Sidak's multiple comparisons test; $^{***}p < 0.001$; $^{**}p < 0.003$; ns, no significant difference ($p > 0.05$).

Homogeneity of Deposition

Control over the amount of aerosol deposited is essential, so too is the aerosol evenly spread over the surface. The sodium fluorescein-LCNPs were aerosolized onto Transwell® insert membranes (area of 1.12 cm^2) at 20–200 µl to determine the deposition's homogeneity. Extraction of the fluorescent intensities of sodium fluorescein across each pixel of the membrane's diameter provided a quantitative analysis that was normalized for comparison (as indicated). The sub-200-nm particles are evenly spread across the Transwell® membranes, as quantified by the trend in the normalized intensity data in **Figures 6A–D**. The heat maps of each individual membrane depict the whole spatial deposition and dictate greater heat spots toward the center of the membranes that spread toward the edges.

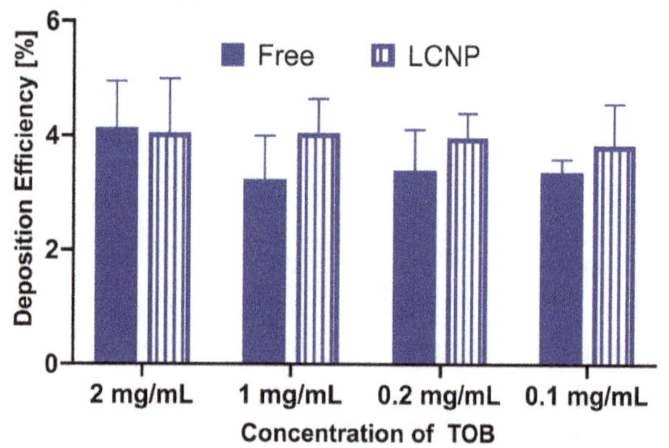

FIGURE 5 | Comparison of deposition efficiency of free and LCNP encapsulated tobramycin (TOB), either as a free solution or in LCNPs after nebulizing 200 µl with Aerogen® Pro nebulizer and nebulization chamber into 24-well plates. Data represented as mean ± standard deviation, $N = 9$ (of three experiments). Two-way ANOVA, Sidak's multiple comparisons test. No significant difference ($p > 0.05$) was found between the groups.

The visual representation suggests an increase in the spread of the particles across the membrane from 20 up to 200 µl, which does not correlate to a difference in spatial homogeneity from the (normalized) quantified data. While the smaller invested volumes have overall lower proportions of red areas, this may reflect the lower dose deposited compared with the higher volumes. There was no statistical difference ($p = 0.945$) between the normalized mean across the diameter, indicating similarities in the homogenous spatial distribution from all four doses. The mean deposition across the diameter was consistent across all volumes invested, normalized to 1.04, 1.02, 1.08, and 1.07 AU for 20, 50, 100, and 200 µl, respectively, indicative of a consistent maximum dose of the compound that was spread homogenously across the membrane. On average, the SD between samples was 7, 12, 10, and 9%, respectively, for 20–200 µl of investment. Even though 10 × more mass is invested, the SD did not severely change and further highlighted the device's robustness depositing spatially even pre-metered doses.

Deposition on Epithelial Cells Is Well Tolerated

To demonstrate that the nebulization-deposition maneuver itself with the new device is not noxious to pulmonary epithelial cells, either 20 or 200 µl of PBS was nebulized on the widely used human bronchial epithelial cell line Calu-3, which forms tight monolayers at ALI conditions (Foster et al., 2000; Schneider-Daum et al., 2019). The cells did not show any loss of viability as measured by LDH release (**Figure 7A**). The TEER as an indicator for the epithelial barrier function remained unchanged as well (**Figure 7B**).

DISCUSSION

Here, we describe a new, custom-designed device intended for aerosol deposition into single Transwell® inserts for drug delivery

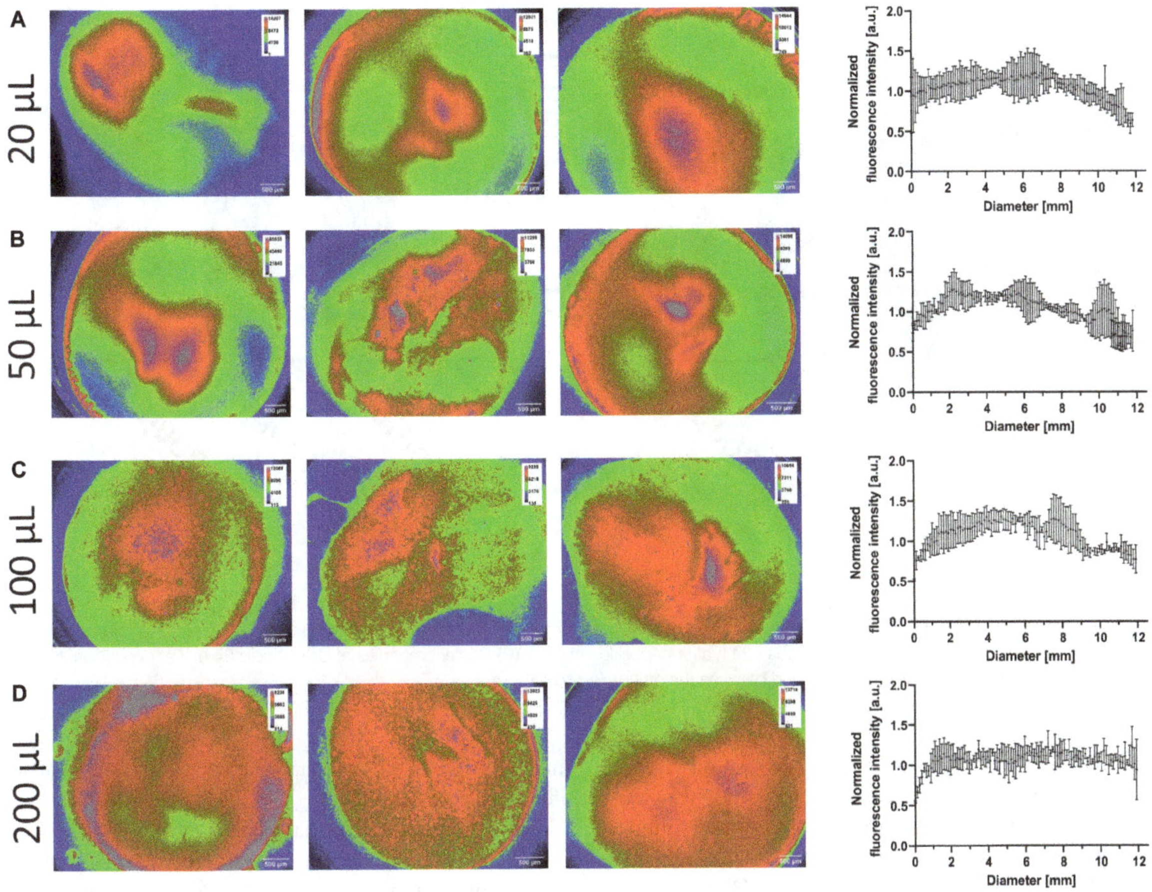

FIGURE 6 | Homogeneity of deposition. Sodium fluorescein-liquid crystalline nanoparticles (LCNPs) were nebulized onto Transwell® insert membranes as described in the section "Materials and Methods." **(A–D)** Representative fluorescent micrographs of the membranes (from the bottom up), where the highest fluorescence intensities are color-coded as red and the lowest as blue. The fluorescence intensities per pixel were extracted across the center of the membrane. The individual intensities (correlated to the mean intensity) were normalized to arbitrary 1 and plotted against the diameter of the membrane. *N* = 3, data are reported as mean with standard deviation, where every 25th data point is shown for clarity. a.u, Arbitrary units.

applications of *in vitro* cell culture models. It consists of a tapered cylinder design, which is very compact and connects to commonly used nebulizers (**Figure 1**). The Aeroneb® Lab nebulizer produces an aerosol cloud into the device that enables a precise and reproducible deposition of a pre-metered dose into the respective well (**Figure 1B**). The device can be used for single experiments nebulizing one dose on one or more inserts, or the device can be employed to deposit more than one dose on one insert. Due to its low price, many devices can be used without the necessity to clean them during time-critical experiments, as there are examples in the literature comparing many substances instead of using only single agents (Meindl et al., 2015; Röhm et al., 2017; Barosova et al., 2020).

There are two commercially available devices from Vitrocell® Systems that also allow for single insert exposure using an Aeroneb® Lab nebulizer and a cloud-settling principle for dose-controlled aerosol delivery, as comparable with the one presented here. These include 1) the Vitrocell® Cloud MAX and (2) the so-called "Starter Kit." However, both systems differ significantly from the device described here, as they offer extensive technical features such as an integrated microbalance to determine the post-metered dose and are significantly more costly. The "Starter Kit" design is comparable with the Cloud Systems with a rectangular aerosol-cell exposure system (Lenz et al., 2014). Rather than exposing an entire well plate with several Transwell® inserts at a time, the chamber is smaller (ca. 1 L) to expose a single Transwell® insert (Di Cristo et al., 2020; Vitrocell® Cloud Systems, 2020). The former, the Vitrocell® Cloud MAX, had been introduced a few months ago, and its performance has been described for a prototype version in the literature (Cei et al., 2020). Its exposure chamber has a compact cylindrical design with roughly comparable dimensions to the device reported here (40–60 mm height, diameter ca. 20 mm) tailored toward providing just enough space for one 6-well Transwell® insert (or a smaller-sized insert), with a settling time of ca. 1 min. The bottom part of the cylindrical chamber is not tapered to a diameter of 12 mm (12-well Transwell® insert), and the Transwell® insert has to be put into a base module for exposure. The Vitrocell® Cloud MAX system comes with three or six exposure units arranged in parallel.

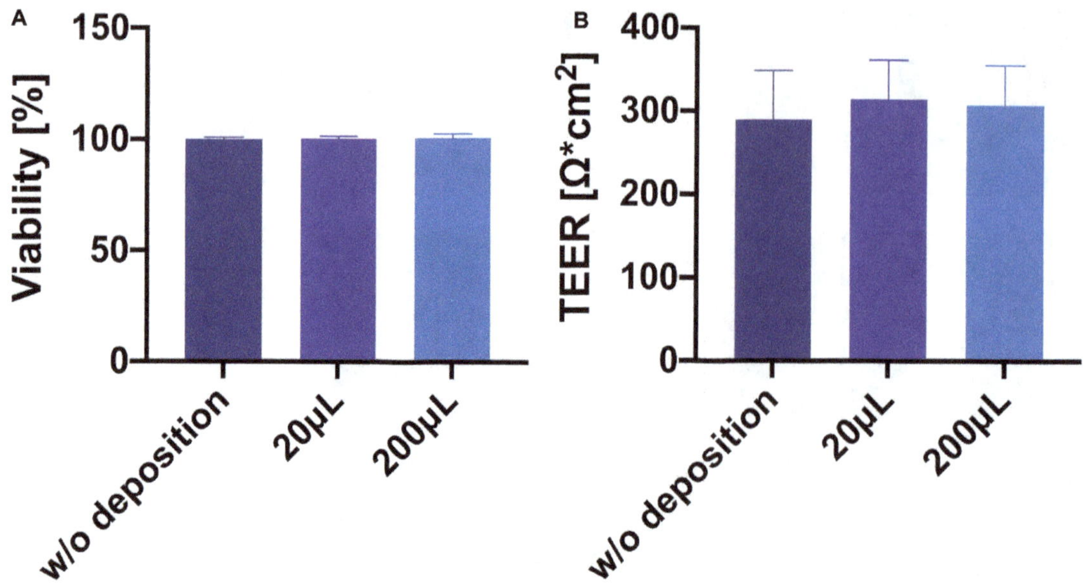

FIGURE 7 | Deposition of phosphate-buffered saline (PBS) on Calu-3 cells grown in Transwell® inserts is well tolerated. **(A)** Viability of Calu-3 cells [Lactate dehydrogenase (LDH), see section "Materials and Methods"] 24 h after deposition of PBS. **(B)** Barrier properties of Calu-3 cells 24 h after deposition. $N = 9$ of three individual experiments. No significant difference was found between the groups ($p > 0.05$).

Despite some commonalities with existing deposition systems, the crucial advantage of the cost-effective and straightforward custom-made device presented here is the precise ability to control and predetermine the exact deposited dose achieved, as would be done in the clinic (Dolovich and Dhand, 2011). The deposited dose increases linearly with the invested volume (**Figure 3A**), where micro-sized volumes can be efficiently deposited and do not differ between drugs or pharmaceutical formulations. The system also allows for consecutive dosing to the cells for any invested volume (**Figures 2A,B**). Thus, the simple design and the low-cost production of the present device allow for reproducible drug deposition as an aerosol *in vitro*.

While a deposition efficiency of about 4% may appear relatively low, it is sufficient for performing meaningful *in vitro* studies, where the amount of compound needed is much smaller than for *in vivo* studies. By increasing the settling time, higher deposition efficiencies can be achieved (**Figure 2**). Still, we recommend using only 30 s, as the deposition efficiency is not significantly higher ($p = 0.60$). It is more important that the absolute dose is well controlled, as widely observed with our device. In comparable studies with the Vitrocell® Cloud MAX system prototype version, a drug delivery efficiency of 52% was reported, albeit for a six-well Transwell® insert (Cei et al., 2020). By extrapolating these data to smaller inserts/wells, it may be expected that for 12-well Transwell® inserts, the delivery efficiency is about 4.5-fold lower (ca. 12% delivery efficiency), since the surface area of a 12-well Transwell® insert is about 4.5 times less than a six-well Transwell® insert. By using a similar nebulizer and the ALICE/Vitrocell® Cloud system, a deposition efficacy of about 17% was reported (Lenz et al., 2014), but this refers to the simultaneous deposition of an entire six-well plate and needs to be divided by the respective number of wells, which equates to an approximate 3% deposition efficiency per well.

Moreover, Di Cristo et al. (2020) have also recently used the newer Vitrocell® Starter Kit, investing 125 µl of a 1 mg/ml particle suspension. From these data, one can calculate a deposition efficiency per well (1.12 cm^2) by dividing the deposited amount by the invested amount, yielding an efficiency of 0.64% per well (1.12 cm^2). This value, which is lower than what we report in the present study, is likely attributable to the larger space that the cloud is nebulized in and the larger surface area for deposition, which is the space around the insert and the walls of the device.

None of the previous studies further investigated the fraction of the lost aerosol during the nebulization process. In this study, it was hypothesized that most of the aerosol lands in the cylinder device. Indeed, with elevating the nebulized dose, more than half of the substance deposits in the cylinder [46% (20 µl) vs. 64% (200 µl)]. This finding explains the already mentioned upper limit of possible nebulized volume (see section Effects of Concentration, Settling Time, and Repeated Deposition). Nebulization of more than 200 µl leads to condensing drops to fall, foiling the intended use at ALI conditions. Regardless, as long as it remains consistent, the deposition of aerosol droplets on the device's walls is not a clinically relevant problem in practice. By gently wiping the device with (sterile) tissues, repeated nebulization-deposition maneuvers can be done in a row. According to the deposition efficiencies, the total maximum volume deposited onto the wells/inserts was never more than 8 µl, challenging to spread evenly using a pipette without touching the cells.

As could be expected, the deposition of aerosolized saline was well tolerated by commonly used Calu-3 cells, which is in concordance with comparable devices following the same principle, as there are no impaction forces or drying processes (Lenz et al., 2009). The device is usable under sterile experimental circumstances, as it is easily cleanable with ethanolic disinfectant and can be autoclaved with steam. Both LDH release and TEER values show no differences to the control that was not deposited with PBS at either 20 or 200 μl after 24 h (**Figure 7**). Epithelial cells and the biological absorption barrier formed by their tight junctions must not be harmed following deposition, especially when creating infected or inflamed models and then treated. The spatial distribution snapshot demonstrates an almost-even distribution of the aerosol, as represented in **Figure 6**, across 20–200 μl of invested dose and further suggests that cell cultures will be exposed to an even dose.

Here, we have visually shown and quantified the fluorescent intensity of nanoparticles deposited onto Transwell® membranes. The precise spatial distribution was observed on a non-wetted membrane that was not tampered with during the nebulization and imaging processes. The particles are homogeneously spread from the quantification of the normalized fluorescent intensity across the membrane's diameter. This is in agreement with other devices, such as ALICE, which produced a spatially homogenous spread of zinc oxide nanoparticles (Lenz et al., 2009), while in ALI cell culture conditions, the membrane may be wetted from the basolateral compartment and lining fluid of the cells, and this would lead to a greater spread of the aerosol over time. Our snapshot dictates that the aerosol spreads evenly on a dry membrane and does not need to rely on the surface's wettability. Comparatively, the naturally dried membrane may have resulted in small amounts of crystal formation from the deposited dose resulting in some small artifacts in the micrographs. The consistent ca. 10% SD of the deposited dose across all invested volumes tends to be higher than that of other reports from the Vitrocell® Cloud systems (Ding et al., 2020); however, it may be indicative of the fluorescent microscopy imaging technique as opposed to quartz crystal microbalance quantification. In any case, the device deposits a robust, spatially homogenous dose.

The present paper describes a straightforward device, in both manufacture and use, that enables reproducible deposition (4.8% relative SD) of pre-metered doses of aerosolized drugs on pulmonary *in vitro* cell cultures grown at ALI conditions. With this device, volume-defined amounts of solubilized drugs and pharmaceutical aerosol formulations can be deposited precisely on wells. The distribution of the deposited mass of free drug could be analyzed throughout the whole system. As expected, the deposition, when using this device on cell culture inserts, does not interfere with cell viability and epithelial barrier function. It is easy to clean, cost-efficient, and easily transferable to the bench. It can be customized to connect to any nebulizer and is the only device that could be completely produced using 3D printers, a technology that is employed universally at most universities in the world. Therefore, it can provide a valuable tool for studying the effects of aerosolized drugs and nanoscale delivery systems on *in vitro* pulmonary cell culture models.

AUTHOR CONTRIBUTIONS

JH performed the experiments and wrote the manuscript. CT performed the LCNP experiments, including the data analysis of deposition efficiency and spatial deposition of the aerosol and revising the manuscript. PC helped in the setup and design of the deposition chamber and technical questions and in revising the manuscript. XM and FG had the initial idea of producing the cylinder, planned the concept, and developed the device. CC-W advised on experiments and strategy and helped to create the manuscript and to enhance it. C-ML provided help in planning the experiments and supervised, creating, and enhancing the manuscript. All authors contributed to the article and approved the submitted version.

ACKNOWLEDGMENTS

We gratefully thank Rudolf Richter (Workshop, Department of Physical Chemistry and Didactics of Chemistry, Saarland University) for support in technical planning, construction of the device, and providing the scheme for **Figure 1A**; Pascal Paul for his help in conducting some of the deposition experiments; and Petra König and Jana Westhues for their support in cell cultures.

REFERENCES

Aerogen® (2020). *Aerogen Pro. Descubra Aerogen Pro*. Available online at: https://www.aerogen.com/de/aerogen-produkte/aerogen-pro/ (accessed September 2, 2020)

Altube, M. J., Cutro, A., Bakas, L., Morilla, M. J., Disalvo, E. A., and Romero, E. L. (2017). Nebulizing novel multifunctional nanovesicles: the impact of macrophage-targeted-pH-sensitive archaeosomes on a pulmonary surfactant. *J. Mater. Chem. B* 5, 8083–8095. doi: 10.1039/c7tb01694h

Barosova, H., Maione, A. G., Septiadi, D., Sharma, M., Haeni, L., Balog, S., et al. (2020). Use of EpiAlveolar lung model to predict fibrotic potential of multiwalled carbon nanotubes. *ACS Nano* 14, 3941–3956. doi: 10.1021/acsnano.9b06860

Bastacky, J., Lee, C. Y. C., Goerke, J., Koushafar, H., Yager, D., Kenaga, L., et al. (1995). Alveolar lining layer is thin and continuous: low-temperature scanning electron microscopy of rat lung. *J. Appl. Physiol.* 79, 1615–1628. doi: 10.1152/jappl.1995.79.5.1615

Blank, F., Rothen-Rutishauser, B. M., Schurch, S., and Gehr, P. (2006). An optimized in vitro model of the respiratory tract wall to study particle cell interactions. *J. Aerosol Med.* 19, 392–405. doi: 10.1089/jam.2006.19.392

Brandenberger, C., Mühlfeld, C., Ali, Z., Lenz, A. G., Schmid, O., Parak, W. J., et al. (2010). Quantitative evaluation of cellular uptake and trafficking of plain and polyethylene glycol-coated gold nanoparticles. *Small* 6, 1669–1678. doi: 10.1002/smll.201000528

Bur, M., Huwer, H., Muys, L., and Lehr, C.-M. (2010). Drug transport across pulmonary epithelial cell monolayers. *J. Aerosol Med. Pulm. Drug Deliv.* 23, 119–127. doi: 10.1089/jamp.2009.0757

Bur, M., Rothen-Rutishauser, B., Huwer, H., and Lehr, C. M. (2009). A novel cell compatible impingement system to study in vitro drug absorption from dry powder aerosol formulations. *Eur. J. Pharm. Biopharm.* 72, 350–357. doi: 10.1016/j.ejpb.2008.07.019

Cei, D., Doryab, A., Lenz, A., Schröppel, A., Mayer, P., Burgstaller, G., et al. (2020). Development of a dynamic in vitro stretch model of the alveolar interface with aerosol delivery. *Biotechnol. Bioeng.* 118, 690–702. doi: 10.1002/bit.27600

Chortarea, S., Barosova, H., Clift, M. J. D., Wick, P., Petri-Fink, A., and Rothen-Rutishauser, B. (2017). Human asthmatic bronchial cells are more susceptible to subchronic repeated exposures of aerosolized carbon nanotubes at occupationally relevant doses than healthy cells. *ACS Nano* 11, 7615–7625. doi: 10.1021/acsnano.7b01992

Cooney, D. J., Kazantseva, M., and Hickey, A. J. (2004). Development of a size-dependent aerosol deposition model utilising human airway epithelial cells for evaluating aerosol drug delivery. *ATLA Altern. Lab. Anim.* 32, 581–590. doi: 10.1177/026119290403200609

Cultex® Technology (2020). *Leading the Field in Quality and Expertise.* Available online at: https://www.cultex-technology.com/products/ (accessed September 1, 2020)

D'Angelo, I., Costabile, G., Durantie, E., Brocca, P., Rondelli, V., Russo, A., et al. (2018). Hybrid lipid/polymer nanoparticles for pulmonary delivery of siRNA: development and fate upon in vitro deposition on the human epithelial airway barrier. *J. Aerosol Med. Pulm. Drug Deliv.* 31, 170–181. doi: 10.1089/jamp.2017.1364

Di Cristo, L., Grimaldi, B., Catelani, T., Vázquez, E., Pompa, P. P., and Sabella, S. (2020). Repeated exposure to aerosolized graphene oxide mediates autophagy inhibition and inflammation in a three-dimensional human airway model. *Mater. Today Bio* 6:100050. doi: 10.1016/j.mtbio.2020.100050

Ding, Y., Weindl, P., Lenz, A. G., Mayer, P., Krebs, T., and Schmid, O. (2020). Quartz crystal microbalances (QCM) are suitable for real-time dosimetry in nanotoxicological studies using Vitrocell® Cloud cell exposure systems. *Part. Fibre Toxicol.* 17:44. doi: 10.1186/s12989-020-00376-w

Dolovich, M. B., and Dhand, R. (2011). Aerosol drug delivery: developments in device design and clinical use. *Lancet* 377, 1032–1045. doi: 10.1016/S0140-6736(10)60926-9

Ehrmann, S., Schmid, O., Darquenne, C., Rothen-Rutishauser, B., Sznitman, J., Yang, L., et al. (2020). Innovative preclinical models for pulmonary drug delivery research. *Expert Opin. Drug Deliv.* 17, 463–478. doi: 10.1080/17425247.2020.1730807

Foster, K. A., Avery, M. L., Yazdanian, M., and Audus, K. L. (2000). Characterization of the Calu-3 cell line as a tool to screen pulmonary drug delivery. *Int. J. Pharm.* 208, 1–11. doi: 10.1016/S0378-5173(00)00452-X

Fraunhofer P.R.I.T® Systems (2020). *P.R.I.T. Professionelle In-Vitro Technologien* Available online at: https://www.prit-systems.de/de/home.html (accessed October 27, 2020)

Frijns, E., Verstraelen, S., Stoehr, L. C., Van Laer, J., Jacobs, A., Peters, J., et al. (2017). A novel exposure system termed NAVETTA for in vitro laminar flow electrodeposition of nanoaerosol and evaluation of immune effects in human lung reporter cells. *Environ. Sci. Technol.* 51, 5259–5269. doi: 10.1021/acs.est.7b00493

Graef, F., Richter, R., Fetz, V., Murgia, X., De Rossi, C., Schneider-Daum, N., et al. (2018). In vitro model of the gram-negative bacterial cell envelope for investigation of anti-infective permeation kinetics. *ACS Infect. Dis.* 4, 1188–1196. doi: 10.1021/acsinfecdis.7b00165

He, R. W., Gerlofs-Nijland, M. E., Boere, J., Fokkens, P., Leseman, D., Janssen, N. A. H., et al. (2020). Comparative toxicity of ultrafine particles around a major airport in human bronchial epithelial (Calu-3) cell model at the air–liquid interface. *Toxicol. In Vitro* 68:104950. doi: 10.1016/j.tiv.2020.104950

Hein, S., Bur, M., Kolb, T., Muellinger, B., Schaefer, U. F., and Lehr, C. M. (2010). The Pharmaceutical Aerosol Deposition Device on Cell Cultures (PADDOCC) in vitro system: design and experimental protocol. *ATLA Altern. Lab. Anim.* 38, 285–295. doi: 10.1177/026119291003800408

Hein, S., Bur, M., Schaefer, U. F., and Lehr, C. M. (2011). A new Pharmaceutical Aerosol Deposition Device on Cell Cultures (PADDOCC) to evaluate pulmonary drug absorption for metered dose dry powder formulations. *Eur. J. Pharm. Biopharm.* 77, 132–138. doi: 10.1016/j.ejpb.2010.10.003

Hiemstra, P. S., Grootaers, G., van der Does, A. M., Krul, C. A. M., and Kooter, I. M. (2018). Human lung epithelial cell cultures for analysis of inhaled toxicants: lessons learned and future directions. *Toxicol. In Vitro* 47, 137–146. doi: 10.1016/j.tiv.2017.11.005

Hittinger, M., Barthold, S., Siebenbürger, L., Zäh, K., Gress, A., Guenther, S., et al. (2017). "Proof of concept of the Vitrocell® dry powder chamber: a new in vitro test system for the controlled deposition of aerosol formulations," in *Proceedings of the Europe Respiratory Drug Delivery 2017 Scientific Conference* (Antibes), 283–288.

Inhalation Sciences (2020). *Technical Specifications.* Available online at: https://inhalation.se/products/technical-specifications/ (accessed September 1, 2020).

Jeannet, N., Fierz, M., Schneider, S., Künzi, L., Baumlin, N., Salathe, M., et al. (2016). Acute toxicity of silver and carbon nanoaerosols to normal and cystic fibrosis human bronchial epithelial cells. *Nanotoxicology* 10, 279–291. doi: 10.3109/17435390.2015.1049233

Lacroix, G., Koch, W., Ritter, D., Gutleb, A. C., Larsen, S. T., Loret, T., et al. (2018). Air-liquid interface in vitro models for respiratory toxicology research: consensus workshop and recommendations. *Appl. In Vitro Toxicol.* 4, 91–106. doi: 10.1089/aivt.2017.0034

Lenz, A. G., Karg, E., Lentner, B., Dittrich, V., Brandenberger, C., Rothen-Rutishauser, B., et al. (2009). A dose-controlled system for air-liquid interface cell exposure and application to zinc oxide nanoparticles. *Part. Fibre Toxicol.* 6:32. doi: 10.1186/1743-8977-6-32

Lenz, A. G., Stoeger, T., Cei, D., Schmidmeir, M., Semren, N., Burgstaller, G., et al. (2014). Efficient bioactive delivery of aerosolized drugs to human pulmonary epithelial cells cultured in air-liquid interface conditions. *Am. J. Respir. Cell .Mol. Biol.* 51, 526–535. doi: 10.1165/rcmb.2013-0479OC

Loret, T., Peyret, E., Dubreuil, M., Aguerre-Chariol, O., Bressot, C., le Bihan, O., et al. (2016). Air-liquid interface exposure to aerosols of poorly soluble nanomaterials induces different biological activation levels compared to exposure to suspensions. *Part. Fibre Toxicol.* 13:58. doi: 10.1186/s12989-016-0171-3

Meindl, C., Stranzinger, S., Dzidic, N., Salar-Behzadi, S., Mohr, S., Zimmer, A., et al. (2015). Permeation of therapeutic drugs in different formulations across the airway epithelium in vitro. *PLoS One* 10:e0135690. doi: 10.1371/journal.pone.0135690

Metz, J. K., Scharnowske, L., Hans, F., Schnur, S., Knoth, K., Zimmer, H., et al. (2020). Safety assessment of excipients (SAFE) for orally inhaled drug products. *Altex* 37, 275–286. doi: 10.14573/altex.1910231

Paur, H. R., Cassee, F. R., Teeguarden, J., Fissan, H., Diabate, S., Aufderheide, M., et al. (2011). In-vitro cell exposure studies for the assessment of nanoparticle toxicity in the lung-A dialog between aerosol science and biology. *J. Aerosol Sci.* 42, 668–692. doi: 10.1016/j.jaerosci.2011.06.005

Pulskamp, K., Diabaté, S., and Krug, H. F. (2007). Carbon nanotubes show no sign of acute toxicity but induce intracellular reactive oxygen species in dependence on contaminants. *Toxicol. Lett.* 168, 58–74. doi: 10.1016/j.toxlet.2006.11.001

Röhm, M., Carle, S., Maigler, F., Flamm, J., Kramer, V., Mavoungou, C., et al. (2017). A comprehensive screening platform for aerosolizable protein formulations for intranasal and pulmonary drug delivery. *Int. J. Pharm.* 532, 537–546. doi: 10.1016/j.ijpharm.2017.09.027

Rothen-Rutishauser, B., Mühlfeld, C., Blank, F., Musso, C., and Gehr, P. (2007). Translocation of particles and inflammatory responses after exposure to fine particles and nanoparticles in an epithelial airway model. *Part. Fibre Toxicol.* 4:9. doi: 10.1186/1743-8977-4-9

Schneider-Daum, N., Carius, P., Horstmann, J., and Lehr, C.-M. (2019). "Cell- and tissue-based (reconstituted) 2D In vitro models to study drug transport processes across the air-blood barrier," in *Pharmaceutical Inhalation Aerosol Technology*, eds A. J. Hickey and S. Da Rocha (Boca Raton, FL: CRC Press), 627–651.

Tannenbaum, J., and Bennett, B. T. (2015). Russell and Burch's 3Rs then and now: the need for clarity in definition and purpose. *J. Am. Assoc. Lab. Anim. Sci.* 54, 120–132.

Thorn, C. R., Clulow, A. J., Boyd, B. J., Prestidge, C. A., and Thomas, N. (2020). Bacterial lipase triggers the release of antibiotics from digestible liquid crystal nanoparticles. *J. Control. Release* 319, 168–182. doi: 10.1016/j.jconrel.2019.12.037

Upadhyay, S., and Palmberg, L. (2018). Air-liquid interface: relevant in vitro models for investigating air pollutant-induced pulmonary toxicity. *Toxicol. Sci.* 164, 21–30. doi: 10.1093/toxsci/kfy053

Vitrocell® Cloud Systems (2020). *Vitrocell® Cloud For The Exposure to Liquid Aerosols.* Available online at: https://www.vitrocell.com/inhalation-toxicology/exposure-systems/vitrocell-cloud-system (accessed October 27, 2020)

6

Organ-on-a-Chip: Opportunities for Assessing the Toxicity of Particulate Matter

Jia-Wei Yang [1,2†], Yu-Chih Shen [2,3†], Ko-Chih Lin [1,2], Sheng-Jen Cheng [1,2], Shiue-Luen Chen [1,2], Chong-You Chen [1,2], Priyank V. Kumar [4], Shien-Fong Lin [1,2], Huai-En Lu [5] and Guan-Yu Chen [1,2,6*]*

[1] Department of Electrical and Computer Engineering, College of Electrical and Computer Engineering National Chiao Tung University, Hsinchu, Taiwan, [2] Institute of Biomedical Engineering, College of Electrical and Computer Engineering, National Chiao Tung University, Hsinchu, Taiwan, [3] Ph.D. Degree Program of Biomedical Science and Engineering, National Chiao Tung University, Hsinchu, Taiwan, [4] School of Chemical Engineering, University of New South Wales, Sydney, NSW, Australia, [5] Bioresource Collection and Research Center, Food Industry Research and Development Institute, Hsinchu, Taiwan, [6] Department of Biological Science and Technology, National Chiao Tung University, Hsinchu, Taiwan

***Correspondence:**
Huai-En Lu
hel@firdi.org.tw
Guan-Yu Chen
guanyu@nctu.edu.tw

† These authors have contributed equally to this work

Recent developments in epidemiology have confirmed that airborne particulates are directly associated with respiratory pathology and mortality. Although clinical studies have yielded evidence of the effects of many types of fine particulates on human health, it still does not have a complete understanding of how physiological reactions are caused nor to the changes and damages associated with cellular and molecular mechanisms. Currently, most health assessment studies of particulate matter (PM) are conducted through cell culture or animal experiments. The results of such experiments often do not correlate with clinical findings or actual human reactions, and they also cause difficulty when investigating the causes of air pollution and associated human health hazards, the analysis of biomarkers, and the development of future pollution control strategies. Microfluidic-based cell culture technology has considerable potential to expand the capabilities of conventional cell culture by providing high-precision measurement, considerably increasing the potential for the parallelization of cellular assays, ensuring inexpensive automation, and improving the response of the overall cell culture in a more physiologically relevant context. This review paper focuses on integrating the important respiratory health problems caused by air pollution today, as well as the development and application of biomimetic organ-on-a-chip technology. This more precise experimental model is expected to accelerate studies elucidating the effect of PM on the human body and to reveal new opportunities for breakthroughs in disease research and drug development.

Keywords: particulate matter, air pollution, respiratory health, cardiovascular effects, organ-on-a-chip

INTRODUCTION

With the development of epidemiology in recent years, scientists have confirmed that airborne particulate matter (PM) is directly associated with respiratory pathology and mortality (Kim et al., 2018; Khaniabadi et al., 2019). For every 10 $\mu g/m^3$ increase in PM_{10} concentration, respiratory system-related mortality increases by 0.58% (Analitis et al., 2006), and for every 10 $\mu g/m^3$ increase in $PM_{2.5}$, the incidence of respiratory-system related diseases increases by 2.07% (Zanobetti et al., 2009). These studies indicate that impaired lung function also increases the incidence and mortality of cardiopulmonary disease (Zanobetti et al., 2009; de Oliveira et al., 2012). In addition to the problem of increased risk of respiratory disease caused by compromised lung function, PM may also increase the incidence of lung cancer (Raaschou-Nielsen et al., 2016). In a large-scale study conducted in the United States with a sample of 188,699 non-smokers, each 10 $\mu g/m^3$ increase in $PM_{2.5}$ concentrations increased lung cancer-related mortality by 15–27% (Turner et al., 2011). Although PM is a global concern, severe air pollution episodes are often associated with industrialization, and urbanization. As China's rapid economic growth, several recent studies paid attentions to frequent air pollution episodes (Li et al., 2016; Lin et al., 2018). The air quality statistics report of Beijing from 2013 to 2015 shows that the 2 year average $PM_{2.5}$ concentrations from 69 to 89 $\mu g/m^3$ and the daily average concentrations ranged from 3 to 437 $\mu g/m^3$ (Batterman et al., 2016). These studies have shown that it is imperative to address the harmful effects of PM on the human body, in addition to traditionally known respiratory diseases such as asthma and chronic obstructive pulmonary disease (COPD) (Hopke et al., 2019). The incidence of cardiopulmonary disease and lung cancer are also associated with a high mortality rate (Hamanaka and Mutlu, 2018). Therefore, it is essential to quickly and accurately elucidate the effects of PM on the human body, determine the causes of diseases, and formulate response strategies.

PARTICULATE MATTER AND RESPIRATORY SYSTEM

PM is one of the most important components of air pollution that affects human health and disease. It is classified based on the relative size, which is defined in terms of aerodynamic equivalent diameter (AED), not directly by the diameter of their actual particles. In other words, the size of the actual particles is converted into an equivalent diameter having the same aerodynamic properties (Raabe, 1976). PM can be divided into three AED levels based on the deposition and penetration ability of the particles in the human respiratory system: $\leq$ 10 μm, $\leq$ 2.5 μm, and $\leq$0.1 μm (PM_{10}, $PM_{2.5}$, and $PM_{0.1}$, respectively) (**Figure 1A**). Particles with AED diameters >10 μm have a relatively small half-life in suspension and are mostly filtered by the nasal and upper respiratory tract, so researchers have classified PM >10 μm into three categories: (i) coarse PM ($PM_{2.5-10}$), (ii) fine PM ($PM_{0.1-2.5}$), and (iii) ultrafine PM ($PM_{0.1}$) (Anderson et al., 2012).

Although the effects of PM exposure depend on individual physical characteristics, such as the pattern and rate of breathing, weight, and age, the size of the particles has been identified as a direct cause of health problems (Brown et al., 2013). Generally, the smaller the particles, the faster they penetrate and deposit in the deeper levels of the respiratory system. In nasal breathing, cilia and mucous membranes are very effective in filtering most particles larger than 10 μm in diameter. Because of the rapid deposition of PM with larger particle size, they tend to remain in the trachea or bronchi (upper respiratory tract). They initially accumulate in the nose and throat, and the body will eliminate these invasive PM through some reactive processes such as sneezing and coughing. Up to now, particles <10 μm in diameter are considered to have the greatest impact on human health, and because of their high penetration ability, they can evade the protective mechanisms of the upper respiratory tract and enter the alveoli deep in the lungs (Löndahl et al., 2006; Kim et al., 2015). Computer simulations have shown that particles with diameters between 1 and 10 μm are primarily deposited in the nasopharyngeal and laryngeal of upper airway regions, and particles with diameters between 1 and 100 nm are deposited in the lower bronchial and alveolar region, where gas exchange occurs (Tsuda et al., 2013) (**Figure 1B**). However, particles smaller than 1 μm tend to behave like gas molecules, so it is extremely easy for them to penetrate into the alveoli and affect gas exchange in the lungs and even penetrate the barrier of the lungs and enter the circulatory system, further migrating to other cells, tissues, or circulatory and metabolic systems and leading to serious health problems (**Table 1**).

Currently, there have been many studies on the biological mechanism and effects of PM on the respiratory system (Xing et al., 2016), which primarily involve the following aspects: (1) Functional injury caused by free radical peroxidation. Studies have shown that free radicals, metals, and organic components in $PM_{2.5}$ can induce the free radical formation, cause oxidation of lung cells, and also cause the production of reactive oxygen species (ROS), resulting in DNA damage and cell death (Donaldson et al., 1996; Lodovici and Bigagli, 2011). (2) Imbalance of intracellular calcium regulation (calcium homeostasis). Calcium ion is a physiological index of cell function regulation. However, free radical and ROS reactions induced by $PM_{2.5}$ can cause abnormal intracellular calcium concentrations, which lead to apoptosis and necrosis (Li et al., 2015; Al Hanai et al., 2019). (3) Inflammatory injury. This is also the most extensive part of current studies. $PM_{2.5}$ can cause significant immune responses and inflammation in lung cells (Nadeau et al., 2010; He et al., 2017). These inflammatory responses to Th1 and Th2 triggered by Toll-like receptor (TLRs) pathways can lead to activation of neutrophils, T cells, and alveolar macrophages, which is also associated with asthma and COPD (Nemmar et al., 2013) (**Figure 1C**). Although studies on PM and its biological mechanisms are currently ongoing, an important future research direction is to elucidate the inflammatory response to PM in the lungs.

PARTICULATE MATTER AND CARDIOVASCULAR EFFECTS

With the development of epidemiology in recent years, scientists have validated the effects of long-term PM exposure on the respiratory system. PM can penetrate deep into the trachea and bronchi and can even deposit in alveolar tissue. Hydroxyl radicals (·OH) produced from reactive oxygen species (ROS) through activated metals are the main factors that cause oxidative damage to DNA. If damaged DNA is not repaired in a timely

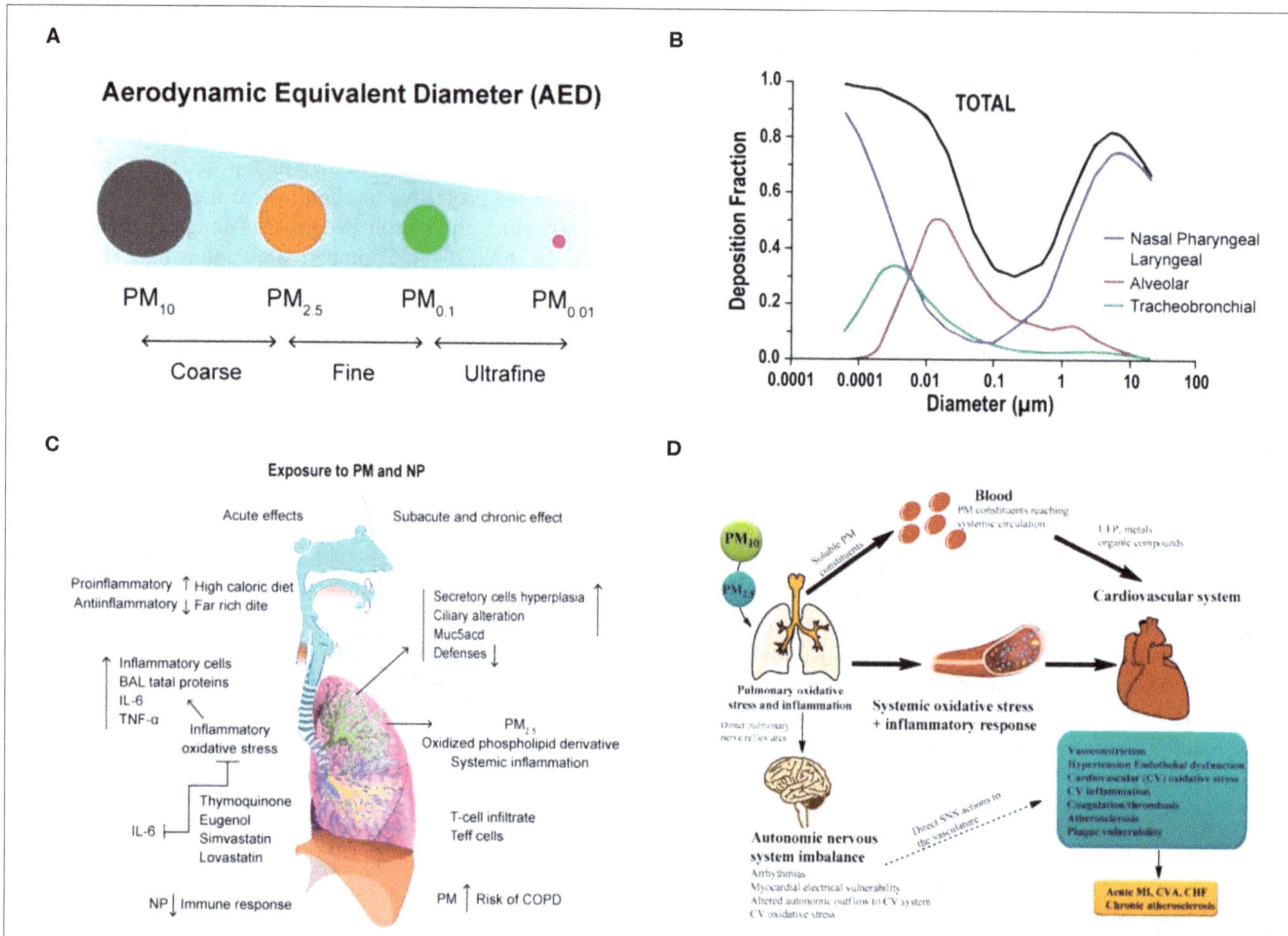

FIGURE 1 | The transport and health effects of PM in human lung and cardiovascular. **(A)** Classification of PM size by aerodynamic equivalent diameter (AED). **(B)** PM deposition curves in the extrathoracic, bronchial, and alveolar regions for adult humans. Reproduced with permission from Tsuda et al. (2013). **(C)** The schematization of the immune responses and inflammation in lung cells by inhaled PM. Reproduced with permission from Nemmar et al. (2013). **(D)** There are three main hypotheses that PM can cause biological pathways for cardiovascular impairment. Reproduced with permission from Ngoc et al. (2018).

matter, it can induce cancer or lead to other irreversible damage (Valavanidis et al., 2005). Environmental exposure to this fine PM not only causes respiratory disease but also affects heart rate, blood pressure, vascular tone, blood coagulation, and formation of atherosclerotic lesions (Suwa et al., 2002; Bennett et al., 2018; Huang et al., 2018). In addition, there is a positive correlation between fine PM and the incidence and mortality of cardiopulmonary disease. The World Health Organization (WHO) reported that 3.7 million deaths in 2012 were due to air pollution, which accounted for 6.7% of deaths worldwide. Of these, 16% were deaths due to lung cancer, 11% were due to chronic obstructive pulmonary disease and associated diseases, 29% were due to heart disease and stroke, and about 13% were due to respiratory infections. In addition, fine PM in the air that is inhaled into the lungs can translocate to the bloodstream and be transported to the blood vessels and the heart, which can induce arrhythmia and reduce myocardial contractility and coronary blood flow (Nemmar et al., 2003). The possible mechanisms for cardiopulmonary risk following inhalation of fine PM into the lungs can be roughly classified into three groups: (1) Stimulating the production of inflammatory factors: inducing the secretion of inflammatory factors such as cytokines, activated immune cells, platelets, and endothelin, from basal cells in the lungs (Kido et al., 2011; Tsai et al., 2012). (2) Translocation of PM: toxic effects caused by translocation of PM or its components to the circulatory system (Nemmar et al., 2002). (3) Neuroendocrine disorders: the balance of the autonomic nervous system or heart rate is affected by the binding of PM to receptors located on the lungs or nerves (Ngoc et al., 2018; Snow et al., 2018) (**Figure 1D**).

Du *et al.* summarized recent research results on short- and long-term exposure to $PM_{2.5}$ (Du et al., 2016). The results show that every 10 $\mu g/m^3$ increase in short-term $PM_{2.5}$ exposure concentration increases overall mortality and cardiovascular-related mortality by 0.4–1.0%, while every 10 $\mu g/m^3$ increase in long-term exposure increases overall mortality by 10% and cardiovascular-related mortality by 3–76%. With respect to various cardiovascular diseases, $PM_{2.5}$ has the greatest impact on coronary heart disease, moderate impact on heart failure and stroke, and the smallest impact on peripheral vascular diseases and arrhythmia. Because these risk factors not only cause a sharp increase in the risk of cardiovascular disease, and the metabolic syndrome secondary to it is closely associated with some of the most significant causes of death worldwide, including increased risk of Alzheimer's disease, Parkinson disease, dementia, and stroke (Fu et al., 2019). Although the true pathogenic mechanism is currently unknown and the impairment of cardiopulmonary function due to fine PM is due to a complex series of effects, the establishment of an *in vitro* model that represents the human body in a large number of studies is an urgent need. It is expected that establishing an *in vitro* model of cardiopulmonary function will yield new possibilities and opportunities for understanding the hazards and influencing mechanisms associated with environmental engineering and human health.

TABLE 1 | Effects of PM on the human respiratory system.

Diameter (μm)	Distribution characteristics	Effects on human physiology
PM_{10}	Deposits in nose and throat	Can cause allergic rhinitis, cough, asthma, and other symptoms
$PM_{2.5-10}$	Deposits in upper nasal cavity and deep respiratory tract	Causes fibrous paralysis, bronchial mucus hypersecretion, and mucosal gland hyperplasia leading to reversible bronchospasm, inhibits deep breathing and spreading to bronchi
$PM_{2.5}$	Less than 10% deposits in bronchi, ~20–30% deposits in lungs	Can cause chronic bronchitis, bronchiole expansion, pulmonary edema, bronchial fibrosis, or other symptoms
$PM_{0.1}$	Deposits inside alveolar tissue	Promotes significant increase in macrophages in the lungs, causes emphysema and alveolar destruction

ASSESSMENT FOR BIOLOGICAL TOXICITY OF FINE PARTICULATE MATTER

Epidemiological and clinical studies have linked exposure to fine PM to adverse health outcomes, which may also be associated with increased mortality and morbidity in various cardiopulmonary diseases. Despite much evidence of the effects of PM on human health, the causes of physiological responses and the changes and damage to cellular and molecular mechanisms have not yet been fully explained. There are currently two main methods for elucidating the mechanisms of PM toxicity (Fröhlich and Salar-Behzadi, 2014; Yang et al., 2017) (**Figure 2A**). One is the use of *in vivo* animal models to evaluate the effects of fine PM on the respiratory and cardiovascular systems (**Figure 2B**). The other type is *in vitro* cell experiment models (**Figure 2C**); the use of various *in vitro* models has proven valuable for studying the molecular and cellular mechanisms behind different physiological effects more deeply.

Studies using animal models have demonstrated the effects of fine PM exposure on different organs and the incidence of different diseases. With respect to acute reactions, most studies have focused on inflammatory responses, and relatively few researchers have investigated specific responses to disease (Hong et al., 2016; Wang H. et al., 2017). Conversely, with respect to chronic reactions, a large number of disease-related findings have been reported, including DNA damage, lung parenchyma

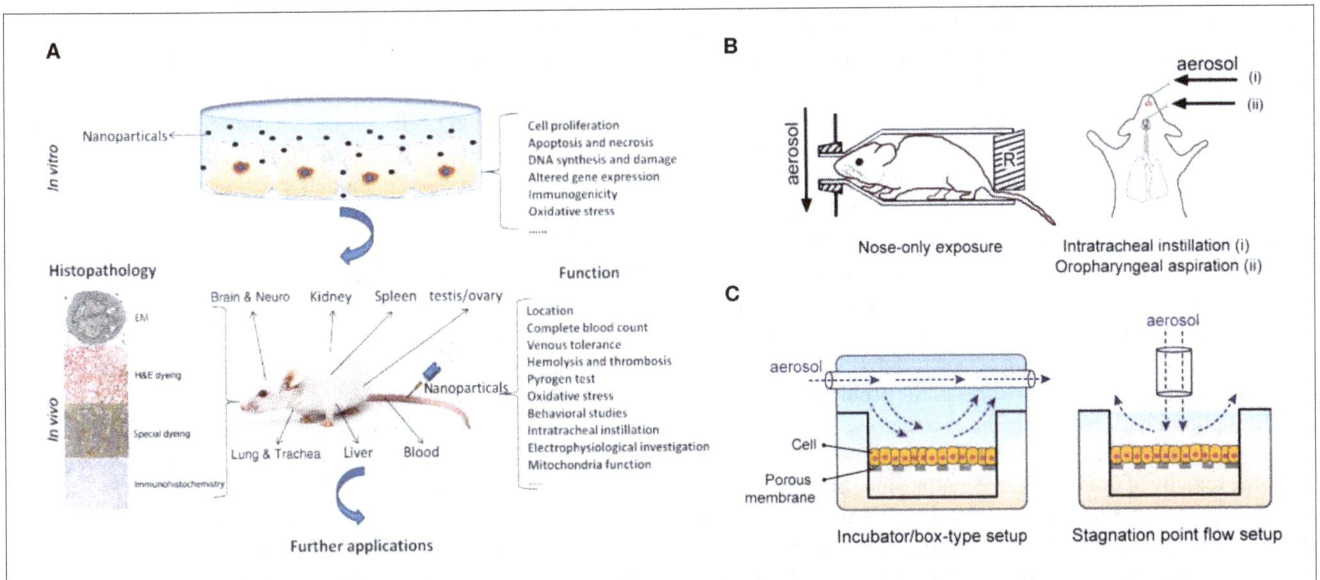

FIGURE 2 | Two main methods for elucidating the mechanisms of PM toxicity. **(A)** *In vitro* and *in vivo* toxicity assessment of PM. Reproduced with permission from Yang et al. (2017). **(B)** *In vitro* animal experiments exposed to aerosols mainly include nose exposure, intratracheal instillation, and oropharyngeal aspiration. Reproduced with permission from Fröhlich and Salar-Behzadi (2014). **(C)** Air–liquid interface (ALI) *in vitro* models for investigating respiratory research.

damage, pulmonary fibrosis, and granuloma formation (Xu et al., 2013; Shadie et al., 2014). Meanwhile, because *in vitro* models have demonstrated that cell experiments are the most suitable model for investigating mechanisms of toxicity, such as initiation events for inflammatory effects or genotoxicity, these data cannot be explained because of genetic differences in animal experiments (Wang J. et al., 2017). In view of this, the genotoxicity and biological indicators linking disease and cancer have been clearly recognized in particular, but this is still a challenge in other applications, which also includes further elucidation of the mechanism of fine PM toxicity in humans (Vawda et al., 2013).

Although current knowledge does not fully understand the health effects of PM exposure, studies over the past decade have suggested the potential cytotoxicity. It has been observed in cell studies that PM stimulation has caused cell viability decline, cell death, ultrastructural disruptions, genetic toxicity (mutagenicity and DNA damage), and oxidative stress (Peixoto et al., 2017). These mechanisms involved in the inflammatory response, including the up-regulation of cytokines downstream of the caspase cascade and the kinase pathway, the up-regulation of metal-redox sensitive transcription factors NF-κβ and AP-1 (Øvrevik et al., 2015). In addition, the PM also increases inflammatory mediator-related gene expression and protein secretion, such as TNF-α, IL-1β, IL-8, IL-6, and MCP-1 (Fuentes-Mattei et al., 2010; Ryu et al., 2019). On the other hand, similar reactions have been observed in animal experiments, showing DNA damage, oxidative stress and inflammatory mediator-related protein secretion and recruitment of inflammatory cells in many organs (de Oliveira et al., 2018). In addition, many studies have shown association between exposure to PM and chronic diseases. These adverse health effects include asthma, chronic obstructive pulmonary disease (COPD), atherosclerosis, diabetes and allergic sensitization (Guo et al., 2018; Li et al., 2018).

Mammalian cell culture studies are often used as the first step in toxicity evaluation, cell-based studies are still greatly limited with respect to the complex structures of physiological mechanisms in humans, and it is impossible to simulate the complex conditions and the interrelated physiological information of the entire organism. Animal experiments play an important role in PM research, where they allow *in vivo* toxicological testing by exposing animals to various PM environments via the oral and dermal routes. Although animals can inhale PM and develop comprehensive systemic outcomes, there is often a large difference between mechanistic and genetic indicator data and clinical outcomes. This is primarily due to differences among species and their physiological functions, such as differences in respiratory rate between experimental mice and humans (Curbani et al., 2019), as well as the problems of genetics, low throughput, high cost, and ethical concerns.

As yet, there is currently no ideal experimental model for study the toxicity of fine particulate matter since both *in vitro* and *in vivo* models have limitations. Notably, the interpretation of chronic toxicity studies is relatively lacking of information, which requires consideration of whether the information obtained from animal studies is similar to human responses. This issue may be expected to be overcome through the advancement of biotechnology and biomedical engineering technologies, thereby obtaining a useful *in vitro* model that allow long-term cultivation of functional responses that express the human organ. In addition, due to the diversity and regional differences of PM composition, how to systematically study the toxicology of PM on the human body (including single components and the interaction between components) is also the focus of future research (Jia et al., 2017; Park et al., 2018).

ORGANS-ON-CHIPS

With respect to the effects of PM exposure on the human body, many studies have demonstrated the relationship between PM and health risk, but further understanding of the mechanisms of human toxicity is still lacking. The problems faced are derived from the major differences in genes and structures between the species used in animal experiments and humans. Although biomimetic technology experiments are the most appropriate model for investigating mechanisms of toxicity, only a complete description and definition of genotoxicity and indicators between disease and cancer have been made at present, and other aspects are still being researched. In this field, improving the representativeness of *in vitro* experiments and strengthening the reference value of data has become important issues in research. This topic has been discussed by other authors (Vanderburgh et al., 2017; Ahadian et al., 2018; Costa and Ahluwalia, 2019). Developments and progress in biomimetic technology will bring unlimited potential for breaking through the research bottlenecks faced in this field.

To resolve the great differences between animal experiments and clinical trials, techniques have been developed in recent years for construction of organs-on-chips, with the goal of replacing animal experiments and achieving more accurate and reliable preclinical data (Alépée et al., 2014; Zhang et al., 2017, 2018) (**Figure 3A**). Currently, organ-on-a-chip development mostly relies on materials with high biocompatibility for construction of a 3D microenvironment suitable for cell growth so that cells can establish cell-to-cell interactions that are not possible in most 2D cell culture environments, to observe the phenomena of simulated organs more accurately. In particular, this new organ-on-a-chip models provide unlimited potential to replicate critical tissue-tissue responses by reconstructing dynamic physiological forces, cellular microenvironments, and 3D structures of human organ. The development of organ-on-chips and in-depth descriptions have been heatedly discussed in other reviews (Rothbauer et al., 2018; Nawroth et al., 2019) (**Figure 3B**). In addition, when combined with the "induced pluripotent stem cell (iPSCs)" technique in somatic cells, it is possible to successfully differentiate individualized target tissues of interest without traumatizing the organs. Researchers have successfully integrated various iPSC-derived cells with organ-on-chips, such as blood vessels-on-chip, a blood–brain barrier-on-chip and heart-on-chip systems. The different methods for creating organ-on-chips using stem cells also have been described in depth by other groups (Geraili et al., 2018; Jodat et al., 2018; Cochrane et al., 2019).

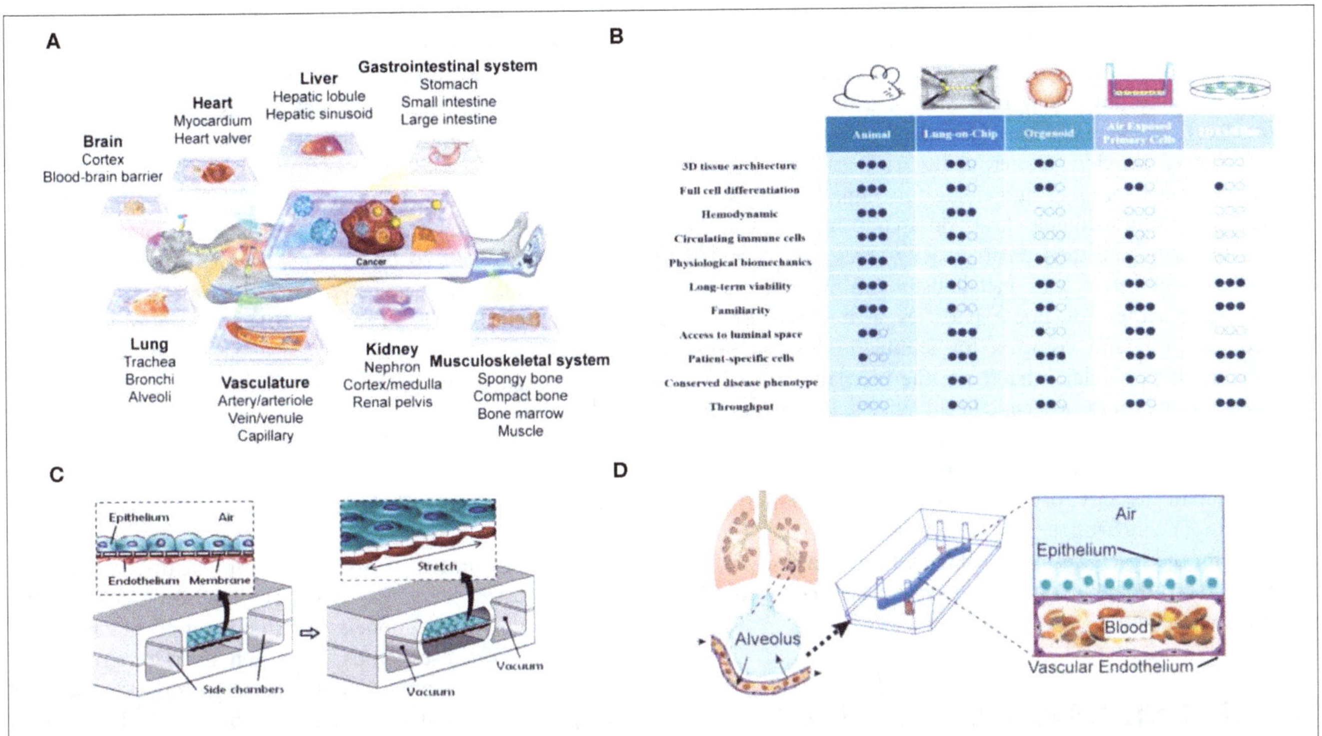

FIGURE 3 | Organs-on-chips technology for tissue model development. **(A)** Organs-on-chips platform provides an *in vitro* model of various organs. Reproduced with permission from Zhang et al. (2017). **(B)** Comparison of experimental strategies for current *in vitro*, *in vivo*, and Organs-on-chips models. Adapted with permission from Nawroth et al. (2019). **(C)** A lung-on-a-chip microdevice reproduce human physiological respiratory movements. Reproduced with permission from Huh et al. (2010). **(D)** Construction of a lung-on-a-chip with tissue/organ-level physical microstructure and microenvironment. Reproduced with permission from Jain et al. (2018).

LUNG-ON-A-CHIP

Although different organs-on-chips have their own requirements, applications associated with the respiratory tract are always very strong. For example, when the lungs are infected by fine PM, bacteria, or viruses, white blood cells accumulate, and the mucus produced block the airway. These processes are difficult to observe in animals and further highlight the importance of developing lung-on-a-chip technology. The Wyss Institute at Harvard University has been a worldwide pioneer in the development of *in vitro* organ-on-a-chip, and the lung-on-a-chip they developed was the first in the world (Huh et al., 2010) (**Figures 3C,D**). It is entirely based on polydimethylsiloxane (PDMS) material, with an upper and a lower layer of channels separated by a porous membrane coated with extracellular matrix. In its internal structure, the upper layer consists of alveolar epithelial cells that allow gases to pass through, and the lower layer consists of microvascular epithelial cells that allow white blood cells to pass through, thus simulating lung function. In 2016, Benam et al. used this technology to test smoking and non-smoking conditions, and confirmed that using the lung-on-a-chip yielded experimental results that were closer to clinical physiological and inflammatory reactions compared with those from animal experiments, and previously undiscovered biomarkers that were even more accurate were found and analyzed (Benam et al., 2016a). At the same time, other teams have developed lung chip models with different design structures and physiological responses (Fishler et al., 2015; Fishler and Sznitman, 2016; Humayun et al., 2018; Stucki et al., 2018; Khalid et al., 2020). The lung-on-a-chip have been developed to demonstrate their importance in drug development and disease models, but still have several practical challenges must be overcome if such devices are to be used in toxicology research and application (Low and Tagle, 2017; Wu et al., 2020). The aim of overcoming these challenges is to improve the usability of these devices and to simulate metabolism in the human body more accurately.

HEART-ON-A-CHIP

In addition, evidence from animal studies has shown that nanoparticles can cross the alveolar-capillary barrier and subsequently deposit in extrapulmonary organs such as the vasculature and heart (Choi et al., 2010). Using specific organ chips, such as heart-on-a-chip to investigate the toxicity of PM may also have great potential value. The heart-on-a-chip is mainly used to study electrical stimulation (Xiao et al., 2014), cardiac electrophysiology (Sidorov et al., 2017) and disease models (Wang et al., 2014). Marsano et al. recently established heart-on-a-chip platform integrates mechanical stress and 3D matrix microenvironment, showing better differentiation and electromechanical coupling of the iPSC-derived cardiomyocyte (Marsano et al., 2016). Liu *et al.* demonstrated the latest bioelectronic heart-on-a-chip model, which can regulate the concentration of oxygen through the microfluidic channel, and integrated bioelectronic devices to successfully monitor the cardiac electrophysiology responses to acute hypoxia (Liu et al., 2020). These examples fully demonstrate that heart-on-a-chip may provide greater ability to recapitulation the cellular microenvironment and tissue function. In the future, it is expected that suitable heart-on-a-chip models can be selected to investigate the human toxicity investigation of PM deposition, penetration and metabolism, but it is necessary to consider whether to choose particles with corresponding size, composition and complex for stimulation or exposure assessment. Of particular interest are the mechanisms of PM-mediated toxicity on the systemic health effects. In recent years, with the gradual advancement of multi-organ chips technology, it is expected to provide more clues to accelerate the clarification of the human toxicity of PM deposition, penetration and metabolism (Yuancheng et al., 2018; Carvalho et al., 2019), especially for the specific examples of lung- heart- on chip model, which could be used to investigate the systemic toxicology of PM into the human body.

OPPORTUNITIES AND CHALLENGES

It is worth mentioning that the organ-on-a-chip not only shows the application value in research, but also the establishment of related companies has started to appear in the past 5 years (Mastrangeli et al., 2019), such as TissUse GmbH, Emulate, Inc., MIMETAS Inc., Nortis, Inc., AlveoliX AG., Hesperos Inc.. In addition, the U.S. Food and Drug Administration (FDA) announced in April 2017 that it had signed a multi-year cooperation agreement with Emulate Inc. (spinoff from the Wyss Institute for Biologically Inspired Engineering at Harvard University), and will begin a series of trials using organ-on-a-chip technology to develop a testing platform for toxicological safety assessment (Isoherranen et al., 2019). These results demonstrate the potential of applying organ-on-a-chip systems to human health assessments. In the future, the organ-on-a-chip technology is able to integrate stem cell technology, microenvironment and personalization parameters (e.g., breathing pattern, heart rate, substance abuse, etc.) to allow the construction of models of different genders, regions, ages, and diseases to minute minor physiological differences, thereby promoting the development of precision health (van den Berg et al., 2019).

Despite the progress made with organ-on-a-chip models, there remains a question that the organ-level functional replication is limited by the source of cells. In the case of pulmonary alveolar model, the aspect of long-term culture of primary human alveolar type I and type II epithelial cells is particularly challenging limitation (Shiraishi et al., 2019; Weiner et al., 2019). Therefore, the organ-on-a-chip technology faces limited availability and the inability to expand primary cells, requiring the establishment of cell cultures directly from donors and patients, which will increase the cost of experiments and the difficulty of popularizing the technology. On the other hand, the most organ-on-a-chip are made of PDMS due to their high biocompatibility, oxygen permeability, and transparency. The PDMS chip devices can directly match conventional cell culture incubators and biological microscopes. However, a large amount of protein molecules will be adsorbed on the surface of PDMS (Wong and Ho, 2009; Gokaltun et al., 2017), which results in that the supplement or stimulating substance of the cell culture cannot fully interact with the cells. To avoid adsorption of non-specific proteins, some teams have used polylactic acid (PLA) (Ongaro et al., 2020), poly (methyl methacrylate) (PMMA) (Nguyen et al., 2019), polystyrene (PS) (Lee et al., 2018), and polycarbonate (PC) (Henry et al., 2017), and more advantages and limitations of PDMS materials also have been introduced in detail by other teams (Halldorsson et al., 2015; Gokaltun et al., 2017).

MULTI-ORGAN CHIPS

With the development of organs-on-chips in the past decade, the establishment of single types of organ-on-a-chip or the development of disease models on a chip has gradually matured. Although the organ-on-chips have seen great progress, it is not enough to rely on a simulation single organ model for a comprehensive understanding due to the highly complex interactions between human organs. In 2004, Dr. Shuler and colleagues first proposed the concept of reproducing human physiological functions in chip devices (Sin et al., 2004). The increasing demand for *in vitro* models, chips integrating multiple organs have become a major topic in recent years, and they also represent a major step forward in organ-on-a-chip technology (**Figure 4A**). Currently, chips capable of representing multiple organs in an integrated manner and fully and accurately simulating human tissue are still being developed (Skardal et al., 2017; Oleaga et al., 2018; Boos et al., 2019; Sung et al., 2019; Zhao et al., 2019). For example, a new model for physiological pharmacokinetics (PKs) and pharmacodynamics (PDs) has successfully predicted the clinical patient data of cisplatin PDs. This model is linked through fluidically coupled vascularized organ chips to investigate PK and PD parameters of oral and injectable drugs (Herland et al., 2020). It is worth noting that the experiments of this model have reached an automated system through robotic fluidic coupling of multiple organ chips, and maintained the long-term culture of organ-specific functions for 3 weeks (Novak et al., 2020). The automated multi-organ chip system integrated with high-throughput screening has the potential to improve the prediction of drugs (or other foreign substances) absorption, distribution, metabolism, excretion and toxicity for clinical trials.

As another example, the device in a recent study mainly integrates four tissues—liver, heart, muscle, and neurons (Oleaga et al., 2016). It is composed of the liver (which serves to process drug metabolites and drug processes drugs or prodrugs), heart (which is the most important organ in the human body), skeletal muscle (which is responsible for glucose storage levels in the body), and neurons (which represent a particularly sensitive cell system). After culturing this system in a continuous flow environment for 14 days, its feasibility and

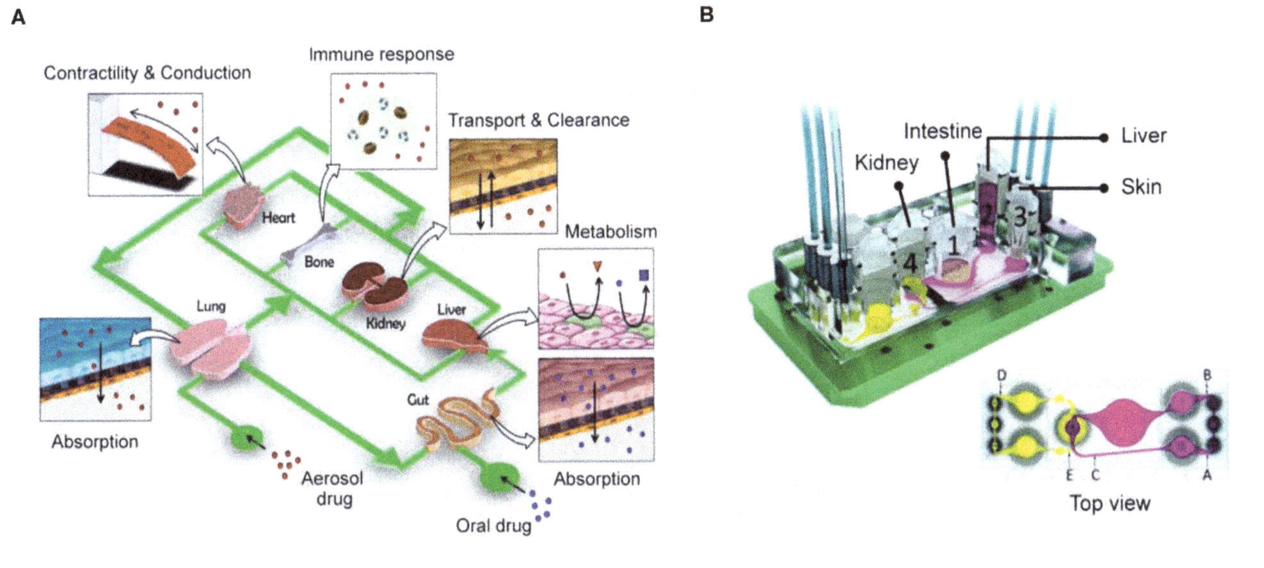

FIGURE 4 | Integrate multi-organ chip platforms to create complex interactions between human organs. **(A)** The design concept of the human body chip. One of the most promising *in vitro* system for replicating the systemic responses of human body. Reproduced with permission from Huh et al. (2011). **(B)** Four-organs-on-a-chip system employed intestine, liver, skin, and kidney tissue that proportionately simulated the physiological environment of the human body. Reproduced with permission from Maschmeyer et al. (2015).

functionality were demonstrated, and because the cells used in the system were primary cells and cells derived from iPSCs, they exhibited the exchange of metabolites and signaling molecules. In addition, by measuring heart rate, muscle contractility, neuroelectrophysiology, and production of liver albumin and urea, it served as an accurate model for predicting toxicity in multiple human organs. In another study, Maschmeyer et al. integrated pre-formed bowel and skin models into a hepatic spheroid and renal epithelial barrier tissue model, establishing a microchannel system that could support the functions of four types of organs in a co-culture over a long period of 1 month (Maschmeyer et al., 2015) (**Figure 4B**). In addition, this four-organs-on-a-chip system employed a structure that more proportionately simulated the physiological fluid and tissue environment of the human body. It simulated drug absorption and metabolism in the small intestine, metabolism by the liver, and excretion by the kidneys, which are all key factors that determine the efficacy and safety of drug treatments. These systems allow us to further understand metabolic and genetic analyses and provide an alternative to systemic toxicity testing. In addition, these examples demonstrate that integrated multi-organ chips are an important part in the ability to simulate complex reactions and interactions between tissues, whether in drug testing, toxicological screening, or construction of organ-on-a-chip models.

Therefore, integrating multi-organ chips are expected to replace the inadequacies of traditional *in vitro* models, promoting studies of the effects of air pollution on the body and the early development of drugs, as these devices are designed to mimic the physiological structure of internal organs and interactions with soluble metabolites, thereby achieving *in vitro* the interactive effects between organs. However, current multi-organ chip models are mainly used for systemic processes of oral and injectable drugs, but lacks models for PM inhalation. In a recent human inhalation study, Miller et al. investigated the transport behavior of gold nanoparticle inhaled into the lung (Miller et al., 2017). The results showed that the blood and urine of the volunteers still found gold nanoparticle after 3 months of exposure, indicating systemic retention and delayed urinary excretion. This study clearly understands the ability of inhaled nanoparticles to penetrate lung tissue, but investigating the interactions between human organs, especially for the cardiopulmonary system remains a challenge. Based on the most direct impact of PM on cardiopulmonary function, in the future, it is urgent to form an integrated platform by connecting the organ chips of the lung and heart in the future. Even PM gas can be exposed to such a platform for discussion. It is hoped that the cardiopulmonary function model established *in vitro* can be used to obtain new possibilities and opportunities for PM analysis, so that it can more effectively clarify the impact of PM on the human body *in vitro* and find out the causes of cardiopulmonary diseases.

OUTLOOK

In addition to well-known respiratory diseases such as COPD, fine PM in the air that is inhaled into the lungs are translocated to the bloodstream and transported to the blood vessels and heart, where they induce arrhythmia, reduce myocardial contractility, and reduce coronary blood flow, thereby increasing the incidence and mortality of cardiopulmonary diseases. Related studies have shown that the harmful effects of fine PM on health may reach an uncontrollable point by 2030. Therefore, it is essential to quickly and accurately elucidate their effects on the

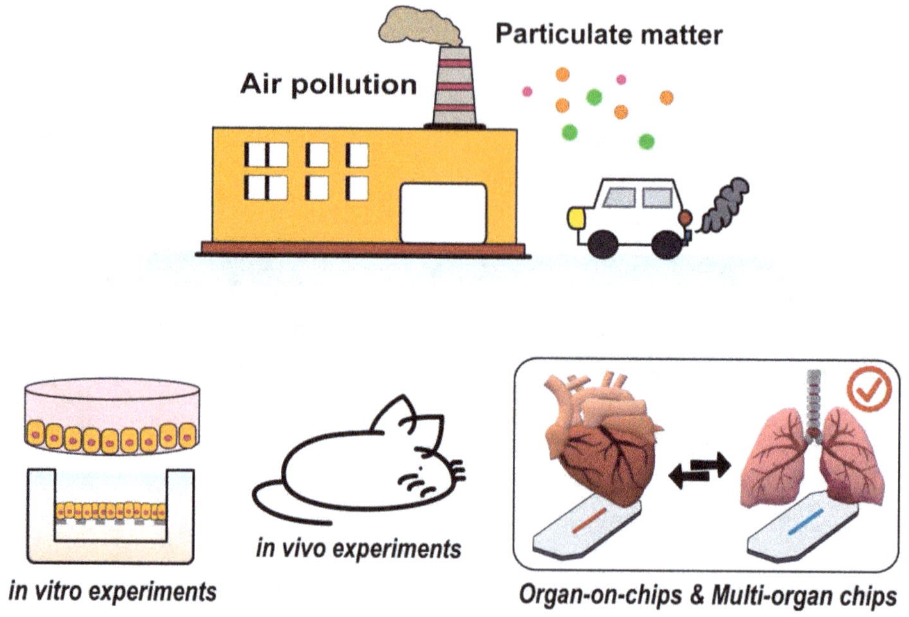

FIGURE 5 | The potential value of organ-on-a-chip biomimetic technology for PM toxicity. Its 3D microenvironment and biomimetic circulating air/liquid dynamic environment are expected to be used for PM health assessment.

human body, determine the causes of disease, and formulate response strategies.

Although epidemiological and clinical studies have produced much evidence of the effects of fine PM on human health, it has not yet been fully explained how physiological responses and cellular and molecular mechanisms of change and injury are caused. Currently, most health evaluation studies of fine PM are conducted through cell culture or animal experiments. Cell-based studies are still greatly limited compared to the complex structures of physiological mechanisms in humans, and it is impossible to simulate the complex conditions and the interrelated physiological information of the entire organism. Animal experiments play an important role in studies on fine PM, where they allow *in vivo* toxicological testing by exposing animals to various fine PM environments via the oral and dermal routes. Although animals can inhale fine PM and develop comprehensive systemic outcomes, there is often a large difference between mechanistic and genetic indicator data and clinical outcomes. This is primarily due to differences among species and their physiological functions, such as differences in respiratory rate between experimental mice and humans, as well as the problems of genetics, low throughput, high cost, and ethical concerns. These reasons have caused difficulty when investigating the causes of air pollution and associated human health hazards, the analysis of biomarkers, and the development of future pollution control strategies. Organ-on-a-chip biomimetic technology will bring unlimited potential for breaking through the bottlenecks faced in previous studies.

Reviewing the current development of organ-on-chips, most research focuses on drug development and disease models (Huh et al., 2012; Esch et al., 2015; Benam et al., 2016b). Except for the toxicological applications of lung-on-a-chip and cigarette smoking, other integrated studies related to environmental PM have not been extensive. According to previous reviews (see the section on Particulate matter and respiratory system and Particulate matter and cardiovascular effects), there are several clues worthy of attention such as DNA damage, inflammatory injury and PM translocation. For these research topics, it is believed that there is a great opportunity to obtain more undiscovered information by applying current organ-on-chips and multi-organ chips technology. For example, DNA damage and inflammatory injury could refer to related research on drug toxicity testing, translocation of PM could refer to related research on nanoparticle drug delivery, and further research on chronic toxicology could refer to the multi-organ chips model with PKs and PDs parameters. On the other hand, organ-on-a-chip systems have been shown to be closer to clinical physiology and inflammatory response, compared to traditional experimental model approaches. It has the potential to be a useful *in vitro* model for investigating the relationship between PM and related diseases. Therefore, the successful development of *in vitro* chips for simulating organs is a necessary avenue toward modern assessment of the health effects of air pollution. Its rapid and efficient screening capabilities are expected to help governmental agencies and the clinical sector move toward the correct policy and drug development routes, reduce costs, and significantly shorten the process of drug and foreign substance toxicity testing (Ronaldson-Bouchard and Vunjak-Novakovic, 2018).

The technology is still evolving from single organ to multi-organ chips, it is expected to be realized as a long-term and highly active cardiopulmonary chip. Its 3D microenvironment and more biomimetic cyclic dynamic environment combined with fine PM are expected to be applied to health evaluation, physiological indicators, creation of cardiopulmonary disease models, and drug testing. This more precise experimental model is expected to replace existing cell culture or animal experiments and accelerate studies elucidating the effect of fine PM on the human body (**Figure 5**).

AUTHOR CONTRIBUTIONS

All authors contributed toward conceptualization, preparation, and validation of the manuscript.

REFERENCES

Ahadian, S., Civitarese, R., Bannerman, D., Mohammadi, M. H., Lu, R., Wang, E., et al. (2018). Organ-on-a-chip platforms: a convergence of advanced materials, cells, and microscale technologies. *Adv. Healthcare Mater.* 7:1700506. doi: 10.1002/adhm.201700506

Al Hanai, A. H., Antkiewicz, D. S., Hemming, J. D. C., Shafer, M. M., Lai, A. M., Arhami, M., et al. (2019). Seasonal variations in the oxidative stress and inflammatory potential of PM2.5 in Tehran using an alveolar macrophage model: the role of chemical composition and sources. *Environ. Int.* 123, 417–427. doi: 10.1016/j.envint.2018.12.023

Alépée, N., Bahinski, A., Daneshian, M., De Wever, B., Fritsche, E., Goldberg, A., et al. (2014). State-of-the-art of 3D cultures (organs-on-a-chip) in safety testing and pathophysiology. *ALTEX* 31, 441–477. doi: 10.14573/altex140 6111

Analitis, A., Katsouyanni, K., Dimakopoulou, K., Samoli, E., Nikoloulopoulos, A. K., Petasakis, Y., et al. (2006). Short-term effects of ambient particles on cardiovascular and respiratory mortality. *Epidemiology* 17, 230–233. doi: 10.1097/01.ede.0000199439.57655.6b

Anderson, J. O., Thundiyil, J. G., and Stolbach, A. (2012). Clearing the air: a review of the effects of particulate matter air pollution on human health. *J. Med. Toxicol.* 8, 166–175. doi: 10.1007/s13181-011-0203-1

Batterman, S., Xu, L., Chen, F., Chen, F., and Zhong, X. (2016). Characteristics of PM(2.5) concentrations across Beijing during 2013-2015. *Atmos. Environ.* 145, 104–114. doi: 10.1016/j.atmosenv.2016.08.060

Benam, K. H., Novak, R., Nawroth, J., Hirano-Kobayashi, M., Ferrante, T. C., Choe, Y., et al. (2016a). Matched-comparative modeling of normal and diseased human airway responses using a microengineered breathing lung chip. *Cell Syst.* 3, 456–466.e454. doi: 10.1016/j.cels.2016.10.003

Benam, K. H., Villenave, R., Lucchesi, C., Varone, A., Hubeau, C., Lee, H.-H., et al. (2016b). Small airway-on-a-chip enables analysis of human lung inflammation and drug responses *in vitro*. *Nat. Methods* 13, 151–157. doi: 10.1038/nmeth.3697

Bennett, B. A., Spannhake, E. W., Rule, A. M., Breysse, P. N., and Tankersley, C. G. (2018). The acute effects of age and particulate matter exposure on heart rate and heart rate variability in Mice. *Cardiovasc. Toxicol.* 18, 507–519. doi: 10.1007/s12012-018-9461-3

Boos, J. A., Misun, P. M., Michlmayr, A., Hierlemann, A., and Frey, O. (2019). Microfluidic multitissue platform for advanced embryotoxicity testing *in vitro*. *Adv. Sci.* 6:1900294. doi: 10.1002/advs.201900294

Brown, J. S., Gordon, T., Price, O., and Asgharian, B. (2013). Thoracic and respirable particle definitions for human health risk assessment. *Part. Fibre Toxicol.* 10:12. doi: 10.1186/1743-89 77-10-12

Carvalho, M. R., Barata, D., Teixeira, L. M., Giselbrecht, S., Reis, R. L., et al. (2019). Colorectal tumor-on-a-chip system: a 3D tool for precision onco-nanomedicine. *Sci. Adv.* 5:eaaw1317. doi: 10.1126/sciadv.aaw1317

Choi, H. S., Ashitate, Y., Lee, J. H., Kim, S. H., Matsui, A., Insin, N., et al. (2010). Rapid translocation of nanoparticles from the lung airspaces to the body. *Nat. Biotechnol.* 28, 1300–1303. doi: 10.1038/ nbt.1696

Cochrane, A., Albers, H. J., Passier, R., Mummery, C. L., van den Berg, A., Orlova, V. V., et al. (2019). Advanced *in vitro* models of vascular biology: human induced pluripotent stem cells and organ-on-chip technology. *Adv. Drug Deliv. Rev.* 140, 68–77. doi: 10.1016/j.addr.2018. 06.007

Costa, J., and Ahluwalia, A. (2019). Advances and current challenges in intestinal *in vitro* model engineering: a digest. *Front. Bioeng. Biotechnol.* 7:144. doi: 10.3389/fbioe.2019.00144

Curbani, F., de Oliveira Busato, F., Marcarini do Nascimento, M., Olivieri, D. N., and Tadokoro, C. E. (2019). Inhale, exhale: why particulate matter exposure in animal models are so acute? Data and facts behind the history. *Data Brief.* 25:104237. doi: 10.1016/j.dib.2019.104237

de Oliveira, A. A. F., de Oliveira, T. F., Dias, M. F., Medeiros, M. H. G., Di Mascio, P., Veras, M., et al. (2018). Genotoxic and epigenotoxic effects in mice exposed to concentrated ambient fine particulate matter (PM2.5) from São Paulo city, Brazil. *Part. Fibre Toxicol.* 15:40. doi: 10.1186/s12989-018-0276-y

de Oliveira, B. F. A., Ignotti, E., Artaxo, P., do Nascimento Saldiva, P. H., Junger, W. L., and Hacon, S. (2012). Risk assessment of PM2.5 to child residents in Brazilian Amazon region with biofuel production. *Environ. Health* 11:64. doi: 10.1186/1476-069X-11-64

Donaldson, K., Beswick, P. H., and Gilmour, P. S. (1996). Free radical activity associated with the surface of particles: a unifying factor in determining biological activity? *Toxicol. Lett.* 88, 293–298. doi: 10.1016/0378-4274(96)03752-6

Du, Y., Xu, X., Chu, M., Guo, Y., and Wang, J. (2016). Air particulate matter and cardiovascular disease: the epidemiological, biomedical and clinical evidence. *J. Thorac. Dis.* 8, E8–E19. doi: 10.3978/j.issn.2072-1439.2015.11.37

Esch, E. W., Bahinski, A., and Huh, D. (2015). Organs-on-chips at the frontiers of drug discovery. *Nat. Rev. Drug Discov.* 14, 248–260. doi: 10.1038/nrd4539

Fishler, R., Hofemeier, P., Etzion, Y., Dubowski, Y., and Sznitman, J. (2015). Particle dynamics and deposition in true-scale pulmonary acinar models. *Sci. Rep.* 5:14071. doi: 10.1038/srep14071

Fishler, R., and Sznitman, J. (2016). A microfluidic model of biomimetically breathing pulmonary acinar airways. *J. Vis. Exp.* 9:53588. doi: 10.3791/ 53588

Fröhlich, E., and Salar-Behzadi, S. (2014). Toxicological assessment of inhaled nanoparticles: role of *in vivo, ex vivo, in vitro,* and *in silico* studies. *Int. J. Mol. Sci.* 15, 4795–4822. doi: 10.3390/ijms15034795

Fu, P., Guo, X., Cheung, F. M. H., and Yung, K. K. L. (2019). The association between PM2.5 exposure and neurological disorders: a systematic review and meta-analysis. *Sci. Total Environ.* 655, 1240–1248. doi: 10.1016/j.scitotenv.2018.11.218

Fuentes-Mattei, E., Rivera, E., Gioda, A., Sanchez-Rivera, D., Roman-Velazquez, F. R., and Jimenez-Velez, B. D. (2010). Use of human bronchial epithelial cells (BEAS-2B) to study immunological markers resulting from exposure to PM(2.5) organic extract from Puerto Rico. *Toxicol. Appl. Pharmacol.* 243, 381–389. doi: 10.1016/j.taap.2009.12.009

Geraili, A., Jafari, P., Hassani, M. S., Araghi, B. H., Mohammadi, M. H., Ghafari, A. M., et al. (2018). Controlling differentiation of stem cells for developing personalized organ-on-chip platforms. *Adv. Healthc. Mater.* 7:1700426. doi: 10.1002/adhm.201700426

Gokaltun, A., Yarmush, M. L., Asatekin, A., and Usta, O. B. (2017). Recent advances in nonbiofouling PDMS surface modification strategies applicable to microfluidic technology. *Tech. Singap. World Sci.* 5, 1–12. doi: 10.1142/S2339547817300013

Guo, C., Zhang, Z., Lau, A. K. H., Lin, C. Q., Chuang, Y. C., Chan, J., et al. (2018). Effect of long-term exposure to fine particulate matter on lung function decline and risk of chronic obstructive pulmonary disease in Taiwan: a longitudinal, cohort study. *Lancet Planet. Health* 2, e114–e125. doi: 10.1016/S2542-5196(18)30028-7

Halldorsson, S., Lucumi, E., Gómez-Sjöberg, R., and Fleming, R. M. T. (2015). Advantages and challenges of microfluidic cell culture in polydimethylsiloxane devices. *Biosens. Bioelectro.* 63, 218–231. doi: 10.1016/j.bios.2014.07.029

Hamanaka, R. B., and Mutlu, G. M. (2018). Particulate matter air pollution: effects on the cardiovascular system. *Front. Endocrinol.* 9:680. doi: 10.3389/fendo.2018.00680

He, F., Liao, B., Pu, J., Li, C., Zheng, M., Huang, L., et al. (2017). Exposure to ambient particulate matter induced COPD in a rat model and a description of the underlying mechanism. *Sci. Rep.* 7:45666. doi: 10.1038/srep45666

Henry, O. Y. F., Villenave, R., Cronce, M. J., Leineweber, W. D., Benz, M. A., and Ingber, D. E. (2017). Organs-on-chips with integrated electrodes for trans-epithelial electrical resistance (TEER) measurements of human epithelial barrier function. *Lab Chip.* 17, 2264–2271. doi: 10.1039/C7LC00155J

Herland, A., Maoz, B. M., Das, D., Somayaji, M. R., Prantil-Baun, R., Novak, R., et al. (2020). Quantitative prediction of human pharmacokinetic responses to drugs via fluidically coupled vascularized organ chips. *Nat. Biomed. Eng.* 4, 421–436. doi: 10.1038/s41551-019-0498-9

Hong, Z., Guo, Z., Zhang, R., Xu, J., Dong, W., Zhuang, G., et al. (2016). Airborne fine particulate matter induces oxidative stress and inflammation in human nasal epithelial cells. *Tohoku J. Exp. Med.* 239, 117–125. doi: 10.1620/tjem.239.117

Hopke, P. K., Croft, D., Zhang, W., Lin, S., Masiol, M., Squizzato, S., et al. (2019). Changes in the acute response of respiratory diseases to PM2.5 in New York State from 2005 to 2016. *Sci. Total Environ.* 677, 328–339. doi: 10.1016/j.scitotenv.2019.04.357

Huang, W., Wang, L., Li, J., Liu, M., Xu, H., Liu, S., et al. (2018). Short-term blood pressure responses to ambient fine particulate matter exposures at the extremes of global air pollution concentrations. *Am. J. Hypertens.* 31, 590–599. doi: 10.1093/ajh/hpx216

Huh, D., Hamilton, G. A., and Ingber, D. E. J. T. (2011). From 3D cell culture to organs-on-chips. *Trends Cell Biol.* 21, 745–754. doi: 10.1016/j.tcb.2011.09.005

Huh, D., Leslie, D. C., Matthews, B. D., Fraser, J. P., Jurek, S., Hamilton, G. A., et al. (2012). A human disease model of drug toxicity–induced pulmonary edema in a lung-on-a-chip microdevice. *Sci. Transl. Med.* 4:159ra147. doi: 10.1126/scitranslmed.3004249

Huh, D., Matthews, B. D., Mammoto, A., Montoya-Zavala, M., Hsin, H. Y., and Ingber, D. E. (2010). Reconstituting organ-level lung functions on a chip. *Science* 328, 1662–1668. doi: 10.1126/science.1188302

Humayun, M., Chow, C.-W., and Young, E. W. K. (2018). Microfluidic lung airway-on-a-chip with arrayable suspended gels for studying epithelial and smooth muscle cell interactions. *Lab Chip.* 18, 1298–1309. doi: 10.1039/C7LC01357D

Isoherranen, N., Madabushi, R., and Huang, S.-M. (2019). Emerging role of organ-on-a-chip technologies in quantitative clinical pharmacology evaluation. *Clin. Transl. Sci.* 12, 113–121. doi: 10.1111/cts.12627

Jain, A., Barrile, R., van der Meer, A., Mammoto, A., Mammoto, T., De Ceunynck, K., et al. (2018). Primary human lung alveolus-on-a-chip model of intravascular thrombosis for assessment of therapeutics. *Clin. Pharmacol. Ther.* 103, 332–340. doi: 10.1002/cpt.742

Jia, Y.-Y., Wang, Q., and Liu, T. (2017). Toxicity Research of PM(2.5) Compositions *in vitro*. *Int. J. Environ. Res. Public Health.* 14:232. doi: 10.3390/ijerph14030232

Jodat, Y. A., Kang, M. G., Kiaee, K., Kim, G. J., Martinez, A. F. H., Rosenkranz, A., et al. (2018). Human-derived organ-on-a-chip for personalized drug development. *Curr. Pharm. Des.* 24, 5471–5486. doi: 10.2174/1381612825666190308150055

Khalid, M. A. U., Kim, Y. S., Ali, M., Lee, B. G., Cho, Y.-J., and Choi, K. H. (2020). A lung cancer-on-chip platform with integrated biosensors for physiological monitoring and toxicity assessment. *Biochem. Eng. J.* 15:107469. doi: 10.1016/j.bej.2019.107469

Khaniabadi, Y. O., Sicard, P., Takdastan, A., Hopke, P. K., Taiwo, A. M., Khaniabadi, F. O., et al. (2019). Mortality and morbidity due to ambient air pollution in Iran. *Clin. Epidemiol. Glob. Health* 7, 222–227. doi: 10.1016/j.cegh.2018.06.006

Kido, T., Tamagawa, E., Bai, N., Suda, K., Yang, H.-H. C., Li, Y., et al. (2011). Particulate matter induces translocation of IL-6 from the lung to the systemic circulation. *Am. J. Respir. Cell Mol. Biol.* 44, 197–204. doi: 10.1165/rcmb.2009-0427OC

Kim, D., Chen, Z., Zhou, L.-F., and Huang, S.-X. (2018). Air pollutants and early origins of respiratory diseases. *Chronic Dis. Transl. Med.* 4, 75–94. doi: 10.1016/j.cdtm.2018.03.003

Kim, K.-H., Kabir, E., and Kabir, S. (2015). A review on the human health impact of airborne particulate matter. *Environ. Int.* 74, 136–143. doi: 10.1016/j.envint.2014.10.005

Lee, Y., Choi, J. W., Yu, J., Park, D., Ha, J., Son, K., et al. (2018). Microfluidics within a well: an injection-molded plastic array 3D culture platform. *Lab Chip.* 18, 2433–2440. doi: 10.1039/C8LC00336J

Li, G., Fang, C., Wang, S., and Sun, S. (2016). The effect of economic growth, urbanization, and industrialization on fine particulate matter (PM2.5) concentrations in China. *Environ. Sci. Technol.* 50, 11452–11459. doi: 10.1021/acs.est.6b02562

Li, R., Kou, X., Geng, H., Xie, J., Yang, Z., Zhang, Y., et al. (2015). Effect of ambient PM2.5 on lung mitochondrial damage and fusion/fission gene expression in rats. *Chem. Res. Toxicol.* 28, 408–418. doi: 10.1021/tx5003723

Li, T., Hu, R., Chen, Z., Li, Q., Huang, S., Zhu, Z., et al. (2018). Fine particulate matter [PM(2.5)]: the culprit for chronic lung diseases in China. *Chronic Dis. Transl. Med.* 4, 176–186. doi: 10.1016/j.cdtm.2018.07.002

Lin, Y., Zou, J., Yang, W., and Li, C.-Q. (2018). A review of recent advances in research on PM2.5 in China. *Int. J. Environ. Res. Public Health.* 15:438. doi: 10.3390/ijerph15030438

Liu, H., Bolonduro, O. A., Hu, N., Ju, J., Rao, A. A., Duffy, B. M., et al. (2020). Heart-on-a-chip model with integrated extra- and intracellular bioelectronics for monitoring cardiac electrophysiology under acute hypoxia. *Nano Lett.* 20, 2585–2593. doi: 10.1021/acs.nanolett.0c00076

Lodovici, M., and Bigagli, E. (2011). Oxidative stress and air pollution exposure. *J. Toxicol.* 2011:487074. doi: 10.1155/2011/487074

Löndahl, J., Pagels, J., Swietlicki, E., Zhou, J., Ketzel, M., Massling, A., et al. (2006). A set-up for field studies of respiratory tract deposition of fine and ultrafine particles in humans. *J. Aerosol Sci.* 37, 1152–1163. doi: 10.1016/j.jaerosci.2005.11.004

Low, L. A., and Tagle, D. A. (2017). Organs-on-chips: progress, challenges, and future directions. *Exp. Biol. Med. (Maywood)* 242, 1573–1578. doi: 10.1177/1535370217700523

Marsano, A., Conficconi, C., Lemme, M., Occhetta, P., Gaudiello, E., Votta, E., et al. (2016). Beating heart on a chip: a novel microfluidic platform to generate functional 3D cardiac microtissues. *Lab Chip.* 16, 599–610. doi: 10.1039/C5LC01356A

Maschmeyer, I., Lorenz, A. K., Schimek, K., Hasenberg, T., Ramme, A. P., Hübner, J., et al. (2015). A four-organ-chip for interconnected long-term co-culture of human intestine, liver, skin and kidney equivalents. *Lab Chip.* 15, 2688–2699. doi: 10.1039/C5LC00392J

Mastrangeli, M., Millet, S., and van den Eijnden-van Raaij, J. (2019). Organ-on-chip in development: towards a roadmap for organs-on-chip. *ALTEX* 36, 650–668. doi: 10.14573/altex.1908271

Miller, M. R., Raftis, J. B., Langrish, J. P., McLean, S. G., Samutrtai, P., Connell, S. P., et al. (2017). Inhaled nanoparticles accumulate at sites of vascular disease. *ACS Nano.* 11, 4542–4552. doi: 10.1021/acsnano.6b08551

Nadeau, K., McDonald-Hyman, C., Noth, E. M., Pratt, B., Hammond, S. K., Balmes, J., et al. (2010). Ambient air pollution impairs regulatory T-cell function in asthma. *J. Allergy Clin. Immunol.* 126, 845–852.e810. doi: 10.1016/j.jaci.2010.08.008

Nawroth, J. C., Barrile, R., Conegliano, D., van Riet, S., Hiemstra, P. S., and Villenave, R. (2019). Stem cell-based lung-on-chips: the best of both worlds? *Adv. Drug Deliv. Rev.* 140, 12–32. doi: 10.1016/j.addr.2018.07.005

Nemmar, A., Hoet, P. H. M., Dinsdale, D., Vermylen, J., Hoylaerts, M. F., and Nemery, B. (2003). Diesel exhaust particles in lung acutely enhance experimental peripheral thrombosis. *Circulation* 107, 1202–1208. doi: 10.1161/01.CIR.0000053568.13058.67

Nemmar, A., Hoet, P. H. M., Vanquickenborne, B., Dinsdale, D., Thomeer, M., Hoylaerts, M. F., et al. (2002). Passage of inhaled particles into the blood circulation in humans. *Circulation* 105, 411–414. doi: 10.1161/hc0402.104118

Nemmar, A., Holme, J. A., Rosas, I., Schwarze, P. E., and Alfaro-Moreno, E. (2013). Recent advances in particulate matter and nanoparticle toxicology: a review of the *in vivo* and *in vitro* studies. *BioMed. Res. Int.* 2013:279371. doi: 10.1155/2013/279371

Ngoc, L. T. N., Kim, M., Bui, V. K. H., Park, D., and Lee, Y.-C. (2018). Particulate matter exposure of passengers at bus stations: a review. *Int. J. Environ. Res. Public Health.* 15:E2886. doi: 10.3390/ijerph15122886

Nguyen, T., Jung, S. H., Lee, M. S., Park, T.-E., Ahn, S. K., and Kang, J. H. (2019). Robust chemical bonding of PMMA microfluidic devices to porous PETE membranes for reliable cytotoxicity testing of drugs. *Lab Chip.* 19, 3706–3713. doi: 10.1039/C9LC00338J

Novak, R., Ingram, M., Marquez, S., Das, D., Delahanty, A., Herland, A., et al. (2020). Robotic fluidic coupling and interrogation of multiple vascularized organ chips. *Nat. Biomed. Eng.*4, 407–420.

Oleaga, C., Bernabini, C., Smith, A. S. T., Srinivasan, B., Jackson, M., McLamb, W., et al. (2016). Multi-organ toxicity demonstration in a functional human *in vitro* system composed of four organs. *Sci. Rep.* 6:20030. doi: 10.1038/srep20030

Oleaga, C., Riu, A., Rothemund, S., Lavado, A., McAleer, C. W., Long, C. J., et al. (2018). Investigation of the effect of hepatic metabolism on off-target cardiotoxicity in a multi-organ human-on-a-chip system. *Biomaterials* 182, 176–190. doi: 10.1016/j.biomaterials.2018.07.062

Ongaro, A. E., Giuseppe, D. D., Kermanizadeh, A., Crespo, A. M., Mencatti, A., Ghibelli, L., et al. (2020). Polylactic is a sustainable, low absorption, low autofluorescence alternative to other plastics for microfluidic and organ-on-chip applications. *Anal. Chem.* 92, 6693–6701. doi: 10.1021/acs.analchem.0c00651

Øvrevik, J., Refsnes, M., Låg, M., and Holme, J. A., Schwarze, P.E. (2015). Activation of proinflammatory responses in cells of the airway mucosa by particulate matter: oxidant- and non-oxidant-mediated triggering mechanisms. *Biomolecules* 5, 1399–1440. doi: 10.3390/biom5031399

Park, M., Joo, H. S., Lee, K., Jang, M., Kim, S. D., Kim, I., et al. (2018). Differential toxicities of fine particulate matters from various sources. *Sci. Rep.* 8:17007. doi: 10.1038/s41598-018-35398-0

Peixoto, M. S., de Oliveira Galvão, M. F., and de Batistuzzo Medeiros, S. R. (2017). Cell death pathways of particulate matter toxicity. *Chemosphere* 188, 32–48. doi: 10.1016/j.chemosphere.2017.08.076

Raabe, O. G. (1976). Aerosol aerodynamic size conventions for inertia! sampler calibration. *J. Air Pollut. Control Assoc.* 26, 856–860. doi: 10.1080/00022470.1976.10470329

Raaschou-Nielsen, O., Beelen, R., Wang, M., Hoek, G., Andersen, Z. J., Hoffmann, B., et al. (2016). Particulate matter air pollution components and risk for lung cancer. *Environ. Int.* 87, 66–73. doi: 10.1016/j.envint.2015.11.007

Ronaldson-Bouchard, K., and Vunjak-Novakovic, G. (2018). Organs-on-a-chip: a fast track for engineered human tissues in drug development. *Cell Stem Cell.* 22, 310–324. doi: 10.1016/j.stem.2018.02.011

Rothbauer, M., Zirath, H., and Ertl, P. (2018). Recent advances in microfluidic technologies for cell-to-cell interaction studies. *Lab Chip.* 18, 249–270. doi: 10.1039/C7LC00815E

Ryu, Y. S., Kang, K. A., Piao, M. J., Ahn, M. J., Yi, J. M., Hyun, Y.-M., et al. (2019). Particulate matter induces inflammatory cytokine production via activation of NFκB by TLR5-NOX4-ROS signaling in human skin keratinocyte and mouse skin. *Redox Biol.* 21:101080. doi: 10.1016/j.redox.2018.101080

Shadie, A. M., Herbert, C., and Kumar, R. K. (2014). Ambient particulate matter induces an exacerbation of airway inflammation in experimental asthma: role of interleukin-33. *Clin. Exp. Immunol.* 177, 491–499. doi: 10.1111/cei.12348

Shiraishi, K., Nakajima, T., Shichino, S., Deshimaru, S., Matsushima, K., and Ueha, S. (2019). *In vitro* expansion of endogenous human alveolar epithelial type II cells in fibroblast-free spheroid culture. *Biochem. Biophys. Res. Commun.* 515, 579–585. doi: 10.1016/j.bbrc.2019.05.187

Sidorov, V. Y., Samson, P. C., Sidorova, T. N., Davidson, J. M., Lim, C. C., and Wikswo, J. P. (2017). I-wire heart-on-a-chip i: three-dimensional cardiac tissue constructs for physiology and pharmacology. *Acta Biomater.* 48, 68–78. doi: 10.1016/j.actbio.2016.11.009

Sin, A., Chin, K. C., Jamil, M. F., Kostov, Y., Rao, G., and Shuler, M. L. (2004). The design and fabrication of three-chamber microscale cell culture analog devices with integrated dissolved oxygen sensors. *Nat. Rev. Mol. Cell Biol.* 20, 338–345. doi: 10.1021/bp034077d

Skardal, A., Murphy, S. V., Devarasetty, M., Mead, I., Kang, H.-W., Seol, Y.-J., et al. (2017). Multi-tissue interactions in an integrated three-tissue organ-on-a-chip platform. *Sci. Rep.* 7:8837. doi: 10.1038/s41598-017-08879-x

Snow, S. J., Henriquez, A. R., Costa, D. L., and Kodavanti, U. P. (2018). Neuroendocrine regulation of air pollution health effects: emerging insights. *Toxicol. Sci.* 164, 9–20. doi: 10.1093/toxsci/kfy129

Stucki, J. D., Hobi, N., Galimov, A., Stucki, A. O., Schneider-Daum, N., Lehr, C.-M., et al. (2018). Medium throughput breathing human primary cell alveolus-on-chip model. *Sci. Rep.* 8:14359. doi: 10.1038/s41598-018-32523-x

Sung, J. H., Wang, Y. I., Narasimhan Sriram, N., Jackson, M., Long, C., Hickman, J. J., et al. (2019). Recent advances in body-on-a-chip systems. *Anal. Chem.* 91, 330–351. doi: 10.1021/acs.analchem.8b05293

Suwa, T., Hogg, J. C., Quinlan, K. B., Ohgami, A., Vincent, R., and van Eeden, S. F. (2002). Particulate air pollution induces progression of atherosclerosis. *J. Am. Coll. Cardiol.* 39, 935–942. doi: 10.1016/S0735-1097(02)01715-1

Tsai, D.-H., Amyai, N., Marques-Vidal, P., Wang, J.-L., Riediker, M., Mooser, V., et al. (2012). Effects of particulate matter on inflammatory markers in the general adult population. *Part. Fibre Toxicol.* 9:24. doi: 10.1186/1743-8977-9-24

Tsuda, A., Henry, F. S., and Butler, J. P. (2013). Particle transport and deposition: basic physics of particle kinetics. *Compr. Physiol.* 3, 1437–1471. doi: 10.1002/cphy.c100085

Turner, M. C., Krewski, D., C., Arden Pope, I., Chen, Y., Gapstur, S. M., et al. (2011). Long-term ambient fine particulate matter air pollution and lung cancer in a large cohort of never-smokers. *Am. J. Respir. Crit. Care Med.* 184, 1374–1381. doi: 10.1164/rccm.201106-1011OC

Valavanidis, A., Fiotakis, K., Bakeas, E., and Vlahogianni, T. (2005). Electron paramagnetic resonance study of the generation of reactive oxygen species catalysed by transition metals and quinoid redox cycling by inhalable ambient particulate matter. *Redox Rep.* 10, 37–51. doi: 10.1179/135100005X 21606

van den Berg, A., Mummery, C. L., Passier, R., and van der Meer, A. D. (2019). Personalised organs-on-chips: functional testing for precision medicine. *Lab Chip.* 19, 198–205. doi: 10.1039/C8LC00827B

Vanderburgh, J., Sterling, J. A., and Guelcher, S. A. (2017). 3D printing of tissue engineered constructs for *in vitro* modeling of disease progression and drug screening. *Ann. Biomed. Eng.* 45, 164–179. doi: 10.1007/s10439-016-1640-4

Vawda, S., Mansour, R., Takeda, A., Funnell, P., Kerry, S., Mudway, I., et al. (2013). Associations between inflammatory and immune response genes and adverse respiratory outcomes following exposure to outdoor air pollution: a HuGE systematic review. *Am. J. Epidemiol.* 179, 432–442. doi: 10.1093/aje/kwt269

Wang, G., McCain, M. L., Yang, L., He, A., Pasqualini, F. S., Agarwal, A., et al. (2014). Modeling the mitochondrial cardiomyopathy of Barth syndrome with induced pluripotent stem cell and heart-on-chip technologies. *Nat. Med.* 20, 616–623. doi: 10.1038/nm.3545

Wang, H., Song, L., Ju, W., Wang, X., Dong, L., Zhang, Y., et al. (2017). The acute airway inflammation induced by PM2.5 exposure and the treatment of essential oils in Balb/c mice. *Sci. Rep.* 7:44256. doi: 10.1038/srep44256

Wang, J., Huang, J., Wang, L., Chen, C., Yang, D., Jin, M., et al. (2017). Urban particulate matter triggers lung inflammation via the ROS-MAPK-NF-κB signaling pathway. *J. Thorac. Dis.* 9, 4398–4412. doi: 10.21037/jtd.2017.09.135

Weiner, A. I., Jackson, S. R., Zhao, G., Quansah, K. K., Farshchian, J. N., Neupauer, K. M., et al. (2019). Mesenchyme-free expansion and transplantation of adult alveolar progenitor cells: steps toward cell-based regenerative therapies. *NPJ Regen. Med.* 4:17. doi: 10.1038/s41536-019-0080-9

Wong, I., and Ho, C.-M. (2009). Surface molecular property modifications for poly(dimethylsiloxane) (PDMS) based microfluidic devices. *Microfluid. Nanofluidics.* 7, 291–306. doi: 10.1007/s10404-009-0443-4

Wu, Q., Liu, J., Wang, X., Feng, L., Wu, J., Zhu, X., et al. (2020). Organ-on-a-chip: recent breakthroughs and future prospects. *Biomed. Eng. Online* 19:9. doi: 10.1186/s12938-020-0752-0

Xiao, Y., Zhang, B., Liu, H., Miklas, J. W., Gagliardi, M., Pahnke, A., et al. (2014). Microfabricated perfusable cardiac biowire: a platform that mimics native cardiac bundle. *Lab Chip.* 14, 869–882. doi: 10.1039/C3LC51123E

Xing, Y. F., Xu, Y. H., Shi, M. H., and Lian, Y. X. (2016). The impact of PM2.5 on the human respiratory system. *J. Thorac. Dis.* 8, E69–E74. doi: 10.3978/j.issn.2072-1439.2016.01.19

Xu, X., Jiang, S. Y., Wang, T.-Y., Bai, Y., Zhong, M., Wang, A., et al. (2013). Inflammatory response to fine particulate air pollution exposure: neutrophil versus monocyte. *PLoS ONE* 8:e71414. doi: 10.1371/journal.pone.0071414

Yang, Y., Qin, Z., Zeng, W., Yang, T., Cao, Y., Mei, C., et al. (2017). Toxicity assessment of nanoparticles in various systems and organs. *Nanotechnol. Rev.* 6:279. doi: 10.1515/ntrev-2016-0047

Yuancheng, L., Kai, Z., Xiao, L., and Yu Shrike, Z. (2018). Blood-vessel-on-a-chip platforms for evaluating nanoparticle drug delivery systems. *Curr. Drug Metab.* 19, 100–109. doi: 10.2174/1389200218666170925114636

Zanobetti, A., Franklin, M., Koutrakis, P., and Schwartz, J. (2009). Fine particulate air pollution and its components in association with cause-specific emergency admissions. *Environ. Health* 8:58. doi: 10.1186/1476-069X-8-58

Zhang, B., Korolj, A., Lai, B. F. L., and Radisic, M. (2018). Advances in organ-on-a-chip engineering. *Nat. Rev. Mater.* 3, 257–278. doi: 10.1038/s41578-018-0034-7

Zhang, Y. S., Zhang, Y.-N., and Zhang, W. (2017). Cancer-on-a-chip systems at the frontier of nanomedicine. *Drug Discov. Today* 22, 1392–1399. doi: 10.1016/j.drudis.2017.03.011

Zhao, Y., Kankala, R. K., Wang, S.-B., and Chen, A.-Z. (2019). Multi-organs-on-chips: towards long-term biomedical investigations. *Molecules* 24:675. doi: 10.3390/molecules24040675

7

Kinetic Analysis of Label-Free Microscale Collagen Gel Contraction using Machine Learning-Aided Image Analysis

*Cameron Yamanishi[1,2], Eric Parigoris[1,2] and Shuichi Takayama[1,2]**

[1] Wallace H. Coulter Department of Biomedical Engineering, Georgia Institute of Technology, Atlanta, GA, United States,
[2] The Parker H. Petit Institute of Bioengineering and Bioscience, Georgia Institute of Technology, Atlanta, GA, United States

Correspondence:
Shuichi Takayama
takayama@gatech.edu

Pulmonary fibrosis is a deadly lung disease, wherein normal lung tissue is progressively replaced with fibrotic scar tissue. An aspect of this process can be recreated *in vitro* by embedding fibroblasts into a collagen matrix and providing a fibrotic stimulus. This work expands upon a previously described method to print microscale cell-laden collagen gels and combines it with live cell imaging and automated image analysis to enable high-throughput analysis of the kinetics of cell-mediated contraction of this collagen matrix. The image analysis method utilizes a plugin for FIJI, built around Waikato Environment for Knowledge Analysis (WEKA) Segmentation. After cross-validation of this automated image analysis with manual shape tracing, the assay was applied to primary human lung fibroblasts including cells isolated from idiopathic pulmonary fibrosis patients. In the absence of any exogenous stimuli, the analysis showed significantly faster and more extensive contraction of the diseased cells compared to the healthy ones. Upon stimulation with transforming growth factor beta 1 (TGF-β1), fibroblasts from the healthy donor showed significantly more contraction throughout the observation period while differences in the response of diseased cells was subtle and could only be detected during a smaller window of time. Finally, dose-response curves for the inhibition of collagen gel contraction were determined for 3 small molecules including the only 2 FDA-approved drugs for idiopathic pulmonary fibrosis.

Keywords: pulmonary fibrosis, collagen contraction, fibroblasts, phenotypic assay, aqueous two-phase systems, machine learning

INTRODUCTION

Pulmonary fibrosis is a deadly lung disease, characterized by an aberrant wound healing response (Ahluwalia et al., 2014). Healthy lung parenchyma is progressively replaced with fibrotic scar tissue, reducing patients' lung capacity and often leading to death. Although progress has been made in understanding disease mechanisms, treatment options are limited to merely slowing the decline of lung function (Maher and Strek, 2019). Part of the difficulty in studying pulmonary fibrosis arises from the complex interplay between different cell types, mechanics, genetics, and the microenvironment (Ahluwalia et al., 2014; Barkauskas and Noble, 2014; Borensztajn et al., 2014; Betensley et al., 2016). Phenotypic assays, which can measure more holistic responses than gene or protein expression assays, are an important, complementary set of tools to understand cell and tissue processes (Yamanishi et al., 2019).

One of the classic phenotypic assays for pulmonary fibrosis is the collagen gel contraction assay (Bell et al., 1979). In this assay, fibroblasts are embedded into a collagen gel, which is detached from the surface of its container – usually a microplate well. Activated fibroblasts remodel the collagen gel, macroscopically shrinking the gel in a process similar to wound closure. Despite the assay's utility and reliability in cell lines, the behavior of primary lung fibroblasts can be more subtle and difficult to detect (Campbell et al., 2012; Cui et al., 2016; Jin et al., 2019). These differences arise, as primary cells have variable initial states and sensitivities to stimulation. Primary cells present additional challenges, as they have limited growth capacity. Furthermore, the throughput has previously been low, as the collagen gel contraction assay traditionally requires the user to manually detach each gel from the edges of the well with a pipet tip (Bell et al., 1979). Measurement of the contracting area has also been manual, with pictures taken daily and images traced by hand (**Figure 1A**). While some collagen contraction assays have been adapted to a 96-well format (Kondo et al., 2004; Mohan and Bargagna-Mohan, 2016; Zhang et al., 2019), these higher-throughput assays have not been universally adopted due to challenges of manual detachment and image analysis. While several techniques have been developed for automated segmentation of label-free spheroid images (Rodday et al., 2011; Chen et al., 2014), these multicellular structures generally have high contrast compared to the media; cell-laden hydrogels have lower contrast, thereby requiring more modern image analysis algorithms.

To address these issues, we explore methods to increase the throughput of the assay and incorporate high frequency imaging. Our lab has previously developed a high-throughput collagen microgel bioprinting technique that does not require manual gel detachment and demonstrated its effectiveness with cell lines (Moraes et al., 2013). In this assay, evaporation of the small microgel during the gelation process is prevented by mixing the collagen and cells with an aqueous solution of dextran (DEX), which forms an aqueous two-phase system (ATPS) with an aqueous solution of polyethylene glycol (PEG). Collagen mostly remains within the DEX phase as it gels (Singh and Tavana, 2018), while the PEG phase provides an aqueous buffer, containing the collagen and limiting evaporation. This approach may be applicable to a variety of other hydrogel systems, however, our work here focuses on collagen. In this study, we extend the ATPS collagen bioprinting technique through automated imaging and image analysis (**Figure 1B**) to examine contraction kinetics of normal vs. diseased primary human lung fibroblasts, particularly in the context of anti-fibrotic drugs. Furthermore, this high frequency of sampling aids in distinguishing the more subtle differences in primary cells, compared to the cell lines used in our initial proof of concept study (Moraes et al., 2013).

MATERIALS AND METHODS

Cell Culture

Normal human lung fibroblasts (NHLF, lot 0000655309, 56 year-old male) and idiopathic pulmonary fibrosis human lung fibroblasts (IPF, lot 0000627840, 52 year-old male) were purchased from Lonza (Walkersville, MD). These primary cells were cultured in complete Fibroblast Growth Medium (FGM-2, Lonza) and used from passages 2–5. For collagen gel contraction assays, cells were passaged into FGM-2, without serum (FGM-SF), then seeded into collagen gels the following day where they were collected at ~75% confluence.

Collagen Microgel Contraction Assay

Collagen microgel contraction assays were seeded as previously described (Moraes et al., 2013). 96-well round bottom microplates were filled with 100 μL per well of 6% (w/w) PEG, MW 35,000 (Sigma) dissolved in serum-free DMEM (Gibco) with 10% distilled water (Gibco) to adjust for osmotic pressure. This plate was warmed to 37°C in a 5% CO_2 incubator. A collagen-dextran mixture was prepared on ice, consisting of 6% (w/w) DEX T500 (Sigma), 2 mg/mL Type I bovine skin collagen (Advanced Biomatrix), and 5 mM NaOH (Sigma) to neutralize the collagen. This mixture was mixed by pipetting up and down on ice, with care taken to avoid introducing bubbles. The mixture was kept on ice while cells were prepared for seeding. Cells were washed with PBS (Gibco), then trypsinized with 0.05% Trypsin (Gibco). After the cells lifted, they were quickly diluted in FGM-SF and centrifuged at 200 × g, 5 min, room temperature. After aspirating the supernatant, cells were resuspended in 1 mL FGM-SF and counted. Appropriate volumes of resuspended cells were centrifuged again and resuspended in DMEM. The cells were then mixed 1:1 with the collagen mixture to generate a 1 mg/mL collagen, 3% DEX solution. The collagen-DEX-cell suspension was transferred to a 96-well plate for seeding, where the DEX-cell suspension would be seeded into the wells containing PEG, as in **Figure 1B**.

Liquid Handling and Imaging

As in our previous publication (Moraes et al., 2013), a Cybio FeliX liquid handler (Analytik Jena) was used to prepare collagen microgel plates (see **Supplementary File** for liquid handler script).

Collagen microgels were incubated and imaged using an Incucyte S3 (Sartorious) in-incubator microscope system. The Incucyte S3 performs auto-focus on each well of the microplate. 4x brightfield images were acquired at 1 h intervals for 2 days, then at 6 h intervals for the next 6 days.

Drug Response Studies

Cell-laden collagen microgels were stimulated with or without 10 ng/mL TGF-β1 (R&D Systems) and anti-fibrotic drugs: nintedanib (Selleck Chem), pirfenidone (Selleck Chem), and the focal adhesion kinase inhibitor PF 431396 (Tocris) at specified concentrations. These collagen microgels were imaged over 8 days to monitor contraction. To determine the half maximal inhibitory concentration (IC50), the area under the curve (AUC) of the area over time graph was calculated for each individual gel as a parameter of overall contractility. These values were normalized, such that a gel with no contraction would have a normalized AUC of 100%. These contraction responses were fit

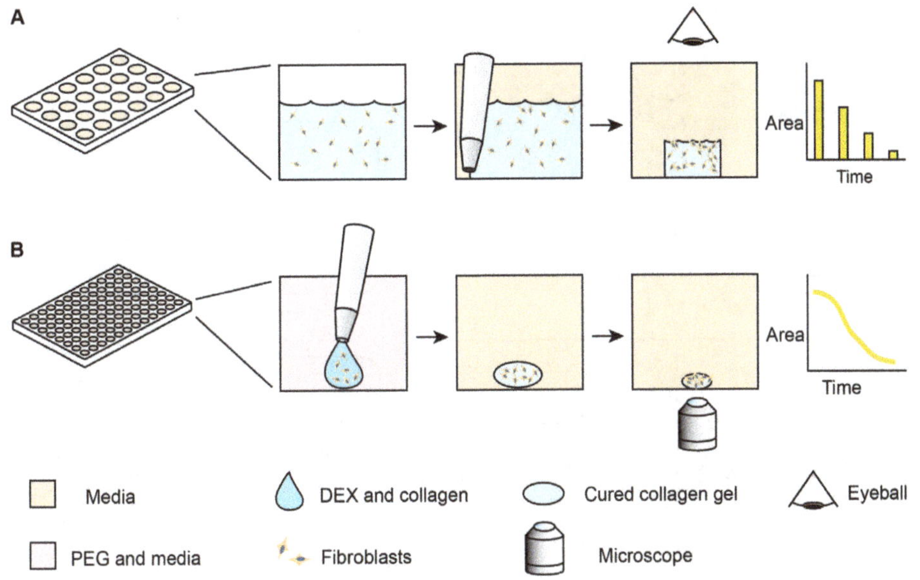

FIGURE 1 | Comparison of standard collagen contraction assay with high-throughput ATPS method presented here. **(A)** Overview of traditional collagen contraction assay in a 24-well plate. After seeding fibroblasts in a collagen matrix, the gels are individually detached from the well and imaged at discrete time intervals. **(B)** In the ATPS collagen contraction assay, DEX and collagen droplets containing fibroblasts are mixed with PEG and media in 96-well plates. This creates a microgel in the center of the well, thereby eliminating the need for individual gel removal from the wall. The PEG and DEX solutions are then washed out, and then imaged every 2 h with an Incucyte microscope.

to sigmoidal curves using the scipy module in python (Virtanen et al., 2020), using Eq. 1:

$$Response = A + \frac{100 - A}{1 + 10^{(\log(x) - \log(C))*B}} \quad (1)$$

where A is the extent of contraction in the control condition, B is the Hill Coefficient, and C is the IC50.

Image Processing

Collagen microgel areas were quantified using three methods: manual, Incucyte, and trainable WEKA segmentation. For manual quantification, gel perimeters were traced using ImageJ and areas were measured. For Incucyte quantification, images were segmented using the built-in Incucyte 2019A segmentation software from the Spheroid Module. In the trainable WEKA segmentation plugin from FIJI (ImageJ) (Arganda-Carreras et al., 2017), 1–10 representative microgel images were annotated and used to train the classifier. We wrote a new plugin (see **Supplementary File**) to iterate through a folder of images exported from the Incucyte 2019A software, apply the WEKA classifier, run quality checks, measure areas, and generate a .csv file containing areas, well positions, and times. Further analyses were performed using the pandas module in python (McKinney, 2010).

Statistical Analysis

For the comparison between manual and algorithm measurements of gel areas, the Pearsons correlation coefficient was calculated. The differences between gel contraction for +/− TGF-β1 conditions at the indicated time points were analyzed using multiple *t*-tests with a Bonferroni correction and a 95% confidence interval. Lastly, standard deviations for parameter estimates of the IC50 values in the drug dose response studies were acquired from the covariance matrix of the model fit (scipy.optimize.curve_fit module in Python).

RESULTS

Validation and Optimization of Machine Learning Image Processing

To quantify collagen microgel area, we initially examined the built-in Incucyte segmentation software. However, the software performed poorly with microplate imperfections (i.e., - plate scratches) and gels at early time points, when they are relatively translucent (data not shown). We next examined WEKA Trainable Segmentation, a machine learning plugin included in the open source image processing program, FIJI (ImageJ). **Figure 2** shows the process for training the WEKA Segmentation classifier. After loading an image sequence into FIJI and selecting Trainable WEKA Segmentation, the background area is manually identified with the cursor and marked as Class 1. Gel areas are similarly marked as Class 2. After training a classifier, additional annotations can be added to revise the classifier until it performs adequately. Once a satisfactory classifier has been found, it is saved for future use (**Figures 2A–C**).

To analyze large sets of images exported from the Incucyte in-incubator microscope, a FIJI plugin was written (**Supplementary File**). This plugin uses the built-in Trainable WEKA Segmentation plugin to apply the saved classifier to each

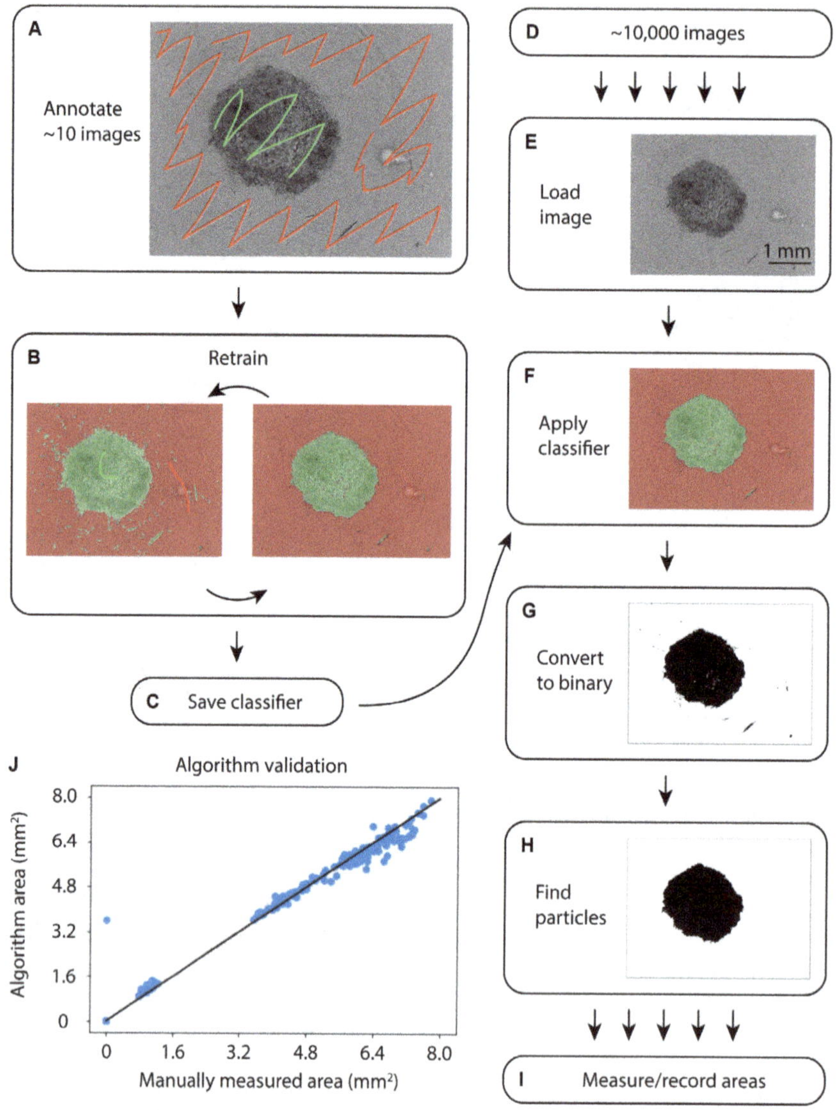

FIGURE 2 | Overview of WEKA segmentation. **(A)** First, the training set of ~10 images is annotated, clearly indicating the collagen gel and microwell plate background. **(B)** The classifier is retrained until it performs adequately. **(C)** After ensuring appropriate performance, the classifier is saved. **(D)** Approximately 10,000 images are acquired from the Incucyte microscopy system. **(E)** Images are loaded into FIJI and **(F)** the classifier created in **(A–C)** is applied. **(G)** The images are converted to binary and **(H)** particles are selected. **(I)** Finally, the area of each gel is measured and recorded. **(J)** Correlation plot of WEKA Segmentation and manual area annotation, showing a linear relationship.

image in a directory, as in **Figures 2D–I**. Following classification, the image was converted to binary and the largest particle was found using the built-in particles function. Areas and metadata were then recorded.

During initial testing on an Intel^{TM} Core® i7-7700 CPU at 3.60 GHz, classification of a single image took 15 s. Further exploration revealed that smaller training sets enabled faster classification. The iterative training process in **Figure 2** allowed for fine-tuning small training sets to achieve accurate segmentation without sacrificing speed.

To validate the automated image analysis algorithm, 300 images of microgels from early and late time points were manually annotated for comparison of area measurements. A strong correlation of 0.990 (Pearsons) with manual area measurements was achieved (**Figure 2J**).

Collagen Microgel Contractions Kinetics

We examined the performance of the ATPS collagen microgel contraction assay with NHLF and IPF responses to TGF-β1 stimulation at a high dose (10 ng/mL) using our automated seeding, washing, and image processing system. The NHLF had both slower baseline contraction and slower TGF-β1 activated contraction compared to IPF, as expected. However, we only tested cells from one patient of each category, so conclusions about biological differences between patients are not justified from this study alone. TGF-β1 induced a moderate increase in

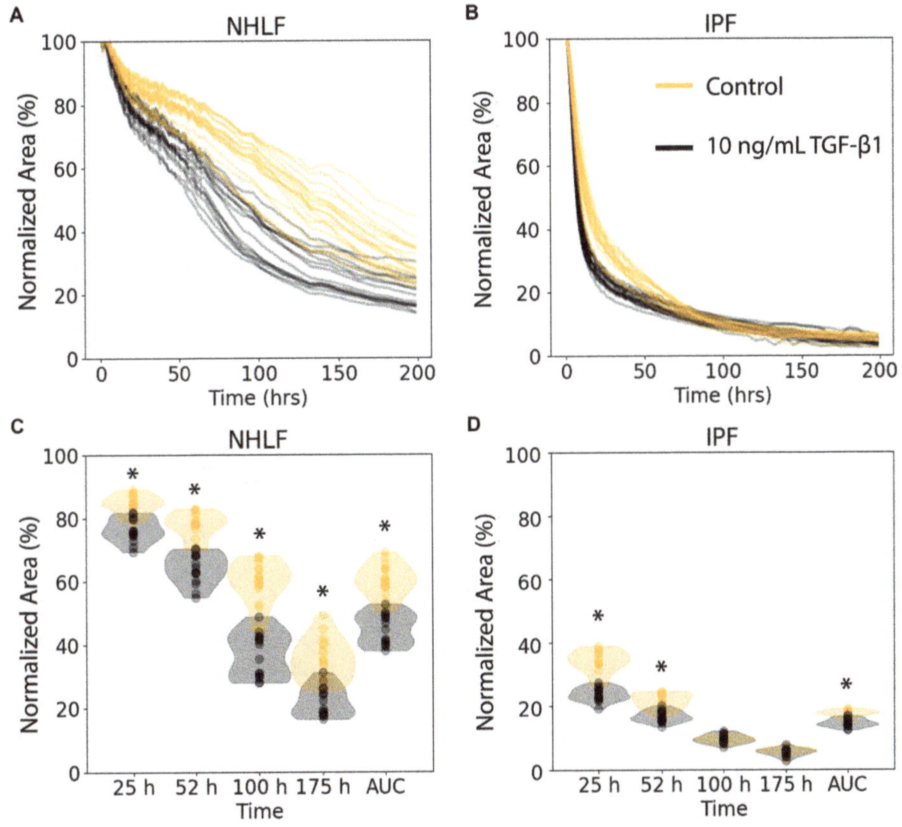

FIGURE 3 | Collagen microgel contraction kinetics and use of an aggregate statistic to distinguish contraction behavior depending on imaging timepoint. **(A)** Normalized area of collagen gels over time for NHLF and **(B)** IPF cells. Each line represents an individual gel. Orange curves are for control samples, and black curves are for cells stimulated with 10 ng/ml TFG-β1. **(C)** Contraction of NHLF and **(D)** IPF cells in response to stimulation with 10 ng/mL TGF-β1. The ability to discern a difference in response depends on the timepoint at which measurements are made. However, the area under the curve more readily and consistently reflects these differences. $n = 15$ per condition. *$p < 0.05$ between the +/− TGF-β1 conditions on multiple t-tests with a Bonferroni correction.

the rate of contraction for both cell types, as shown in **Figure 3**. **Figures 3A,B** show the area of each collagen gel (NHLF and IPF, respectively) as it contracts over time, normalized to that gel's initial area. The same data is shown again in **Figures 3C,D**, but with violin plots to convey the distribution. For the NHLF cells, multiple t-tests with Bonferroni correction indicated significant differences with a 95% confidence interval between groups (presence or absence of TGF-β1) at each of the selected time points – 25, 52, 100, and 175 h, as well as using the area under the curve aggregated data. However, the IPF cells only showed significantly different responses to TGF-β1 at the early time points (25 and 52 h) and with the area under the curve.

Examination of Anti-fibrotic Drugs

We next assessed the ability of known anti-fibrotic drugs to inhibit contraction of collagen microgels. Using a concentration range of 32 nM to 500 μM, we analyzed the dynamic contraction of collagen microgels with NHLF and IPF cells, both with and without 10 ng/mL TGF-β1. For these studies, we selected the two FDA-approved fibrosis therapeutics, nintedanib (pan-kinase inhibitor) and pirfenidone (mechanism still unclear). Additionally, we examined the focal adhesion kinase (FAK) inhibitor, PF 431396 (**Figures 4A–D** and **Supplementary Figures 1–3**).

Dose response curves were fit for normalized area measurements at each time point (**Supplementary Figure 4**). In comparison to the high variance seen at individual time points, dose response curves for area under the curve measurements incorporated kinetic data, generating narrower standard deviations of the parameter estimate for IC50, as seen in **Figure 4E**. The IC50 values for each drug and cell condition are shown for AUC measurements in **Figure 4E** and for each individual time point in **Supplementary Figure 4**. The IC50 values for AUC measurements are also listed in **Supplementary Table 1**. Both the FAK inhibitor (PF 431396) and nintedanib showed efficacy across the cell and stimulation type, while pirfenidone did not achieve 50% effect within the range of concentrations tested.

DISCUSSION

In this work, we added automated image acquisition and analysis to our group's prior development of an ATPS collagen microgel contraction assay (Moraes et al., 2013). We also analyzed normal

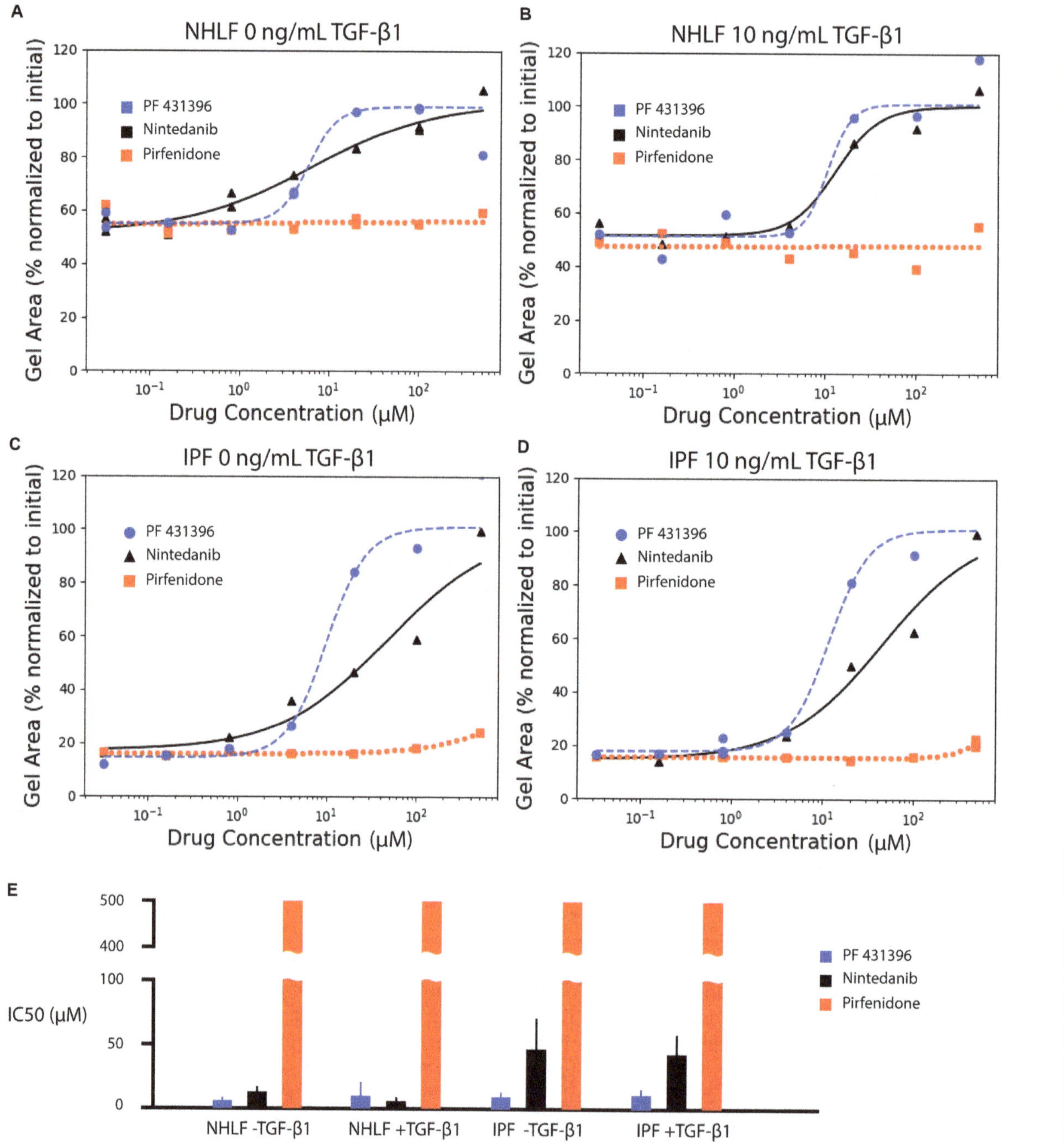

FIGURE 4 | Effect of anti-fibrotic drugs (nintedanib and pirfenidone) and focal adhesion kinase inhibitor (PF 431396) on collagen contraction of NHLF cells without **(A)** and with **(B)** 10 ng/mL TGF-β1, and IPF cells without **(C)** and with **(D)** 10 ng/mL TGF-β1. The fitted parameters for IC50 are plotted in **(E)**. Error bars are the standard deviation of the parameter estimate.

and diseased primary human lung fibroblasts, whereas we had previously analyzed only fibroblast immortalized cell lines. Our previous work focused on the miniaturization of the ATPS collagen microgel contraction assay, opening the possibility for more effective mass transport of agonists and antagonists to the cells (Moraes et al., 2013). The addition of automated imaging and subsequent analysis in this report enabled higher throughput, as well as kinetic analysis of the collagen microgel contraction. Due to the translucent properties of the collagen microgels, the built-in image analysis software in the Incucyte was unable to accurately detect the collagen gels. This shortcoming was addressed by implementing WEKA Segmentation through a custom Jython plugin for FIJI. The WEKA Segmentation reliably yielded measurements matching those found by manually tracing the outlines of the collagen gels, indicating that the WEKA Segmentation was a sufficient tool for image processing. The automated image acquisition and analysis enabled an order of magnitude higher frequency of imaging compared to the standard daily measurement. This temporal analysis unveiled the rapid initial contraction seen in IPF-sourced fibroblasts.

For downstream analysis, it is useful to aggregate the data from an individual contraction time course into a single metric. Although some individual time points are useful to detect the increased contraction in response to TGF-β1, much of the kinetic information is lost. Therefore, we used the area under the curve to aggregate the rate of contraction for each individual gel into a single metric.

Consistent with literature reports (Jin et al., 2019), pirfenidone has little effect below 500 μM, but mildly inhibits contraction at 500 μM in all conditions (**Supplementary Figure 1**). Previous examinations of pirfenidone to modulate fibroblast behavior *in vitro* have required concentrations of 500 μM or higher to see statistically significant suppression of α-SMA and collagen (Nakayama et al., 2008; Conte et al., 2014). However, 500 μM was selected as the high concentration for these studies due to the requirement for high concentrations of dimethyl sulfoxide (DMSO) necessary to achieve pirfenidone concentrations above 500 μM. In this study, the DMSO concentration was kept at 0.1%. None of the concentrations of pirfenidone tested in this study produced a half maximal inhibition of contraction (**Figure 4**).

In contrast, nintedanib exhibits a dose-dependent inhibition of contraction in all cell conditions tested (**Supplementary Figure 2**). Areas of collagen microgels were normalized to their initial area. Interestingly, the inhibition of microgel contraction was largely independent of TGF-β1 for both NHLF and IPF. After a rapid initial contraction, the area reduction dramatically slowed after ~1 day in culture for both cell types (Rangarajan et al., 2016). Our study is the only *in vitro* study to obtain IC50 values for nintedanib in NHLF and IPF cells with and without TGF-β1 in side-by-side studies. We do note that in the few *in vitro* studies that do report IC50, that those values were lower - 144 nM for inhibition of α-SMA in IPF cells (Wollin et al., 2014) and a conference abstract that notes 73 nM for inhibition of PDGF-stimulated collagen gel contraction with NHLF (Wollin et al., 2016). IC50, however, is not a fundamental constant but rather a convenient, assay-specific measure of potency. Thus, comparison of values across different experiments must be made with caution (Kalliokoski et al., 2013).

Lastly, the focal adhesion kinase (FAK) inhibitor, PF 431396, inhibited contraction at concentrations above 4 μM for all cell types, as shown in **Supplementary Figure 3**. Although FAK inhibition is not a widely used drug target due to many off-target effects, this experiment does corroborate previous reports indicating that NHLF contraction of collagen gels requires FAK stimulation (Liu et al., 2010; Epa et al., 2015).

These are, to our knowledge, the first reports of dose response for inhibition of TGF-β1 stimulated collagen gel contraction of primary human fibroblasts by pirfenidone, nintedanib, and PF 431396. While these results nicely demonstrate the technical capabilities, this proof-of-concept drug comparison study is limited with regards to biological conclusions by the small number of replicates and cells from just two donors.

CONCLUSION

We have extended the ATPS microgel contraction assay with live-cell imaging to uncover differential phenotypic behavior of primary cells, whereas our previous methods were limited to cell lines. Because contraction is a time-dependent process, a higher sampling frequency (e.g., every hour vs. the more common every 12–24 h) can provide richer information. We assessed and optimized an automated image segmentation algorithm using WEKA machine learning to measure the areas of 10,000 collagen gel images with high temporal resolution. The assay provides added convenience and throughput, making it appropriate for secondary screening assays and dose response studies. Lastly, we report dose response characteristics for two FDA approved drugs: nintedanib, pirfenidone, as well as the FAK inhibitor, PF 431396 with healthy and diseased primary human fibroblasts, each with and without TGF-β1 activation. The calculated IC50 values confirm previous reports of lower potency for pirfenidone relative to nintedanib. This assay could provide useful phenotypic data to aid secondary and tertiary drug screens, as well as high-throughput information about primary cell behavior in basic research on fibroblast contraction.

AUTHOR CONTRIBUTIONS

CY and ST conceptualized the project idea. CY performed experiments. All authors contributed to writing the manuscript.

ACKNOWLEDGMENTS

We thank Prof. Louise Hecker for helpful discussions.

REFERENCES

Ahluwalia, N., Shea, B. S., and Tager, A. M. (2014). New therapeutic targets in idiopathic pulmonary fibrosis. Aiming to rein in runaway wound-healing responses. *Am. J. Respir. Crit. Care Med.* 190, 867–878. doi: 10.1164/rccm.201403-0509PP

Arganda-Carreras, I., Kaynig, V., Rueden, C., Eliceiri, K. W., Schindelin, J., Cardona, A., et al. (2017). Trainable weka segmentation: a machine learning tool for microscopy pixel classification. *Bioinformatics* 33, 2424–2426. doi: 10.1093/bioinformatics/btx180

Barkauskas, C. E., and Noble, P. W. (2014). Cellular mechanisms of tissue fibrosis. 7. New insights into the cellular mechanisms of pulmonary fibrosis. *Am. J. Physiol. Cell Physiol.* 306, C987–C996. doi: 10.1152/ajpcell.00321.2013

Bell, E., Ivarsson, B., and Merrill, C. (1979). Production of a tissue-like structure by contraction of collagen lattices by human fibroblasts of different proliferative potential in vitro. *Proc. Natl. Acad. Sci. U.S.A.* 76, 1274–1278. doi: 10.1073/pnas.76.3.1274

Betensley, A., Sharif, R., and Karamichos, D. (2016). A systematic review of the role of dysfunctional wound healing in the pathogenesis and treatment of idiopathic pulmonary fibrosis. *J. Clin. Med.* 6:2. doi: 10.3390/jcm6010002

Borensztajn, K., Crestani, B., and Kolb, M. (2014). Idiopathic pulmonary fibrosis: from epithelial injury to biomarkers-insights from the bench side. *Respiration* 86, 441–452. doi: 10.1159/000357598

Campbell, J. D., McDonough, J. E., Zeskind, J. E., Hackett, T. L., Pechkovsky, D. V., Brandsma, C. A., et al. (2012). A gene expression signature of emphysema-related lung destruction and its reversal by the tripeptide GHK. *Genome Med.* 4:67. doi: 10.1186/gm367

Chen, W., Wong, C., Vosburgh, E., Levine, A. J., Foran, D. J., and Xu, E. Y. (2014). High-throughput image analysis of tumor spheroids: A user-friendly software application to measure the size of spheroids automatically and accurately. *J. Vis. Exp.* e51639. doi: 10.3791/51639

Conte, E., Gili, E., Fagone, E., Fruciano, M., Iemmolo, M., and Vancheri, C. (2014). Effect of pirfenidone on proliferation, TGF-β-induced myofibroblast differentiation and fibrogenic activity of primary human lung fibroblasts. *Eur. J. Pharm. Sci.* 58, 13–19. doi: 10.1016/j.ejps.2014.02.014

Cui, H., Banerjee, S., Xie, N., Ge, J., Liu, R. M., Matalon, S., et al. (2016). MicroRNA-27a-3p is a negative regulator of lung fibrosis by targeting myofibroblast differentiation. *Am. J. Respir. Cell Mol. Biol.* 54, 843–852. doi: 10.1165/rcmb.2015-0205OC

Epa, A. P., Thatcher, T. H., Pollock, S. J., Wahl, L. A., Lyda, E., Kottmann, R. M., et al. (2015). Normal human lung epithelial cells inhibit transforming growth factor-β induced myofibroblast differentiation via prostaglandin E2. *PLoS One* 10:e0135266. doi: 10.1371/journal.pone.0135266

Jin, J., Togo, S., Kadoya, K., Tulafu, M., Namba, Y., Iwai, M., et al. (2019). Pirfenidone attenuates lung fibrotic fibroblast responses to transforming growth factor-β1. *Respir. Res.* 20, 1–14. doi: 10.1186/s12931-019-1093-z

Kalliokoski, T., Kramer, C., Vulpetti, A., and Gedeck, P. (2013). Comparability of mixed IC_{50} Data - a statistical analysis. *PLoS One* 8:e61007. doi: 10.1371/journal.pone.0061007

Kondo, S., Kagami, S., Urushihara, M., Kitamura, A., Shimizu, M., Strutz, F., et al. (2004). Transforming growth factor-β1 stimulates collagen matrix remodeling through increased adhesive and contractive potential by human renal fibroblasts. *Biochim. Biophys. Acta Mol. Cell Res.* 1693, 91–100. doi: 10.1016/j.bbamcr.2004.05.005

Liu, F., Mih, J. D., Shea, B. S., Kho, A. T., Sharif, A. S., Tager, A. M., et al. (2010). Feedback amplification of fibrosis through matrix stiffening and COX-2 suppression. *J. Cell Biol.* 190, 693–706. doi: 10.1083/jcb.201004082

Maher, T. M., and Strek, M. E. (2019). Antifibrotic therapy for idiopathic pulmonary fibrosis: time to treat. *Respir. Res.* 20:205. doi: 10.1186/s12931-019-1161-4

McKinney, W. (2010). "Data structures for statistical computing in python," in *Proceedings of the. 9th Python Scicence*, Vol. 445, Austin, TX, 51–56. doi: 10.25080/Majora-92bf1922-00a

Mohan, R., and Bargagna-Mohan, P. (2016). *The Use of Withaferin A to Study Intermediate Filaments*, 1st Edn. Amsterdam: Elsevier Inc.

Moraes, C., Simon, A. B., Putnam, A. J., and Takayama, S. (2013). Aqueous two-phase printing of cell-containing contractile collagen microgels. *Biomaterials* 34, 9623–9631. doi: 10.1016/j.biomaterials.2013.08.046

Nakayama, S., Mukae, H., Sakamoto, N., Kakugawa, T., Yoshioka, S., Soda, H., et al. (2008). Pirfenidone inhibits the expression of HSP47 in TGF-β1-stimulated human lung fibroblasts. *Life Sci.* 82, 210–217. doi: 10.1016/j.lfs.2007.11.003

Rangarajan, S., Kurundkar, A., Kurundkar, D., Bernard, K., Sanders, Y. Y., Ding, Q., et al. (2016). Novel mechanisms for the antifibrotic action of nintedanib. *Am. J. Respir. Cell Mol. Biol.* 54, 51–59. doi: 10.1165/rcmb.2014-0445OC

Rodday, B., Hirschhaeuser, F., Walenta, S., and Mueller-Klieser, W. (2011). Semiautomatic growth analysis of multicellular tumor spheroids. *J. Biomol. Screen.* 16, 1119–1124. doi: 10.1177/1087057111419501

Singh, S., and Tavana, H. (2018). Collagen partition in polymeric aqueous two-phase systems for tissue engineering. *Front. Chem.* 6:379. doi: 10.3389/fchem.2018.00379

Virtanen, P., Gommers, R., Oliphant, T. E., Haberland, M., Reddy, T., Cournapeau, D., et al. (2020). SciPy 1.0: fundamental algorithms for scientific computing in Python. *Nat. Methods* 17, 261–272. doi: 10.1038/s41592-019-0686-2

Wollin, L., Maillet, I., Quesniaux, V., Holweg, A., and Ryffel, B. (2014). Antifibrotic and anti-inflammatory activity of the tyrosine kinase inhibitor nintedanib in experimental models of lung fibrosiss. *J. Pharmacol. Exp. Ther.* 349, 209–220. doi: 10.1124/jpet.113.208223

Wollin, L., Schuett, J., Ostermann, A., and Herrmann, F. (2016). "The effect of nintedanib on platelet derived growth factor-stimulated contraction of human primary lung fibroblasts," in *Proceedings of the American Thoracic Society International Conference Abstracts A73. LUNG FIBROSIS: NEW DIRECTIONS TO INFORM THE FUTURE*, (New York, NY: American Thoracic Society).

Yamanishi, C., Robinson, S., and Takayama, S. (2019). Biofabrication of phenotypic pulmonary fibrosis assays. *Biofabrication* 11:032005. doi: 10.1088/1758-5090/ab2286

Zhang, T., Day, J. H., Su, X., Guadarrama, A. G., Sandbo, N. K., Esnault, S., et al. (2019). Investigating fibroblast-induced collagen gel contraction using a dynamic microscale platform. *Front. Bioeng. Biotechnol.* 7:196. doi: 10.3389/fbioe.2019.00196

8

Metabolic Glycoengineering Enables the Ultrastructural Visualization of Sialic Acids in the Glycocalyx of the Alveolar Epithelial Cell Line hAELVi

Raphael Brandt[1], Sara Timm[2], Jacob L. Gorenflos López[3,4], Jubilant Kwame Abledu[5], Wolfgang M. Kuebler[5,6], Christian P. R. Hackenberger[3,4], Matthias Ochs[1,2,6] and Elena Lopez-Rodriguez[1]*

[1] Institute of Functional Anatomy, Charité – Universitätsmedizin Berlin, Berlin, Germany, [2] Core Facility Electron Microscopy, Charité – Universitätsmedizin Berlin, Berlin, Germany, [3] Department Chemical Biology, Leibniz-Forschungsinstitut für Molekulare Pharmakologie (FMP), Berlin, Germany, [4] Department of Chemistry, Humboldt Universität zu Berlin, Berlin, Germany, [5] Institute of Physiology, Charité-Universitätsmedizin Berlin, Berlin, Germany, [6] German Center for Lung Research (DZL), Berlin, Germany

***Correspondence:**
Raphael Brandt
raphael.brandt@charite.de

The glycocalyx—a plethora of sugars forming a dense layer that covers the cell membrane—is commonly found on the epithelial surface of lumen forming tissue. New glycocalyx specific properties have been defined for various organs in the last decade. However, in the lung alveolar epithelium, its structure and functions remain almost completely unexplored. This is partly due to the lack of physiologically relevant, cost effective *in vitro* models. As the glycocalyx is an essential but neglected part of the alveolar epithelial barrier, understanding its properties holds the promise to enhance the pulmonary administration of drugs and delivery of nanoparticles. Here, using air-liquid-interface (ALI) cell culture, we focus on combining metabolic glycoengineering with glycan specific electron and confocal microscopy to visualize the glycocalyx of a recently immortalized human alveolar epithelial cell line (hAELVi). For this purpose, we applied different bioorthogonal labeling approaches to visualize sialic acid—an amino sugar that provides negative charge to the lung epithelial glycocalyx—using both fluorescence and gold-nanoparticle labeling. Further, we compared mild chemical fixing/freeze substitution and standard cytochemical electron microscopy embedding protocols for their capacity of contrasting the glycocalyx. In our study, we established hAELVi cells as a convenient model for investigating human alveolar epithelial glycocalyx. Transmission electron microscopy revealed hAELVi cells to develop ultrastructural features reminiscent of alveolar epithelial type II cells (ATII). Further, we visualized extracellular uni- and multilamellar membranous structures in direct proximity to the glycocalyx at ultrastructural level, indicating putative interactions. The lamellar membranes were able to form structures of higher organization, and we report sialic acid to be present within those. In conclusion, combining metabolite specific glycoengineering with ultrastructural localization presents an innovative method with high potential to depict the molecular distribution of individual components of the alveolar epithelial glycocalyx and its interaction partners.

Keywords: glycocalyx, sialic acid, electron microscopy, metabolic glycoengineering, bioorthogonal labeling, alveolar epithelium, hAELVi, huAELVi

INTRODUCTION

The Alveolar Lining Layer as Integral Part of the Blood-Air-Barrier

The lung alveolar epithelium constitutes the first cell lining that atmospheric oxygen has to pass for oxygen uptake in the lungs. Thus, its morphology needs to meet criteria for optimal gas exchange. While the majority of the alveolar epithelial surface is comprised of extended alveolar epithelial type I cells (ATI) whose flattened architecture allows for efficient gas exchange, the majority of alveolar epithelial cells belongs to the smaller alveolar epithelial type II cells (ATII) (Hsia et al., 2016). The multifunctional ATII are cuboidal in shape, have important secretory capacity and are further considered as proliferative precursors capable of differentiation into ATI, most notably upon lung injury (Matthay et al., 2019).

During exhalation, physically relevant pressure differences put the smaller alveoli at constant risk of collapse. Keeping the alveoli homogeneously open in all states of respiration is a function that has been attributed to a continuous liquid lining layer covering the alveolar epithelium. The alveolar lining layer comprises two phases: a liquid hypophase and an upper film composed of a lipid-protein mixture called lung surfactant (surface active agent) (Pattle, 1955). Surfactant is best known for its ability to cause a surface-dependent decrease of surface tension at the air-liquid interface, which prevents collapse of the alveolar space, especially during exhalation. Extending its biophysical mode of action, additional functions have been attributed to surfactant, including a role in immunomodulation (Wright, 2005; Han and Mallampalli, 2015). Surfactant has been in the center of fruitful translational research for the last decades (Owen et al., 2017), resulting in beneficial pharmaceutical treatments for preterm children born at a stadium of immature lung development.

The Alveolar Glycocalyx—Little Is Known

The underlying liquid hypophase acts as a space for assembly and recycling of surfactant precursor and degradation products, respectively, but also consists of an apical sugar-rich cell surface coat called the glycocalyx. The latter has recently been proposed to interact with surfactant components (Ochs et al., 2020). The epithelial surface of lumen forming organs is characteristically rich in glycocalyx, providing overlapping but also highly tissue specific functions. The chemical complexity of the glycocalyx is immense, as are the different glycans forming it (Mockl, 2020). Not only the order at which different monosaccharides can be combined to form poly-antennary polymers of different lengths is of relevance, but also the types of glycosidic bonds covalently linking the chain of monosaccharides. Two monosaccharides can be linked *via* glycosidic bonds between the anomeric hydroxyl of the first unit, and either one of several possible hydroxyl groups of the second, which vastly increases the combinatory potential (Laine, 1994). In addition, chemical modifications such as oxidation of hydroxyl groups, sulfation, N-acetylation, sialylation, to name a few, extend the spectrum of potential functional properties of glycans, for instance by adding specific charges. Given this steric and chemical complexity and its position at the cell periphery, not only the structural organization but also the regulatory potential of the glycocalyx is increasingly recognized in the field (Varki, 2017). Sialic acids serve as receptors for the attachment of many viruses to host cells (Matrosovich et al., 2015) and have been shown to determine pulmonary endothelial barrier integrity (Cioffi et al., 2012). Also, exposure to cigarette smoke was shown to influence levels of sialylation in an alveolar epithelial cancer cell model (Wielgat et al., 2018).

Despite upcoming interest in the glycocalyx of the alveolar epithelium, its structure and functions remain largely unexplored (reviewed in Ochs et al., 2020). This is first, attributable to the lack of physiologically relevant and cost effective *in vitro* models. Secondly, traditional methods to study biological systems are of limited use when studying the glycocalyx (reviewed by Mockl, 2020). Thirdly, the focus of research of the alveolar lining layer had strictly been on surfactant over the last decades, thereby neglecting the glycocalyx.

Using Metabolic Glycoengineering to Label Sialic Acids

Metabolic glycoengineering (MGE) is a method used to modify glycan structures by treating cells with unnatural derivatives of monosaccharides. Especially, sialic acid modification using *N*-acetyl-mannosamine (ManNAc) derivatives have become a standard methodology (Wratil et al., 2016). Sialic acids are nonose monosaccharides primarily found as terminal components of glycans. They play crucial roles in cellular processes such as extrinsic and intrinsic cell-cell communication as well as in defense (Schauer and Kamerling, 2018). MGE is based on the promiscuity in the sialic acid biosynthesis pathway and has enabled the introduction of a variety of bioorthogonal reporters into the sialic acid component. For the incorporation of azides, acetylated *N*-azidoacetyl-mannosamine (Ac_4ManNAz) developed by the Bertozzi group is the most prominent example (Jacobs et al., 2000; Baskin et al., 2007; Moller et al., 2011). After entering the cell, non-specific esterases cleave the acetyl groups and ManNAz is processed by the promiscuous enzymes of the sialic acid biosynthesis pathway (**Figure 1A**) to CMP-Neu-5-Az. The latter is used by sialic acid transferases in the Golgi to modify the glycans of glycoproteins by adding Neu-5-Az (Wratil et al., 2016). The glycosylated proteins become, for the most part, tethered to the cell surface.

The introduction of azides to the cell surface *via* MGE enables the employment of bioorthogonal reactions for the specific labeling *in vitro* and *in vivo*, which do otherwise not interact with the biochemistry of the cells (Baskin et al., 2007; Kenry and Liu, 2019). Here, we employed this method

---

Abbreviations: ATI, alveolar epithelial type I cell; ATII, alveolar epithelial type II cell; BTTAA, 2-(4-((Bis((1-(*tert*-butyl)-1*H*-1,2,3-triazol-4-yl)methyl)amino)methyl)-1*H*-1,2,3-triazol-1-yl)acetic acid; CuAAC, Cu(I) catalyzed azide-alkyne cycloaddition; DBCO, dibenzocyclooctyne; EM, electron microscopy; GNP, gold nanoparticles; LaDy, mixture of lanthanum and dysprosium; LSM, laser scanning microscopy; MGE, metabolic glycoengineering; PEG, polyethylene glycol; RT, room temperature; SPAAC, strain-promoted-azide-alkyne cycloaddition; THPTA, Tris((1-hydroxy-propyl-1H-1,2,3-triazol-4-yl)methyl)amine.

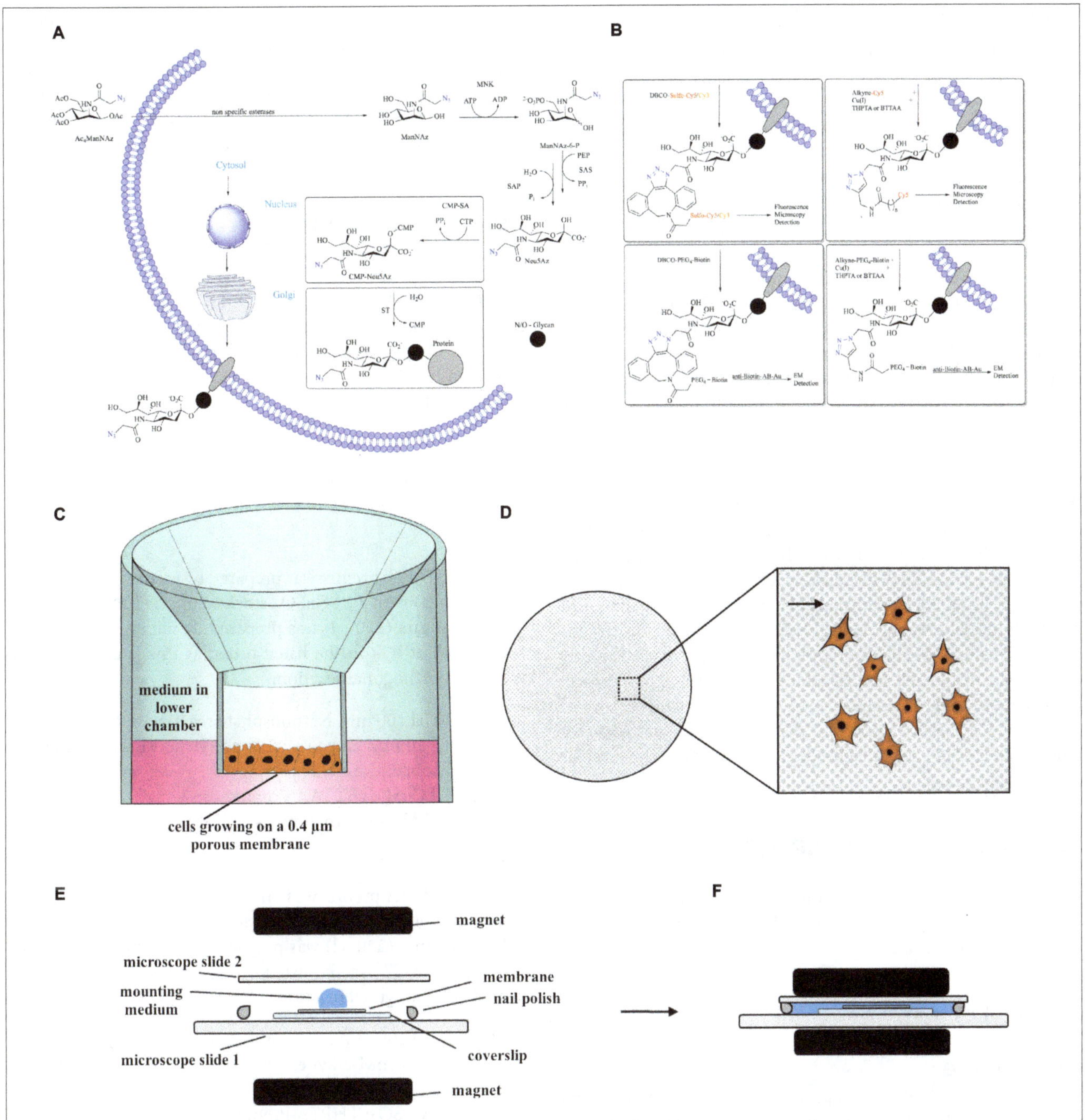

FIGURE 1 | (A) Introduction of Ac_4ManNAz to the sialic acid biosynthesis pathway. **(B)** Different approaches of labeling azide-modified sialic acid that were successfully applied in this study and the and the method of detection. These encompass biorthogonal reactions via CuAAC or copper-free SPAAC linked to fluorophores or biotin, enabling either fluorescence microscopy or, upon immunogold labeling using antibodies against biotin, electron microscopy. **(C)** Scheme showing cells growing at ALI using a transwell membrane inset that is placed in a well of a 12-well plate filled with medium. **(D)** Scheme of the membrane as seen from the top. Large Inset displays higher magnification of the porous membrane with plated cells. Arrowhead points to a 0.4 µm pore. **(E,F)** Schematic visualization of the embedding procedure used for fluorescence microscopy. The magnets are applied carefully in order to flatten the membrane.

by bioorthogonally reacting azide-containing sialic acids obtained from ManNAz with alkynes linked to fluorophores or biotin. The latter was subsequently detected by anti-biotin-antibodies coupled to gold nanoparticles (anti-Biotin-AB-Au). We applied two bioorthogonal labeling approaches: Cu(I) catalyzed azide-alkyne cycloaddition (CuAAC) with THPTA or BTTAA (see Abbreviations list for chemical names) as stabilizing additives or strain-promoted-azide-alkyne cycloaddition (SPAAC), which is copper-free and uses cyclooctynes such as dibenzocyclooctyne (DBCO) (**Figure 1B**).

Visualizing the Glycocalyx—Electron Microscopy as a Method of Choice

The alveolar lining layer has an average height of 200 nm in rat lungs (Bastacky et al., 1995). The size of the glycocalyx, which constitutes the bottom part of the lining layer, is therefore regularly below the diffraction limit of light (~250 nm). Thus, conventional optical microscopy is limited in accurately assessing glycocalyx dimensions, and resolving fine structures below 25 nm can exclusively be performed by electron microscopy (EM) methods. EM requires elaborate sample preparation, and there is ongoing debate if and how the required treatments affect the ultrastructural preservation of the glycocalyx (Ebong et al., 2011; Hegermann et al., 2016; Chevalier et al., 2017). Furthermore, the molecular identity of glycans is not depicted by conventional EM, despite dynamic progress in this regard (Broecker et al., 2015).

Here, we overcame some of these limitations by combining MGE with EM sample preparation based on mild chemical fixation followed by freeze substitution (FS) and postembedding immunogold labeling to determine sialic acid localization within the glycocalyx of alveolar epithelial cells at ultrastructural resolution. This is not only a methodically achievement in itself but also guides interpretation of MGE-based light microscopy imaging. We compared the ultrastructural preservation of the glycocalyx upon FS to conventional and glycan labeling EM protocols, the latter using Alcian blue. In addition, our work adds new insights into specific morphological features of the recently developed hAELVi cell line (Kuehn et al., 2016), e.g. microvilli dense regions and extracellular membranous structures, both of which show a marked sialic acid distribution. In summary, we established hAELVi cells as a model for the study of the alveolar epithelial glycocalyx.

MATERIALS AND EQUIPMENT

A list of reagents and equipment required for cell culture, confocal and electron microscopy preparation is provided in **Table 1**.

METHODS

Cell Culture

The immortalized alveolar epithelial cell line hAELVi was purchased from InSRCEENneX (Braunschweig, Germany). Cells were cultured on flasks or 12-well-plates that had been precoated for 2 h with a commercial coating solution harboring extracellular matrix components (Inscreenex, Braunschweig, Germany). Cells were seeded at a density of 6,000 or 8,000 cells/cm^2 and passaged every 3 or 4 days. Medium (huAEC + Primocin 100 μg/ml) was exchanged every 2–3 days.

For experiments, cells between passage 12 and 26 have been used. Experiments were performed at an air-liquid-interface (ALI): the cell suspension (50 μl) was seeded on top of a transwell membrane system that had been precoated for 2 h, and 200–250 μl medium was added to the bottom compartment (**Figures 1C,D**). Medium in the bottom compartment was carefully exchanged every 2–3 days using a pipette. In order to visualize confluent cell layers, cells were seeded at a density of 6.000 cells/cm^2 and grown for 14 days. In order to visualize cells in the exponential growth phase, cells were seeded at 8.000 cells/cm^2 and grown for 3 days. Cells labeled with Alcian blue (see below) were grown for 3 and 10 days, respectively, and were seeded at 8.000 cells/cm^2.

Metabolic Glycoengineering

A summarized evaluation of different MGE concentrations and conditions applied in this study is provided in **Table 2**. Cells were fed with $Ac_4ManNAz$ or DMSO control (max. 0.1%). After incorporation of $Ac_4ManNAz$, the cells were washed twice on the membrane using 50 μl DPBS, 3% BSA and subsequently, the orthogonal reaction was performed using CuAAC or SPAAC protocols.

CuAAC

CuAAC with either BTTAA or THPTA was performed according to manufacturer's instruction with minor modifications.

BTTAA

A $CuSO_4$: BTTAA premix was prepared by mixing 70 μl BTTAA stock (50 mM) with 7 μl $CuSO_4$ stock solution (100 mM) at RT.

The final mix (220 μl) was prepared by mixing the following reagents (all at RT) in the listed order, as this is critical for an efficient bioorthogonal reaction:

148.28 μl 100 mM Na-phosphate reaction buffer.
1.32 μl 10 mM alkyne-Cy5 or acetylene-PEG_4-Biotin stock (final concentration 60 μM).
48.4 μl $CuSO_4$: BTTAA Premix.
22 μl 1M Na-ascorbate stock solution.

THPTA

A $CuSO_4$: THPTA premix was prepared by mixing 20 μl THPTA stock (250 mM) with 10 μl $CuSO_4$ stock solution (100 mM) at RT.

The final mix (220 μl) was prepared by mixing the following reagents (all at RT) in the listed order, as this is critical for an efficient bioorthogonal reaction:

183.48 μl 100 mM Na-phosphate reaction buffer.
1.98 μl 10 mM alkyne-Cy5 stock final concentration (60 μM).
13.2 μl $CuSO_4$: THPTA Premix.
22 μl 1M Na-ascorbate stock solution.

Whenever lower concentrations of the alkyne were used, a reciprocal amount of Na-phosphate buffer was added to achieve a volume of 220 μ l.

For (ultimately futile) attempts to label with alkyne-gold, the following two final mixes using alkyne-gold in a 1:19 dilution (for BTTAA) or 1:9 dilution (for THPTA) were prepared:

75.6 μl 100 mM Na-phosphate reaction buffer.
6 μl alkyne-gold.
26.4 μl $CuSO_4$: BTTAA Premix.
12 μl 1M Na-ascorbate stock solution.

TABLE 1 | List of materials and chemicals used in this study.

Material/Equipment	Manufacturer
×60 objective silicon oil-immersion, 1.35 N.A., 0.15 mm W.D.	Olympus, Tokyo, Japan
15 ml falcon tubes, G028-BC	Corning, Wiesbaden, Germany
50 ml falcons falcon tubes, G027-GC	Corning, Wiesbaden, Germany
6.5 mm transwell with 0.4 µm pore polyester membrane insert, 3470	Corning, Wiesbaden, Germany
Acetone	Roth, Karlsruhe, Germany
Acetylene-PEG4-Biotin, CLK-TA105-25	Jena Bioscience, Jena, Germany
AFS2	Leica, Wetzlar, Germany
Alcian Blue	Sigma-Aldrich, St. Louis, United States
Alkyne-Cy5	Jena Bioscience, Jena, Germany
Anti-fade fluorescence mounting medium – aqueous, fluoroshield	Abcam, ab104135
BSA-c	Aurion, Wageningen, Netherlands
BTTAA, CLK-067	Jena Bioscience, Jena, Germany
BX61 confocal LSM, diode laser 405 nm/647 nm	Olympus, Tokyo, Japan
Cacodylate	Serva, Heidelberg, Germany
Copper grids	Plano, Wetzlar, Germany
Coverslips 24 × 50 mm, 631-0146	VWR International, Darmstadt, Germany
CuAAC reaction ligand test kit (THPTA and BTTAA based), CLK-075	Jena Bioscience, Jena, Germany
CuSO4, CLK-MI004	Jena Bioscience, Jena, Germany
DBCO-Sulfo-Cy3, CLK-A140	Jena Bioscience, Jena, Germany
DBCO-Sulfo-Cy5, CLK-A130	Jena Bioscience, Jena, Germany
DBCO-PEG4-Biotin, CLK-A105P4	Jena Bioscience, Jena, Germany
Diamond Knife	Diatome, Nidau, Switzerland
DPBS w/o calcium and magnesium, Gibco 14190250	Thermo Fischer Scientific, Waltham, MA, United States
DPBS w/o calcium and magnesium, D8537	Sigma-Aldrich, St. Louis, United States
EM blocking solution, SKU 905.002	Aurion, Wageningen, Netherlands
Epon	Serva, Heidelberg, Germany
Falcon 24-well clear flat bottom TC-treated multiwell cell culture plate, 353047	Corning, Wiesbaden, Germany
Falcon 25 cm^2 rectangular canted neck cell culture flask with vented cap 353109	Corning, Wiesbaden, Germany
Falcon 75 cm^2 rectangular canted neck cell culture flask with vented cap, 353136	Corning, Wiesbaden, Germany
FluoView FV1000 V4.2 software	Olympus, Tokyo, Japan
Glutaraldehyde	Serva, Heidelberg, Germany
Goat-anti-biotin, 10 nm gold nanoparticles, SKU 110.088	Aurion, Wageningen, Netherlands
Gold nanoparticles, alkyne function, 0.05% Au 15 nm, GP15-AK-1	Nanocs, New York, United States
hAELVi cells	InSCREENeX, Braunschweig, Germany
HEPES buffer	Merck Millipore, Darmstadt, Germany
huAEC coating solution, INS-SU-1018	InSCREENeX, Braunschweig, Germany
huAEC medium, INS-ME-1013	InSCREENeX, Braunschweig, Germany
Lead citrate	Merck Millipore, Darmstadt, Germany
Lowicryl HM20	Electron Microscopy Sciences, Hatfield, United States
Methanol	Roth, Karlsruhe, Germany
Na-Ascorbate, CLK-MI005	Jena Bioscience, Jena, Germany
Nickel grids	Plano, Wetzlar, Germany
OsO4	Electron Microscopy Sciences, Hatfield, United States
Paraformaldehyde	Electron Microscopy Sciences, Hatfield, United States
Phosphotungstic acid	Merck Millipore, Darmstadt, Germany
Primocin, ant-pm-05	Invivogen, Toulouse, France
Slow scan 2K CCD camera	TRS, Moorenweis, Germany
Sucrose	Roth, Karlsruhe, Germany
THPTA, CLK-1010	Jena Bioscience, Jena, Germany
Ultramicrotome	Leica, Wetzlar, Germany
Uranyl acetate	Serva, Heidelberg, Germany
Zeiss Leo 906 electron microscope	Carl Zeiss, Oberkochen, Germany

TABLE 2 | Summary of the different MGE experimental setups performed in this study and the corresponding outcome regarding signal-to-noise ratio.

Ac4ManNAz	Alkyne	Stabilizing agent	Signal to noise ratio	Microscopy
48 h 20 μM	Alkyne-Cy5 40 μM	THPTA	Excellent	LSM
24 h 20 μM	Alkyne-Cy5 40 μM	BTTAA	Excellent	LSM
24 h 20 μM	Alkyne-Cy5 60 μM	BTTAA	Excellent	LSM
24 h 50 μM	Alkyne-Cy5 40 μM	BTTAA	Excellent	LSM
24 h 50 μM	Alkyne-Cy5 60 μM	BTTAA	Excellent	LSM
48 h 20 μM	Alkyne-Cy5 40 μM	BTTAA	Excellent	LSM
72 h 50 μM	DBCO-Sulfo-Cy3 20 μM	N/A	Good	LSM
48 h 50 μM	DBCO-Sulfo-Cy5 60 μM	N/A	Good	LSM
48 h 50 μM	DBCO-Sulfo-Cy5 20 μM	N/A	Good	LSM
48 h 50 μM	DBCO-Sulfo-Cy5 6 μM	N/A	Mediocre	LSM
72 h 50 μM	Alkyne-gold 0.005%	BTTAA	No signal detectable	EM
72 h 50 μM	Alkyne-gold 0.001%	BTTAA	No signal detectable	EM
72 h 50 μM	Acetylene-PEG4-biotin 40 μM	BTTAA	Excellent	EM
72 h 50 μM	Acetylene-PEG4-biotin 60 μM	BTTAA	Excellent	EM
72 h 50 μM	DBCO-PEG4-biotin 60 μM	N/A	Excellent	EM

or

133.4 μl 100 mM Na-phosphate reaction buffer.
23 μl alkyne-gold.
50.6 μl $CuSO_4$: THPTA Premix.
23 μl 1M Na-ascorbate stock solution.

In addition, a mix using alkyne-gold in a 1:49 dilution was tested—to exclude the possibility that the biorthogonal reactions failed due to inappropriate buffer concentrations. However, also using that dilution we could not detect any gold nanoparticles (data not shown).

The final alkyne mix (50 μl per transwell) was pipetted on top of the cells and incubated at 37°C for 30 min.

SPAAC

SPAAC was performed using either DBCO-Sulfo-Cy5, DBCO-Sulfo-Cy3 or DBCO-PEG_4-Biotin:

DBCO-"X" was diluted in DPBS, 1% FBS to the required final concentration. The solution (50 μl per transwells) was added on top of the cells and incubated at 37°C for 1 h.

Fluorescence Microscopy Sample Preparation

Cells were washed once using 50 μl DPBS, 3% BSA before fixation. Cells were fixed with DPBS containing 4% paraformaldehyde for 15 min at 37°C. To this end, the fixative was added to the top (100 μl) and bottom compartment (500 μl). Subsequently, cells were washed three times using DPBS on a shaker. Cells were counterstained using 0.1% DAPI in DPBS for ~10 min on a shaker in the dark. After washing twice with DPBS, the transwell membrane harboring the cells was cut out with fine scissors and mounted on a glass slide using liquid mounting medium (**Figure 1E**). Two small magnets were applied to the glass slide and the coverslip, opposing each other, in order to gently flatten the membrane (**Figures 1E,F**). This step is critical for visualizing the cell layer as otherwise the transwell membrane tends to get embedded tangentially and appears wavy. The embedded transwells were visualized by confocal laser scanning microscopy using a BX61 (Olympus) and a × 60 objective, silicon oil-immersion, 1.35 N.A., 0.15 mm W.D. Both, Cy5 and DAPI were excited using a multi-argon laser (405 nm/633 nm). Cy3 was excited using a helium-neon laser (559 nm). Images were acquired with FluoView FV1000 V4.2 software using the preconfigured settings for DAPI, Cy3 and Cy5, respectively.

Transmission Electron Microscopy (TEM) Sample Preparation

For standard cytochemical fixation/Epon embedding, cells were washed twice using 50 μl DPBS, 3% BSA and once using 50μl DPBS. After washing, cells were fixed by adding 0.15 M HEPES buffer containing 1.5% paraformaldehyde and 1.5% glutaraldehyde for at least 3 h (up to 24 h) at 4°C. To this end, fixative was added to the top (100 μl) and bottom compartment (500 μl). Post fixation was performed using 1% OsO_4 in 0.1 M cacodylate buffer at RT for 2 h, followed by incubation in half-saturated aqueous uranyl acetate over night at 4°C. After dehydration in a graded acetone series, samples were transferred to Epon resin. Ultrathin sections (70 nm) were prepared using an ultramicrotome equipped with a diamond knife, collected on pioloform-coated copper grids and subsequently stained with lead citrate according to Reynolds (Reynolds, 1963).

In order to stain cell-surface glycans, Alcian blue was optionally added to the fixative (0.15%) and to every subsequently applied solution (0.075%) until 70% acetone was reached within the graded series.

For freeze substitution and immunogold labeling, cells were fixed using a mixture of 4% paraformaldehyde and 0.1% glutaraldehyde in 0.2 M HEPES buffer. After cryoprotective infiltration using 2.3 M sucrose in PBS, cells were frozen in liquid nitrogen and transferred to a freeze substitution system (AFS2, Leica, Wetzlar, Germany). Freeze substitution was performed at −90°C using methanol containing 0.5% uranyl acetate at −90°C. Subsequently, samples were embedded in Lowicryl HM20 at

−45°C (Fehrenbach and Ochs, 1998). Ultrathin sections (70 nm) were collected on pioloform-coated nickel grids and used for immunogold labeling.

Sections were floated on drops of 50 mM glycine, 0.1% BSA-c in PBS (PH 7.4) for 20 min and subsequently blocked for 30 min using blocking solution (Aurion, Wageningen, Netherlands). After a washing step in incubation buffer (0.1% BSA-c in PBS), sections were labeled for 90 min at RT using an antibody against Biotin, conjugated with 10 nm gold particles, diluted 1:30 in incubation buffer Finally, the sections were rinsed in incubation buffer (six times) and PBS (three times), fixed with 2.5% glutaraldehyde in PBS and treated with an aqueous solution of 4% uranyl acetate and 1% phosphotungstic acid (5 min). Finally, grids were washed three times in distilled water.

Grids were examined on a Zeiss Leo 906 electron microscope at 80 kV acceleration voltage, and electron micrographs were recorded using a slow scan 2K CCD camera (TRS, Moorenweis, Germany).

RESULTS

Visualization of Sialic Acid by Fluorescence Microscopy

For visualization of sialic acid as part of the alveolar epithelial glycocalyx, we used the recently established human alveolar epithelial cell line hAELVi, derived from immortalized primary alveolar epithelial cells. Mimicking the physiological situation in the alveolar space, we grew hAELVi cells at an air-liquid-interface (ALI) using polyethylene transwell membranes (Ø0.4 μm pore size) that had been coated with extracellular matrix components. After 2 weeks, hAELVi cells form a dense layer that display intact barrier function (Kuehn et al., 2016). We fed hAELVi cells with Ac_4ManAz (20 μM) for 48 h, an unnatural precursor metabolite of the sialic acid biosynthesis pathway. Metabolically labeled sialic acids were finally visualized by chemical linkage to alkyne-Cy5 (40 μM, 30 min) in a Co(I) catalyzed azide-alkyne click chemistry reaction (CuAAC) along with THPTA as a helper substance. Subsequently, cells were fixed, counterstained with DAPI and the membrane was cut and mounted for laser scanning microscopy (LSM). Fourteen days old cells presented with intense plasma membrane staining which allowed the visualization of microvilli (**Figures 2A,B**). The staining was particularly pronounced at the apical (luminal) cell surface (**Figure 2A**, see cross-section projection). As expected, cells that had been fed with DMSO control did not display any detectable Cy5 staining (**Figure 2C**), highlighting the specificity of CuAAC. Of note, DAPI gathers within the 0.4 μM pores of the polyethylene membrane leading to artificial staining of the basal pores, which are, however, clearly distinguishable in size from the cell nuclei (**Figure 2D**). Another potential pitfall concerns the embedding of the membrane that tends to corrugate within the mounting medium impairing planar scanning. We overcame this issue by sandwiching the mounted membrane between two small magnets.

Next, we tested different concentrations of Ac_4ManAz (20–50 μM) and alkyne-Cy5 (40–60 μM) in 3 days old hAELVi cells using BTTAA as a helper substance of CuAAC (**Supplementary Figure S1**). We confirmed excellent signal-to-noise ratio even at low concentrations, respectively. When visualized 3 days after plating, hAELVi cells were less confluent, larger in shape and formed long filopodia (thin protrusions) that extended up to ~100 μm, often spanning from cell to cell. Although present, microvilli were less frequently seen.

In addition to visualizing the glycocalyx using CuAAC, we also performed copper-free strain-promoted azide-alkyne cycloaddition (SPAAC) using DBCO-Sulfo-Cy3 (**Supplementary Figure S2**) or DBCO-Sulfo-Cy5 (not shown). DBCO-based cycloaddition overcomes the potential cytotoxicity of copper making it suitable for long term *in vitro* and *in vivo* live-cell imaging at the expense of higher background staining due to non-specific binding to thiol groups. We found best and very acceptable signal-to-noise ratio when cells were fed with at least 50 μM Ac_4ManAz and stained with 20 μM DBCO-Sulfo-fluorophore. Considerable background was detected within single apoptotic cells as defined by highly condensed chromatin and fragmented nuclei (**Supplementary Figure S2D**). Of interest, in addition to regular cell membrane staining, we occasionally detected intensely stained structures of tubular appearance forming an extracellular meshwork (**Supplementary Figure S2B**).

Visualization of Sialic Acid Could Not Be Achieved Using Alkyne-Gold Nanoparticles

In order to investigate the distribution of sialic acid in more detail, we decided to combine metabolic glycoengineering with ultrastructural analyses providing resolution at the single molecule level. To this end, we fed hAELVi cells with $Ac_4ManNAz$, but replaced alkyne-Cy5 by a solution of alkyne-gold nanoparticles for detectability by EM. Subsequently, cells were fixed, embedded and contrasted using an EPON-based electron microscopy protocol that had been optimized for ultrastructural preservation of lung tissue.

To our disappointment, we could not detect any gold nanoparticles although cells treated in parallel for confocal microscopy stained effectively (**Supplementary Figure S3**). We consider that the inevitable dilution (1:9) of the alkyne-gold solution during reagent preparation—which leads to a final concentration of 0.005% (w/v) of gold nanoparticles corresponding to calculated 0.93 nM alkyne-gold—is probably too low for efficient detection. This may become particular limiting in EM, as ultrathin sections contain far less labeled molecules per section when compared to an optical section plane in confocal microscopy.

Alcian Blue Enhances a Standard EM Protocol for Visualization of the Glycocalyx

Despite the expected good ultrastructural preservation of intracellular structures, we noticed that the Epon embedding protocol performed poorly in visualizing the glycocalyx in general (**Figures 3A,B**). In order to evaluate whether the basic protocol either leads to the complete decomposition of the glycocalyx

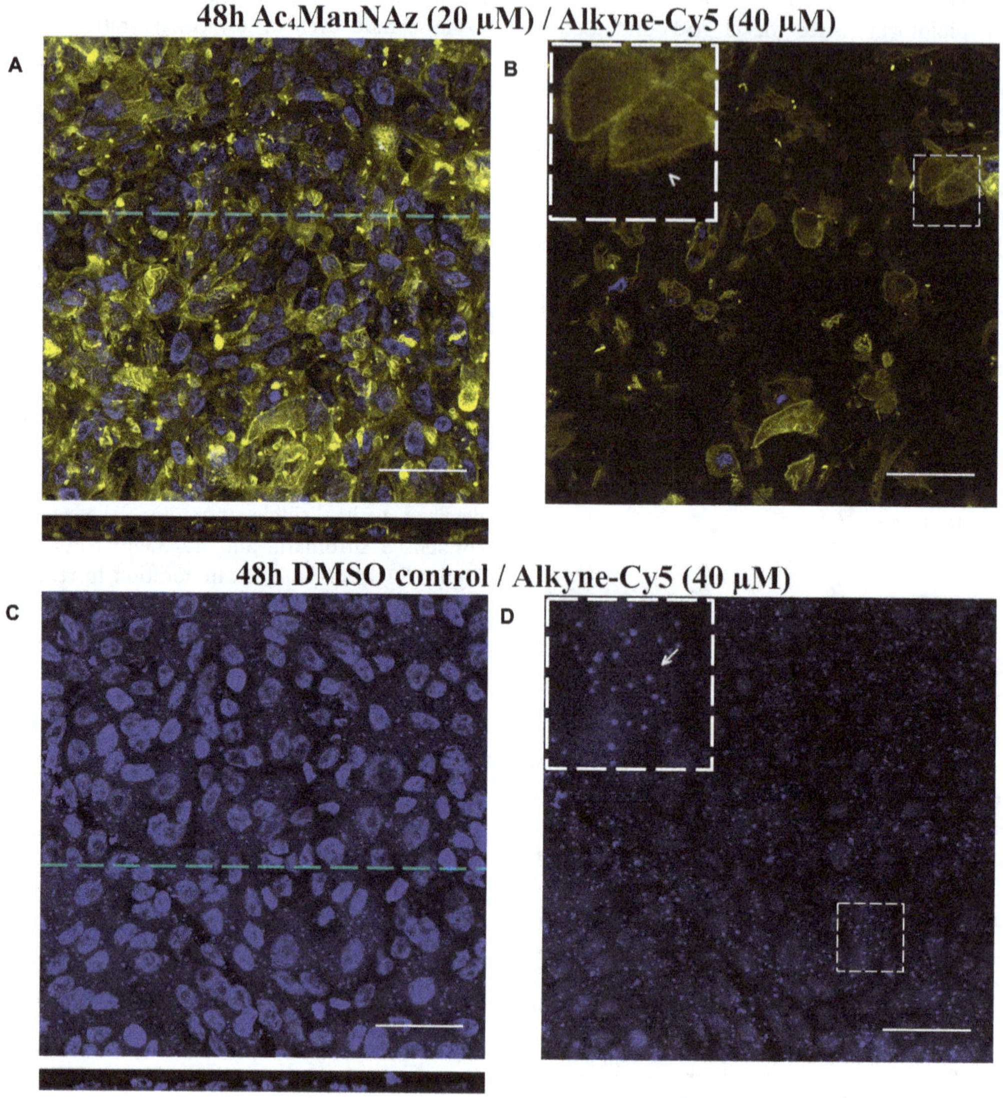

FIGURE 2 | LSM micrographs of hAELVi cells that have been grown for 14 days after seeding. Cells have been fed for 48 h with $Ac_4ManNAz$ (20 µM) or DMSO control and stained with alkyne-Cy5 (40 µM) using Cu(I) stabilizing helper THPTA. **(A)** Full z-stack projection of hAELVI cells. Dashed line indicates position of the corresponding cross-section plane. **(B)** Single section plane of **(A)** at the apical side of the cells shows membranous staining. Inset shows apical part of two cells at higher magnification. Arrowhead points to longitudinally oriented microvilli, while the fine dots covering most of the apical cell bodies (asterisk) represent transversally oriented microvilli. **(C)** Full z-stack projection of hAELVi cells fed with DMSO control display no alkyne-Cy5 staining indicating specificity of the staining. **(D)** Single section of **(C)** at a very basal position. The inset displays a higher magnification. The arrow points to the 0.4 µm pores of the transwell membrane which stain, because DAPI accumulates in the pores and cannot be washed out efficiently. Scale bars: 50 µm. Cross sections are scaled in *z*-axis by factor 3 to provide better visibility.

or simply fails in contrasting it sufficiently, we added Alcian blue during fixation and sample processing as it has previously been used in enhancing labeling of the glycocalyx by non-specific binding to glycosaminoglycans (Ruggeri et al., 1975; Singh et al., 2007). Indeed, adding Alcian blue to our Epon embedding protocol contrasted the glycocalyx as visualized by the typical ramifying structures (up to ~150 nm in length) emerging on top of the plasma membrane, especially in microvilli-rich domains (**Figures 3C,D**). However, when we compared our EPON-embedding to a freeze-substitution protocol using Lowycryl HM20 (HM20), we found the latter to preserve the network structure of the glycocalyx in more detail, even in the absence of additional labeling agents (**Figures 3E,F**).

Visualization of Sialic Acid by Combining MGE With a Biotin/AB-Gold Labeling Approach in a Freeze-Substitution Protocol

As HM20 based freeze-substitution technically allows for post-embedding antibody staining, we decided to modify the alkyne click chemistry reaction in favor of a combined click-chemistry

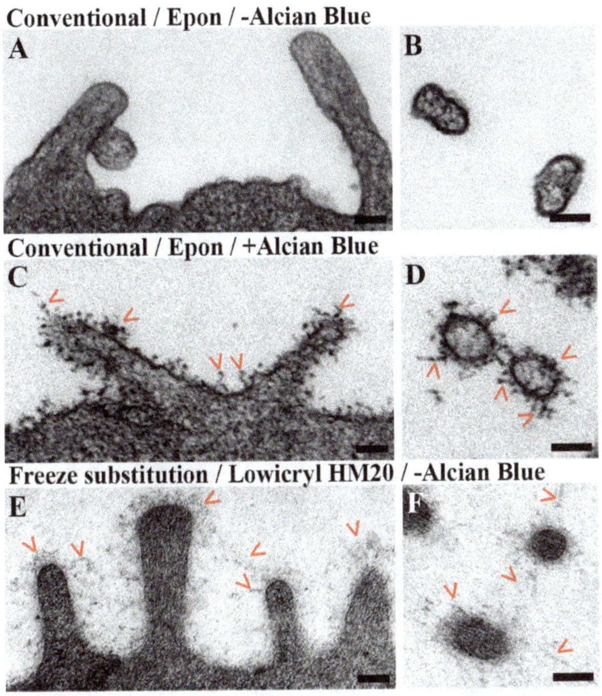

FIGURE 3 | Visualization of glycocalyx in electron micrographs of hAELVi cells using different EM procedures. **(A,B)** Chemically fixed and EPON embedded hAELVi cells 3 days after seeding. **(A)** Longitudinally, **(B)** transversally sectioned microvilli poorly displayed any ultrastructurally recognizable glycocalyx labeling. **(C,D)** Addition of Alcian blue labels glycocalyx as branching structures in **(C)** longitudinally and **(D)** transversally sectioned microvilli. **(E,F)** Mild chemical fixation and freeze substitution of 14 days old hAELVi cells resolves a fine, interconnected network structure around **(E)** longitudinally and **(F)** transversally sectioned microvilli. Scale bars: 100 nm.

antibody-based approach. For this purpose, we labeled cells with Acetylene-PEG$_4$-Biotin (CuAAC), before fixation and subsequent freeze substitution using HM20. After sectioning, we applied an antibody against biotin linked to a gold nanoparticle (anti-Biotin-AB-Au). This strategy successfully detected labeled sialic acid molecules at an ultrastructural level with high specificity (**Figure 4** and **Supplementary Figures S4, S5**). We confirmed the results in an SPAAC setting using DBCO-PEG$_4$-Biotin and the same antibody (**Supplementary Figure S6**).

Anti-Biotin-AB-Au specifically colocalized with the network structures of the glycocalyx, i.e., within close proximity to the plasma membrane (up to ~200 nm). Similar to our findings from confocal microscopy, labeled sialic acid as well as glycocalyx was most prominent around microvilli. Around sectioned microvilli (**Figure 4B** and **Supplementary Figure S5A**) and along the membrane (**Supplementary Figure S5**), we could detect sialic acid frequently localized at the distal end of glycan structures, corresponding to a terminal position.

In close proximity to the microvilli, we could further detect unilamellar and multilamellar membranous structures (**Figure 5**). Those often appeared to be attached to the fine glycan network of the glycocalyx (**Figures 5A,C,D**). Upon labeling of sialic acid, such areas were positive for gold nanoparticles (**Figure 5A**). Furthermore, we detected gold nanoparticles deeply within the lamellar structures, and this was notably in the absence of structurally visible colocalizing glycocalyx networks (**Figure 5B**). Some of the multilamellar structures adopted signs of a higher degree of organization (**Figure 5B**, Inset).

Cells fed with DMSO control displayed glycocalyx as well as uni- and multilamellar structures, yet in neither of those we could detect attaching gold nanoparticles, demonstrating the specificity of anti-Biotin-AB-Au labeling (**Figures 5C,D**).

DISCUSSION

In the last decades, glycan biology has made considerable progress in systematically applying established techniques in combination with newly emerging tools (Varki, 2017). For surface labeling of distinct species of sialic acids, sugarbinding lectins have been proven successful in light- and electron microscopy (Taatjes et al., 1988; Sata et al., 1991; Langereis et al., 2015). However, lectins rely on multivalency of their ligands as their single-site affinity is typically poor (Kiessling and Grim, 2013; Taylor et al., 2015). Thus, lectin binding tends to reflect the presence of closely clustered residues, inflicting bias in terms of sensitivity and quantification. In contrast to lectin based approaches, labeling of sialic acids originating from Ac$_4$ManNAz (**Figure 1A**) first, allows for single molecular analysis independent of ligand multivalency and second, enables the study of all types of sialic acids present on the surface, independent of the sub-entity of sialic acids for which lectins are specific. Interestingly, acetylated 4-Azido-ManNAc as an alternative to Ac$_4$ManNAz has been shown to integrate predominantly into sialic acids of O-glycans (Moller et al., 2012). Thus, MGE has also potential to label distinct sialic acid subspecies with certain specificity. Regarding single-molecule detection methods of glycans, there is a current lack of studies using *in vitro* or even *in vivo* settings (Lakshminarayanan et al., 2018). Super-resolution microscopy has been applied to study surface glycans (Letschert et al., 2014; Chen et al., 2016), and achieves a resolution of ~20 nm, which is at the edge of being suitable for visualizing protein complexes (ribosome: >80 proteins = 25 nm). This resolution is, however, still not sufficient for analysis of single glycan residues.

The herein established combination of MGE and EM proved suitable to overcome several of the before mentioned limitations, thus allowing for the first time for visualization of specific alveolar epithelial glycocalyx components at the single molecule level. Yet, care should be taken when utilizing MGE labeling in quantitative approaches, as the rate of metabolic incorporation of the labeled precursors has to be taken into consideration.

So far, glycocalyx-like structures of hAELVi cells have been previously demonstrated in one published electron micrograph of a hAELVi/THP-1 co-culture system (Kletting et al., 2018). In this study, the surface coat was non-specifically visualized around microvilli of hAELVi cells that seemingly interacted with THP-1 cells by a protocol using chemical fixation followed by Epon embedding and a combination of osmium and ferrocyanide

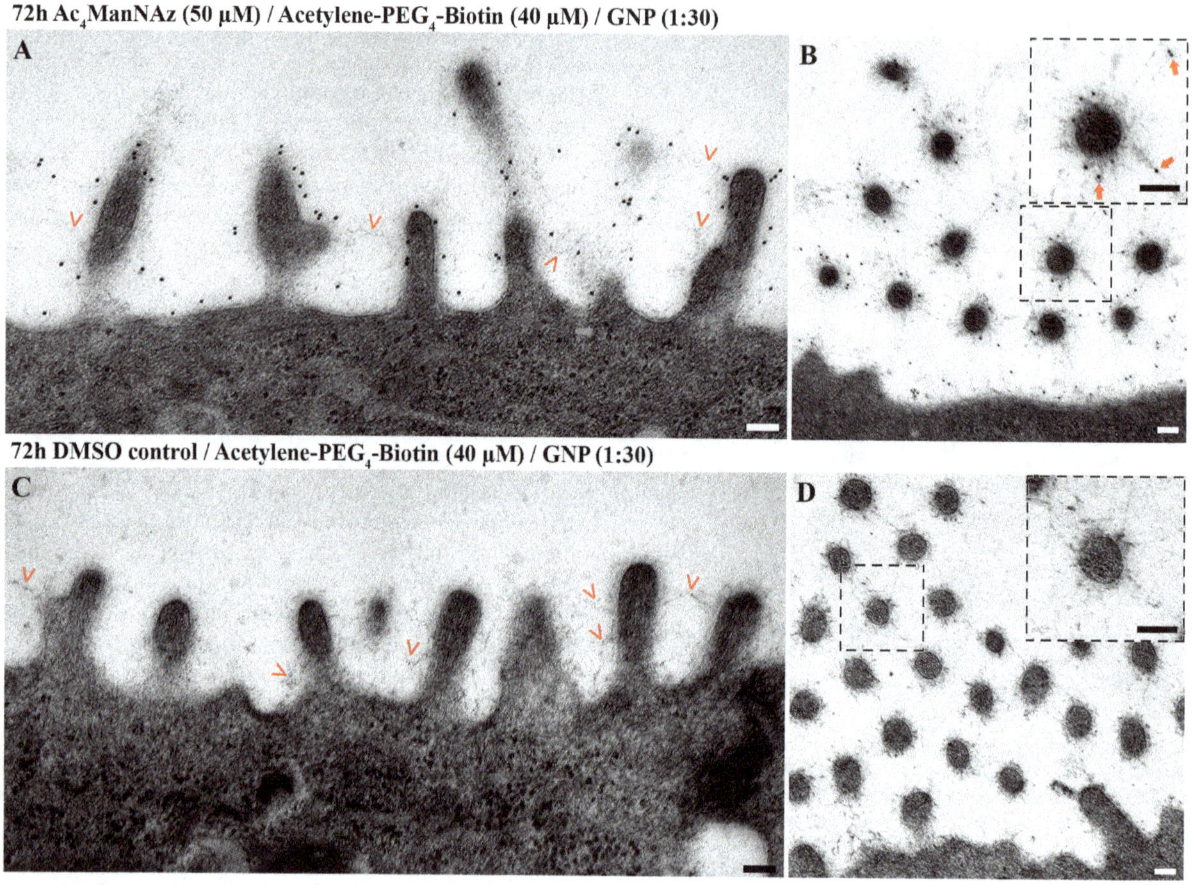

FIGURE 4 | Gold nanoparticles label sialic acid and colocalize with glycocalyx on the plasma membrane and around microvilli. Electron micrographs of hAELVi cell samples prepared using mild chemical fixation and subsequent FS. Micrographs show 14 days old cells fed **(A,B)** with Ac$_4$ManNAz (50 µM) or **(C,D)** DMSO control for 72 h before reacting with Acetylene-PEG$_4$-Biotin (40 µM). Postembedding, antibodies against biotin (dilution 1:30) linked to 10 nm gold nanoparticles were applied. Microvilli sectioned **(A)** longitudinally and **(B)** transversally display extensive labeling with gold nanoparticles within the glycocalyx. Those often colocalize at the distal end of branched filamentous structures **(B)**. Cells fed with DMSO control display no attached gold nanoparticles at the membrane, at **(C)** longitudinally and **(D)** transversally sectioned microvilli despite presence of glycocalyx networks, indicating specificity of the labeling. Scale bars: 100 nm. Insets: Large insets derive from micrographs recorded at higher magnification. Arrowheads: arrowheads point to fuzzy material on top of the plasma membrane that represents glycocalyx.

treatment. Ferrocyanide, which was not used in the present study, had previously been reported to be able to trace the glycocalyx of liver and renal cortex when applied in appropriate concentrations (Neiss, 1984). In our hands, hAELVi cells showed a staining pattern comparable to Kletting et al. (2018) when adding Alcian blue to our Epon embedding protocol (**Figure 3**), thus independently validating the presence of cell surface glycans. Alcian blue has positive charges, and is therefore able to bind to various acidic sugars when applied at low osmolarity conditions, most importantly sulfated and sialyated residues but also non-sulfated hyaluronic acid (Danes et al., 1970; Mohos and Skoza, 1970; Hayat, 1993). Upon binding, it typically forms particles (2–3 nm) with variable contrast, that can arrange in rods or chains, which showed a subtle degree of branching in our study. As such, we could improve a regular chemical fixation/Epon embedding method that was originally optimized for ultrastructural preservation of lung alveoli but not suitable to visualize the glycocalyx of hAELVi cells, with the purpose of labeling glycan structures non-specifically.

As described in the introduction, there is ongoing debate in the field, how the type of fixation, subsequent dehydration steps and chemical labeling reagents affects the preservation of the glycocalyx. Recently, it was hypothesized that dehydration rather than fixing is critically in terms of volume collapse of the glycocalyx as chemical fixation/dehydration versus cryofixation/freeze-substitution (which includes dehydration) resulted in comparable heights within lung- and heart vessels that were perfused with lanthanum and dysprosium (LaDy) for chemical labeling of the glycocalyx (Hempel et al., 2020). In this study, the authors then tried visualizing the glycocalyx of vessels by combining cryofixation and low-dose x-ray tomography (SXT), a methodology requiring a synchrotron but no dehydration step. However, this method provided not enough contrast for the glycocalyx to be detected without additional chemical labeling. Adding the latter (LaDy) prior to cryofixation/SXT partly overcame this issue but was not suitable to resolve any structural details due to its very high absorbance of x-rays. Despite, the authors indirectly estimated the height of

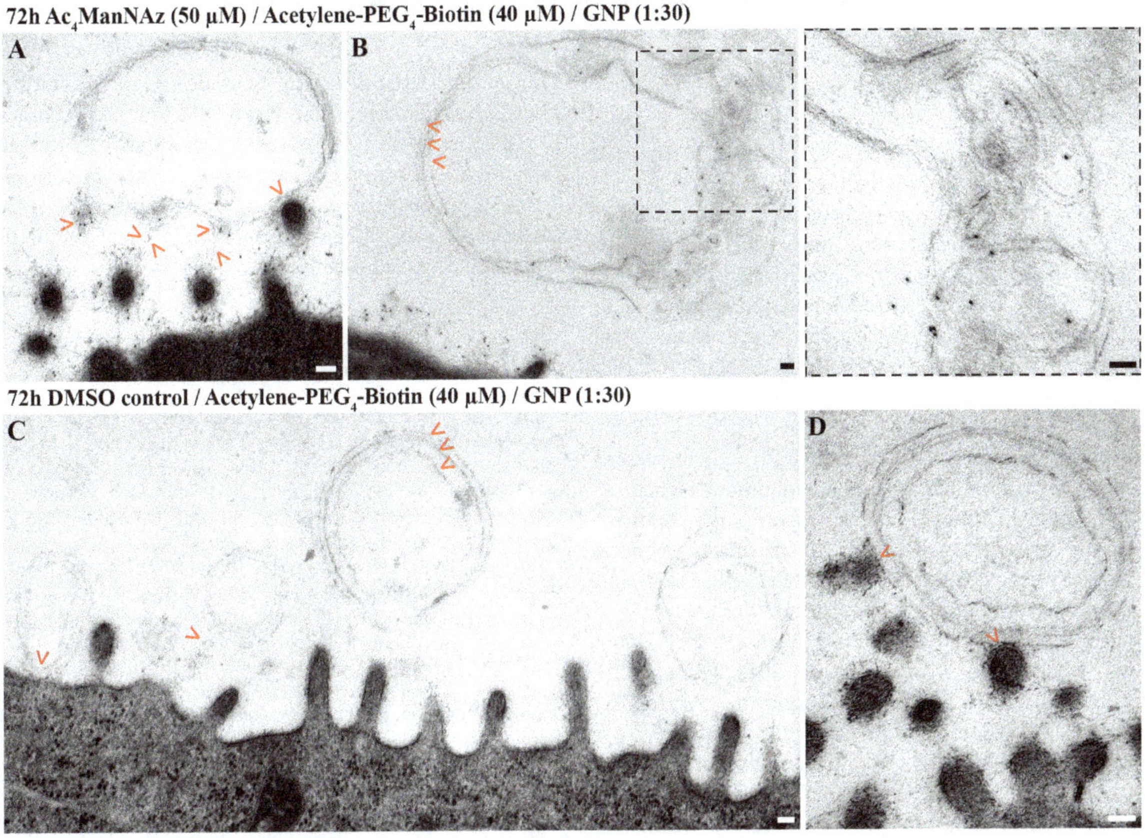

FIGURE 5 | hAELVi cells secrete lamellar membranous structures that interact with microvilli and were labeled for sialic acid. Electron micrographs of hAELVi cells prepared using a mild chemical fixation and subsequent FS. Micrographs show 14 days old cells that had been fed **(A,B)** with Ac_4ManNAz (50 µM) or **(C,D)** DMSO control for 72 h before reacting with Acetylene-PEG$_4$-Biotin (40 µM). Postembedding, antibodies against biotin (dilution 1:30) linked to 10 nm gold nanoparticles were applied. **(A)** Microvilli sectioned transversally interacting with multilamellar membranous structure. Gold nanoparticle labeling is displayed at the zone of contact (arrowheads). **(B)** Multilamellar membranous material forming higher ordered structures in close proximity to the plasma membrane. Arrowheads point to three lamellae, respectively. Inset: Large inset derives from micrograph recorded at higher magnification and shows gold nanoparticles within the multilamellar structure, which are devoid of obvious glycocalyx-like fibrous material. **(C)** In cells treated with DMSO control, attached gold particles are neither visible around the microvilli nor at or within the secreted lamellar membranous structures (arrowheads) indicating specificity of the labeling. **(D)** Micrograph recorded at higher magnification. Arrowheads point to the contact zone between a multilamellar membranous structure and multiple microvilli, apical of cells treated with DMSO control. Scale bars: 100 nm.

the glycocalyx by measuring the distance between the endothelial plasma membrane and trapped erythrocytes and found larger dimensions as compared to dehydration depending methods.

Here, we present the first ultrastructural analysis of the hAELVi cell glycocalyx based on a mild chemical fixation with subsequent freeze substitution procedure (**Figure 4** and **Supplementary Figures S4, S5**). Our freeze substitution protocol is devoid of additional glycan labeling chemicals (like LaDy or Alcian blue) and allowed for a more unbiased representation of the glycocalyx ultrastructure. According to previous findings (Reipert et al., 2018), our results show freeze substituted cells presenting with a fine, fuzzy surface coat (height up to ~200 nm), slightly exceeding dimensions found for Alcian blue labeling (up to ~150 nm). Albeit fainter in contrast, the network structure generally displayed a higher degree of complexity and interconnectivity.

We detected antibody-linked gold nanoparticles specifically bound to metabolically labeled sialic acid throughout the glycocalyx of the plasma membrane, using CuAAC (**Figure 4** and **Supplementary Figures S4, S5**) and SPAAC (**Supplementary Figure S6**), respectively. Importantly, we could localize gold particles at the end of branched filaments (**Figure 4B Supplementary Figure S5**), which correlates with the biochemically defined terminal position of sialic acid at the end of glycoconjugates (Varki et al., 2015). This prompts us to argue, that the preservation of the glycocalyx using our freeze substitution procedure holds promise to reflect the ultrastructural architecture to a reasonable extent. Our findings thus indicate that the combination of MGE with our freeze substitution protocol preserved a plausible representation of the glycocalyx that is unbiased of additional glycan stabilizing chemicals while equally providing molecular identity to the labeled structures in alveolar epithelial cells for the first time.

The recently established hAELVi cell line has been described as a model for ATI cells, although molecular characterization has been first, limited to the expression of a few marker genes and second, not been performed using cells harvested at ALI (Kuehn et al., 2016). After 13–14 days of culture at ALI, we report extensive formation of microvilli and a well-marked glycocalyx, both structural features more prevalent in ATII cells (Brooks, 1969; Adamson and Bowden, 1970; Roth, 1973; Mason, 2006; Ochs et al., 2020). Thus, the differentiation fate of the cell line might depend on the applied culture conditions. Of note, a comprehensive ultrastructural and molecular characterization is beyond the scope of the present study which focuses on establishing methods of glycocalyx visualization in alveolar epithelial cells. At the moment, there is ongoing refinement of hAELVi cell culture medium aiming to improve the physiological properties of the model (Tobias May, InSRCEENneX GmbH, personal communication, 28th September 2020).

Our ultrastructural analysis revealed hAELVi cells to present uni- and more complex multilamellar membranous structures (**Figure 5**). We regularly observed these structures to be in direct contact with the glycocalyx on top of the plasma membrane. Previous work studying interactions between surfactant and specific glycocalyx components has been limited to the proteoglycan hyaluronan (Lu et al., 2005; Taeusch et al., 2005; Wang et al., 2006; Lopez-Rodriguez et al., 2013; Dong et al., 2020). By combining MGE and EM, we found the extracellular lamellar structures to be enriched in sialic acids (**Figure 5**). We thus can hypothesize, that either glycolipids or glycoproteins are present in these lamellar structures. Notably, glycoproteins in alveolar spaces such as surfactant protein A (SP-A) (Munakata et al., 1982; White et al., 1985; Haagsman et al., 1991; Berg et al., 2000)contain sialic acid. Recently, glycans on surfactant protein D (SP-D), isolated from human amniotic fluid, were similarly reported to be sialylated (Arroyo et al., 2020). Future work will focus on characterizing the membranous material secreted by hAELVi cells in more detail, potentially opening novel model qualities for this cell line.

In summary, we established hAELVi cells as a model to study the alveolar epithelial cell glycocalyx and report a combination of tools for its ultrastructural characterization with molecular identity. As MGE is applicable for *in vivo* studies, this approach will facilitate the identification of the evolutionary developed functionalities of the so far scarcely investigated alveolar epithelial glycocalyx, its role in the interaction with surfactant components in the lining layer, and alterations upon onset of diseases.

AUTHOR CONTRIBUTIONS

EL-R, RB, ST, and MO evolved study design and conception and contributed to data interpretation. RB and ST performed the experiments. RB, JG, and ST wrote the manuscript. CH contributed to providing material. WK and JK offered constructive suggestions for the research. EL-R, CH, WK, and JK contributed to script revision. All authors approved to the final version.

ACKNOWLEDGMENTS

The authors thank Petra Schrade (Core Facility Electron Microscopy, Charité), John Horn (EM sample preparation), and Kerstin Riskowsky (LSM sample preparation) (both, Institute of Functional Anatomy, Charité) for excellent technical assistance. The authors also thank Prof. Imre Vida and Paul Turko (both, Institute of Integrative Neuroanatomy, Charité) for providing unlimited access to their confocal microscope.

SUPPLEMENTARY MATERIAL

Supplementary Figure 1 | LSM micrographs of hAELVi cells 3 days after seeding. Cells have been fed for 24 h with different concentrations of Ac_4ManNAz (20 μM, 60 μM, or DMSO control) and stained with alkyne-Cy5 using Cu(I) stabilizing helper BTTAA. **(A)** 20 μM Ac_4ManNAz, 40 μM alkyne-Cy5, laser intensity (LI) 2%, **(B)** 20 μM Ac_4ManNAz, 60 μM alkyne-Cy5, LI 2%, **(C)** 50 μM Ac4ManNAz, 40 μM alkyne-Cy5, LI 1%, **(D)** 50 μM Ac_4ManNAz, 60 μM alkyne-Cy5, LI 1%, **(E)** 60 μM alkyne-Cy5 LI 1%, **(F)** 60 μM alkyne-Cy5 LI 2%. Yellow channel: alkyne-Cy5, blue channel: DAPI. Laser intensities indicated for yellow channels. Scale bars: 50 μ m.

Supplementary Figure 2 | LSM micrographs of hAELVi cells that have been grown for 14 days after seeding. Cells have been fed for 72 h with Ac_4ManNAz (50 μM) and stained with DBCO-Sulfo-Cy3 (20 μM) in a SPAAC. **(A)** Full z-stack projection of hAELVI cells. Dashed line indicates position of the corresponding cross-section plane. **(B)** Single section plane of **(A)** at an apical position of the cells. Inset displays a higher magnification. The arrowhead points to an intensely stained structure (compare also to cross section plane of **A**) at the apical side of a cell that forms a tubular meshwork. **(C)** Full z-stack projection of hAELVI cells fed with DMSO control display minor background staining. **(D)** Single section plane of **(C)**. Inset displays a higher magnification. The arrow points to a dying cell with fragmented nuclei and highly condensed chromatin which displays considerable amount of unspecific DBCO-Sulfo-Cy5 staining. Scale bars: 50 μm. Cross sections are scaled in z-axis by factor 3 to provide better visibility.

Supplementary Figure 3 | hAELVi cells that have been grown for 14 days after seeding. Cells, seeded the same day, had been fed with Ac_4ManNAz (20 μM) for 48 h **(A–C)** or 50 μM for 72 h **(D)** and labeled with alkyne-Cy5 (40 μM) **(A–C)** or alkyne-gold (0.005%) **(D)** using CuAAC stabilizing helper substance BTTAA. **(A)** Full z-stack projection of hAELVi cells. Dashed line indicates position of the corresponding cross-section plane. **(B)** Single section plane of **(A)** at the apical side of the cells shows membranous staining. Inset shows apical part of cells at higher magnification. Brackets points to longitudinally oriented microvilli, while the fine dots covering most of the apical cell bodies represent transversally oriented microvilli. **(C)** Full z-stack projection of hAELVi cells fed with DMSO control display no alkyne-Cy5 staining indicating specificity of the staining using CuAAC. **(D)** Electron micrograph of chemically fixed and EPON embedded cells showing longitudinally sectioned microvilli that display no gold nanoparticles labeling around the microvilli or other parts of the plasma membrane indicating failing labeling efficiency using alkyne-gold. Scale bars LSM: 50 μm. Cross sections are scaled in z-axis by factor 3 to provide better visibility. Scale bars EM: 100 nm.

Supplementary Figure 4 | Sialic acid labeling of the glycocalyx on plasma membrane and around microvilli using CuAAC and gold nanoparticles. Electron micrograph (freeze substitution protocol) of 14 days old hAELVi cells fed **(A,B)** with Ac_4ManNAz (50 μM) or **(C,D)** DMSO control for 72 h before reacting with Acetylene-PEG_4-Biotin (60 μM). Postembedding, antibodies against biotin (dilution 1:30) linked to 10 nm gold nanoparticles were applied. Microvilli sectioned **(A)** longitudinally and **(B)** transversally show extensive labeling by gold nanoparticles, colocalizing with extracellular fuzzy material that exhibit network-like

structures. Cells fed with DMSO control display no attached gold nanoparticles at the membrane, at **(C)** longitudinally or **(D)** transversally sectioned microvilli despite presence of glycocalyx networks, indicating specificity of the labeling.
Scale bars: 100 nm.

Supplementary Figure 5 | Sialic acid labeling of the glycocalyx around microvilli **(A)** and on plasma membrane **(B,C)** using CuAAC and gold nanoparticles. Electron micrograph (freeze substitution protocol) of 14 days old hAELVi cells fed with Ac_4ManNAz (50 μM) for 72 h before reacting with Acetylene-PEG_4-Biotin (40 μM). Postembedding, antibodies against biotin (dilution 1:30) linked to 10 nm gold nanoparticles were applied. Note that a large proportion of gold nanoparticles appears to be localized at the distal end of glycan structures. Scale bars: 100 nm.

Supplementary Figure 6 | Labeling of sialic acid around the plasma membrane of microvilli using SPAAC and gold nanoparticles. Electron microscopy using freeze substitution protocol of 14 days old hAELVi cells fed **(A)** with Ac_4ManNAz (50 μM) or **(B)** DMSO control for 72 h before reacting with DBCO-PEG_4-Biotin (60 μM). Postembedding, antibodies against biotin (dilution 1:30) linked to 10 nm gold nanoparticles were applied. Scale bars: 100 nm.

REFERENCES

Adamson, I. Y., and Bowden, D. H. (1970). The surface complexes of the lung. A cytochemical partition of phospholipid surfactant and mucopolysaccharide. *Am. J. Pathol.* 61, 359–376. doi: 10.1007/978-1-4757-5806-1_11

Arroyo, R., Echaide, M., Wilmanowski, R., Martin-Gonzalez, A., Batllori, E., Galindo, A., et al. (2020). Structure and activity of human surfactant protein D from different natural sources. *Am. J. Physiol. Lung. Cell Mol. Physiol.* 319, L148–L158.

Baskin, J. M., Prescher, J. A., Laughlin, S. T., Agard, N. J., Chang, P. V., Miller, I. A., et al. (2007). Copper-free click chemistry for dynamic in vivo imaging. *Proc. Natl. Acad. Sci. U.S.A.* 104, 16793–16797. doi: 10.1073/pnas.0707090104

Bastacky, J., Lee, C. Y., Goerke, J., Koushafar, H., Yager, D., Kenaga, L., et al. (1995). Alveolar lining layer is thin and continuous: low-temperature scanning electron microscopy of rat lung. *J. Appl. Physiol.* 79, 1615–1628. doi: 10.1152/jappl.1995.79.5.1615

Berg, T., Leth-Larsen, R., Holmskov, U., and Hojrup, P. (2000). Structural characterisation of human proteinosis surfactant protein A. *Biochim. Biophys. Acta* 1543, 159–173. doi: 10.1016/s0167-4838(00)00184-9

Broecker, F., Anish, C., and Seeberger, P. H. (2015). Generation of monoclonal antibodies against defined oligosaccharide antigens. *Methods Mol. Biol.* 1331, 57–80. doi: 10.1007/978-1-4939-2874-3_5

Brooks, R. E. (1969). Ruthenium red stainable surface layer on lung alveolar cells; electron microscopic interpretation. *Stain. Technol.* 44, 173–177. doi: 10.3109/10520296909063346

Chen, J., Gao, J., Zhang, M., Cai, M., Xu, H., Jiang, J., et al. (2016). Systemic localization of seven major types of carbohydrates on cell membranes by dSTORM imaging. *Sci. Rep.* 6:30247.

Chevalier, L., Selim, J., Genty, D., Baste, J. M., Piton, N., Boukhalfa, I., et al. (2017). Electron microscopy approach for the visualization of the epithelial and endothelial glycocalyx. *Morphologie* 101, 55–63. doi: 10.1016/j.morpho.2017.04.001

Cioffi, D. L., Pandey, S., Alvarez, D. F., and Cioffi, E. A. (2012). Terminal sialic acids are an important determinant of pulmonary endothelial barrier integrity. *Am. J. Physiol. Lung. Cell Mol. Physiol.* 302, L1067–L1077.

Danes, B. S., Scott, J. E., and Bearn, A. G. (1970). Further studies on metachromasia in cultured human fibroblasts – staining of glycosaminoglycans (Mucopolysaccharides) by alcian blue in salt solutions. *J. Exp. Med.* 132, 765–774. doi: 10.1084/jem.132.4.765

Dong, Y., Arif, A. A., Guo, J., Ha, Z., Lee-Sayer, S. S. M., Poon, G. F. T., et al. (2020). CD44 loss disrupts lung lipid surfactant homeostasis and exacerbates oxidized lipid-induced lung inflammation. *Front. Immunol.* 11:29. doi: 10.3389/fimmu.2020.00029

Ebong, E. E., Macaluso, F. P., Spray, D. C., and Tarbell, J. M. (2011). Imaging the endothelial glycocalyx in vitro by rapid freezing/freeze substitution transmission electron microscopy. *Arterioscler. Thromb. Vasc. Biol.* 31, 1908–1915. doi: 10.1161/atvbaha.111.225268

Fehrenbach, H., and Ochs, M. (1998). "Studying lung ultrastructure," in *Methods in Pulmonary Research*, eds S. Uhlig and A. E. Taylor (Basel: Birkhäuser), 429–454. doi: 10.1007/978-3-0348-8855-4_17

Haagsman, H. P., Elfring, R. H., Van Buel, B. L., and Voorhout, W. F. (1991). The lung lectin surfactant protein A aggregates phospholipid vesicles via a novel mechanism. *Biochem. J.* 275(Pt 1), 273–276. doi: 10.1042/bj2750273

Han, S., and Mallampalli, R. K. (2015). The role of surfactant in lung disease and host defense against pulmonary infections. *Ann. Am. Thorac. Soc.* 12, 765–774. doi: 10.1513/annalsats.201411-507fr

Hayat, M. A. (1993). *Stains and Cytochemical Methods*. New York, NY: Plenum Press.

Hegermann, J., Lunsdorf, H., Ochs, M., and Haller, H. (2016). Visualization of the glomerular endothelial glycocalyx by electron microscopy using cationic colloidal thorium dioxide. *Histochem. Cell Bio.* 145, 41–51. doi: 10.1007/s00418-015-1378-3

Hempel, C., Kapishnikov, S., Perez-Berna, A. J., Werner, S., Guttmann, P., Pereiro, E., et al. (2020). The need to freeze-dehydration during specimen preparation for electron microscopy collapses the endothelial glycocalyx regardless of fixation method. *Microcirculation* 27:e12643.

Hsia, C. C., Hyde, D. M., and Weibel, E. R. (2016). Lung structure and the intrinsic challenges of gas exchange. *Compr. Physiol.* 6, 827–895. doi: 10.1002/cphy.c150028

Jacobs, C. L., Yarema, K. J., Mahal, L. K., Nauman, D. A., Charters, N. W., and Bertozzi, C. R. (2000). Metabolic labeling of glycoproteins with chemical tags through unnatural sialic acid biosynthesis. *Methods Enzymol.* 327, 260–275. doi: 10.1016/s0076-6879(00)27282-0

Kenry, and Liu, B. (2019). Bio-orthogonal click chemistry for in vivo bioimaging. *Trends Chem.* 1, 763–778. doi: 10.1016/j.trechm.2019.08.003

Kiessling, L. L., and Grim, J. C. (2013). Glycopolymer probes of signal transduction. *Chem. Soc. Rev.* 42, 4476–4491. doi: 10.1039/c3cs60097a

Kletting, S., Barthold, S., Repnik, U., Griffiths, G., Loretz, B., Schneider-Daum, N., et al. (2018). Co-culture of human alveolar epithelial (hAELVi) and macrophage (THP-1) cell lines. *ALTEX* 35, 211–222. doi: 10.14573/altex.1607191

Kuehn, A., Kletting, S., De Souza Carvalho-Wodarz, C., Repnik, U., Griffiths, G., Fischer, U., et al. (2016). Human alveolar epithelial cells expressing tight junctions to model the air-blood barrier. *ALTEX* 33, 251–260.

Laine, R. A. (1994). A calculation of all possible oligosaccharide isomers both branched and linear yields 1.05 x 10(12) structures for a reducing hexasaccharide: the Isomer Barrier to development of single-method saccharide sequencing or synthesis systems. *Glycobiology* 4, 759–767. doi: 10.1093/glycob/4.6.759

Lakshminarayanan, A., Richard, M., and Davis, B. G. (2018). Studying glycobiology at the single-molecule level. *Nat. Rev. Chem.* 2, 148–159. doi: 10.1038/s41570-018-0019-5

Langereis, M. A., Bakkers, M. J., Deng, L., Padler-Karavani, V., Vervoort, S. J., Hulswit, R. J., et al. (2015). Complexity and diversity of the mammalian sialome revealed by nidovirus virolectins. *Cell Rep.* 11, 1966–1978. doi: 10.1016/j.celrep.2015.05.044

Letschert, S., Gohler, A., Franke, C., Bertleff-Zieschang, N., Memmel, E., Doose, S., et al. (2014). Super-resolution imaging of plasma membrane glycans. *Angew. Chem. Int. Ed.* 53, 10921–10924. doi: 10.1002/anie.201406045

Lopez-Rodriguez, E., Cruz, A., Richter, R. P., Taeusch, H. W., and Perez-Gil, J. (2013). Transient exposure of pulmonary surfactant to hyaluronan promotes structural and compositional transformations into a highly active state. *J. Biol. Chem.* 288, 29872–29881. doi: 10.1074/jbc.m113.493957

Lu, K. W., Goerke, J., Clements, J. A., and Taeusch, H. W. (2005). Hyaluronan decreases surfactant inactivation in vitro. *Pediatr. Res.* 57, 237–241. doi: 10.1203/01.pdr.0000150726.75308.22

Mason, R. J. (2006). Biology of alveolar type II cells. *Respirology* 11(Suppl.), S12–S15.

Matrosovich, M., Herrler, G., and Klenk, H. D. (2015). Sialic acid receptors of viruses. *Top. Curr. Chem.* 367, 1–28. doi: 10.1007/128_2013_466

Matthay, M. A., Zemans, R. L., Zimmerman, G. A., Arabi, Y. M., Beitler, J. R., Mercat, A., et al. (2019). Acute respiratory distress syndrome. *Nat. Rev. Dis. Primers* 5:18.

Mockl, L. (2020). The emerging role of the mammalian glycocalyx in functional membrane organization and immune system regulation. *Front. Cell Dev. Biol.* 8:253. doi: 10.3389/fcell.2020.00253

Mohos, S. C., and Skoza, L. (1970). Histochemical demonstration and localization of sialoproteins in the glomerulus. *Exp. Mol. Pathol.* 12, 316–323. doi: 10.1016/0014-4800(70)90063-8

Moller, H., Bohrsch, V., Bentrop, J., Bender, J., Hinderlich, S., and Hackenberger, C. P. R. (2012). Glycan-specific metabolic oligosaccharide engineering of C7-substituted sialic acids. *Angew. Chem. Int. Ed.* 51, 5986–5990. doi: 10.1002/anie.201108809

Moller, H., Bohrsch, V., Lucka, L., Hackenberger, C. P., and Hinderlich, S. (2011). Efficient metabolic oligosaccharide engineering of glycoproteins by UDP-N-acetylglucosamine 2-epimerase/N-acetylmannosamine kinase (GNE) knock-down. *Mol. Biosyst.* 7, 2245–2251. doi: 10.1039/c1mb05059a

Munakata, H., Nimberg, R. B., Snider, G. L., Robins, A. G., Van Halbeek, H., Vliegenthart, J. F., et al. (1982). The structure of the carbohydrate units of the 36K glycoprotein derived from the lung lavage of a patient with alveolar proteinosis by high resolution 1H-NMR spectroscopy. *Biochem. Biophys. Res. Commun.* 108, 1401–1405. doi: 10.1016/s0006-291x(82)80062-4

Neiss, W. F. (1984). Electron staining of the cell surface coat by osmium-low ferrocyanide. *Histochemistry* 80, 231–242. doi: 10.1007/bf00495771

Ochs, M., Hegermann, J., Lopez-Rodriguez, E., Timm, S., Nouailles, G., Matuszak, J., et al. (2020). On top of the alveolar epithelium: surfactant and the glycocalyx. *Int. J. Mol. Sci.* 21:3075. doi: 10.3390/ijms21093075

Owen, L. S., Manley, B. J., Davis, P. G., and Doyle, L. W. (2017). The evolution of modern respiratory care for preterm infants. *Lancet* 389, 1649–1659. doi: 10.1016/s0140-6736(17)30312-4

Pattle, R. E. (1955). Properties, function and origin of the alveolar lining layer. *Nature* 175, 1125–1126. doi: 10.1038/1751125b0

Reipert, S., Goldammer, H., Richardson, C., Goldberg, M. W., Hawkins, T. J., Hollergschwandtner, E., et al. (2018). Agitation modules: flexible means to accelerate automated freeze substitution. *J. Histochem. Cytochem.* 66, 903–921. doi: 10.1369/0022155418786698

Reynolds, E. S. (1963). The use of lead citrate at high pH as an electron-opaque stain in electron microscopy. *J. Cell Biol.* 17, 208–212. doi: 10.1083/jcb.17.1.208

Roth, J. (1973). Ultrahistochemical demonstration of saccharide components of complex carbohydrates at the alveolar cell surface and at the mesothelial cell surface of the pleura visceralis of mice by means of concanavalin A. *Exp. Pathol.* 8, 157–167.

Ruggeri, A., Dell'orbo, C., and Quacci, D. (1975). Electron microscopic visualization of proteoglycans with Alcian Blue. *Histochem. J.* 7, 187–197. doi: 10.1007/bf01004562

Sata, T., Roth, J., Zuber, C., Stamm, B., and Heitz, P. U. (1991). Expression of Alpha-2,6-linked sialic-acid residues in neoplastic but not in normal human colonic mucosa – a lectin-gold cytochemical study with sambucus-nigra and maackia-amurensis lectins. *Am. J. Pathol.* 139, 1435–1448.

Schauer, R., and Kamerling, J. P. (2018). Exploration of the sialic acid world. *Adv. Carbohydr. Chem. Biochem.* 75, 1–213. doi: 10.1016/bs.accb.2018.09.001

Singh, A., Satchell, S. C., Neal, C. R., Mckenzie, E. A., Tooke, J. E., and Mathieson, P. W. (2007). Glomerular endothelial glycocalyx constitutes a barrier to protein permeability. *J. Am. Soc. Nephrol.* 18, 2885–2893. doi: 10.1681/asn.2007010119

Taatjes, D. J., Roth, J., Peumans, W., and Goldstein, I. J. (1988). Elderberry bark lectin gold techniques for the detection of Neu5ac (Alpha-2,6) Gal galnac sequences – applications and limitations. *Histochem. J.* 20, 478–490. doi: 10.1007/bf01002646

Taeusch, H. W., De La Serna, J. B., Perez-Gil, J., Alonso, C., and Zasadzinski, J. A. (2005). Inactivation of pulmonary surfactant due to serum-inhibited adsorption and reversal by hydrophilic polymers: experimental. *Biophys. J.* 89, 1769–1779. doi: 10.1529/biophysj.105.062620

Taylor, M. E., Drickamer, K., Schnaar, R. L., Etzler, M. E., and Varki, A. (2015). "Discovery and classification of glycan-binding proteins," in *Essentials of Glycobiology*, eds A. Varki, R. D. Cummings, J. D. Esko, P. Stanley, G. W. Hart, M. Aebi, et al. (New York, NY: Cold Spring Harbor), 361–372.

Varki, A. (2017). Biological roles of glycans. *Glycobiology* 27, 3–49. doi: 10.1093/glycob/cww086

Varki, A., Schnaar, R. L., and Schauer, R. (2015). "Sialic acids and other nonulosonic acids," in *Essentials of Glycobiology*, eds A. Varki, R. D. Cummings, J. D. Esko, P. Stanley, G. W. Hart, M. Aebi, et al. (New York, NY: Cold Spring Harbor), 179–195.

Wang, X., Sun, Z., Qian, L., Guo, C., Yu, W., Wang, W., et al. (2006). Effects of hyaluronan-fortified surfactant in ventilated premature piglets with respiratory distress. *Biol. Neonate* 89, 15–24. doi: 10.1159/000088194

White, R. T., Damm, D., Miller, J., Spratt, K., Schilling, J., Hawgood, S., et al. (1985). Isolation and characterization of the human pulmonary surfactant apoprotein gene. *Nature* 317, 361–363. doi: 10.1038/317361a0

Wielgat, P., Trofimiuk, E., Czarnomysy, R., Holownia, A., and Braszko, J. J. (2018). Sialylation pattern in lung epithelial cell line and siglecs expression in monocytic THP-1 cells as cellular indicators of cigarette smoke – induced pathology in vitro. *Exp. Lung. Res.* 44, 167–177. doi: 10.1080/01902148.2018.1461959

Wratil, P. R., Horstkorte, R., and Reutter, W. (2016). Metabolic glycoengineering with N-Acyl side chain modified mannosamines. *Angew. Chem. Int. Ed.* 55, 9482–9512. doi: 10.1002/anie.201601123

Wright, J. R. (2005). Immunoregulatory functions of surfactant proteins. *Nat. Rev. Immunol.* 5, 58–68. doi: 10.1038/nri1528

9

In situ-Like Aerosol Inhalation Exposure for Cytotoxicity Assessment using *Airway-on-Chips* Platforms

Shani Elias-Kirma, Arbel Artzy-Schnirman, Prashant Das, Metar Heller-Algazi, Netanel Korin and Josué Sznitman*

Department of Biomedical Engineering, Technion – Israel Institute of Technology, Haifa, Israel

Correspondence:
Josué Sznitman
sznitman@bm.technion.ac.il

Lung exposure to inhaled particulate matter (PM) is known to injure the airway epithelium via inflammation, a phenomenon linked to increased levels of global morbidity and mortality. To evaluate physiological outcomes following PM exposure and concurrently circumvent the use of animal experiments, *in vitro* approaches have typically relied on traditional assays with plates or well inserts. Yet, these manifest drawbacks including the inability to capture physiological inhalation conditions and aerosol deposition characteristics relative to *in vivo* human conditions. Here, we present a novel *airway-on-chip* exposure platform that emulates the epithelium of human bronchial airways with critical cellular barrier functions at an air–liquid interface (ALI). As a proof-of-concept for *in vitro* lung cytotoxicity testing, we recapitulate a well-characterized cell apoptosis pathway, induced through exposure to 2 μm airborne particles coated with αVR1 antibody that leads to significant loss in cell viability across the recapitulated airway epithelium. Notably, our *in vitro* inhalation assays enable simultaneous aerosol exposure across multiple airway chips integrated within a larger bronchial airway tree model, under physiological respiratory airflow conditions. Our findings underscore *in situ*-like aerosol deposition outcomes where patterns depend on respiratory flows across the airway tree geometry and gravitational orientation, as corroborated by concurrent numerical simulations. Our *airway-on-chips* not only highlight the prospect of realistic *in vitro* exposure assays in recapitulating characteristic local *in vivo* deposition outcomes, such platforms open opportunities toward advanced *in vitro* exposure assays for preclinical cytotoxicity and drug screening applications.

Keywords: pulmonary, airway, organ-on-chip, *in vitro*, human primary cells, inhalation, aerosol, cytotoxicity

INTRODUCTION

With a vast and highly vascularized surface optimized for gas exchange (Grotberg, 2011; Janssen et al., 2016), the lungs constitute the largest organ directly exposed to the external environment. As such, the lungs are vulnerable to a breadth of threats associated with occupational (Leggat et al., 2007) and environmental (Brulle and Pellow, 2006) hazards. In particular, exposure to inhaled airborne particulate matter (PM) represents a global health problem due to adverse cardiovascular and respiratory outcomes linked to increased morbidity and mortality (Anderson et al., 2012; Kim et al., 2015; Conibear et al., 2018; Wu et al., 2018). To protect the body from continuous exposure to foreign PM, and also pathogens and other toxic chemicals (Bals and Hiemstra, 2004), the lungs' luminal surface is populated with a confluent, uninterrupted epithelial cell carpet that exists as a continuum across the airway tree (Daniels and Orgeig, 2003). In the conducting airways specifically, epithelial cells are covered with an extracellular periciliary lining (Button et al., 2012) itself immersed under a mucus layer present at an air–liquid interface (ALI) (Fahy and Dickey, 2010). Briefly, the secretion of mucus by goblet and club cells (Barnes et al., 2003; Lai et al., 2008; Fahy and Dickey, 2010; Whitsett, 2018), in combination with ciliated cells, contributes to airway clearance (Janssen et al., 2016) by trapping (Stannard and O'Callaghan, 2006) inhaled particles and pathogens (e.g., bacteria) depositing on the pulmonary epithelium. This complex cellular environment requires a well-differentiated bronchial epithelium that constitutes the conducting airways' innate defense mechanisms and maintains pulmonary homeostasis.

In an effort to evaluate physiological outcomes following PM exposure and its association with diseases (e.g., COPD; Anderson et al., 2012), *in vivo* animal experiments have been traditionally pursued. For example, *in vivo* studies have demonstrated that pulmonary exposure to PM causes lung inflammation and oxidative stress (Inoue et al., 2006; Nemmar et al., 2009, 2011). Nemmar et al. (2009) showed that 24 h post intratracheal instillation of diesel exhaust particles, the influx of macrophages and neutrophils in broncho-alveolar mice lavages was elevated. Despite such progress, *in vivo* animal studies remain contentious due to critical differences in anatomy, immune systems, and inflammatory responses compared with humans (Benam et al., 2015), thereby raising the need for more relevant platforms for evaluation (Bueters et al., 2013). To overcome such drawbacks and uncover cellular mechanisms in which PM toxicity affects the respiratory system, *in vitro* studies with cell cultures have been actively sought (Paur et al., 2011; Nemmar et al., 2013; Drasler et al., 2017). In particular, ALI conditions can be recapitulated by culturing cells on the apical side of a porous membrane using for instance commercially available Transwell inserts; such setups are indeed critical in striving to mimic physiologically relevant characteristics of the bronchial airway lumen, including for example mucus secretion (Grainger et al., 2006; Lin et al., 2007). Furthermore, capturing biological airway responses specific to humans following PM exposure to toxins (Mustafiz et al., 2015) calls for the use of human primary cells (Skardal et al., 2016) in an effort to overcome ongoing limitations with animal studies. Although the aforementioned macroscopic *in vitro* approaches reproduce some of the cellular functions of the human pulmonary environment, both true-scale anatomical airway features and physiological (air) flow conditions are still widely absent from existing *in vitro* exposure assays. Such drawbacks continue to restrict *in vitro* setups from addressing faithfully the physical aerosol transport determinants leading to PM deposition along the inhalation route. Since direct *in vivo* human exposure studies are ethically controversial, the development of realistic *in vitro* human exposure assays is thus desired to advance our understanding of inflammation and disease following harmful PM exposure under realistic *in situ* inhalation conditions.

Over the past decade, *organ-on-chips* have gained momentum in laying the foundations for constructing attractive *in vitro* models that mimic more realistically physiologically relevant organ functions in humans (Nesmith et al., 2014; Abaci et al., 2015; Bovard et al., 2018; Ronaldson-Bouchard and Vunjak-Novakovic, 2018; Shirure et al., 2018). Such platforms allow *in vitro* examinations within micro-devices lined with human cells, thereby fostering new physiological insights, in both health and disease, complementary to current tools available for diagnostics and conventional *in vitro* approaches (Tenenbaum-Katan et al., 2018). Specifically, lung-related models have been devised to mimic the human alveolar–capillary interface and stimulate inflammatory responses *in vitro* (Huh et al., 2010, 2012; Artzy-Schnirman et al., 2019b). For example, Huh et al. (2010) demonstrated the importance of using cyclic mechanical strain, which accentuates toxic and lung inflammatory responses to silica nanoparticles, associated with the development of vascular leakage, which leads to pulmonary edema. In parallel, Benam et al. (2015) reconstituted a human lung *small airway-on-a-chip* model by co-culturing both endothelium cells and epithelial tissue from healthy individuals and COPD patients to model human lung inflammatory disorders. In addition, using the *small airway-on-a-chip* model connected to a smoking instrument, Benam et al. (2016) established a platform to study a patient-specific response to inhaled smoke. Punde et al. (2015) showed protein-induced lung inflammation and emphasized the need of using flow, which allows reconstituting the blood vessel–tissue interface for *in vitro* assays, and by that improve pre-clinical studies. Together with other recent efforts (Douville et al., 2011; Nesmith et al., 2014; Stucki et al., 2014; Li et al., 2015; Hassell et al., 2017; Humayun et al., 2018), these studies have brought tremendous progress in lung research but are still widely limited to platforms with a single airway channel, thus short of mimicking the complexity of the conducting airway tree. This is especially critical when exploring the fate of inhaled aerosols where the coupling between respiratory airflows and lung anatomy is known to modulate particle deposition outcomes (Kleinstreuer and Zhang, 2010; Fishler et al., 2015; Koullapis P.G. et al., 2018).

Motivated by the critical need to deliver *in vitro* platforms that mimic more closely physiological inhalation conditions of human lung exposure with characteristic *in situ*-like deposition outcomes (Artzy-schnirman et al., 2019a), we have established a novel inhalation assay integrated with an *airway-on-chip* platform comprising three-generational bronchial airways cultured with a differentiated human bronchial epithelium. Specifically, such *in vitro* inhalation assay reproduces mechanistically faithful aerosol transport determinants leading to airway deposition at a functional epithelial barrier. As a proof-of-concept, we characterize PM toxicity whereby we recapitulate a well-characterized apoptosis pathway (Agopyan et al., 2003, 2004). One of the better-known pathways in which PM affects human airway cytotoxicity is mediated by receptors which induce cell apoptosis (Becker et al., 1996; Holian et al., 1998), including importantly the Vanilloid (i.e., VR1) receptor (Agopyan et al., 2003). Seminal *in vitro* studies using primary cells have shown that 48 h post PM particle stimulation the level of apoptotic cells is elevated by activation of such VR1 receptor (Agopyan et al., 2004). Here, apoptosis is induced through exposure to 2-μm airborne particles coated by αVR1 antibody; an aerosol size known to deposit in the small bronchi and bronchioles (Bair, 1989; Stahlhofen et al., 1989; Hinds, 1999). Importantly, our *in vitro* inhalation assays deliver aerosols simultaneously across four *airway-on-chips* integrated within a larger conductive airway tree model to explore *in situ*-like aerosol deposition outcomes under physiological respiratory airflows and for various gravitational orientations. Given that current cytotoxicity assays are still widely based on either non-physiological liquid installations of PM suspensions (Hittinger et al., 2017) or alternatively direct spraying at an ALI (Blank et al., 2006; Lenz et al., 2014; Röhm et al., 2017), our *airway-on-chip* exposure setup is part of steadfast efforts (Artzy-schnirman et al., 2019a) leading toward a new generation of advanced *in vitro* lung toolkits for human inhalation toxicity assays.

MATERIALS AND METHODS

Airway-on-Chip

Device Design

The design of the proposed *airway-on-chips* consists of a planar, symmetric airway tree spanning three generations (with a total of four outlets), as schematically shown in **Figure 1a**. Individual airways consist of lumens of semi-circular cross-sections (chosen as a result of the need for a porous membrane for cell culture, see below) where dimensions, summarized in **Table 1**, are based on morphometric measurements representative of a typical human adult lung, following the seminal works of Weibel et al. (1963) and Horsfield et al. (1971). Note that our *in vitro* platform broadly mimics small bronchial branches of the conducting zone, with airway diameters <2.5 mm, along with an idealized constant planar bifurcating angle of 60° across all generations (Ménache et al., 2008). In line with recent *lung-on-chip* designs limited to single airway channels, the present design allows to culture cells at ALI conditions together with access for inhalation airflows through the apical compartment using a syringe pump (see below).

Device Fabrication

The model negative is 3D printed in house via stereo-lithography (Formlabs, Form 2). The mould is used as a master template for polydimethylsiloxane (PDMS) casting. PDMS was mixed with a curing agent (Dow Corning) at a 10:1 weight ratio, poured on the template and baked for 4 h at ~65°C. Cured PDMS was subsequently pealed from the mould and punched using a biopsy punch of 1 mm size (Miltex, 3331) to create inlet and outlets. Next, a 10 μm thick polyethylene terephthalate (PET) membrane with 0.4 μm pore size (Corning, CLS3450) was bonded to the PDMS model and channels were irreversibly sealed. Upon seeding cells on the apical side of the PET membrane, the model is placed above a medium reservoir (i.e., basal side). The completed assembly of the platform is presented in **Figure 1b**.

Aerosol Exposure Experiments

Particle Preparation

Following an established protocol, 2 μm monodispersed polystyrene (PS) particles [FluoSpheres Carboxylate-Modified microspheres, Red Fluorescent (580/605), 2% solid F8826, Thermo Scientific] were coupled to αVR1 antibody (Baker et al., 2019) (Abcam, ab3487)/bovine serum albumin (BSA; MP Biomedicals, 160069) in phosphate-buffered saline (PBS; Sigma-Aldrich, D8537), respectively, using a two-step *EDC/Sulfo NHS Covalent Coupling Procedure* (Merck, 2015) (Merck Millipore). Such protocol yields 2 μm monodispersed PS particles conjugated with αVR1 antibody/BSA. Briefly, after 15 min sonication, 250 μl PS particles were suspended in 250 μl of 50 mM MES buffer solution (pH 6). The suspension was vortexed and centrifuged at 3000 × *g* for 5 min at 4°C. This washing procedure was repeated three times. Next, 12 μl of 200 mM EDC reagent solution and 120 μl of 200 mM Sulfo-NHS reagent solution were added to the particle suspension with 250 μl of MES buffer. The suspension was vortexed and mixed gently in a vertically rotating plate for 30 min at room temperature (RT), followed by three washes with 1 ml MES buffer. Next, 33 μl of αVR1 antibody (1 mg/ml)/100 μl of BSA (1 mg/ml), respectively, were added to the particles with 1 ml MES buffer, vortexed and mixed gently in a vertically rotating plate for 3 h at RT. The suspension was washed from the unreacted protein using a spin down centrifugation cycle (the supernatant was kept for protein content analysis), and the particles were suspended in 1 ml MES buffer and 15 μl of ethanolamine to quench the reaction. Finally, the particles were washed three times using 1 ml blocking buffer [containing 0.5% (w/v) casein in MES buffer], and three times with 1 ml of PBS. The particles were kept at 4°C until used for an experiment. To assess qualitatively the PS-VR1 conjugation, particles were incubated for 1 h at RT with secondary antibody Alexa Fluor 488 anti-rabbit, before confocal microscopy imaging of fluorescent immunostaining was performed on the conjugated particles (**Supplementary Figure S2**).

Aerosol Exposure Assay

The present *in vitro* aerosol exposure assays strive to recapitulate *in situ*-like inhalation conditions. In a first step, aerosol exposure assays were conducted in the absence of cells to characterize *in vitro* aerosol transport determinants and examine solely aerosol deposition patterns inside the devices. Subsequently, the identical protocol was implemented to explore cytotoxicity on the epithelium. Briefly, a monodispersed aerosol was produced by aerosolization (Fishler et al., 2015) of PBS-suspended 2 μm red fluorescent PS microspheres conjugated to αVR1 antibody (as described above) using an aerosol generator (TSI, 3076) with air as the gas source and subsequently drying the PBS droplets using two consecutive diffusion driers (TSI, 3062). The rationale for selecting such particle size follows as 2 μm represents a good candidate for aerosol deposition in the deep tracheobronchial (TB) regions (Bair, 1989; Stahlhofen et al., 1989; Hinds, 1999). To avoid aggregate formation prior to the

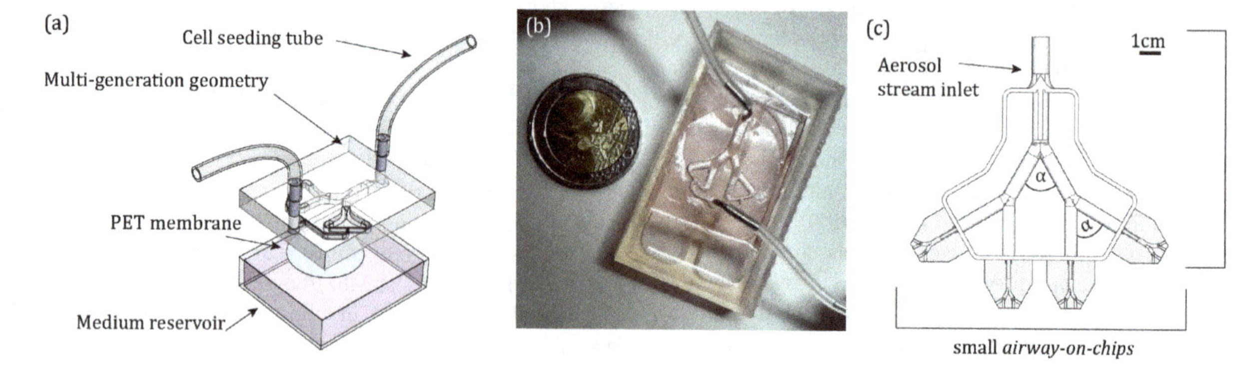

FIGURE 1 | Design of the *airway-on-chip* platform and its integration for aerosol inhalation exposure assays. **(a)** Computer-aided drawing (CAD) schematic of the device including the airway tree model (apical side), a porous PET membrane (gray circle) separating the bottom reservoir for medium (basal side). **(b)** Photograph of the assembled device. **(c)** CAD schematic of the custom-designed 3D airway tree connector which allows to simultaneously perform experiments across four individual *airway-on-chip* devices (shown in gray), and control the orientation of gravity during an exposure assay, with bifurcating angle of $\alpha = 60°$ (**Supplementary Figure S1**).

TABLE 1 | Dimensions of the *airway-on-chip* platform.

Generation	Length (mm)	Diameter (mm)
1	6.59	2.20
2	5.55	1.68
3	3.58	1.25

deposition assays, the microspheres were first sonicated in a water bath for 20 min. Next, the 2 μm PS particles were diluted in distilled water to a concentration of 1×10^7 particle/ml for aerosol exposure, while for the cell viability assay in the cultured *airway-on-chips*, particles were diluted in PBS to a concentration of 4.55×10^8 particle/ml (see the section "Results"). The aerosol flow was fed through an antistatic tube where the flow rate was controlled by a pinch valve. To deliver a physiologically relevant exposure assay, the flow rate was further reduced by splitting the main aerosol stream into four paths integrated within a custom-designed conducting 3D airway tree model that approximately mimics mid-bronchial generations in an average adult human lung (Ménache et al., 2008; **Figure 1c** and **Supplementary Figure S1**).

Using the 3D airway connecting model enables to simultaneously perform $n = 4$ *airway-on-chip* experiments, directly integrated within an anatomically inspired conducting airway tree. The overall flow rate selected was 0.2 l/min, as measured using a flow meter (TSI, 4100) at the aerosol generator outlet; the ensuing flow rate at the entrance of each (four) device was 0.05 l/min, i.e., corresponding to physiological airflow conditions representative of flow phenomena in small bronchial airways. Specifically, we replicate quiet breathing conditions (Pedley, 2003; Sznitman, 2013), such that the characteristic Reynolds numbers (Re) range between approximately 22 and 10 across the three generations of the *airway-on-chip*, where $Re = ud/\nu$ and represents the relative magnitude of the inertial forces to viscous forces (i.e., ν is the kinematic viscosity of air, u is the characteristic mean airflow velocity in each generation of diameter d).

In each experiment, four *airway-on-chip* devices are positioned in a horizontal orientation relative to gravity and directly tight-fitted to the four outlets of the 3D airway tree connector along the streamwise flow direction (see **Figure 1c** and **Supplementary Figure S1**). Unlike cell seeding via the top of the device (**Figures 1a,b**), this design ensures anatomical continuity and thereby adequate respiratory airflows during aerosol exposure assays. Note that the influence of gravity, and thus particle deposition, can be modified with the present design by changing the device position relative to the connector's outlet (**Supplementary Figure S3**). Each exposure assay was conducted for 30 min in an effort to yield representative ensemble depositions of aerosols and in parallel compare these with numerical simulation (see the section "Results"); in the case of cell viability assays a continuous exposure was conducted for 5 min. Note that here, constant steady-state inhalation flow conditions are mimicked, giving rise to fully developed laminar flow conditions; the range of Re across the 3D airway connector ranges approximately between Re ~ 50–22, in line with physiological respiratory conditions (Pedley, 2003; Sznitman, 2013).

To quantify ensuing aerosol deposition patterns, the models were subsequently imaged under microscopy using an inverted fluorescent microscope (Nikon eclipse Ti) at 20× magnification. A resulting single, high-resolution image of the complete *airway-on-chips* was obtained by tiling multiple images where the location of each deposited fluorescent particle was identified by locating local intensity maxima (ImageJ).

Numerical Simulations

Computational Fluid Dynamics Simulations

In an effort to interpret the underlying physical aerosol transport determinants governing deposition outcomes and further compare the experimentally obtained particle deposition patterns, *in silico* flow simulations were carried out using a commercial software (Fluent 18.2, ANSYS Inc.) that solves the mass and momentum (i.e., Navier–Stokes) equations numerically. An airway model identical to the *airway-on-chip* design was first discretized with tetrahedral cell elements using the original CAD model and subsequently refined and converted into a polyhedral mesh (Inthavong et al., 2019). Flow convergence tests were conducted on three different mesh sizes, ranging between 240,000 and 660,000 polyhedral cells in size. A final mesh consisting of approximately 540,000 polyhedral cells was selected for flow simulations. To accurately mimic experimental conditions, a steady-state, fully developed velocity profile was imposed at the model inlet. A no-slip boundary condition was implemented at the walls, and any particles impacting the walls were assumed to be deposited. All four outlets were set to identical, zero-pressure outlet conditions. Given the relatively low-Reynolds-number regime (Re << 100), a laminar solver was chosen to simulate airflows. A SIMPLE pressure–velocity coupling scheme with least squares cell-based gradient discretization, second-order for pressure and second-order upwind scheme for momentum was implemented.

Particle Deposition Simulations

We simulated ~6,400 monodisperse 2 μm diameter PS particles (ρ_p = 1.05 g/cm^3), tracked using a Lagrangian one-way coupled, steady-state discrete phase model. As particle mass flow through a cross-section may be assumed proportional to flow rate, particles were seeded at the inlet with a quasi-parabolic initial distribution using a truncated normal probability density function. For such particle size, the main forces governing transport are viscous drag (i.e., low-Re Stokes drag) and gravitational sedimentation; that is Brownian motion, electrostatic charge, or other forces are neglected (Koullapis et al., 2016). Locations of the deposited particles on the bottom wall (analogous to the apical side of the PET membrane) were extracted and identified according to airway branch generation.

Cell Culture

Cell Culture Maintenance

In the footsteps of recent small *airway-on-chip* models led by Benam et al. (2015), Normal Human Bronchial Epithelial (NHBE) cells (Lonza, CC-2540S) were cultured under immersed conditions with B-ALI growth medium (Lonza, 00193516) and 50% of supplemented BEGM SingleQuots (Lonza, CC-4175) in a tissue culture T75-flask (TPP, 90025). The medium was changed every second or third day until cells reached ~90% confluency. A Trypsin–EDTA solution (Lonza, CC-5034) was then used to detach cells from culture dishes. Thereafter, cells were used for experiments as described in detail below. Cells were incubated at 37°C in a humidified atmosphere containing 5% CO_2. Cells were cultured up to passage (Rayner et al., 2019) four; mycoplasma controls were performed routinely using MycoAlert mycoplasma detection kit (Lonza, BELT07-218) without exhibiting infection.

Air–Liquid Interface (ALI)

For *airway-on-chip* cultures, 1.8 × 10^5 NHBE cells (in 135 μl medium) were seeded on top of the apical side of a 0.03 mg/ml collagen type I coated (Corning, 354236) PET membrane inside the devices, and 1 ml of medium was added to the basal compartment. For Transwell inserts culture (Corning, CLS3470), 5 × 10^4 NHBE cells (in 200 μl medium) were seeded on a collagen type I-coated PET membrane inside inserts, and 500 μl of medium was added to the basal compartment. Both cell cultures on chip and on inserts were first conducted under immersed conditions with B-ALI growth complete medium and 1% Antibiotic Antimycotic Solution (Sigma-Aldrich, A5955). By day 4 the NHBE culture was exposed to air (i.e., ALI) by removing the medium from the apical side of the *airway-on-chip* devices and the inserts, respectively. B-ALI differentiation medium (StemCell, 05001) was introduced in the basal chamber of the devices and inserts, respectively. Differentiated NHBE cell cultures were imaged under microscopy starting from day 21 after exposure to ALI.

Imaging

Scanning Electron Microscopy

Samples were washed three times with PBS and fixed in primary fixative buffer [1% para formaldehyde (PFA) and 2% GA in 0.1 M NaP pH 7.4 and 3% sucrose] for 60 min at RT. Following three washes with 0.1 M cacodylate buffer (pH 7.4) samples were fixed with 1% Osmium tetroxide in 0.1 M cacodylate buffer for 15 min at RT. Next, samples were dehydrated through a graded ethanol series and further processed by critical point drying and sputter coating with chromium (5 nm). Images were acquired with a Zeiss ULTRA plus field emission scanning electron microscope (SEM).

Mucus Visualization

Following perfusion of PBS, NHBE cells were fixed within the devices and inserts using 4% PFA (Sigma–Aldrich, 47608) for 20 min at RT and were washed again three times with PBS. For detection of glycoproteins typically present in mucus (Leonard et al., 2010; Lechanteur et al., 2018), samples were treated with 10 mg/ml alcian Blue 8G× (Sigma–Aldrich, A5268) in 3% acetic acid (1% w/v) for 15 min at RT and were washed three times with PBS. Images were then acquired with a light inverted microscope (Nikon Eclipse TS100) at 10×.

Immunofluorescence Microscopy

Directly after cell fixation using 4% PFA, cells were treated with 0.05% Triton X-100 (Sigma–Aldrich, T8787) for 3 min at RT to increase membrane permeability and were blocked for non-specific binding using 2% BSA for 1 h at RT. For F-actin staining, NHBE cells were incubated with Alexa Fluor 568 Phalloidin (ThermoFisher Scientific, A12380) diluted with PBS (ratio of 1:200) for 40 min at RT. For DAPI nucleic acid staining cells were incubated with DAPI solution (ThermoFisher Scientific, D1306), diluted with PBS (ratio of 1:400) for 5 min at RT. For tight junction proteins, Zonula occludens-1 (ZO1), cells were incubated with the primary antibodies rabbit anti-ZO1 (ThermoFisher Scientific, 617300) diluted with PBS (ratio of 1:200) overnight at 4°C, followed by incubation with secondary antibody Alexa Fluor 488 anti-rabbit (Jackson ImmunoResearch, 111-545-144), diluted with PBS (ratio of 1:400) for 1 h at RT. After each step, cells were washed three times with PBS. Finally, confocal microscopy imaging of fluorescent immunostaining was performed (Nikon Eclipse Ti with spinning disk, Yokogawa, Japan).

Apoptosis Quantification

Following 5–8 days under immersed conditions, NHBE cells in the devices were exposed for 5 min to the PS-αVR1 particles and then incubated for 48 h. To ensure that apoptosis resulted solely from the exposure assay, the response of two control groups was monitored: (i) NHBE cells treated with airflow and (ii) cells exposed to PS-BSA particles (without the αVR1 antibody). To quantify apoptosis, following 48 h of incubation, cells were fully harvested using a Trypsin–EDTA solution, collected and then incubated with Alexa Fluor 488 conjugated Annexin V (Abcam, ab14085) in the dark for 5 min at RT. The cells were then imaged using an imaging flow cytometer (Amnis, ImageStreamX Mark II) at 40×. As a positive control, the NHBE cells' apoptotic response was measured over time following exposure to αVR1 antibody. Briefly, 5×10^4 NHBE cells per well were seeded in a 96-well plate (Nunc, 167008). Two days after seeding, medium containing 0.66 μM αVR1 antibody was added, followed by incubation of 24 and 48 h. Next, apoptotic cells were stained using Annexin V (see details above), and imaging of fluorescent immunostaining was performed. In parallel, as an additional positive control, we checked the toxicity effects of PS-VR1 particles using NHBE cells which were seeded on top of an insert for 7 days under immersed conditions, followed by incubation of 48 h with PS-BSA and PS-VR1 in a particle:cell ratio of 1:50. Finally, confocal imaging of fluorescent immunostaining was performed.

Particles Toxicity Assays

To ensure that apoptosis was due to the exposure assay using αVR1 antibody, a toxicity test was first performed. Briefly, 5×10^4 NHBE cells per well were seeded in a 96-well plate; 2 days following seeding, medium containing 2 μm PS-BSA particles with particle:cell ratios of 5:1, 2.5:1, 1:1, 1:2.5, 1:5, 1:10, 1:100, and 1:200 were added, respectively. NHBE cells were returned for 48 h incubation. Next, a cell viability reagent (almarBlue; Bio-Rad, BUF012A) with 10% volume in culture medium was added to each well followed by 4 h incubation. Finally, absorbance measurements were performed using a plate reader (Varioskan LUX, ThermoFisher Scientific) at 570 and 600 nm wavelengths, respectively. Each test was repeated independently three times. As a positive control, medium containing 2 μm PS-VR1 particles with a particle:cell ratio of 1:100 was added in the same experiment and a viability assay using almarBlue was performed.

Statistical Analysis

A student's t-test (two-tailed) was used to determine the level of significance among different experiments device. Error bars are presented as the standard error and asterisks indicating significance in the figures correspond to $p < 0.05$, 0.005, and 0.001 shown as *, **, and ***, respectively.

RESULTS AND DISCUSSION

To emulate a small conducting airway environment in view of cytotoxicity exposure evaluations, we designed a tree-like device featuring two planar, symmetric branching airway channels, broadly resembling the anatomy of small bronchial airways of an average adult lung (**Figures 1a,b**). The device consists of three layers (see the section "Materials and Methods"), including the apical side of the PDMS airway tree, in which the two small punches (1 mm in diameter) first allow to seed the pulmonary cells on top of the PET membrane (10 μm thick with 0.4 μm pores size). The PET membrane is bonded to the bottom PDMS compartment and sealed above by the airway channels. This permeable membrane allows nutrient supply from the medium in the reservoir and prevents cell leakage to the basal side. Notably, our custom design allows to culture the seeded pulmonary cells at ALI conditions; a necessary condition for adequate differentiation (Grainger et al., 2006; Lin et al., 2007). Our design mimics the *in vivo* environment by combining a 3D true scale pulmonary tree geometry with realistic airflow conditions and recapitulating *in situ*-like aerosol inhalation exposure to the deep TB regions of the lungs.

Aerosol Inhalation Exposure Assay

We first explore deposition patterns of inhaled aerosols during the inhalation maneuver and present ensemble deposition patterns for 2 μm particles on the bottom surface of the *airway-on-chips* (i.e., PET membrane). Such results follow a steady (i.e., constant flow rate) inhalation aerosol exposure assay across the anatomically realistic 3D airway connector (**Supplementary Figure S1**). Devices were exposed for 30 min to a steady stream of aerosols at a controlled flow rate matching physiological airflow conditions representative of small bronchial (with an entrance flow rate of Q = 0.05 l/min). We recall that our inhalation assays omit the oscillatory nature of respiratory flows and instead focus on inhalation phenomena. We recently explored in *in silico* simulations particle deposition occurring during inhalation and exhalation phases across extensive deep lung models (Koullapis P.G. et al., 2018) and assessed the contribution of each phase, respectively. Here, rather, the focus of the present proof-of-concept lies in recapitulating for the first time real mechanistic deposition determinants of inhaled aerosols within *lung-on-chip* platforms.

To mimic the hydrophilic environment of the bronchial lumen surrounded by mucus, we used collagen-coated devices (0.03 mg/ml collagen type I); we recall that in view of quantifying solely mechanistic aerosol transport characteristics devices are first void of epithelium. **Figure 2A** presents ensemble results of particle deposition patterns inside the *airway-on-chips* under physiological airflow conditions; the color-coded heat map quantifies particle concentration, defined as the number of neighboring particles within a 0.5 mm radius (results are normalized by the highest concentration in the tree). We begin by observing a heterogeneous deposition pattern with high particle concentrations along the centerline of each generation compared to the peripheral areas (i.e., nearer the airway side walls), in line with Poiseuille velocity profiles characteristics at such Re. When examining the average particle density (defined as the average number of deposited particles in each branch, normalized by the branch's surface area) as shown in **Figure 2B**, a consistent monotonic decrease in particle density is apparent with each deeper generation as

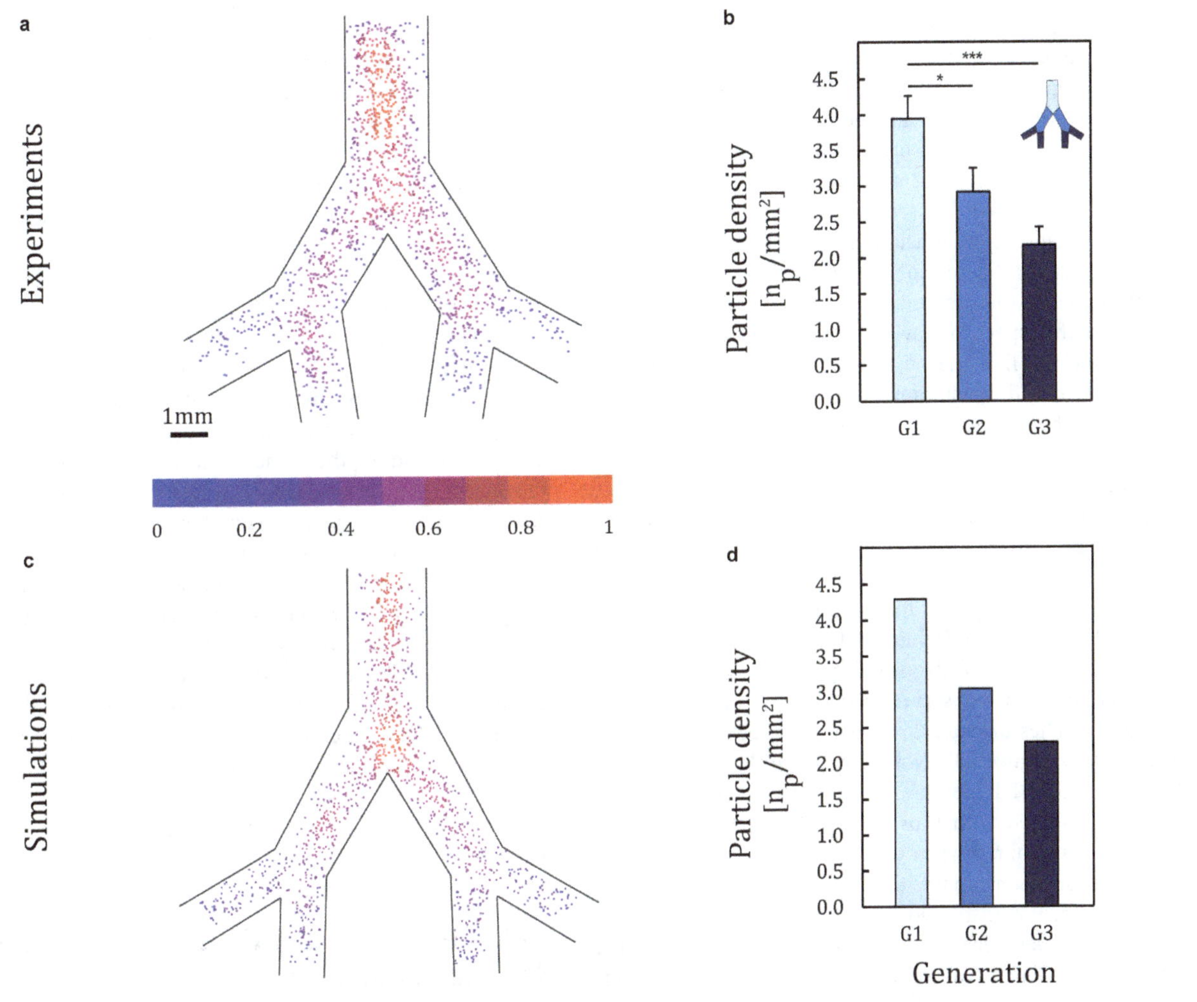

FIGURE 2 | Particle deposition patterns following exposure. Two micrometers of PS particles were aerosolized into the *airway-on-chips* in a horizontal position with respect to gravity at physiological airflow conditions corresponding to quiet breathing. **(a)** Ensemble deposition patterns imaged under fluorescence microscopy (n = 8 models). The color-coded heat map quantifies particle concentration, defined as the number of neighboring particles within an 0.5 mm radius (results are normalized by the highest concentration in the tree). **(b)** Histogram of particle deposition density quantifying the average particle number in each generation normalized by airway area (mm^2). Error bars represent the standard error. Asterisks indicate significance corresponding to $p < 0.05$, 0.001 shown as * and ***, respectively. Corresponding **(c)** aerosol deposition patterns and **(d)** histograms of deposition density obtained from *in silico* CFD simulations.

anticipated in the deep TB lung regions (Zhang et al., 2009). Namely, average particle density is observed to decrease by nearly half between the first and third generation, with a mean of 3.9 particles/mm^2 in generation 1 (G1) compared to 2.2 particles/mm^2 in generation 3 (G3). With our current design and exposure assay, we were able to reproduce spatial particle deposition density gradients across the airway trees and mimic anticipated *in situ* situations. Demonstrating this ability in a proof-of-concept holds ramifications for future cytotoxicity as well as drug screening assays (e.g., inhalation therapy), where local deposition patterns and thereby concentrations hotspots (Imai et al., 2012; Hofemeier and Sznitman, 2015; Islam et al., 2017), can lead to various differences in local inflammatory responses and disease onset. Such feature lies beyond reach using traditional assays (e.g., Transwell) or conversely straight channels.

To date, direct *in vivo* exposure studies of aerosol deposition have focused mainly on olfactory and upper trachea-bronchial regions in both animals (Gerde et al., 1991; Petitot et al., 2013) and humans (Cheng et al., 1996), with little explorations in the small bronchi and bronchioles. In addition, since *in vivo* data are conducted mostly with 2D gamma scintigraphy, the resolution of current imaging modalities remains inadequate to quantify deposition at small scales (Koullapis P. et al., 2018). Such limitations have driven the appeal of *in vitro-in silico* based strategies to deliver insight into deposition determinants. To date, however, efforts have been focused mainly on upper airways (Byron et al., 2010; Carrigy et al., 2014) with few studies exploring deposition endpoints in the mid- to small-bronchi. For example, Fishler et al. (2015) characterized the deposition of PS particles (i.e., 0.2–1 μm in diameter) in an *acinus-on-chip* platform and correlated findings *in silico*. In the footsteps of such endeavors, computational fluid dynamics (CFD) simulations were presently sought to gain quantitative insight into the deposition mechanisms at play. Results exhibit strong consistency when compared with the experimentally obtained deposition patterns (**Figures 2C,D**), with a maximum difference of 8% between experimental and numerical results. Notably, the deposition of 2 μm particles in small bronchi is principally governed by sedimentation, in line with the general understanding of inhalation aerosol deposition theory (Zhang et al., 2009). Dimensional analysis (see **Supplementary Material**) supports that deposition patterns under a horizontal orientation with respect to gravity are the result of the coupling between convective flow (i.e., viscous drag) along the streamwise airway direction and gravitational sedimentation in the normal direction, thereby giving rise to gradients in deposition density along each generation.

In addition, our *in vitro* exposure platform allows to examine the effect of gravity on ensuing deposition patterns by changing the orientation of the *airway-on-chips* (see **Supplementary Material**). Briefly, models were attached at a 45° tilt with respect to gravity and were exposed for 30 min to aerosolized 2 μm particles under physiological inhalation airflows. A decrease in the total number of deposited particles on the bottom PET membrane was observed as well as higher particle density in branches oriented lower with respect to gravity (see **Supplementary Figure S3**). Note that due to the imaged plane of the device (i.e., PET membrane), only deposited particles are identified (compared with those deposited on the PDMS side walls). Altogether, our *in vitro* exposure assays capture realistic aerosol transport determinants that still remain widely absent in more traditional PM instillations or direct spraying techniques (Blank et al., 2006; Lenz et al., 2014; Röhm et al., 2017) on plates and inserts. Furthermore, our *airway-on-chips* highlight for the first time that exposure assays can be configured to explore localized deposition effects, capturing for example deposition outcomes pertinent to regional lung lobes (e.g., upper versus lower lobes) that span broad orientation angles across the chest cavity (Sauret et al., 2002).

Reconstituting a Bronchial Epithelium on Chip

To reconstitute an epithelial cell population lining the conducting airways (e.g., ciliated and secretory cells), primary NHBE cells originating from healthy human bronchi (biopsy) were seeded on the apical side of the ALI device (**Figure 3a**). Although the use of primary cells is limited by difficulties in sample isolation, the small number of cells that can be produced and the large variation between different donors (Skardal et al., 2016), such strategy represents a well-acknowledged *in vitro* approach in mimicking generic airway models (Rayner et al., 2019) that capture the *in vivo* environment; a point advocated in recent *airway-on-chip* designs (Benam et al., 2015). By using NHBE cells, we have thus followed a similar approach, including the recent work of Bovard et al. (2018) who developed a *lung/liver-on-a-chip* platform with NHBE cells to study the toxicity of inhaled aerosols. Moreover, many studies have used such cells as an airway model to study cell exposure to ambient air pollution (Becker et al., 2005), using traditional assays with Transwell inserts. Among other, Wu et al. (2001) studied the expression of IL-8 through the activation of the EGF receptor signaling after NHBE cells were exposed to environmental PM.

To evaluate differentiation, following 21 days at ALI conditions, we visualized mucus secretion from the differentiated cells using SEM as shown in **Figure 3b**, where mucus microstructure is similar to that observed in previous lungs mucus studies (Schuster et al., 2013). Since washing off the mucus layer from the epithelial culture could potentially damage the differentiated NHBE cells (i.e., ciliated and secretory cells), we have reverted to SEM imaging of the epithelium layer that was seeded on top of an insert and cultured at an ALI for 21 days (**Supplementary Figure S4a**), in parallel to those within the devices and under the same growth conditions. As a control, the undifferentiated NHBE cells were also investigated using SEM imaging (**Supplementary Figures S4c,d**) to emphasize the fundamental changes in morphology. In addition, we visualized specific glycoproteins, present in mucus (**Figure 3c**; see **Supplementary Figure S4f** for staining control). A confluent cell monolayer was observed by staining the whole device for F-actin, as shown in **Figure 3d**, and cell nuclei (**Figure 3e** represents an inset of the white square in **Figure 3d**). Finally, to assess the barrier formation in the chip, expression of one of the tight junction proteins (i.e., ZO1) was examined (**Figure 3f**). In parallel, for control, each of the cells passages was seeded on an insert under the same growth conditions (see for example **Supplementary Figure S4**).

Cell Viability Assay Following PM-Like Aerosol Exposure

Next, we explored the influence of PM-like particles on the NHBE cells cultured inside the device for cytotoxicity evaluation. To mimic the toxic characteristics of a PM group [e.g., oil fly ash (Agopyan et al., 2004), soils dust (Veranth et al., 2006), and coal fly ash (Deering-Rice et al., 2016) among others], we chose to simulate a well-known ligand that activates the Vanilloid receptor by preparing PM-like particles consisting of a PS-core conjugated to αVR1 antibodies (see the section "Particle Preparation"). We note that this activation can induce diverse biological cascades, including the release of pro-inflammatory cytokines such as IL-6, IL-8, and TNFα (Veronesi et al., 1999). Here, in a proof-of-concept, we specifically chose to demonstrate one well-known apoptosis pathway in the footsteps of previous studies (Agopyan et al., 2003, 2004).

The conjugation of the αVR1 antibody to the PS particles (i.e., PS-VR1) was confirmed by incubating the PS-VR1 with a secondary antibody (**Supplementary Figure S2**). As previously shown *in vitro*, the binding of the αVR1 antibody to the VR1 receptor, which is expressed on the epithelial surface, induces an apoptosis pathway (Agopyan et al., 2003, 2004). Thus, a qualitative measurement of the apoptotic response as a function of time of the NHBE cells after a αVR1 antibody stimulation was first performed using an Annexin V staining which stains for cells that enter the

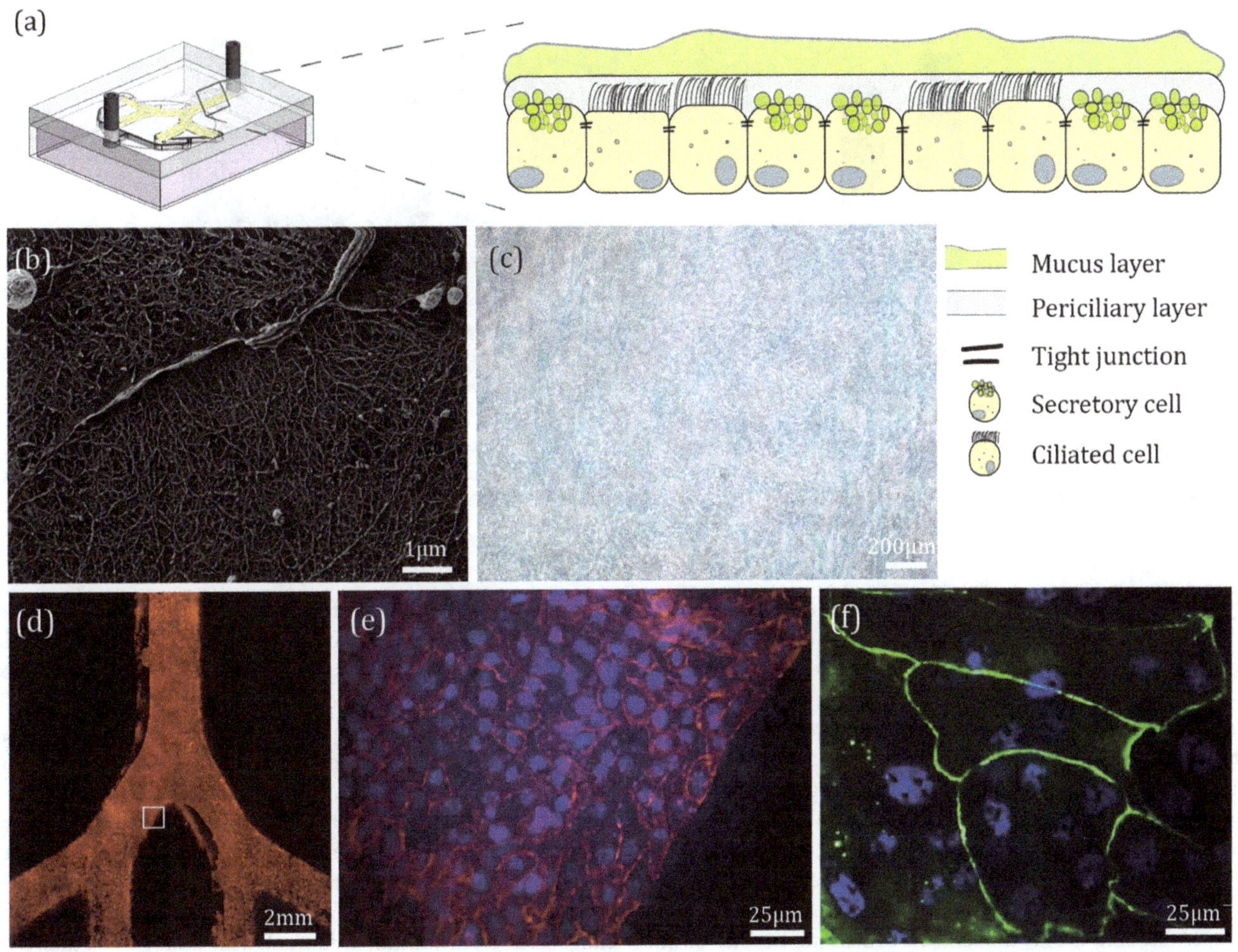

FIGURE 3 | Epithelial barrier reconstitution inside *airway-on-chips*. **(a)** Schematic illustration of the bronchial epithelium environment and the general differentiated cellular make-up. **(b)** Following device fabrication, NHBE cells were seeded on the apical side of the PET membrane under immersed conditions for 4 days, then cultured at ALI conditions for 21 days. Shown here is a scanning electron microscope (SEM) image of the mucus layer covering NHBE cells. **(c)** After 21 days at ALI conditions, NHBE cells were stained for glycoproteins typically present in mucus. **(d)** NHBE cells were cultured for 7 days under immersed conditions, then stained for F-actin. **(e,f)** After 21 days at ALI conditions, NHBE cells were stained for F-actin (red), ZO1 (green), and cell nuclei (blue).

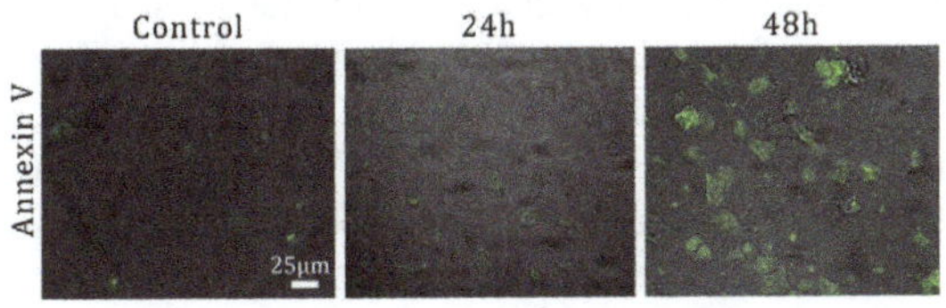

FIGURE 4 | Examination of αVR1 antibody effect on NHBE cells over time. The apoptotic response over time for αVR1 antibody on NHBE cells was investigated as a positive control. 5×10^4 NHBE cells per well are seeded in a 96-well plate. Two days after seeding, medium containing 0.66 μM αVR1 antibody was added, followed by incubation of 24 and 48 h. Next, apoptotic cells were stained using Annexin V (see the section "Apoptosis Quantification"), and imaging of fluorescent immunostaining was performed.

apoptotic pathway. Following an incubation period of 48 h, an increase in the apoptotic cell population was observed (**Figure 4**). As a positive control, to demonstrate the influence of our PM-like particles on the NHBE cells, cells were incubated with PS-BSA and PS-VR1, in a particle:cell ratio of 1:50, for an incubation period of 48 h. A qualitative measurement of the apoptotic cells was performed using Annexin V staining (**Supplementary Figure S5**) showing an increase in apoptotic cells which were incubated with the PS-VR1 particles, compared to control (incubation with PS-BSA particles). In addition, the PS toxicity level was assessed by titration of the PS-BSA particles which were incubated for 48 h with NHBE cells in a range of particles:cells ratios (**Supplementary Figure S6a**). A decrease in cell viability was detected starting from a particles:cells ratio of 5:1 (the selected ratio is ~1:500). The PS-VR1 toxicity effect was evaluated via viability assay following an incubation period of 48 h with NHBE cells in a particles:cells ratio of 1:100, resulting in a decrease in viability (**Supplementary Figure S6b**). This comprehensive examination allows us to refer to the manufactured PS-VR1 as PM-like particles, in line with seminal

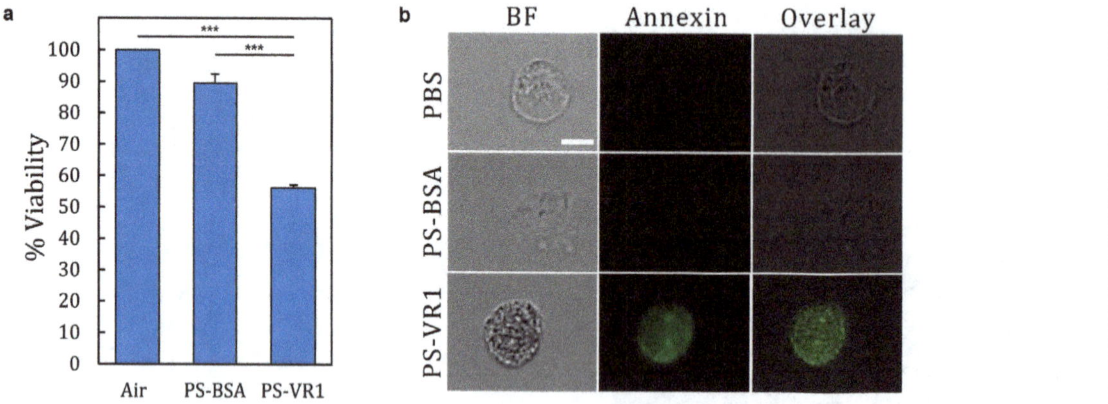

FIGURE 5 | Viability and apoptosis assay following NHBE cell exposure to PM-like particles. **(a)** Following inhalation exposure assays, *airway-on-chip* devices were returned to the incubator for 48 h prior to conducting a viability assay. The presented results are normalized to the air exposure, representing 100% viability (n = 4 for each treatment). **(b)** Single cell imaging using Annexin V staining which stained apoptotic cells with green (BF corresponds to bright field). Error bar represent the standard error and asterisks indicate significance ($p < 0.001$ shown as ***).

in vitro studies using traditional macroscopic assays on plate (Agopyan et al., 2003, 2004).

Our developed *in situ*-like airway exposure platform is suitable for diverse applications in the field of human inhalation toxicity *in vitro*. As a proof-of-concept, our *airway-on-chips* were exposed to harmful PM-like particles and their effect on the human bronchial epithelium was monitored. Following previous studies (Agopyan et al., 2003, 2004), cells were grown under immersed conditions and only exposed to air during the specific exposure assay. Prior to the exposure assay, cells were grown inside the *airway-on-chips* until confluency was reached (5–8 days following seeding). The models were then taken out of the incubator and connected to the larger conducting 3D airway model (**Figure 1c**) where a 5 min inhalation exposure was performed inside the biological hood (at RT). Next, the devices were placed back at the incubator for 48 h incubation (see the section "Materials and Methods"). Experiments were carried out for three independent exposure protocols: air, PS-BSA, and PS-VR1, respectively, using four replicates. Viability measurements were then performed 48 h post-exposure, as shown in **Figure 5A**. The final percentage viability was normalized to the averaged value of the measurements for the air exposed group (defined as 100% viability). Our results indicate that the PS-BSA treatment was not toxic to the cells with around 90% viability. In contrast to the PS-BSA particles, the exposure to PS-VR1 particles led to a stark reduction in cell viability down to around 50% with standard error of 1.04%, demonstrating the high potency of PS-VR1 as an apoptosis inducer.

As the viability assay measures the level of the cellular metabolite and is not directly correlated with the level of apoptotic cells, a complementary assay was furthermore performed using Annexin V staining. The complete monolayer of cultured NHBE cells was trypsinized and harvested from the model, and was then incubated with Annexin V staining, followed by single cell imaging (see the section "Apoptosis Quantification") for each group. Here we present in **Figure 5B** a characteristic image for each treatment illustrating the ensuing apoptotic levels; in the bright field (BF) column, single cells exhibiting a circular shape under each treatment show a typical morphology. When staining the cell membrane with Annexin V, only the cells under the PM-like treatment (i.e., PS-VR1) are stained compared with the controls (i.e., air and PS-BSA). This latter procedure further underlines one of the advantages of the present *airway-on-chip* platform; namely the ability to harvest cultured cells post exposure and conduct advanced single cell analyses. Together, these findings reinforce our setup as the first *in situ*-like platform suitable for aerosol exposure assays that combine realistic aerosol transport pathways in the lungs (i.e., from mouth to lumen) with biological toxicity that corroborates biological endpoints discussed in previous studies (Agopyan et al., 2003, 2004).

CONCLUSION

While past efforts with *lung-on-chips* have been widely restricted to simple isolated airway channels, in the present work we have established an advanced *in vitro* platform to recapitulate *in situ*-like aerosol exposure to PM under ALI conditions. Multi-generational *airway-on-chip* devices, mimicking bifurcating airway structures at true scale, were exposed to inhaled aerosols under physiological airflows within an integrated anatomically inspired bronchial airway tree model. Using *in vitro*–*in silico* strategies, our experimental efforts underscore the importance of the small airway tree anatomy and its orientation to gravity in determining mechanistically driven lung deposition outcomes; an important step toward *in vitro* pathways to explore deposition outcomes for various real lung-like deposition scenarios. Such efforts are anticipated to help shed light on inhaled particle deposition in deep airways and mimic more realistically representative *in vivo* deposition outcomes in human lungs with heterogeneous patterns.

Furthermore, we demonstrated the aptitude to culture human primary cells under ALI conditions for 21 days, guaranteeing them to differentiate to ciliated and secretory cells and thereby deliver a functional *in vivo*-like barrier. Such design allows additionally to incorporate in future studies the presence for example of immune cells as well as other co-/multi-cell cultures for specific endpoints. As a proof-of-concept, we manufactured monodisperse particles that mimic PM-induced apoptosis through the activation of the Vanilloid receptor and used two complementary techniques to demonstrate the effect of such harmful PM-like particles on the human bronchial epithelium (i.e., a viability assay and imaging ensuing apoptotic levels). At this stage, our aim was foremost to demonstrate how PS-VR1-conjugated particles deposited under physiological airflow conditions lead to loss of viability of the epithelium via an apoptotic cascade. In future studies, our devices can lend use for example toward physiological-based particle size screens. Future directions include also quantifying the effects of occupational environments on the epithelium barrier as our platform can be leveraged for more general *in vitro* exposure with the potential to expand our current knowledge on the mechanisms in which the PM injure the bronchial epithelium.

AUTHOR CONTRIBUTIONS

SE-K conceived the project and devised the experiments, designed the device, performed the experiments, analyzed the data, and wrote the manuscript. AA-S designed the experiments, performed the experiments, and wrote the manuscript. PD and MH-A performed the numerical simulations. NK assisted with manuscript drafting. JS conceived the project, supervised the analyses, and wrote the manuscript.

ACKNOWLEDGMENTS

The authors thank Simon Dorfman for technical assistance and Dr. Rami Fishler, Hikaia Zidan, Nofar Azulay, Eyal Habif, Mendel Kiperman, Moran Levi, and Mark Epshtein for helpful discussions and experimental support. They also thank Dr. Shaulov from the Biomedical Core Facilities (Technion) for technical support with the electron microscopy and Dr. Barak from Life Sciences and Engineering Infrastructure Center, Lorry I. Lokey Interdisciplinary Center (Technion) for technical support with the ImageStream.

REFERENCES

Abaci, H. E., Gledhill, K., Guo, Z., Christiano, A. M., and Shuler, M. L. (2015). Pumpless microfluidic platform for drug testing on human skin equivalents. *Lab Chip* 15, 882–888. doi: 10.1039/c4lc00999a

Agopyan, N., Bhatti, T., Yu, S., and Simon, S. (2003). Vanilloid receptor activation by 2- and 10-μm particles induces responses leading to apoptosis in human airway epithelial cells. *Toxicol. Appl. Pharmacol.* 192, 21–35. doi: 10.1016/S0041-008X(03)00259-X

Agopyan, N., Head, J., Yu, S., and Simon, S. A. (2004). TRPV1 receptors mediate particulate matter-induced apoptosis. *Am. J. Physiol. Lung. Cell Mol Physiol.* 286, L563–L572.

Anderson, J. O., Thundiyil, J. G., and Stolbach, A. (2012). Clearing the air: a review of the effects of particulate matter air pollution on human health. *J. Med. Toxicol.* 8, 166–175. doi: 10.1007/s13181-011-0203-1

Artzy-schnirman, A., Hobi, N., Schneider-daum, N., and Guenat, O. T. (2019a). European journal of pharmaceutics and biopharmaceutics advanced in vitro lung-on-chip platforms for inhalation assays: from prospect to pipeline. *Eur. J. Pharm. Biopharm.* 144, 11–17. doi: 10.1016/j.ejpb.2019.09.006

Artzy-Schnirman, A., Zidan, H., Elias-Kirma, S., Ben-Porat, L., Tenenbaum-Katan, J., Carius, P., et al. (2019b). Capturing the onset of bacterial pulmonary infection in acini-on-chips. *Adv. Biosyst.* 3:1900026. doi: 10.1002/adbi.201900026

Bair, W. J. (1989). Human respiratory tract model for radiological protection: a revision of the icrp dosimetric model for the respiratory system. *Health Phys.* 57, 249–253. doi: 10.1097/00004032-198907001-00032

Baker, C., Rodrigues, T., de Almeida, B. P., Barbosa-Morais, N. L., and Bernardes, G. J. L. (2019). Natural product–drug conjugates for modulation of TRPV1-expressing tumors. *Bioorg. Med. Chem.* 27, 2531–2536. doi: 10.1016/j.bmc.2019.03.025

Bals, R., and Hiemstra, P. S. (2004). Innate immunity in the lung: how epithelial cells fight against respiratory pathogens. *Eur. Respir. J.* 23, 327–333. doi: 10.1183/09031936.03.00098803

Barnes, P. J., Shapiro, S. D., and Pauwels, R. A. (2003). Chronic obstructive pulmonary disease: molecular and cellularmechanisms. *Eur. Respir. J.* 22, 672–688. doi: 10.1183/09031936.03.00040703

Becker, S., Mundandhara, S., Devlin, R. B., and Madden, M. (2005). Regulation of cytokine production in human alveolar macrophages and airway epithelial cells in response to ambient air pollution particles: further mechanistic studies. *Toxicol. Appl. Pharmacol.* 207, 269–275. doi: 10.1016/j.taap.2005.01.023

Becker, S., Soukup, J. M., Gilmour, M. I., and Devlin, R. B. (1996). Stimulation of human and rat alveolar macrophages by urban air particulates: effects on oxidant radical generation and cytokine production. *Toxicol. Appl. Pharmacol.* 141, 637–648. doi: 10.1006/TAAP.1996.0330

Benam, K. H., Villenave, R., Lucchesi, C., Varone, A., Hubeau, C., Lee, H.-H., et al. (2015). Small airway-on-a-chip enables analysis of human lung inflammation and drug responses in vitro. *Nat. Methods* 13, 151–157. doi: 10.1038/nmeth.3697

Benam, K. H., Novak, R., Nawroth, J., Hirano-Kobayashi, M., Ferrante, T. C., Choe, Y., et al. (2016). Matched-comparative modeling of normal and diseased human airway responses using a microengineered breathing lung chip. *Cell Syst.* 456.e4–466.e4. doi: 10.1016/j.cels.2016.10.003

Blank, F., Rothen-Rutishauser, B. M., Schurch, S., and Gehr, P. (2006). An Optimized In Vitro Model Of The Respiratory Tract Wall To Study Particle Cell Interactions. *J. AEROSOL Med.* 19, 392–405. doi: 10.1089/jam.2006.19.392

Bovard, D., Sandoz, A., Luettich, K., Frentzel, S., Iskandar, A., Marescotti, D., et al. (2018). Lab on a Chip A lung/liver-on-a-chip platform for acute and chronic toxicity studies †. *Lab Chip* 18, 3814–3829. doi: 10.1039/c8lc01029c

Brulle, R. J., and Pellow, D. N. (2006). Human health and environmental inequalities. *Annu. Rev. Public Heal.* 27, 103–127. doi: 10.1146/annurev.publhealth.27.021405.102124

Bueters, T., Ploeger, B. A., and Visser, S. A. G. (2013). The virtue of translational PKPD modeling in drug discovery: selecting the right clinical candidate while sparing animal lives. *Drug Discov. Today* 18, 853–862. doi: 10.1016/J.DRUDIS.2013.05.001

Button, B., Cai, L.-H., Ehre, C., Kesimer, M., Hill, D. B., Sheehan, J. K., et al. (2012). A periciliary brush promotes the lung health by separating the mucus layer from airway epithelia. *Science* 337, 937–941. doi: 10.1126/science.1223012

Byron, P. R., Hindle, M., Lange, C. F., Longest, P. W., McRobbie, D., Oldham, M. J., et al. (2010). *In vivo-in vitro* correlations: predicting pulmonary drug deposition from pharmaceutical aerosols. *J. Aerosol Med. Pulm. Drug Deliv.* 23, S59–S69. doi: 10.1089/jamp.2010.0846

Carrigy, N. B., Ruzycki, C. A., Golshahi, L., and Finlay, W. H. (2014). Pediatric *in vitro* and *in silico* models of deposition via oral and nasal inhalation. *J. Aerosol Med. Pulm. Drug Deliv.* 27, 149–169. doi: 10.1089/jamp.2013.1075

Cheng, K.-H., Cheng, Y.-S., Yeh, H.-C., Guilmette, R. A., Simpson, S. Q., Yang, Y.-H., et al. (1996). *In vivo* measurements of nasal airway dimensions and ultrafine aerosol deposition in the human nasal and oral airways. *J. Aerosol Sci.* 27, 785–801. doi: 10.1016/0021-8502(96)00029-8

Conibear, L., Butt, E. W., Knote, C., Arnold, S. R., and Spracklen, D. V. (2018). Residential energy use emissions dominate health impacts from exposure to ambient particulate matter in India. *Nat. Commun.* 9:617. doi: 10.1038/s41467-018-02986-7

Daniels, C. B., and Orgeig, S. (2003). Pulmonary surfactant: the key to the evolution of air breathing. *Physiology* 18, 151–157. doi: 10.1152/nips.01438.2003

Deering-Rice, C. E., Stockmann, C., Romero, E. G., Lu, Z., Shapiro, D., Stone, B. L., et al. (2016). Characterization of transient receptor potential vanilloid-1 (TRPV1) variant activation by coal fly ash particles and associations with altered transient receptor potential ankyrin-1 (TRPA1) expression and asthma . *J. Biol. Chem.* 291, 24866–24879. doi: 10.1074/jbc.M116.746156

Douville, N. J., Zamankhan, P., Tung, Y.-C., Li, R., Vaughan, B. L., Tai, C.-F., et al. (2011). Combination of fl uid and solid mechanical stresses contribute to cell death and detachment in a microfl uidic alveolar model Combination of fluid and solid mechanical stresses contribute to cell death and detachment in a microfluidic alveolar model. *Lab Chip* 11, 557–760. doi: 10.1039/c0lc00251h

Drasler, B., Sayre, P., Steinhäuser, K. G., Petri-Fink, A., and Rothen-Rutishauser, B. (2017). In vitro approaches to assess the hazard of nanomaterials. *NanoImpact* 8, 99–116. doi: 10.1016/j.impact.2017.08.002

Fahy, J. V., and Dickey, B. F. (2010). Airway mucus function and dysfunction. *N. Engl. J. Med.* 363, 2233–2247. doi: 10.1056/NEJMra0910061

Fishler, R., Hofemeier, P., Etzion, Y., Dubowski, Y., and Sznitman, J. (2015). Particle dynamics and deposition in true-scale pulmonary acinar models OPEN. *Sci. Rep.* 5:14071. doi: 10.1038/srep14071

Gerde, P., Cheng, Y. S., and Medinsky, M. A. (1991). *In vivo* deposition of ultrafine aerosols in the nasal airway of the rat. *Toxicol. Sci.* 16, 330–336. doi: 10.1093/toxsci/16.2.330

Grainger, C. I., Greenwell, L. L., Lockley, D. J., Martin, G. P., and Forbes, B. (2006). Culture of calu-3 cells at the air interface provides a representative model of the airway epithelial barrier. *Pharm. Res.* 23, 1482–1490. doi: 10.1007/s11095-006-0255-0

Grotberg, J. B. (2011). Respiratory fluid mechanics. *Phys. Fluids* 23:021301. doi: 10.1063/1.3517737

Hassell, B. A., Goyal, G., Lee, E., Sontheimer-Phelps, A., Levy, O., Chen, C. S., et al. (2017). Human organ chip models recapitulate orthotopic lung cancer growth. Therapeutic Responses, and Tumor Dormancy In Vitro. *Cell Rep.* 21, 508–516. doi: 10.1016/j.celrep.2017.09.043

Hinds, W. C. (1999). *Aerosol Technology: Properties, Behavior, and Measurement of Airborne Particles.* Hoboken, NJ: John Wiley & Sons.

Hittinger, M., Schneider-Daum, N., and Lehr, C.-M. (2017). Cell and tissue-based in vitro models for improving the development of oral inhalation drug products. *Eur. J. Pharm. Biopharm.* 118, 73–78. doi: 10.1016/j.ejpb.2017.02.019

Hofemeier, P., and Sznitman, J. (2015). Revisiting pulmonary acinar particle transport: convection, sedimentation, diffusion, and their interplay. *J. Appl. Physiol.* 118, 1375–1385. doi: 10.1152/japplphysiol.01117.2014

Holian, A., Hamilton, R. F., Morandi, M. T., Brown, S. D., and Li, L. (1998). *Urban Particle-induced Apoptosis and Phenotype Shifts in Human Alveolar Macrophages.* Available at: https://www.ncbi.nlm.nih.gov/pmc/articles/PMC1533042/pdf/envhper00526-0053.pdf (accessed January 15, 2019).

Horsfield, K., Dart, G., Olson, D. E., Filley, G. F., Cumming, G., and Olson, E. (1971). Models of the human bronchial tree. *J. Appl. Physiol. Pri. U.S.A* 31, 207–217. doi: 10.1152/jappl.1971.31.2.207

Huh, D., Leslie, D. C., Matthews, B. D., Fraser, J. P., Jurek, S., Hamilton, G. A., et al. (2012). A human disease model of drug toxicity–induced pulmonary edema in a lung-on-a-chip microdevice. *Sci. Transl. Med.* 4:159ra147. doi: 10.1126/SCITRANSLMED.3004249

Huh, D., Matthews, B. D., Mammoto, A., Montoya-Zavala, M., Hsin, H. Y., and Ingber, D. E. (2010). Reconstituting organ-level lung functions on a chip. *Science* 328, 1662–1668. doi: 10.1126/science.1188302

Humayun, M., Chow, C.-W., and Young, E. W. K. (2018). Microfluidic lung airway-on-a-chip with arrayable suspended gels for studying epithelial and smooth muscle cell interactions. *Lab Chip* 18, 1298–1309. doi: 10.1039/c7lc01357d

Imai, Y., Miki, T., Ishikawa, T., Aoki, T., and Yamaguchi, T. (2012). Deposition of micrometer particles in pulmonary airways during inhalation and breath holding. *J. Biomech.* 45, 1809–1815. doi: 10.1016/j.jbiomech.2012.04.017

Inoue, K., Takano, H., Sakurai, M., Oda, T., Tamura, H., Yanagisawa, R., et al. (2006). Pulmonary exposure to diesel exhaust particles enhances coagulatory disturbance with endothelial damage and systemic inflammation related to lung inflammation. *Exp. Biol. Med.* 231, 1626–1632. doi: 10.1177/153537020623101007

Inthavong, K., Ma, J., Shang, Y., Dong, J., Chetty, A. S. R., Tu, J., et al. (2019). Geometry and airflow dynamics analysis in the nasal cavity during inhalation. *Clin. Biomech.* 66, 97–106. doi: 10.1016/j.clinbiomech.2017.10.006

Islam, M. S., Saha, S. C., Sauret, E., Gemci, T., and Gu, Y. T. (2017). Pulmonary aerosol transport and deposition analysis in upper 17 generations of the human respiratory tract. *J. Aerosol Sci.* 108, 29–43. doi: 10.1016/j.jaerosci.2017.03.004

Janssen, W. J., Stefanski, A. L., Bochner, B. S., and Evans, C. M. (2016). Control of lung defence by mucins and macrophages: ancient defence mechanisms with modern functions. *Eur. Respir. J.* 48, 1201–1214. doi: 10.1183/13993003.00120-2015

Kim, K.-H., Kabir, E., and Kabir, S. (2015). A review on the human health impact of airborne particulate matter. *Environ. Int.* 74, 136–143. doi: 10.1016/J.ENVINT.2014.10.005

Kleinstreuer, C., and Zhang, Z. (2010). Airflow and particle transport in the human respiratory system. *Annu. Rev. Fluid Mech* 42, 301–334. doi: 10.1146/annurev-fluid-121108-145453

Koullapis, P. G., Hofemeier, P., Sznitman, J., and Kassinos, S. C. (2018). An efficient computational fluid-particle dynamics method to predict deposition in a simplified approximation of the deep lung. *Eur. J. Pharm. Sci.* 113, 132–144. doi: 10.1016/j.ejps.2017.09.016

Koullapis, P., Kassinos, S. C., Muela, J., Perez-Segarra, C., Rigola, J., Lehmkuhl, O., et al. (2018). Regional aerosol deposition in the human airways: the SimInhale benchmark case and a critical assessment of in silico methods. *Eur. J. Pharm. Sci.* 113, 77–94. doi: 10.1016/j.ejps.2017.09.003

Koullapis, P. G., Kassinos, S. C., Bivolarova, M. P., and Melikov, A. K. (2016). Particle deposition in a realistic geometry of the human conducting airways: effects of inlet velocity profile, inhalation flowrate and electrostatic charge. *J. Biomech.* 49, 2201–2212. doi: 10.1016/j.jbiomech.2015.11.029

Lai, S. K., Wang, Y.-Y., and Hanes, J. (2008). Mucus-penetrating nanoparticles for drug and gene delivery to mucosal tissues ☆. *Adv. Drug Deliv. Rev.* 61, 158–171. doi: 10.1016/j.addr.2008.11.002

Lechanteur, A., das Neves, J., and Sarmento, B. (2018). The role of mucus in cell-based models used to screen mucosal drug delivery. *Adv. Drug Deli. Re*124, 50–63. doi: 10.1016/j.addr.2017.07.019

Leggat, P. A., Kedjarune, U., and Smith, D. R. (2007). Occupational health problems in modern dentistry: a review. *Ind. Health* 45, 611–621. doi: 10.2486/indhealth.45.611

Lenz, A.-G., Stoeger, T., Cei, D., Schmidmeir, M., Semren, N., Burgstaller, G., et al. (2014). Efficient bioactive delivery of aerosolized drugs to human pulmonary epithelial cells cultured in air-liquid interface conditions. *Am. J. Respir. Cell Mol. Biol.* 51, 526–535. doi: 10.1165/rcmb.2013-0479OC

Leonard, F., Collnot, E.-M., and Lehr, C.-M. (2010). A three-dimensional coculture of enterocytes, monocytes and dendritic cells to model inflamed intestinal mucosa in vitro. *Mol. Pharm.* 7, 2103–2119. doi: 10.1021/mp1000795

Li, E., Xu, Z., Zhao, H., Sun, Z., Wang, L., Guo, Z., et al. (2015). Macrophages promote benzopyrene-induced tumor transformation of human bronchial epithelial cells by activation of NF-κB and STAT3 signaling in a bionic airway chip culture and in animal models. *Oncotarget* 6, 8900–8913. doi: 10.18632/oncotarget.3561

Lin, H., Li, H., Cho, H.-J., Bian, S., Roh, H.-J., Lee, M.-K., et al. (2007). Air-Liquid Interface (ALI) culture of human bronchial epithelial cell monolayers as an in vitro model for airway drug transport studies. *J. Pharm. Sci.* 96, 341–350. doi: 10.1002/JPS.20803

Ménache, M. G., Hofmann, W., Ashgarian, B., and Miller, F. J. (2008). Airway geometry models of children's lungs for use in dosimetry modeling. *Inhal. Toxicol.* 20, 101–126. doi: 10.1080/08958370701821433

Merck (2015). *Microsphere Coupling – Two-step EDC / Sulfo NHS Covalent Coupling Procedure for Estapor ® Carboxyl-modified Dyed Microspheres.* Kenilworth, NJ: Merck.

Mustafiz, M., Vaughan, A., Stevanovic, S., Morrison, L. E., Mohammad Pourkhesalian, A., Rahman, M., et al. (2015). Removal of organic content from diesel exhaust particles alters cellular responses of primary human bronchial epithelial cells cultured at an air-liquid interface. *J. Environ. Anal. Toxicol.* 5, 100316–100317. doi: 10.4172/2161-0525.1000316

Nemmar, A., Al-Salam, S., Dhanasekaran, S., Sudhadevi, M., and Ali, B. H. (2009). Pulmonary exposure to diesel exhaust particles promotes cerebral microvessel thrombosis: protective effect of a cysteine prodrug l-2-oxothiazolidine-4-carboxylic acid. *Toxicology* 263, 84–92. doi: 10.1016/J.TOX.2009.06.017

Nemmar, A., Al-Salam, S., Zia, S., Marzouqi, F., Al-Dhaheri, A., Subramaniyan, D., et al. (2011). Contrasting actions of diesel exhaust particles on the pulmonary and cardiovascular systems and the effects of thymoquinone. *Br. J. Pharmacol.* 164, 1871–1882. doi: 10.1111/j.1476-5381.2011.01442.x

Nemmar, A., Holme, J. A., Rosas, I., Schwarze, P. E., and Alfaro-Moreno, E. (2013). Recent advances in particulate matter and nanoparticle toxicology: a review of the in vivo and in vitro studies. *Biomed Res. Int.* 2013, 279371. doi: 10.1155/2013/279371

Nesmith, A. P., Agarwal, A., McCain, M. L., and Parker, K. K. (2014). Human airway musculature on a chip: an in vitro model of allergic asthmatic bronchoconstriction and bronchodilation. *Lab Chip* 14, 3925–3936. doi: 10.1039/C4LC00688G

Paur, H. R., Cassee, F. R., Teeguarden, J., Fissan, H., Diabate, S., Aufderheide, M., et al. (2011). In-vitro cell exposure studies for the assessment of nanoparticle toxicity in the lung-A dialog between aerosol science and biology. *J. Aerosol Sci.* 42, 668–692. doi: 10.1016/j.jaerosci.2011.06.005

Pedley, T. J. (2003). Pulmonary fluid dynamics. *Annu. Rev. Fluid Mech.* 9, 229–274. doi: 10.1146/annurev.fl.09.010177.001305

Petitot, F., Lestaevel, P., Tourlonias, E., Mazzucco, C., Jacquinot, S., Dhieux, B., et al. (2013). Inhalation of uranium nanoparticles: respiratory tract deposition and translocation to secondary target organs in rats. *Toxicol. Lett.* 217, 217–225. doi: 10.1016/j.toxlet.2012.12.022

Punde, T. H., Wu, W. H., Lien, P. C., Chang, Y. L., Kuo, P. H., Chang, M. D. T., et al. (2015). A biologically inspired lung-on-a-chip device for the study of protein-induced lung inflammation. *Integr. Biol* 7, 162–169. doi: 10.1039/c4ib00239c

Rayner, R. E., Makena, P., Prasad, G. L., and Cormet-Boyaka, E. (2019). Optimization of normal human bronchial epithelial (NHBE) cell 3D cultures for in vitro lung model studies. *Sci. Rep.* 9:500. doi: 10.1038/s41598-018-36735-z

Röhm, M., Carle, S., Maigler, F., Flamm, J., Kramer, V., Mavoungou, C., et al. (2017). A comprehensive screening platform for aerosolizable protein formulations for intranasal and pulmonary drug delivery. *Int. J. Pharm.* 532, 537–546. doi: 10.1016/j.ijpharm.2017.09.027

Ronaldson-Bouchard, K., and Vunjak-Novakovic, G. (2018). Organs-on-a-chip: a fast track for engineered human tissues in drug development. *Cell Stem Cell* 22, 310–324. doi: 10.1016/j.stem.2018.02.011

Sauret, V., Halson, P. M., Brown, I. W., Fleming, J. S., and Bailey, A. G. (2002). Study of the three-dimensional geometry of the central conducting airways in man using computed tomographic (CT) images. *J. Anat.* 200, 123–134. doi: 10.1046/j.0021-8782.2001.00018.x

Schuster, B. S., Suk, J. S., Woodworth, G. F., and Hanes, J. (2013). Nanoparticle diffusion in respiratory mucus from humans without lung disease. *Biomaterials* 34, 3439–3446. doi: 10.1016/j.biomaterials.2013.01.064

Shirure, V. S., Bi, Y., Curtis, M. B., Lezia, A., Goedegebuure, M. M., Goedegebuure, S. P., et al. (2018). Tumor-on-a-chip platform to investigate progression and drug sensitivity in cell lines and patient-derived organoids. *Lab Chip* 18, 3687–3702. doi: 10.1039/C8LC00596F

Skardal, A., Shupe, T., and Atala, A. (2016). Organoid-on-a-chip and body-on-a-chip systems for drug screening and disease modeling. *Drug Discov. Today* 21, 1399–1411. doi: 10.1016/j.drudis.2016.07.003

Stahlhofen, W., Rudolf, G., and James, A. C. (1989). Intercomparison of Experimental Regional Aerosol Deposition Data. *J. Aerosol Med.* 2, 285–308. doi: 10.1089/jam.1989.2.285

Stannard, W., and O'Callaghan, C. (2006). Ciliary function and the role of cilia in clearance. *J. AEROSOL Med* 19, 110–115. doi: 10.1089/jam.2006.19.110

Stucki, A. O., Stucki, J. D., Hall, S. R. R., Felder, M., Mermoud, Y., Schmid, R. A., et al. (2014). From chip-in-a-lab to lab-on-a-chip: towards a single handheld electronic system for multiple application-specific lab-on-a-chip (ASLOC). *Lab Chip* 15, 1302–1310. doi: 10.1039/c4lc01252f

Sznitman, J. (2013). Respiratory microflows in the pulmonary acinus. *J. Biomech.* 46, 284–298. doi: 10.1016/j.jbiomech.2012.10.028

Tenenbaum-Katan, J., Artzy-Schnirman, A., Fishler, R., Korin, N., and Sznitman, J. (2018). Biomimetics of the pulmonary environment in vitro: a microfluidics perspective. *Biomicrofluidics* 12:042209. doi: 10.1063/1.5023034

Veranth, J. M., Moss, T. A., Chow, J. C., Labban, R., Nichols, W. K., Walton, J. C., et al. (2006). Correlation of in vitro cytokine responses with the chemical composition of soil-derived particulate matter. *Environ. Health Perspect.* 114, 341–349. doi: 10.1289/ehp.8360

Veronesi, B., Oortgiesen, M., Carter, J. D., and Devlin, R. B. (1999). Particulate matter initiates inflammatory cytokine release by activation of capsaicin and acid receptors in a human bronchial epithelial cell line. *Toxicol. Appl. Pharmacol.* 154, 106–115. doi: 10.1006/taap.1998.8567

Weibel, E. R., Cournand, A. F., and Richards, D. W. (1963). *Morphometry of the Human Lung.* Berlin: Springer.

Whitsett, J. A. (2018). Airway epithelial differentiation and mucociliary clearance. *Ann. Am. Thorac. Soc.* 15, S143–S148. doi: 10.1513/AnnalsATS.201802-128AW

Wu, W., Jin, Y., and Carlsten, C. (2018). Inflammatory health effects of indoor and outdoor particulate matter. *J. Allergy Clin. Immunol.* 141, 833–844. doi: 10.1016/J.JACI.2017.12.981

Wu, W., Samet, J. M., Ghio, A. J., and Devlin, R. B. (2001). Activation of the EGF receptor signaling pathway in airway epithelial cells exposed to Utah Valley PM. *Am. J. Physiol. - Lung Cell. Mol. Physiol.* 281, 483–489. doi: 10.1152/ajplung.2001.281.2.l483

Zhang, Z., Kleinstreuer, C., and Kim, C. S. (2009). Comparison of analytical and CFD models with regard to micron particle deposition in a human 16-generation tracheobronchial airway model. *J. Aerosol Sci.* 40, 16–28. doi: 10.1016/j.jaerosci.2008.08.003

10

Low-Frequency Intrapulmonary Percussive Ventilation Increases Aerosol Penetration in a 2-Compartment Physical Model of Fibrotic Lung Disease

*Sandrine Le Guellec[1,2,3], Laurine Allimonnier[1,3], Nathalie Heuzé-Vourc'h[1,3], Maria Cabrera[1,3], Frédéric Ossant[4], Jérémie Pourchez[5], Laurent Vecellio[1,3] and Laurent Plantier[1,3,6]**

[1] INSERM, Research Center for Respiratory Diseases, U1100, Tours, France, [2] DTF Aerodrug, Tours, France, [3] Université de Tours, Tours, France, [4] Inserm U1253, Imagerie et Cerveau, Tours, France, [5] Mines Saint-Etienne, Univ. Lyon, Univ. Jean Monnet, INSERM, U1059 Sainbiose, Centre CIS, Saint-Etienne, France, [6] CHRU de Tours, Service de Pneumologie et Explorations Fonctionnelles Respiratoires, Tours, France

***Correspondence:**
Laurent Plantier
laurent.plantier@univ-tours.fr

In patients with fibrotic pulmonary disease such as idiopathic pulmonary fibrosis (IPF), inhaled aerosols deposit mostly in the less affected region of the lungs, resulting in suboptimal pharmacokinetics of airway-delivered treatments. Refinement of aerosol delivery technique requires new models to simulate the major alterations of lung physiology associated with IPF, i.e., heterogeneously reduced lung compliance and increased airway caliber. A novel physical model of the respiratory system was constructed to simulate aerosol drug delivery in spontaneously breathing (negative pressure ventilation) IPF patients. The model comprises upper (Alberta ideal throat) and lower airway (plastic tubing) models and branches into two compartments (Michigan lung models) which differ in compliance and caliber of conducting airway. The model was able to reproduce the heterogeneous, compliance-dependent reduction in ventilation and aerosol penetration (using NaF as a model aerosol) seen in fibrotic lung regions in IPF. Of note, intrapulmonary percussive ventilation induced a 2–3-fold increase in aerosol penetration in the low-compliance/high airway caliber compartment of the model, demonstrating the responsiveness of the model to therapeutic intervention.

Keywords: pulmonary fibrosis, nebulization, physiology, compliance, aerosol, inhalation

INTRODUCTION

Fibrotic interstitial lung diseases (ILD) are a group of severe chronic non-communicable lung diseases where excessive deposition of abnormal extracellular matrix, in association with epithelial and/or endothelial lesions, results in progressive respiratory failure. Idiopathic pulmonary fibrosis (IPF) is the most common and the most severe idiopathic ILD (King et al., 2011). In IPF, fibrotic lesions follow the heterogeneous "usual interstitial pneumonia" pattern where fibrotic lesions alternate with preserved regions, and predominate in peripheral (supleural) areas.

Current treatments for IPF are unsatisfactory. Although two therapies, pirfenidone and nintedanib, both slow the decline of lung function (Noble et al., 2011; King et al., 2014; Richeldi et al., 2014) and may increase survival (Canestaro et al., 2016), neither drug blocks or reverses the progress of disease and their tolerance is fair at best (Fletcher et al., 2016). There is a need for new drugs and treatment delivery routes for IPF and other ILDs.

IPF is spatially restricted to the lung, making it an ideal candidate disease for the use of topical, i.e., inhaled drugs. Aerosolized delivery through the airways has key advantages over the oral or injected routes for the administration of drugs to the lungs. Aerosolization is non-invasive and provides high therapeutic index. Aerosolized drug delivery is used routinely in patients with airway diseases. By contrast, the inhaled route is not currently used for the treatment of IPF, owing in part to low aerosol deposition in the lung.

IPF is associated with multiple alterations in lung structure with potential to hinder penetration of inhaled aerosols (Plantier et al., 2018). Fibrosis leads to major reductions in lung compliance (Zielonka et al., 2010) which are presumed heterogeneous given the spatial heterogeneity of lesions, and which result in reduced ventilation of the affected regions. Lung compliance is defined by the ratio of change in lung volume (V) over change in the transpulmonary pressure (Ptp). Besides fibrosis of alveolar regions, bronchial lesions may be observed whose nature is debated. Although the total number of airways in reduced in end-stage IPF (Verleden et al., 2020), the number of visible distal airways in increased in lungs with severe IPF (Verleden et al., 2020), while conducting airway volume is increased by 32% in patients with moderate IPF in comparison with control subjects (Plantier et al., 2016) and expiratory airflow is increased (Plantier et al., 2018).

Anatomical and physiological alterations of the respiratory system in IPF may result in altered deposition of inhaled aerosols. Similar total lung deposition, as measured by concentrations in bronchoalveolar lavage fluid (Khoo et al., 2020) or planar scintigraphy (Samuel and Smaldone, 2019), can be achieved in IPF patients as compared to healthy subjects. However, planar scintigraphy images suggest that deposition of micrometric aerosols is not homogenous in some IPF patients, in contrast with healthy subjects (Kanazawa et al., 1993; Khoo et al., 2020). Similarly, deposition of the nanometric aerosol Technegas was patchy and predominated in the upper regions of the lungs, which are typically the less damaged areas in 2 IPF patients (Watanabe et al., 1995). We hypothesize that reduced lung compliance results in reduced penetration and subsequent heterogeneous deposition of inhaled aerosols in IPF.

At present, inhalation devices and protocols allow high aerosol penetration and deposition in ventilated regions, but poor penetration and deposition in the regions of the respiratory system receiving little or no ventilation. The preferential deposition of aerosols in the less damaged areas needs to be overcome for satisfactory spatial targeting of inhaled therapeutics in IPF. It is therefore important to develop optimized aerosolization protocols allowing to target the low compliance alveolar regions in IPF. Models able to simulate IPF lungs under spontaneous ventilation are required to test the efficacy of such protocols.

Acoustic/pulse pressure waves hold potential to increase aerosol delivery in low compliance lungs. Indeed, acoustic waves increase aerosol penetration and deposition in the maxillary sinuses (Durand et al., 2012; Möller et al., 2014; Leclerc et al., 2015; Moghadam et al., 2018). Maxillary sinuses are bone structures, which have near-null compliance and thus receive no ventilation during the respiratory cycle. Multiple experiments established that acoustic waves were most effective in the 100–300 Hz frequency range, close to the resonance frequency of the maxillary sinuses (Durand et al., 2012; Möller et al., 2014; Leclerc et al., 2015; Moghadam et al., 2018).

In light of these elements, we hypothesized (1) that poor penetration of inhaled aerosols in low compliance lung regions could be reproduced in a two-compartment mechanical model of fibrotic lungs under negative-pressure (spontaneous) ventilation and (2) that acoustic pressure waves near the resonance frequency of the model would increase aerosol penetration in the low compliance compartment.

MATERIALS AND METHODS

Construction of a Two-Compartment Model of the Respiratory System

A two-compartment model of the entire respiratory system (schematic in **Figure 1**) was constructed. This model comprised a physical model of the upper airways (Alberta ldealized throat, Copley Scientific, United Kingdom), a plastic tube modeling the subglottic airways down to the 4th bronchial division, and a Y-piece connecting each lung compartment. Each lung compartment included a plastic tube modeling the distal airways, and a mechanical lung model (Michigan Lung Model, Michigan Instruments, United States) modeling the alveolar regions. Each mechanical lung model comprised (1) a first bellows connected to the airway model described above ("active bellows") and (2) a second bellows ("passive bellows"), which was mechanically coupled to the first bellows, and was ventilated using a clinical ventilator (Servo 300, Siemens, Germany). Thus, the first bellows was ventilated under negative pressure, allowing to simulate physiological spontaneous breathing. Airway diameter and bellows compliance could be individually adjusted. To simulate normal lung, in the "Control compartment" airway diameter was 17 mm, and lung compliance was 100 ml/cmH_2O. To simulate fibrotic lung, in the "Experimental compartment" airway diameter was 22 mm, and lung compliance was $\leq$ 100 ml/cmH_2O. Overall, the volumes corresponded to those observed in an adult man. Filters (Anest-Guard, Teleflex, France) were inserted in each compartment, at the junction of the tube modeling the airways and the bellows modeling the alveolar regions.

Distribution of Ventilation in the Model

For characterization of ventilation distribution, the model was actuated under the following ventilator settings: Frequency = 10/min, inspiratory pressure between 5 and

18 cmH_2O, inspiratory time = 2 s. These settings simulate spontaneous breathing in an adult subject. Ventilation of each compartment was measured with spirometers (300 L/min, AD Instruments, Dunedin, New Zealand) inserted in place of the filters (**Figure 1**). In addition, the resonance frequency of the model were measured using a clinical forced oscillations device (Tremoflo, EMKA, France).

NaF Aerosol Delivery and Quantitation of Aerosol Deposition

The model was connected to a jet nebulizer aerosol generator (Atomisor AOHBOX/NL9M, DTF medical, France) at the upper airway opening. This generator delivers an aerosol with 4–5 μm mass median aerodynamic diameter. Inspiratory and expiratory valves were used. For all aerosol delivery experiments, the pulmonary model was actuated with the following ventilator settings to simulate tidal ventilation: Frequency = 10/min, inspiratory time = 2 sec, inspiratory pressure = 5 cmH_2O. Three milliliter of a 2.5% sodium fluoride (NaF) solution were nebulized over 10–15 min. After each nebulization session, the filters were dismounted. The filters were flushed with 30 ml of 2% vol./vol. aqueous total ionic strength adjustment buffer (TISAB) solution (Sigma-Aldrich, St. Louis, MO, United States) and incubated for 3 h at room temperature. NaF was then assayed by electrochemical analysis (SevenGo Pro, Mettler Toledo, United States). The quantity of NaF aerosol deposited in each filter (Control or Experimental) was expressed as a fraction of the initial NaF dose that was loaded in the nebulizer.

Aerosol Distribution in the Model

Aerosol distribution was controlled for each nebulization experiments by dosing all parts of the model. Aerosol deposition was quantitated at the level of the nebulizer chamber, expiratory filter, construct, upper airway (Alberta throat model, trachea tube and Y-piece), and each lung compartment (tubing and filter). Each section was washed with 30–250 ml TISAB and NaF was assayed as described above.

Delivery of Acoustic/Pulse Pressure Waves

To generate acoustic pressure waves in the 20–500 Hz frequency range, sinusoidal signals were generated with VB Generator freeware[1], amplified (t.amp PM40C, Thomann, Germany), and transmitted to a vibration exciter (S-50009, Tira GmbH, Germany). Amplifier gain was set so that acoustic pressure was identical across the frequency range, using a sonometer; 80 dB acoustic waves could be generated at all frequencies. To generate pulse pressure waves in the 1–10 Hz frequency range, a Pegaso (Dima Italia, Italy) intrapulmonary percussion ventilation device was used. IPV devices deliver small volumes of air; the shape of the signal is not sinusoidal (Toussaint et al., 2012). IPV pulse pressure was set at 40 cmH_2O and the inspiratory/expiratory ration was set to 1. In a first set of experiments, the vibration exciter and the IPV device were connected to the nebulizer/valves construct as shown in **Figure 2A**. In a second set of experiments,

[1]VB Audio. 2002. France. http://vincent.burel.free.fr/download/index.htm

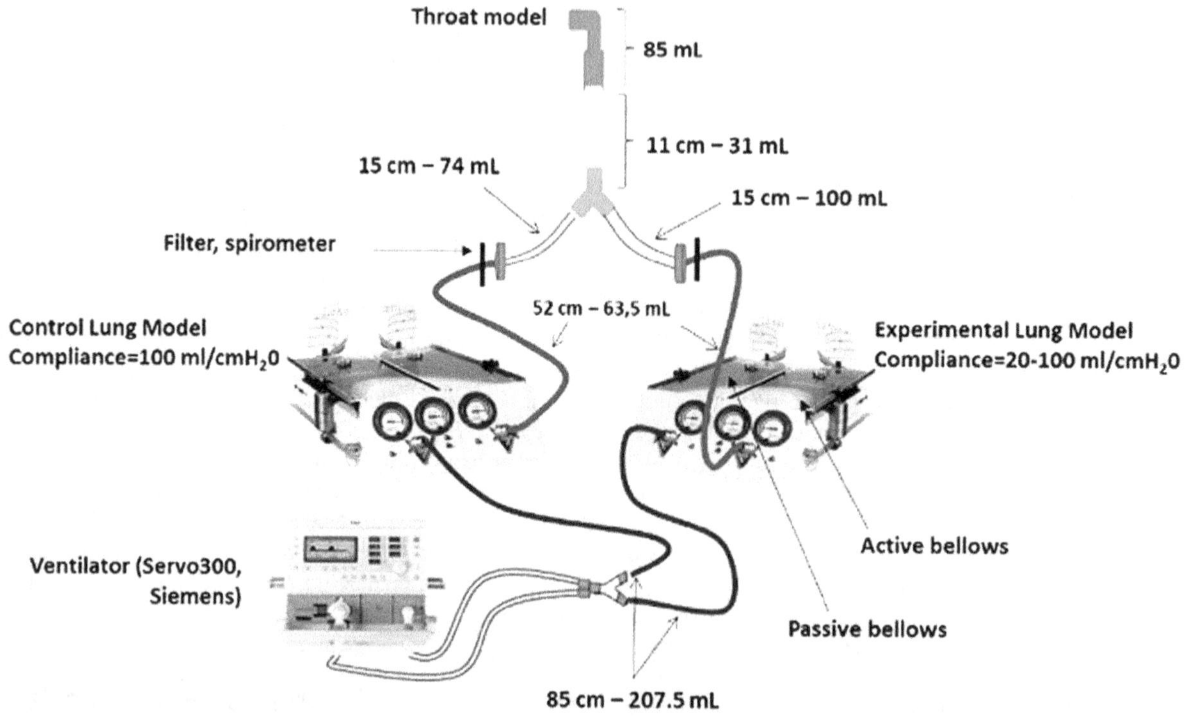

FIGURE 1 | Schematic of the two-compartment model of the respiratory system used to simulate IPF pathophysiology. The length and volume (measured) of corrugated plastic tubing used to model the airways are featured.

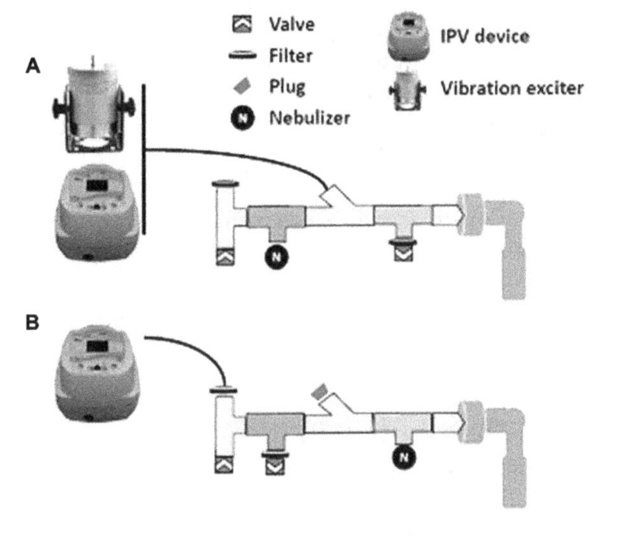

FIGURE 2 | Constructs used for acoustic/pulse pressure wave delivery during nebulization. All constructs are connected to the throat model (right).
(A) Construct used for acoustic wave delivery and initial IPV delivery.
(B) Construct used for multiple-frequency IPV delivery.

the IPV device was connected as shown In **Figure 2B** following optimization experiments. Both high-frequency acoustic waves and low-frequency IPV pulses were delivered to the model for the duration of nebulization.

Statistical Analysis

All data were expressed as means and standard deviations. Group by group comparisons were performed with Student's t-test (2 groups) or ANOVA (more than 2 groups). Paired or unpaired analyses were done as appropriate. Relationships between variables were assessed by linear regression. Prism v5.0 (Graphpad, San Diego, CA, United States) was used for all analyses.

RESULTS

Ventilation and Aerosol Deposition in the Model

Firstly, distribution of ventilation (tidal volume) between the two compartments of the models was assessed. As expected, tidal volume in both compartments of the model was a linear function of the pressure setting on the ventilator, which was applied to the passive bellows of the lung model, and of the compliance setting of the lung model (**Supplementary Figure S1**). For a given level of ventilation pressure and compliance, tidal volume was not significantly different between compartments.

Then, a NaF aerosol was delivered into the model while ventilated, and deposition onto the compartment filters, which assesses aerosol penetration into the respective compartment, was measured. When the compliance of both compartments was set at 100 ml/cmH_2O, aerosol deposition in the Experimental compartment (then characterized only by 33% larger airway) trended to be slightly reduced in comparison with the Control compartment of the model (3.9 $\pm$ 0.5% of the loaded dose vs. 3.0 $\pm$ 0.3%, $p = 0.06$ by paired analysis - **Figure 3A**).

Then, aerosolization experiments were repeated when compliance of the Experimental compartment was decreased to 70, 50, and 30 ml/cmH_2O. As shown in **Figure 3A**, decreasing compliance of the Experimental compartment had two effects. First, an increase in aerosol penetration was observed in the Control compartment; this increase correlated negatively with compliance in the Experimental compartment (R^2 = 0.48, p = 0.012). Second, aerosol penetration decreased in the Experimental condition; this decrease followed a strong linear relationship with compliance ($R^2 = 0.96, p < 0.0001$). Thus, these experiments demonstrated that decreasing lung compliance in one compartment of the system shifted penetration of an inhaled aerosol away from the low compliance compartment and into the compliant compartment. As shown in **Figure 1B**, aerosol penetration in the Experimental compartment was strongly ($R^2 = 0.95$, $p < 0.0001$) associated with tidal volume, supporting the hypothesis that regional reduction in lung compliance and subsequent reduction in local ventilation are key drivers in reducing aerosol deposition in fibrotic lungs.

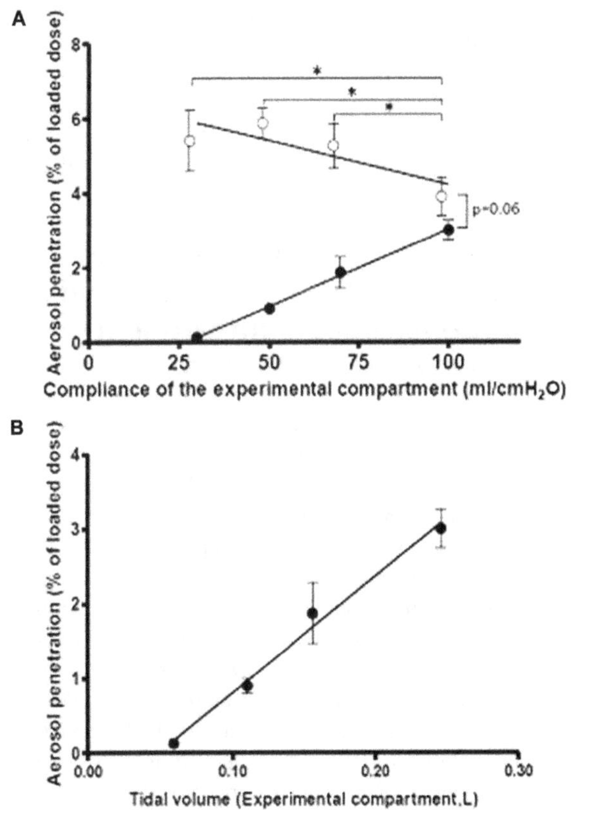

FIGURE 3 | Aerosol deposition in the Control (open circles) and Experimental (filled circles) as a function of **(A)** compliance of the experimental compartment and **(B)** tidal volume in the experimental compartment. Compliance was set at 100 ml/cmH_2O in the Control compartment). $^*p < 0.05$. Regression lines are shown. $N = 3$. Means and SD.

For further experiments, the compliance of the Experimental compartment was set at 50 ml/cmH_2O, so that the model could detect both increases and decreases in aerosol penetration following delivery of acoustic/pulse pressure waves. Oscillometry parameters were determined under this setting. Under these conditions, the resonance frequency of the system was 5 Hz.

20–500 Hz Acoustic Waves Failed to Increase Aerosol Penetration in the Low Compliance Compartment

Audible acoustic waves are known to increase aerosol penetration in the maxillary sinuses (Leclerc et al., 2015). Thus, in a first set of experiments, 80 dB/20–500 Hz acoustic waves were delivered to the nebulizer construct for the duration of nebulization using the construct shown in **Figure 2A**. As shown in **Figure 4A**, audible acoustic waves had no effect on aerosol penetration either in the Control or in the Experimental compartment, and the Experimental/control deposition ratio was unchanged.

In maxillary sinuses, matching acoustic wave frequency with the resonance frequency of the target structures results in increased aerosol deposition (Durand et al., 2012). Because the measured resonance frequency of the model (5 Hz) was much lower than 20 Hz, we raised the hypothesis that low-frequency pressure waves were required to increase aerosol deposition. To deliver such pressure waves, an intra-pulmonary percussion ventilation (IPV) device was used. IPV devices offer important advantages in the context of aerosol deposition in ILD as (1) they are already certified for clinical use in humans including in association with inhaled aerosols, and (2) they have been shown to increase aerosol penetration in a simple one-compartment model independent of compliance (Karashima et al., 2019).

Low-Frequency IPV Pressure Waves Increase Aerosol Penetration Twofold in the Low Compliance Compartment

Initial experiments using IPV (3 Hz, 40 cmH_2O) delivered through the same nebulizer construct as the one used for audible acoustic wave delivery showed, in comparison with absence of pulse pressure waves, (1) that aerosol deposition in both the Control and Experimental compartments was decreased but (2) that the ratio of aerosol deposited in the Experimental/Control compartments increased from 0.16 to 0.41 (**Supplementary Figure S2**). Additional experiments were then conducted to evaluate the effect of IPV (3 Hz) delivered through different nebulizer constructs (**Supplementary Figure S3**). As shown in **Supplementary Figure S4A**, aerosol deposition in the Experimental compartment was increased by IPV (3 Hz) in 2 out of 6 constructs. To verify that the increase in aerosol penetration was IPV-dependent and not only construct-dependent, aerosol penetration was measured in constructs 3 and 4 both with and without IPV (3 Hz). IPV increased aerosol penetration in the Experimental compartment in both constructs (**Supplementary Figure S4B**).

Construct 3 was retained for further experiments where the effect of IPV frequency on aerosol penetration was tested. As shown in **Figure 4B**, low-frequency IPV pressure waves in the 1–3 Hz frequency range increased aerosol penetration in the Experimental compartment. The increase was maximal (twofold) for 1 Hz IPV. By contrast, 10 Hz IPV decreased aerosol penetration in the Experimental compartment. IPV did not significantly increase aerosol penetration in the Control compartment of the model although a trend was present (+29%, $p = 0.08$).

Because low-frequency, high pressure IPV may be uncomfortable in man, an additional experiment was conducted using low-pressure (10 cmH_2O) IPV. As shown in **Figure 5**, 1 Hz, 10 cmH_2O IPV increased aerosol penetration in the Experimental compartment by 121% in comparison with no IPV.

Aerosol Distribution in the Model

In the normal lung model, 97.8 ± 12.1% of aerosol was recovered (**Table 1**). 12 ± 1.7% of aerosol deposited in the respiratory system (including upper airways and lung models) while 85.8 ± 10.6% were recovered outside the model (including nebulizer, expiratory filter and construct). When compliance was reduced in the experimental compartment to simulate IPF, 90.7 ± 7.8% was recovered owing to reduced deposition in both lung and delivery apparatus. Under 1 Hz–40 cmH_2O IPV conditions, 95.5 ± 17.2% of total aerosol was recovered. In addition to a threefold increase of aerosol deposition in the experimental compartment's filter, IPV induced increases in the construct and the throat model, as well as a ~50% decrease in the expiratory filter.

DISCUSSION

In this study, we developed a novel 2-compartment model of the respiratory system simulating fibrotic lung disease, and we showed that heterogeneous reductions in lung compliance resulted in (1) an increase of aerosol penetration in the preserved lung regions and (2) proportionate decreases in tidal volume and aerosol penetration in the less-compliant region. The strength of the associations between lung compliance, tidal volume and aerosol penetration support the hypothesis that reduced lung compliance is the main determinant of reduced aerosol deposition in fibrotic lung regions. Then, we used this model to explore whether acoustic/pulse pressure waves modulated aerosol penetration, and showed that low-frequency intrapulmonary pressure ventilation pulses reliably increased aerosol penetration in the low compliance compartment.

Although the total amount of aerosol-delivered drugs may be similar in patients with fibrotic lung disease and healthy controls at the level of the whole organ (Diaz et al., 2012; Khoo et al., 2020), imaging studies suggest that inhaled aerosols may mainly deposit into the less-affected regions of the lungs and thus presumably miss their cellular targets (Kanazawa et al., 1993; Watanabe et al., 1995). Despite recent demonstration that small aerosol particles (1.5 μm diameter) and polydisperse aerosols should be preferred for IPF patients ("The Topical Study of Inhaled Drug (Salbutamol), 2019 Delivery in Idiopathic Pulmonary Fibrosis. - PubMed - NCBI" n.d.), preferential deposition of aerosols in the less damaged regions needs to be overcome. Optimizing spatial

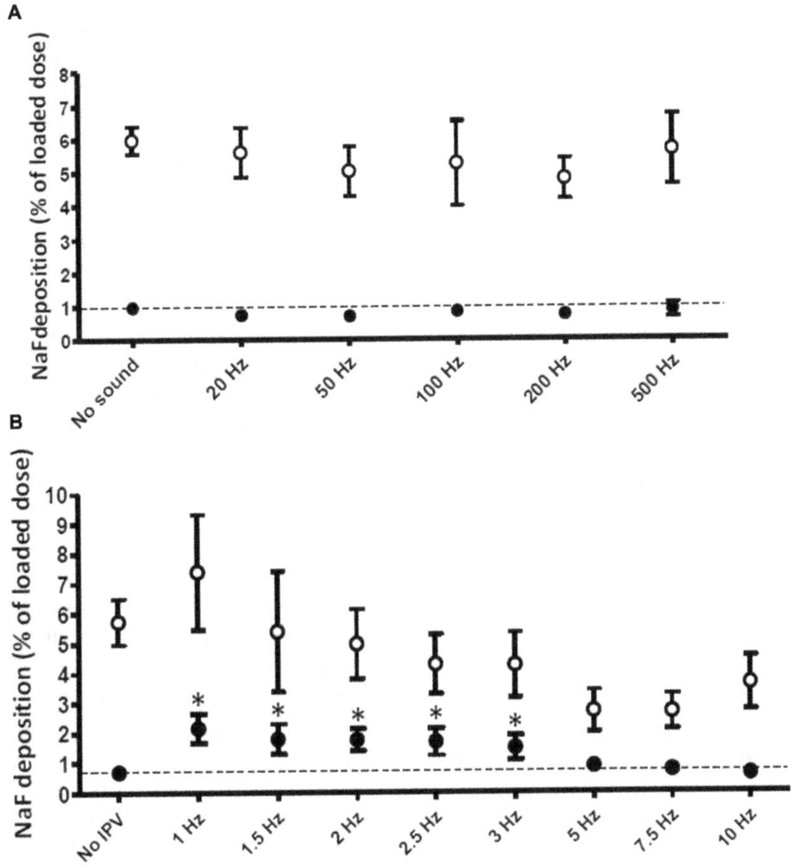

FIGURE 4 | Aerosol deposition in the Control (100 ml/cmH_2O compliance, open circles) and Experimental (50 ml/cmH_2O compliance, filled circles) compartments of the model. **(A)** 20–500 Hz audible acoustic waves (*n* = 3) and **(B)** 1–10 Hz IPV pressure pulses (*n* = 6) were delivered during nebulization. Dotted lines show the control condition (no sound or no IPV). $^*p < 0.05$ vs. no IPV. Means and SD.

targeting is a major challenge to develop inhaled therapies for diseases which, like IPF, are characterized by heterogeneously distributed fibrotic lung lesions.

Experimental models are required to understand the mechanisms driving aerosol penetration and deposition in fibrotic lung disease. To this day, few studies were conducted in the aim of simulating both disease mechanics and aerosol deposition in fibrotic lungs under spontaneous ventilation. Montigaud et al. (2019), developed an *ex vivo* model combining heat-treated porcine lungs and a 3D-printed replica of the human airways. Although this model better simulates a branched airway anatomy, allows to replicate reductions in lung compliance predominating in subpleural regions, and can be used for aerosol deposition studies, it is unwieldy and cannot be reused for multiple experiments. To our knowledge, the mechanical model described herein is the first to offer the possibility to simulate the geometrical and physical characteristics of either mild or severe, restrictive or obstructive (using airflow resistances) lung disease *in vitro*, and to conduct replicated experiments of inhaled drug delivery. The amount of nebulized aerosol that deposited in lower airways of the normal lung model (trachea, Y-piece, bronchi and lung compartments) was approximately 10%, which is similar to observations in healthy volunteers and patients with lung disease during inhalation experiments with jet nebulizer devices (Rau, 2005; Dugernier et al., 2017). This suggests that this new *in vitro* model does simulate *in vivo* aerosol deposition. The main limitation of the mechanical model lies in the fact that it is not clear whether a separate low compliance lung compartment would act the same as isolated low compliance hotspots embedded in otherwise normal lung parenchyma.

Our experiments support that heterogeneous reductions in lung compliance could play a role in the distribution of aerosol penetration in fibrotic lung disease. Indeed, we observed both increased aerosol penetration in the normal-compliance compartment, and reduced aerosol penetration in the reduced-compliance compartment. Although the clinical relevance of this finding remains to be defined, preferential deposition of inhaled drugs to preserved lung regions may result in a reduced therapeutic index and a requirement for higher doses. There is thus a need for inhaled drug delivery methods allowing to increase aerosol penetration and deposition in fibrotic, low compliance lung regions.

The requirement to deliver drugs to low compliance regions of the respiratory system led to the discovery that audible acoustic

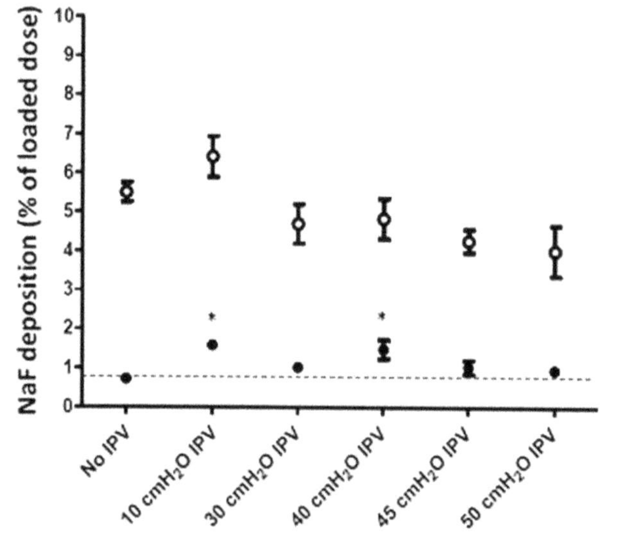

FIGURE 5 | Aerosol deposition in the Control (100 ml/cmH_2O compliance, open circles) and Experimental (50 ml/cmH_2O compliance, filled circles) compartments of the model. Aerosol was delivered with either no IPV or 1 Hz IPV at different pressure levels. *$p < 0.05$ vs. no IPV.

waves enhance deposition of nasally-delivered aerosolized drugs into maxillary sinuses (Möller et al., 2014). By analogy, we hypothesized that acoustic/pressure waves may increase aerosol penetration in the fibrotic lung model. Interestingly, although audible acoustic waves had no effect, contrary to sinus models, low-frequency IPV pulses had a marked effect and increased aerosol penetration threefold. Although the high variance in total mass balance mandates caution in the interpretation of aerosol deposition experiments, the effect of IPV on aerosol deposition in the experimental compartment was highly reproducible. This result is in line with the observation by others that IPV increases penetration of therapeutic aerosols in a single compartment mechanical model of the respiratory system, independent of model compliance (Karashima et al., 2019).

The mechanisms by which pressure pulses, such as those delivered by IPV, increase aerosol penetration remain unknown. These mechanisms can be discussed by analogy with acoustic wave-enhanced delivery of aerosols from the nose to maxillary sinuses, which, like distal airspaces in fibrotic lungs, can be considered a low compliance cavity. A hypothesis is periodic compression of air by acoustic waves, generating bidirectional airflow (Xi et al., 2017). Under this hypothesis, a maximal effect is expected when transmission of the input pressure to the target cavity is maximal, that is, when the frequency of acoustic waves equals the resonance frequency of the target cavity. Indeed, matching soundwave frequency to resonance frequency of the maxillary sinuses (estimated with the Helmhotz resonator model) increases aerosol delivery (Durand et al., 2012; Leclerc et al., 2015), while frequency sweeps bracketing the estimated resonance frequency of the sinus yield optimal results (Moghadam et al., 2018). At variance with the hypothesis that acoustic waves emitted at the resonance frequency of the target may increase aerosol penetration, we observed that audible acoustic waves had no effect. Rather, increased aerosol penetration was observed using low-frequency (≤3 Hz) IPV. Whether it is important that acoustic/pressure pulse frequency is inferior to the resonance frequency of the system (here, 5 Hz) remains to be explored. Interestingly, in a 2-bottle physical model, maximal aerosol penetration aerosol is observed with 100 Hz acoustic waves, while the estimated resonance frequency of the model cavity is 303 Hz (Xi et al., 2017). The mechanisms contributing to IPV-increased aerosol penetration thus remain to fully elucidate. Acoustic radiation pressure, which is well described in the ultrasonic frequency range (Foresti et al., 2013) and is also physically relevant for low-frequency (trending toward 0 Hz) acoustic waves (Löfstedt and Putterman, 1991), may be a candidate mechanism. Importantly, it is unclear how the frequency of the pressure waves that dissipate in the airway relates to the frequency IPV volume/pressure pulses.

TABLE 1 | Mass balance of aerosol deposition experiments.

	Normal lung model (n = 3)	Fibrotic lung model, no IPV (n = 6)		Fibrotic lung model with 1 Hz–40 cmH_2O IPV (n = 6)	
Deposition site	**Deposition**	**Deposition**	***p*-value vs. Normal**	**Deposition**	***p*-value vs. Fibrotic**
Expiratory filter	27.9 ± 6.7%	32.2 ± 4.4%	0.651	17.8 ± 5.3%	**0.001**
Construct	7.1 ± 1.6%	4.8 ± 1.5%	0.530	14.1 ± 4.2%	**0.009**
Nebulizer	50.7 ± 8.0%	45.5 ± 5.9%	0.896	49.1 ± 7.8%	0.509
Alberta throat	1.7 ± 0.3%	0.9 ± 0.3%	**0.009**	4.0 ± 1.1%	**0.002**
Trachea and Y-piece	0.6 ± 0.3%	0.6 ± 0.3%	0.910	0.5 ± 0.1%	0.352
Control bronchus	0.4 ± 0.3%	0.4 ± 0.1%	0.580	0.3 ± 0.2%	0.253
Control compartment	4.6 ± 1.2%	5.5 ± 0.6%	0.578	7.4 ± 1.9%	1.000
Experimental bronchus	0.4 ± 0.3%	0.2 ± 0.1%	0.219	0.2 ± 0.2%	0.079
Experimental compartment	4.4 ± 1.6%	0.7 ± 0.2%	**0.020**	2.2 ± 0.5%	**0.002**
Total	97.8 ± 12.1%	90.7 ± 7.8%	0.899	95.5 ± 17.2%	0.626

Deposition in the normal lung model (compliance of both compartments set at 100 ml/cmH_2O) was compared with the fibrotic lung model (compliance of the Experimental compartment set at 50 ml/cmH_2O) without IPV. Deposition in the fibrotic model with 1 Hz–40 cmH_2O IPV was compared with the fibrotic lung model without IPV. Aerosol was expressed as % of the dose loaded in the nebulizer. p values < 0.05 were shown in bold face.

There is currently great interest in the development of inhaled therapies for IPF and other ILD. Inhaled antifibrotic treatments would represent a key advance in IPF. Although several inhaled drugs were or are currently being evaluated in clinical trials in IPF, such as glutathione (Borok et al., 1991), heparin (Markart et al., 2010), interferon-γ (Diaz et al., 2012), and pirfenidone (Khoo et al., 2020), none has been successful so far.

IPV is a respiratory physiotherapy technique that consists in delivery of small volumes of air into the airways, typically in the 1–10 Hz frequency and 10–50 cmH_2O pressure ranges (Reychler et al., 2018). It is currently used to mobilize secretions, promote lung recruitment and improve gas exchange in chronic conditions such as neuromuscular diseases, cystic fibrosis, and chronic obstructive pulmonary disease. Our observation that low frequency (≤3 Hz) pressure pulses, but not high frequency (>3 Hz) pressure pulses improve aerosol deposition are in line with previous studies. Initial studies into IPV-coupled nebulized delivery in humans were disappointing (Reychler et al., 2004, 2006), although IPV devices were not the same as the one used in our study. In these studies, IPV was delivered at a frequency of 4.2 Hz, higher than the 3 Hz threshold identified in our work. Likewise, bench experiments showed that high-frequency oscillation ventilation (exact frequency not reported) results in reduced lung deposition in comparison with conventional delivery under spontaneous ventilation (Li et al., 2020). Our results suggest that IPV may be repurposed to improve aerosolized drug delivery in the clinic.

Whether low-frequency (≤3 Hz) IPV is a feasible option to improve aerosol delivery to patients with IPF depends on a number of issues, including (1) whether it does improve aerosol delivery to low compliance lung regions *in vivo*, (2) whether it can be tolerated by IPF patients, and (3) whether it is innocuous. Although IPV appears to be well tolerated at frequencies in the order of 4–6 Hz (Nava et al., 2006; Paneroni et al., 2011), whether low-frequency is tolerated for the duration required for nebulized drug delivery remains to explore. Since patient discomfort is associated with IPV pressure, our observation that 10 cmH_2O did increase aerosol penetration in the low-compliance compartment suggests that this method may be usable in patients. Although IPV appears to be generally safe (Paneroni et al., 2011), it is essential to assess whether IPV-associated volutrauma or barotrauma is deleterious in IPF patients. Notably, whether IPV can induce IPF exacerbations will need to be ruled out before clinical application. IPF exacerbations are life-threatening events which can be triggered by medical procedures such as mechanical ventilation and lung surgery (Ryerson et al., 2015). Adverse effects of VPIP are rare in healthy subjects and patients with obstructive lung disease, with cases of pneumothorax and proximal airway obstruction attributed to handling error (Flurin et al., 2009).

CONCLUSION

Using a mechanical model of fibrotic lung disease, we observed that reduced compliance of target lung regions is a critical determinant of aerosol penetration, and thus presumably of aerosol deposition. This finding underscores the need for techniques specifically tailored to enhance delivery of inhaled aerosols to low compliance regions of the lungs, if fibrotic lung disease is to be successfully treated with inhaled therapies. Low-frequency (≤3 Hz) IPV pulses may represent an attractive option to increase aerosol deposition in fibrotic lung regions.

AUTHOR CONTRIBUTIONS

LA, SL, and MC conducted the experiments and analyzed the results. LV, FO, SL, NH-V, and JP provided scientific input into acoustic and pulse wave physics and contributed to the experiment design. LP coordinated the overall project, designed and analyzed experiments, and drafted the manuscript. All authors reviewed and approved the manuscript.

ACKNOWLEDGMENTS

We thank LV medical for providing home ventilators used in preliminary experiments as a loan, and Resmed France for providing the IPV generator as a loan.

SUPPLEMENTARY MATERIAL

FIGURE S1 | Tidal volume in the active bellows, as a function of inspiratory pressure in the passive bellows (as set on the driving respirator) and set compliance. IPV was not used for these measurements. Means of 5 measurements are shown. Standard deviations were close to zero and are not shown.

FIGURE S2 | (A) Aerosol deposition in the Control (100 ml/cmH_2O compliance, open circles) and Experimental (50 ml/cmH_2O compliance, filled circles) compartments of the model. **(B)** Ratio of aerosol deposition in the Experimental and Control compartment. 3 Hz IPV was delivered using the nebulizer construct shown in **Figure 2A**. $^*p < 0.05$.

FIGURE S3 | Nebulizer construct tested for IPV-enhancer aerosol deposition experiments.

FIGURE S4 | Aerosol deposition in the Control (100 ml/cmH_2O compliance, open circles) and Experimental (50 ml/cmH_2O compliance, filled circles) compartments of the model. **(A)** IPV (3 Hz, 40 cmH_2O) was delivered during nebulization, using the 5 constructs shown in **Supplementary Figure S3**. **(B)** Constructs 3 and 4 were used either without or with IPV (3 Hz, 40 cmH_2O).

REFERENCES

Borok, Z., Buhl, R., Grimes, G. J., Bokser, A. D., Hubbard, R. C., and Holroyd, K. J. (1991). Effect of glutathione aerosol on oxidant-antioxidant imbalance in idiopathic pulmonary fibrosis. *Lancet* 338, 215–216. doi: 10.1016/0140-6736(91)90350-x

Canestaro, W. J., Forrester, S. H., Ganesh, R., Lawrence, H., and Devine, B. E. (2016). Drug treatment of idiopathic pulmonary fibrosis: systematic review and network meta-analysis. *Chest* 149, 756–766. doi: 10.1016/j.chest.2015.11.013

Diaz, K. T., Shibu, S., Keith, H., Mario, S., Stephanie, L., and Kristy, B. (2012). Delivery and Safety of Inhaled Interferon-γ in idiopathic pulmonary fibrosis. *J. Aeros. Med. Pulmon Deliv.* 25, 79–87. doi: 10.1089/jamp.2011.0919

Dugernier, J., Michel, H., Rita, V., Virginie, D., Jean, R., and Jean-Bernard, M. (2017). SPECT-CT comparison of lung deposition using a system combining a vibrating-mesh nebulizer with a valved holding chamber and a conventional jet nebulizer: a randomized cross-over study. *Pharm. Res.* 34, 290–300. doi: 10.1007/s11095-016-2061-7

Durand, M., Le Guellec, S., Pourchez, J., Dubois, F., Aubert, G., and Chantrel, G. (2012). Sonic aerosol therapy to target maxillary sinuses. *Eur Ann. Otorhinolaryngol. Head Neck Dis.* 129, 244–250. doi: 10.1016/j.anorl.2011.09.002

Fletcher, S., Mark, G. J., Katherine, S., Giacomo, S., Marshall, B. G., Limbrey, R., et al. (2016). The safety of new drug treatments for idiopathic pulmonary fibrosis. *Expert Opin. Drug Saf.* 15, 1483–1489. doi: 10.1080/14740338.2016.1218470

Flurin, V., Lefrançois, D., Fare, D., Le Manac'h, G., and Colin, D. (2009). [Interest of Percussionator in neuromuscular patients. Eight years experience in three quadriplegic ventilator-dependant children]. *Arch. Pediatr.* 16:758. doi: 10.1016/S0929-693X(09)74140-5

Foresti, D., Majid, N., Mirko, K., Aldo, F., and Poulikakos, D. (2013). Acoustophoretic contactless transport and handling of matter in air. *Proc. Natl. Acad. Sci. U.S.A.* 110, 12549–12554. doi: 10.1073/pnas.1301860110

Kanazawa, M., Suzuki, Y., Ishizaka, A., Hasegawa, N., Fujishima, S., Kawashiro, T., et al. (1993). [Assessment of pulmonary aerosol deposition and epithelial permeability in 99mTc-DTPA inhalation scintigram]. *Nihon Kyôbu Shikkan Gakkai Zasshi* 31, 593–600.

Karashima, T., Yuka, M. K., Miyakawa, K., Nakamura, A., Shimahara, F., and Kamei, H. (2019). Variations in the efficiency of albuterol delivery and intrapulmonary effects with differential parameter settings on intrapulmonary percussive ventilation. *Respir. Care* 64, 502–508. doi: 10.4187/respcare.06348

Khoo, J. K., Montgomery, A. B., Otto, K. L., Surber, M., Faggian, J., and Lickliter, J. D. (2020). A randomized, double-blinded, placebo-controlled, dose-escalation phase 1 study of aerosolized pirfenidone delivered via the PARI investigational EFlow nebulizer in volunteers and patients with idiopathic pulmonary fibrosis. *J. Aerosol Med. Pulmon. Drug Deliv.* 33, 15–20. doi: 10.1089/jamp.2018.1507

King, T. E. Jr., Annie, P., and Selman, M. (2011). Idiopathic pulmonary fibrosis. *Lancet* 378, 1949–1961. doi: 10.1016/S0140-6736(11)60052-4

King, T. E., Bradford, W. Z., Castro-Bernardini, S., Fagan, E. A., Glaspole, I., and Glassberg, M. K. (2014). A phase 3 trial of pirfenidone in patients with idiopathic pulmonary fibrosis. *N. Engl. J. Med.* 370, 2083–2092. doi: 10.1056/NEJMoa1402582

Leclerc, L., Amira, E. M., Navarro, L., Prévôt, N., Durand, M., and Pourchez, J. (2015). Impact of acoustic airflow on intrasinus drug deposition: new insights into the vibrating mode and the optimal acoustic frequency to enhance the delivery of nebulized antibiotic. *Inte. J. Pharm.* 494, 227–234. doi: 10.1016/j.ijpharm.2015.08.025

Li, J., Elshafei, A. A., Gong, L., and Fink, J. B. (2020). Aerosol delivery during continuous high frequency oscillation for simulated adults during quiet and distressed spontaneous breathing. *Respir. Care* 65, 227–232. doi: 10.4187/respcare.07050

Löfstedt, R., and Putterman, S. (1991). Theory of long wavelength acoustic radiation pressure. *J. Acoust. Soc. Am.* 90, 2027–2033. doi: 10.1121/1.401630

Markart, P., Robert, N., Clemens, R., Hundack, L., Wygrecka, M., Korfei, M., et al. (2010). Safety and tolerability of inhaled heparin in idiopathic pulmonary fibrosis. *J. Aerosol Med. Pulmon. Drug Deliv.* 23, 161–172. doi: 10.1089/jamp.2009.0780

Moghadam, S. J., Laurent, N., Lara, L., Hodin, S., and Pourchez, J. (2018). Toward Smart nebulization: engineering acoustic airflow to penetrate maxillary sinuses in chronic rhinosinusitis. *Int. J. Pharm.* 546, 188–193. doi: 10.1016/j.ijpharm.2018.05.039

Möller, W., Schuschnig, U., Bartenstein, P., Meyer, G., Häussinger, K., Schmid, O., et al. (2014). Drug delivery to paranasal sinuses using pulsating aerosols. *J. Aerosol Med. Pulm. Drug Deliv.* 27, 255–263. doi: 10.1089/jamp.2013.1071

Montigaud, Y., Périnel-Ragey, S., Plantier, L., Leclerc, L., Goy, C., and Clotagatide, A. (2019). Development of an ex vivo preclinical respiratory model of idiopathic pulmonary fibrosis for aerosol regional studies. *Sci. Rep.* 9:17949. doi: 10.1038/s41598-019-54479-2

Nava, S., Barbarito, N., Piaggi, G., Mattia, E. D., and Cirio, S. (2006). Physiological response to intrapulmonary percussive ventilation in stable COPD patients. *Respir. Med.* 100, 1526–1533. doi: 10.1016/j.rmed.2006.01.010

Noble, Paul, W., Albera, C., Bradford, W. Z., Costabel, U., Glassberg, M. K., et al. (2011). Pirfenidone in patients with idiopathic pulmonary fibrosis (CAPACITY): two Randomised Trials. *Lancet*377, 1760–1769. doi: 10.1016/S0140-6736(11)60405-4

Paneroni, M., Clini, E., Simonelli, C., Bianchi, L., Antoni, F. D., and Vitacca, M. (2011). Safety and efficacy of short-term intrapulmonary percussive ventilation in patients with bronchiectasis. *Respir. Care* 56, 984–988. doi: 10.4187/respcare.01098

Plantier, L., Aurélie, C., Dinh-Xuan, A. T., Bancal, C., Marchand-Adam, S., and Crestani, B. (2018). Physiology of the lung in idiopathic pulmonary fibrosis. *Eur. Respir. Rev.* 27:170062. doi: 10.1183/16000617.0062-2017

Plantier, L., Debray, M. P., Estellat, C., Flamant, M., Roy, C., Bancal, C., et al. (2016). Increased volume of conducting airways in idiopathic pulmonary fibrosis is independent of disease severity: a volumetric capnography study. *J. Breath Res.* 10:016005. doi: 10.1088/1752-7155/10/1/016005

Rau, J. L. (2005). The inhalation of drugs: advantages and problems. *Respir. Care* 50, 367–382.

Reychler, G., Debier, E., Contal, O., and Audag, N. (2018). Intrapulmonary percussive ventilation as an airway clearance technique in subjects with chronic obstructive airway diseases. *Respir. Care* 63, 620–631. doi: 10.4187/respcare.05876

Reychler, G., Keyeux, A., Cremers, C., Veriter, C., Rodenstein, D. O., and Liistro, G. (2004). Comparison of lung deposition in two types of nebulization: intrapulmonary percussive ventilation vs jet nebulization. *Chest* 125, 502–508. doi: 10.1378/chest.125.2.502

Reychler, G., Wallemacq, P., Rodenstein, D. O., Cumps, J., Leal, T., and Liistro, G. (2006). Comparison of lung deposition of amikacin by intrapulmonary percussive ventilation and jet nebulization by urinary monitoring. *J. Aerosol Med.* 19, 199–207. doi: 10.1089/jam.2006.19.199

Richeldi, L., du Bois, R. M., Raghu, G., Azuma, A., Brown, K. K., Costabel, U., et al. (2014). Efficacy and safety of nintedanib in idiopathic pulmonary fibrosis. *N. Engl. J. Med.* 370, 2071–2082. doi: 10.1056/NEJMoa1402584

Ryerson, C. J., Vincent, C., Brown, K. K., and Collard, H. R. (2015). Acute exacerbation of idiopathic pulmonary fibrosis: shifting the paradigm. *Eur. Respir J.* 46, 512–520. doi: 10.1183/13993003.00419-2015

Samuel, J., and Smaldone, G. C. (2019). Maximizing deep lung deposition in healthy and fibrotic subjects during jet nebulization. *J. Aerosol Med. Pulm. Drug Deliv.* 33, 108–115. doi: 10.1089/jamp.2019.1552

The Topical Study of Inhaled Drug (Salbutamol) (2019). *Delivery in Idiopathic Pulmonary Fibrosis. - PubMed - NCBI. n.d.* Avaliable at: https://www-ncbi-nlm-nih-gov.gate2.inist.fr/pubmed/?term=29409488 (accessed October 19, 2019).

Toussaint, M., Marie-Charlotte, G., Paternotte, S., Soudon, P., and Haan, J. (2012). Intrapulmonary effects of setting parameters in portable intrapulmonary percussive ventilation devices. *Respir. Care* 57, 735–742. doi: 10.4187/respcare.01441

Verleden, S. E., Naoya, T., McDonough, J. E., Vasilescu, D. M., Xu, F., and Wuyts, W. A. (2020). Small airways pathology in idiopathic pulmonary fibrosis: a retrospective cohort study. *Lancet. Respir. Med.* 8, 573–584. doi: 10.1016/S2213-2600(19)30356-X

Watanabe, N., Inoue, T., Tomioka, S., Yamaji, T., and Endo, K. (1995). Discordant findings between Krypton-81m Gas and Tc-99m labeled ultrafine aerosol lung ventilation SPECT in two patients with idiopathic pulmonary fibrosis. *Clin. Nuclear Med.* 20, 315–317. doi: 10.1097/00003072-199504000-00006

Xi, J. X., Xiuhua, A. S., Shannon, P., Dannielle, N., Tianshu, W., and Lehman, M. (2017). Understanding the mechanisms underlying pulsating aerosol delivery to the maxillary sinus: in vitro tests and computational simulations. *Int. J. Pharm.* 520, 254–266. doi: 10.1016/j.ijpharm.2017.02.017

Zielonka, T. M., Demkow, U., Radzikowska, E., Bialas, B., Filewska, M., and Zycinska, K. (2010). Angiogenic activity of sera from interstitial lung disease patients in relation to pulmonary function. *Eur. J. Med. Res.* 15(Suppl. 2), 229–234.

11

Humidified and Heated Cascade Impactor for Aerosol Sizing

Caroline Majoral[1,2], Allan L. Coates[3], Alain Le Pape[1,2] and Laurent Vecellio[1,2]*

[1] INSERM, Research Center for Respiratory Diseases, Tours, France, [2] Université de Tours, Tours, France, [3] Hospital for Sick Children, Toronto, ON, Canada

***Correspondence:**
Laurent Vecellio
vecellio@med.univ-tours.fr

Aerosol sizing is generally measured at ambient air but human airways have different temperature (37°C) and relative humidity (100%) which can affect particle size in airways and consequently deposition prediction. This work aimed to develop and evaluate a new method using cascade impactor to measure particle size at human physiological temperature and humidity (HPTH) taking into account ambient air conditions. A heated and humidified trachea was built and a cascade impactor was heated to 37°C and humidified inside. Four medical aerosols [jet nebulizer, mesh nebulizer, Presurized Metered Dose Inhaler (pMDI), and Dry Powder Inhaler (DPI)] under ambient conditions and at HPTH were tested. MMAD was lower at HPTH for the two nebulizers; it was similar at ambient conditions and HPTH for pMDI, and the mass of particles smaller than 5 μm decreased for DPI at HPTH (51.9 vs. 82.8 μg/puff). In conclusion, we developed a new method to measure particle size at HPTH affecting deposition prediction with relevance. *In vivo* studies are required to evaluate the interest of this new model to improve the precision of deposition prediction.

Keywords: aerosol, cascade impactor, particle, inhalation, size, temperature, humidity

INTRODUCTION

Aerosol particle size is a key parameter for predicting aerosol deposition in the airways of the lungs. Several methods of particle sizing can be used, cascade impactors and lasers being the most common. Cascade impactors offer the major advantage of measuring the aerodynamic diameter of the drug studied.

They are used in different regulatories (ISO 27427, 2012) and pharmacopeias (USP 28-Nf 23, 2005) with a continuous and constant air flow. However, this experimental set up does not take into account the effect of ventilation parameters from the patient which can modify the particle size. Sangwan et al. (2003) has used a low flow cascade impactor (1 L/min) with a breathing machine to mimic patient inhalation. They used clinically relevant breathing patterns to simulate aerosol delivery on the bench recognizing that, during a drug treatment the patient would be breathing a mixture of air at a certain tidal volume and frequency as well as air from the nebulizer and that this degree of ambiant air mixing might influence the final inhaled distribution. Finally in a series of human studies demonstrated the relationship between predicting deposition via bench studies and effects on actual deposition measure particle size at different ventilation conditions. The low flow cascade impactor has the advantage to reduce the impact of air sampling on ventilation parameters and to reduce the particle evaporation effect in standing cloud set up (Solomita and Smaldone, 2009) but it has the unconvenient to collect a small fraction of aerosol which can be different to the aerosol cloud (Vecellio None et al., 2001).

In vitro measurements of aerosol particle size with a cascade impactor are usually made at ambient conditions of temperature and relative humidity (RH).

It has been shown that the temperature of a jet nebulizer outlet can decrease by more than 10°C, leading to evaporation of the droplets when entering the cascade impactor placed at ambient temperature. Previous studies have investigated the effect of temperature on aerosol sizing by cooling the impactor in order to limit droplet evaporation (Stapleton and Finlay, 1998; Kwong et al., 2000; Zhou et al., 2005a; Rao et al., 2010). Several studies have also investigated the effect of ambient air humidity on particle size distribution by sizing the aerosols at several different values of relative humidity (Prokop et al., 1995; Finlay et al., 1997; Nerbrink et al., 2003; Zhou et al., 2005b). However, the human respiratory tract is at 37°C and almost 100%RH (Ferron, 1977; Ferron et al., 1985; O'Doherty and Miller, 1993), which can alter particle size either through evaporation or condensation (i.e., hygroscopic growth) and can therefore affect the relevance of the prediction of deposition in the respiratory tract.

Studies have focused on mathematically modeling heat and water transport in the human respiratory tract (Daviskas et al., 1990; Eisner, 1992; Finlay and Stapleton, 1995; Zhang et al., 2006), or on establishing equations to predict the change in size of hygroscopic inhaled particles (Ferron, 1977; Ferron et al., 1988; Gradon and Podgórski, 1996; Broday and Georgopoulos, 2001; Longest and Hindle, 2012; Boudin et al., 2020). Particle growing in airways has been recently considered as a potential interest to reduce upper airways deposition and increase lung penetration, and deposition when using submicronic aerosols (Longest and Hindle, 2012; Spence et al., 2019). Martin et al. (1988) developed a model for particle sizing composed of a trachea and a cascade impactor at 37°C and either 30%RH or 97.5%RH. However, their model did not duplicate what happens *in vivo*. Instead of humidifying the aerosol after its generation, they humidified and heated the ambient air to 37°C before it entered the model. In fact, when a patient inhales an aerosol, the air he/she breathes comes from the atmosphere and is at ambient conditions of temperature, and humidity. In another study, Bell and Ho (1981) developed an experimental system which mixed a dry monodisperse aerosol with water-saturated air at 37°C at the top of a growth tube. They sized aerosol particles at the exit of this tube using an optical particle counter, thus measuring the geometric diameter, but neither the aerodynamic diameter nor the drug mass contained in the particles.

Consequently, temperature and humidity affect particle size. Particle size modification in airways depends on device and formulation. Different mathematical models have been developed to predict this size modification but they are complex to use. Different experimental measurement methods have been developed to measure *in vitro* aerosol size at 37°C and 100% but they have not measured the size of aerosol drug in realistic ambiant air mixing conditions, i.e., with ambiant temperature and humidity crossing the device and followed by a heating and humidifying just after aerosol delivery.

The purpose of the present study was (1) to develop an *in vitro* cascade impactor measurement method approaching human temperature and humidity with the respect of the ambient air before penetration in the trachea/induction port model, (2) to compare aerosol particle size measured at ambient conditions and at HPTH to evaluate the relevance of our method.

MATERIALS AND METHODS

Materials

Experimental Set Up at Ambient Air

The aerosol were sized using an 8-stage Andersen Cascade Impactor (ACI) (Mark II, Ecomesure, France) operating at 28.3 L/min for nebulizers and pMDI, and operating at 60 L/min for DPI. An artificial trachea for the ACI was created using a coarse screen wrapped with cotton with a heating coil running inside the walls which were then covered with aluminum foil and plastic (**Figure 1**). Absorbent glass fiber filters (Type A/E Glass, Pall Corporation, United States) were used on each plate of the impactor. The trachea was kept dry and not heated, and the cascade impactor was used with dry filters and at ambient temperature (22 ± 3°C; 50 ± 10%RH) (**Figure 2A**).

Experimental Set Up at 37°C and Ambient RH

Same cascade impactor and trachea as described above were used. The trachea was dry and heated to 37°C and the impactor was warmed in a water bath at 37°C. A potentiometer was used to regulate the temperature of the heating coil to 37°C and a temperature sensor was used to measure the temperature of the trachea and of the water bath. The filters on cascade impactor stages were dry so that humidity inside the impactor was the same as that of the ambient air, as the impactor was perfectly watertight (**Figure 2B**).

Experimental Set Up at 37°C and 100% RH

Same cascade impactor and trachea as described above were used. In this experimental set up, the trachea was humidified inside with water and heated to 37°C, and the cascade impactor filters were moistened with 3 mL of water and placed in a water bath at 37°C (**Figure 2C**).

Inhalation Drug Delivery Devices

Different inhalation drug were tested: Jet nebulizer (PariLC Star® with Turbo Boy N® compressor, Pari, Germany) filled with 2 mL of terbutaline (Bricanyl® 5 mg/2 mL, Astra Zeneca, France) or with 2 mL of 1%w/v NaF solution, a vibrating

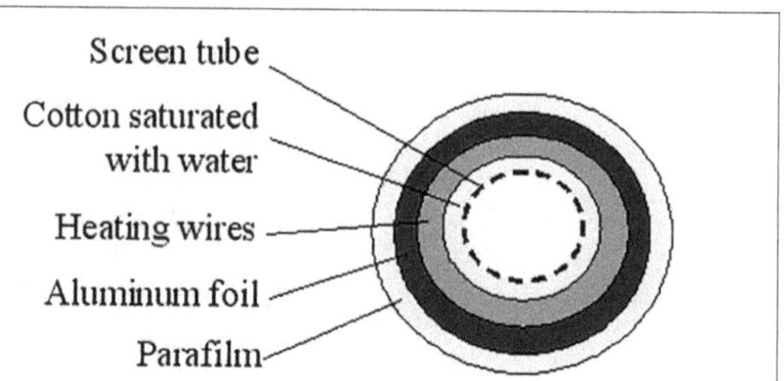

FIGURE 1 | Cross-section of the new trachea.

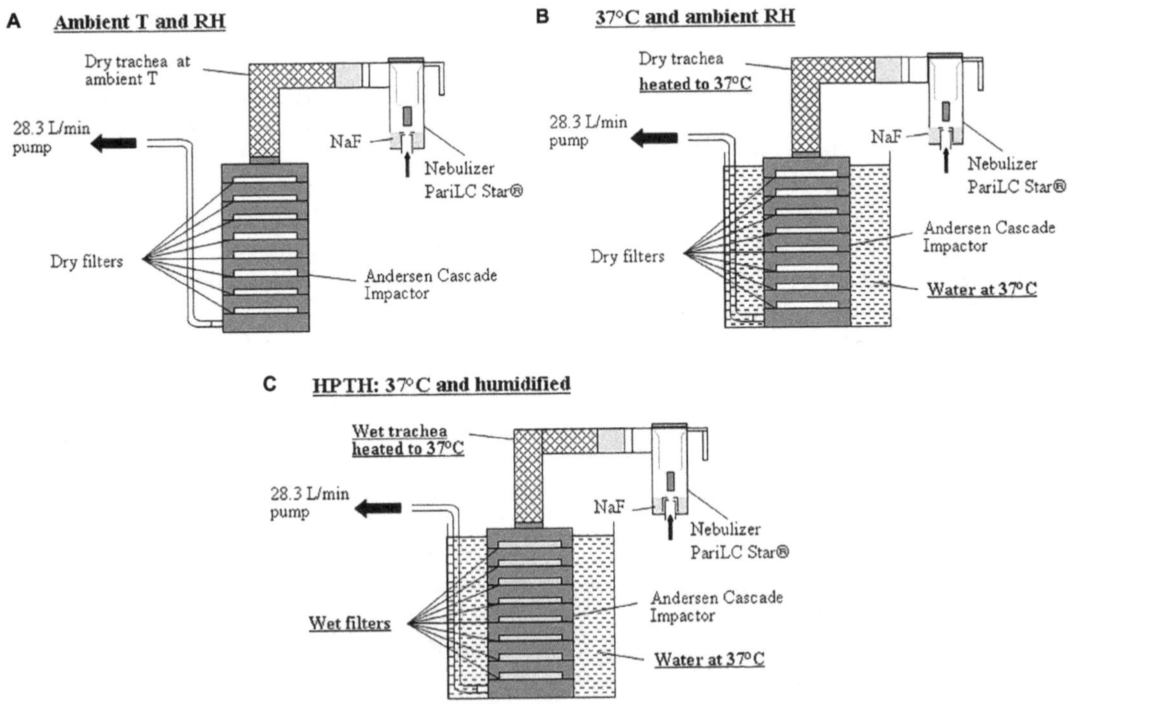

FIGURE 2 | Experimental set-ups using ACI sampling at 28.3 L/min with stage's substrates (filters) for 3 different conditions: **(A)** Aerosol measurement using cascade impactor at ambient temperature and ambient relative humidity. **(B)** Aerosol measurement using cascade impactor in a bath of water at 37°C and ambient relative humidity. **(C)** Aerosol measurement using cascade impactor in a bath of water at 37°C and humidified air inside the trachea model and the cascade impactor using the new trachea and wetted stage's substrates (HPTH: human physiological temperature and humidity).

mesh nebulizer (Aeroneb Go®, Ireland, United States) filled with 2 mL of terbutaline (Bricanyl® 5 mg /2 mL, Astra Zeneca, France), a salbutamol Presurized Metered Dose Inhaler (PMDI) (Ventoline® 100 μg/puff, GlaxoSmithKline, France), and a terbutaline Dry Powder Inhaler (DPI) (Bricanyl® Turbuhaler® 500 μg/puff, Astra Zeneca, France). Only the Pari LC Star® nebulizer with NaF was measured at 37°C-ambiant humidity. Others inhalation drug delivery device were sized at ambient conditions (**Figure 2A**) and at HPTH (**Figure 2C**).

Methods

Experimental Setup Validation

Three milliliter of water were poured onto dry absorbent filters (Type A/E Glass, Pall Corporation, United States) laid on each impactor plate and they were each immediately weighed. The experimental set-up at HPTH described in **Figure 2C** was then carried out, substituting the nebulizer by an absolute filter to limit the risk of air particle contamination on wet filters. The impactor pump, operating at 28.3 L/min, was turned on for 5 min. The impactor was then dismantled and the filters were weighed again. The difference between the weights of the filters before and after the 5 min of sampling corresponded to the quantity of water evaporated inside the impactor during the 5 min. The experiment was performed three times. The relative humidity inside the trachea was measured after its humidification by a humidity measuring stick (Testo, France). Each experiment was carried out in triplicate.

Aerosol Sizing

For the two nebulizers, nebulization was stopped when no more aerosol was produced. After Naf nebulization, each filter and impactor stage were placed in 10 mL of 25% TISAB solution (TISAB IV, Riedel-de Haën, Germany) and was assayed with a fluoride electrode.

After terbutaline nebulization, each filter was placed in a centrifuge tube and each impactor stage was placed in 20 mL of sodium hydroxide 0.1M. The amount of drug was assayed by UV-spectrophotometry (Spectronic Unicam, Helios, United Kingdom). Residual drug mass in nebulizers was measured by drug assay method.

For pMDI, a total of 30 puffs of the were delivered for each experiment. The UV spectrophotometer was calibrated to measure salbutamol, and the filters were processed as described above for the nebulizers.

Terbutaline Turbuhaler® DPI required a 60 L/min pump instead of a 28.3 L/min pump. As the ACI was calibrated at 28.3 L/min, the usual values given for the cut-off diameters were only valid for the impactor operating at 28.3 L/min. The cut-off diameters were determined for a 60 L/min flow rate according to the following formula (Van Oort et al., 1996; Marple et al., 2003):

$$D_{60L/min} = D_{28.3L/min}\sqrt{\frac{28.3}{60}}$$

where $D_{60L/min}$ and $D_{28.3L/min}$ correspond to the cut-off diameters for the ACI operating at 60 and 28.3 L/min respectively.

The values of the cut-off diameters for a flow rate of 28.3 L/min were 9, 5.8, 4.7, 3.3, 2.1, 1.1, 0.7, and 0.4 μm for stages 0–7, respectively. The values of the cut-off diameters for a flow rate of 60 L/min were 6.2, 4.0, 3.2, 2.3, 1.4, 0.8, 0.5, and 0.3 μm for stages 0–7, respectively.

A total of 20 puffs of terbutaline Turbuhaler® DPI were generated for each experiment. The filters were processed as described above for the nebulizers.

Analysis of the Results

NaF aerosol particle size distributions were represented as mass deposited per stages in the cascade impactor. The percentage of recovery from the impactor and the trachea was expressed from the nebulizer load for the nebulizers, the difference from 100% corresponding to the residual volume. The deposition in the trachea was calculated by subtracting (total deposition on the impactor stages + residual volume) from the initial charge for nebulizers, and (total deposition on the impactor stages) from the emitted dose for the PMDI and DPI.

The results were also expressed in terms of Mass Median Aerodynamic Diameter (MMAD), total deposited mass on the stages of the impactor, % recovery from the impactor and the trachea of the nebulizer load for the nebulizers and of the emitted dose for the PMDI and DPI, and mass of particles smaller than 5 μm, also called the respirable mass or fine particle dose and predicting deposited mass in the lungs (Coates et al., 1998; ISO 27427, 2012).

RESULTS

Validation of the Method

A volume of 0.41 ± 0.07 mL of water was evaporated from each filter during the 5 min of sampling. There was no difference between each stage in term of evaporated volume water. These results validated the humidification of the air inside the impactor. The relative humidity inside the trachea after its humidification was superior to 95%, which corresponds to the relative humidity inside the respiratory tract.

Aerosol Sizing at Different Air Temperature and Humidity Conditions

MMAD, total deposited mass on the stages of the ACI and % recovery from the impactor and the trachea of the nebulizer load of 1%w/v NaF aerosol nebulized with PariLC Star® for the three experimental set-ups are summarized in **Table 1**. MMAD equaled 2.6 ± 0.2, 1.3 ± 0.1, and 1.8 ± 0.1 μm for ambient T and RH, 37°C and ambient RH, and HPTH respectively. Total deposited mass on the stages of the impactor was similar for the three experimental set-ups (10.0 ± 0.7, 9.2 ± 0.3, and 9.3 ± 0.7 mg).

Figure 3 shows the deposited mass on impactor stages with NaF aerosol nebulized by PariLC Star® for the three experimental set-ups.

MMAD, total deposited mass on the stages of the ACI, % recovery from the impactor and the trachea of the nebulizer load for the nebulizers and of the emitted dose for the PMDI and DPI, and mass of particles smaller than 5 μm of terbutaline nebulized with PariLC Star® and Aeroneb Go® nebulizers, salbutamol PMDI and terbutaline Turbuhaler® DPI for both ambient conditions and HPTH are summarized in **Table 2**. MMAD values at ambient conditions and HPTH were, respectively, 2.1 ± 0.3 and 1.6 ± 0.1 μm for PariLC Star®, 3.3 ± 0.1 and 2.0 ± 0.2 μm for Aeroneb Go®, 3.1 ± 0.0 and 3.1 ± 0.1 μm for salbutamol PMDI, 3.7 ± 0.0 and 3.2 ± 0.1 μm for terbutaline Turbuhaler® DPI. Total deposited mass on the stages of the impactor was similar at ambient conditions and HPTH for all the devices except for terbutaline Turbuhaler® DPI: it was, respectively, 2.3 ± 0.2 and 2.5 ± 0.3 mg for PariLC Star®, 3.9 ± 0.3 and 3.9 ± 0.3 mg for Aeroneb Go®, 0.6 ± 0.0 and 0.6 ± 0.0 mg for salbutamol PMDI, 2.6 ± 0.2 and 1.5 ± 0.2 mg for terbutaline Turbuhaler® DPI. The mass of particles smaller than 5 μm was also similar at ambient conditions and HPTH for all the devices except for terbutaline Turbuhaler® DPI: it was, respectively, 2.0 ± 0.2 and 2.2 ± 0.2 mg for PariLC Star®, 2.9 ± 0.1 and 2.9 ± 0.2 mg for Aeroneb Go®, 15.8 ± 0.5 μg/puff and 15.8 ± 1.3 μg/puff for salbutamol PMDI, 82.8 ± 8.7 μg/puff and 51.9 ± 3.3 μg/puff for terbutaline Turbuhaler® DPI. **Figure 4** shows the deposited mass on impactor stages with the differents devices at HPTH and ambient air conditions.

DISCUSSION

This study developed an operational method of aerosol sizing at human humidity and temperature conditions and taken into account inhaled air at ambient temperature and humidity. This study has not the objective to be an alternative of regulatories/standard methods but to provide scientific information regarding the effect of temperature and humidity in inhaled condition on particle size and consequently deposition. Standard methods measure particle sizes emitted by the device. Our method has the objective to measure the particle size in the airways.

The first step of the study, consisting in sizing 1%w/v NaF aerosol nebulized with PariLC Star® nebulizer for three intermediate experimental set-ups, highlighted the effect of temperature and humidity on particle size. It demonstrated that MMAD decreased significantly when heating to 37°C as the particles evaporated (2.6 vs. 1.3 μm); it then increased when RH was brought to saturation due to condensation, i.e., hygroscopic growth (1.3 vs. 1.8 μm). The second set-up may have been subjected to a decrease in relative humidity below ambient conditions, and thus conditions in the trachea and cascade impactor for this experimental set-up may have been drier than ambient conditions. The decrease of MMAD when comparing it at ambient temperature and RH and at HPTH (2.6 vs. 1.8 μm) leads to the conclusion that evaporation has more impact than condensation. This may be due to the functioning of the PariLC Star® nebulizer: the air circulates through the interior of the PariLC Star® and becomes saturated with humidity drawn from the large reservoir of solution (Nerbrink et al., 2003), so the air carrying the aerosol is already saturated when it comes out of the nebulizer. Prediction of lung deposition was

TABLE 1 | MMAD, total deposited mass on the stages of the ACI and % recovery from the impactor and the trachea of the nebulizer load of 1%w/v NaF aerosol nebulized with PariLC Star® for the three experimental set-ups [Ambient T and RH; 37°C and ambient RH; 37°C and humidified (HPTH: human physiological temperature and humidity)], expressed as mean ± standard deviation.

	MMAD (μm)	Total deposited mass on the stages of the ACI (mg) (% of the nebulizer load)	% recovery from the trachea of the nebulizer load
(1) Ambient T and RH	2.6 ± 0.2	10.0 ± 0.7 (47 ± 3%)	4 ± 4%
(2) 37°C and ambient RH	1.3 ± 0.1	9.2 ± 0.3 (46 ± 2%)	1 ± 2%
(3) HPTH	1.8 ± 0.1	9.3 ± 0.7 (43 ± 3%)	3 ± 3%

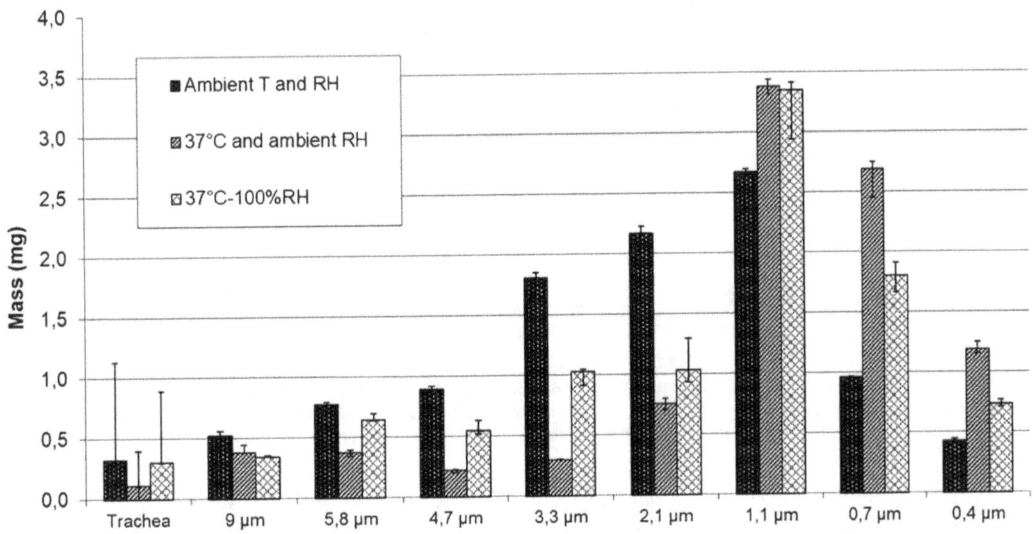

FIGURE 3 | Deposited mass on impactor stages using 1%w/v NaF aerosol nebulized with PariLC Star® for the three conditions of temperature (T) and relative humidity (RH): ambient T and ambient RH; 37°C and ambient RH; 37°C and 100% RH inside the trachea model and the cascade impactor.

TABLE 2 | MMAD, total deposited mass on the stages of the ACI, % recovery from the impactor and the trachea of the nebulizer load for the nebulizers and of the emitted dose for the pMDI and DPI, and mass of particles smaller than 5 μm of terbutaline (5 mg/2 mL) nebulized with PariLC Star and Aeroneb Go® nebulizers, salbutamol pMDI (100 μg/puff) and terbutaline Turbuhaler® DPI (500 μg/puff) for both ambient conditions and 37°C-humidified (HPTH: human physiological temperature and humidity), expressed as mean ± standard deviation.

		MMAD (μm)	Total deposited mass on the stages of the ACI (mg) (% of the nebulizer load or emitted dose)	% recovery from the trachea of the nebulizer load or emitted dose	Mass of particles < 5 μm
PariLC Star (1) + terbutaline	Ambient T and RH	2.1 ± 0.3	2.3 ± 0.2 (43 ± 3%)	6 ± 3%	2.0 ± 0.2 (mg)
	HPTH	1.6 ± 0.1	2.5 ± 0.3 (47 ± 4%)	6 ± 3%	2.2 ± 0.2 (mg)
Aeroneb Go® (2) + terbutaline	Ambient T and RH	3.3 ± 0.1	3.9 ± 0.3 (76 ± 1%)	6 ± 1%	2.9 ± 0.1 (mg)
	HPTH	2.0 ± 0.2	3.9 ± 0.3 (74 ± 5%)	10 ± 5%	2.9 ± 0.2 (mg)
Salbutamol pMDI (3)	Ambient T and RH	3.1 ± 0.0	0.6 ± 0.0 (26 ± 1%)	74 ± 1%	15.8 ± 0.5 (μg/puff)
	HPTH	3.1 ± 0.1	0.6 ± 0.0 (28 ± 2%)	72 ± 2%	15.8 ± 1.3 (μg/puff)
Terbutaline DPI (4)	Ambient T and RH	3.7 ± 0.1	2.6 ± 0.2 (41 ± 3%)	59 ± 3%	82.8 ± 8.7 (μg/puff)
	HPTH	3.2 ± 0.1	1.5 ± 0.2 (25 ± 3%)	75 ± 3%	51.9 ± 3.3 (μg/puff)

(1) jet nebulizer, (2) vibrating mesh nebulizer, (3) presurized metered-dose inhaler (pMDI), (4) dry powder inhaler (DPI).

consequently higher in the peripheral region at HPTH than at ambient conditions (MMAD smaller at HPTH than at ambiant condition), but both conditions (HPTH and ambient) predicted a significant deposition in the pulmonary region (mass of particles < 5 μm). These results could explain why Sangwan et al. (2003) have correlated cascade impaction data with deposition studies

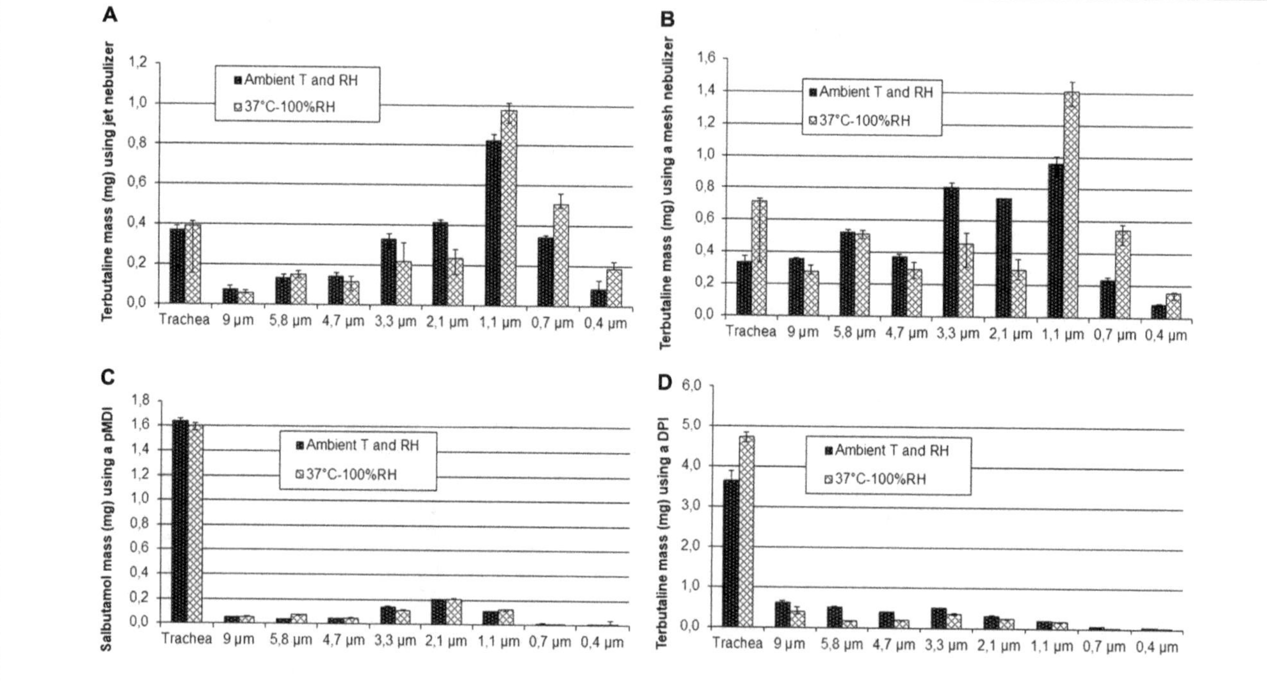

FIGURE 4 | Deposited mass on impactor stages for both ambient conditions and 37°C humidified (HPTH: human physiological temperature and humidity) using the Pari LC Star® jet nebulizer **(A)**, the Aeroneb Go® mesh nebulizer **(B)**, 30 puffs of Ventoline® pMDI **(C)** and 20 puffs of Bricanyl® Turbuhaler® DPI **(D)**.

and found that a more meaningful cut off is 2.5 µm instead of 5 µm. Our work also tested the three main types of device: two nebulizers (a jet nebulizer and a vibrating mesh nebulizer), a PMDI and a DPI. This enabled the behavior of each kind of device to be studied for the two conditions of temperature and humidity (ambient and HPTH), and to determine their respective sensitivity to high temperature and humidity. The comparison of particle size distributions sized at ambient conditions and at HPTH showed that MMAD at HPTH was smaller than at ambient conditions for the two nebulizers (PariLC Star® and Aeroneb Go®) with terbutaline, which is consistent with the results described above for NaF solution aerosolized with PariLC Star®. This indicates that particle evaporation was greater than hygroscopic growth.

An explanation of this low effect of condensation, even with the Aeroneb Go® nebulizer, could be the same as that given by Finlay and Smaldone (1998), who emphasized that much of the understanding of hygroscopic aerosols is based on considering the fate of single droplets which may behave quite differently from the clouds of droplets produced by nebulizers, as it is possible for such clouds to behave in a non-hygroscopic way. Aerosols with large numbers of droplets per unit volume, such as can occur with nebulized aerosols, can actually self-humidify the air around them and thereby prematurely stop hygroscopic size changes. This phenomenon, known as the "two-way coupled effect," occurs when each droplet shrinks only slightly, but the number of droplets is so great that the vapor evaporating off the droplets into the surrounding air causes the air to reach water vapor equilibrium (Finlay, 1998). Thus, the "two-way coupled effect" may stabilize some hygroscopic aerosols against size alteration in the respiratory tract. While the airflow rate of our model was fixed, changing the airflow rate may change the dilution of the aerosol in the air, which could give different results.

This result is consistent with the study of Martin et al. (2005) who observed no significant difference in the evaporation rate of PMDI between dry and humid conditions at 37°C, i.e., PMDI particles did not evaporate more slowly in the presence of high levels of humidity. In their study, the droplets placed at 37°C evaporated under both humid and dry conditions, showing that evaporation was greater than condensation. Another study performed by Martin and Finlay (2005) led to the hypothesis that in humid conditions, PMDI particles initially undergo a rapid evaporation of propellant from residual drug particles which quickly reduces aerosol diameters, then a transient growth of propellant-cooled particles due to condensation of water, followed by a water re-evaporation at a steady, warmer temperature. Thus, given sufficient time, quasi-steady state evaporation of water from PMDI particles may largely negate the initial condensation.

For the nebulizers and the salbutamol PMDI, there was no difference in total drug deposition on the ACI stages between ambient conditions and HPTH, indicating that particles did not grow at the entrance of the trachea (before being impacted on the impactor stages) at HPTH. However, the results obtained for terbutaline Turbuhaler® DPI showed many fewer particles were deposited in the cascade impactor at HPTH than at ambient conditions, indicating that more particles were deposited in the trachea at HPTH. This would mean that at HPTH, particles grew very rapidly at the entrance of the trachea due to condensation, and impacted on the walls of the trachea and the cylinder. As a result, the mass of particles smaller than 5 μm at HPTH was nearly half that under ambient conditions. Terbutaline Turbuhaler® DPI was the only device tested whose particles grew, i.e., underwent more condensation than evaporation. This phenomenon may be explained by the fact that terbutaline Turbuhaler® DPI is a powder, and thus much more subject to hygroscopic growth than a solution. Moisture is well known to affect powder cohesion through capillary force at high relative humidity (Telko and Hickey, 2005; Chan, 2006).

There are clearly some limitations to this study. The flow chosen were constant and did not follow a pattern of breathing. The flow of 28.3 L/min was that recommended for the ACI and has stood the test of time with regard to accuracy. It is also a reasonable approximation of the mean inspiratory flow of an adult (tidal volume 750 mL and inspiratory time of 1.5 s). However, it would be too low to fully activate the DPI device so the flow of 60 L/min was chosen with a mathematical recalculation of the cut points which could have introduced some inaccuracies. This flow would be in the same order of magnitude as that expected from a patient inhaling forcefully from the device. These studies are in contrast to those of where Sangwan et al. (2003); Solomita and Smaldone (2009), Sagalla and Smaldone (2014), and Samuel and Smaldone (2020) used a low flow impactor to sample the aerosol rather than directing the entire output of the device into the impactor. This set up has the advantage to use a pattern of breathing but eliminated the "throat" where, in the present setup, it is expected that most of the changes in particle size occurred. NGI cascade impactor with a lower flow rate at 15 L/min is recommended for nebulizers particle size measurement (ISO 27427, 2012). Our method could be adapted with the NGI cascade impactor. A further issue is that they used either normal saline (Solomita and Smaldone, 2009; Sagalla and Smaldone, 2014) or γ interferon (Sangwan et al., 2003; Samuel and Smaldone, 2020) whereas the focus in the present study was asthma medication and the results suggest that changes in particle size due to exposure to HPTH conditions are specific for individual formulations. Finally, this was an *in vitro* study designed to evaluate temperature and humidity on various asthma medication and their delivery systems and does not have the power of *in vivo* deposition studies (Sangwan et al., 2003; Sagalla and Smaldone, 2014; Samuel and Smaldone, 2020) to predict pulmonary deposition in the face of significant disease.

The overall comparison of the four devices tested predicted a major deposition in the central and peripheral regions of the lung for the nebulizers (PariLC Star® and Aeroneb Go®), and in upper airways for the salbutamol PMDI and the terbutaline Turbuhaler® DPI. Thus PariLC Star® and Aeroneb Go® may allow the desired site of action to be targeted, i.e., the lung, whereas most of the drug delivered by salbutamol PMDI and terbutaline Turbuhaler® DPI may be lost in the upper airways. The high injection speed for the salbutamol PMDI and the 60 L/min sampling flow rate for the terbutaline Turbuhaler® DPI are mainly responsible for this large deposition in the trachea (Newman et al., 1996; Newman, 2003).

In this study, the nebulizers were associated with terbutaline solution. It is essential to consider the "nebulizer + solution to nebulize" couple and not the nebulizer alone, as one nebulizer can produce a different aerosol with different solutions. Results may have been different if another drug had been used. Formulation affects the particle growing/evaporation and consequently deposition prediction.

The potential change in cut-off diameters of the cascade impactor stages at 37°C was taken into account. Particle collection at the impactor stage is governed by the Stokes number. The cut-off diameter of the corresponding stage can be calculated from the Stokes number and depends on air viscosity. Air viscosity is defined by Willeke and Baron (1993), Baron and Willeke (2001):

$$\mu = \frac{\mu(\text{ref}) * (\text{T(ref)} + \text{S})}{\text{T} + \text{S}} * \left(\frac{\text{T}}{\text{T(ref)}}\right)^{3/2}$$

where μ(ref) is the reference air viscosity (183.25 micropoise), T(ref) is the reference temperature (293.15 Kelvin), S is the Sutherland constant (110.4 Kelvin).

When comparing air viscosity at 20°C (ambient temperature) and 37°C, a deviation of 4% was observed. This deviation is not significant compared to the bias between the experiments.

The Stokes number can be defined by Hinds (1999), Willeke and Baron (1993), Baron and Willeke (2001):

$$St = \frac{\rho_p * d_p^2 * Q * C_p}{9 * \mu * W}$$

where ρ_p is the particle density (1,000 kg/m^3), d_p is the particle diameter, Q is the jet velocity, C_p is the slip correction factor, μ is the air viscosity, W is the jet diameter.

For d_p = 3 μm and W = 0.0025 m, a deviation of 2% was observed when comparing air viscosity at 20°C (ambient temperature) and 37°C.

Mathematical models, which can be used to predict aerosol deposition in the respiratory tract, require knowledge of many parameters, including the characteristics of the drug, the aerosol generator and the aerosol itself. As the aerosol particle size has to be known, it seems more relevant to perform the sizing directly at HPTH to predict drug deposition. This is a considerable advantage of the method proposed in this study which allows study of the effect of temperature and humidity on the aerosol generated by the device and not on the device itself, a distinction which is not always clearly made. Moreover, our model is close to human physiological conditions where the air carrying the aerosol came from the ambient atmosphere, which is similar to the clinical setting. The continuous airflow may approximate the deep inhalation for PMDI and DPI, but did not simulate patient breathing for nebulizers. However, this study was an initial step in exploring the potential for hygroscopic growth and other changes to the aerosol that could take place while particle sizing with the ACI. The results obtained in this study for the nebulizers are consistent with the study of Fleming et al. (2006) which showed that alveolar deposition (i.e., small particles) was greater for *in vivo* experiments than for the LUDEP deposition modeling program. Our results could explain this difference. Finally, terbutaline Turbuhaler® DPI was the only device subject to hygroscopic growth, since its mass of particles smaller than 5 μm decreased at HPTH, whereas it did not change for the nebulizers and the salbutamol pMDI.

CONCLUSION

An aerosol sizing at controlled temperature and humidity with the respect of ambient air before aerosol delivery has been developed using a cascade impactor. Using physiological temperature (37°C) and humidity (100%RH) conditions vs. ambient air condition, we observed a decrease of particle size for liquid aerosol produced by nebulizers; no particle size change for PMDI, and a decrease of mass of particle smaller than 5 μm suggesting a rapid particle growing for powder aerosol produced by a DPI. Scintigraphic measurement obtained by Sangwan et al. (2003) support our results obtained with nebulization. *In vivo* deposition studies have to be conducted to evaluate the relevance of this method for aerosol deposition prediction.

AUTHOR CONTRIBUTIONS

CM, AC, and LV conducted experiments and analyzed results. AC, AL, and LV provided scientific input and contributed to experiment design. CM and LV analyzed experiments and drafted the manuscript. AC, AL, and LV designed and coordinated the overall project. All authors contributed to the article and approved the submitted version.

REFERENCES

Baron, P. A., and Willeke, K. (2001). *Aerosol Measurement: Principles, Techniques, and Applications*, 2nd Edn. New York,NY: J Wiley and Sons.

Bell, K. A., and Ho, A. T. (1981). Growth rate measurements of hygroscopic aerosols under conditions simulating the respiratory tract. *J. Aerosol Sci.* 12, 247–254.

Boudin, L., Grandmont, C., Grec, B., Martin, S., Mecherbet, A., and Noël, F. (2020). Fluid-kinetic modelling for respiratory aerosols with variable size and temperature. *ESAIM: Proc. Surv.* 67, 100–119. doi: 10.1051/proc/202067007

Broday, D. M., and Georgopoulos, P. G. (2001). Growth and deposition of hygroscopic particulate matter in the human lungs. *Aerosol Sci. Technol.* 34, 144–159.

Chan, H. K. (2006). Dry powder aerosol delivery systems: current and future research directions. *J. Aerosol Med.* 19, 21–27.

Coates, A. L., MacNeish, C. F., Lands, L. C., Meisner, D., Kelemen, S., and Vadas, E. B. (1998). A comparison of the availability of Tobramycin for inhalation from vented vs unvented nebulizers. *Chest* 113, 951–956.

Daviskas, E., Gonda, I., and Anderson, S. (1990). Mathematical modeling of heat and water transport in human respiratory tract. *J. Appl. Physiol.* 69, 362–372.

Eisner, A. D. (1992). On the coupled mass and energy transport phenomena during breathing of high volume aqueous aerosols. *J. Aerosol Med.* 5, 241–250.

Ferron, G. A. (1977). The size of soluble aerosol particles as a function of the humidity of the air. Application to the human respiratory tract. *J. Aerosol Sci.* 8, 251–267.

Ferron, G. A., Haider, B., and Kreyling, W. G. (1985). A method for the approximation of the relative humidity in the upper human airways. *Bull. Math. Biol.* 47, 565–589.

Ferron, G. A., Kreyling, W. G., and Haider, B. (1988). Inhalation of salt aerosol particles - II. Growth and deposition in the human respiratory tract. *J. Aerosol Sci.* 19, 611–631.

Finlay, W. H. (1998). Estimating the type of hygroscopic behavior exhibited by aqueous droplets. *J. Aerosol Med.* 11, 221–229.

Finlay, W. H., and Smaldone, G. C. (1998). Hygroscopic behaviour of nebulized aerosols: not as important as we thought? *J. Aerosol Med.* 11, 193–195.

Finlay, W. H., and Stapleton, K. W. (1995). The effect on regional lung deposition of coupled heat and mass transfer between hygroscopic droplets and their surrounding phase. *J. Aerosol Sci.* 26, 655–670.

Finlay, W. H., Stapleton, K. W., and Zuberbuhler, P. (1997). Errors in regional lung deposition predictions of nebulized salbutamol sulphate due to neglect or partial inclusion of hygroscopic effects. *Int. J. Pharm.* 149, 63–72.

Fleming, J. S., Epps, B. P., Conway, J. H., and Martonen, T. B. (2006). Comparison of SPECT aerosol deposition data with a human respiratory tract model. *J. Aerosol Med.* 19, 268–278.

Gradon, L., and Podgórski, A. (1996). Deposition of Inhaled Particles: Discussion of Present Modeling Techniques. *J. Aerosol Med.* 9, 343–355.

Hinds, W. C. (1999). *Aerosol Technology., 2nd edition*. New York,NY: J Wiley and Sons.

Hindle, M., and Longest, P. W., (2012). Condensational growth of combination drug-excipient submicrometer particles for targeted high efficiency pulmonary delivery: evaluation of formulation and delivery device. *J. Pharm. Pharmacol.* 64, 1254–1263. doi: 10.1111/j.2042-7158.2012.01476.x

ISO 27427. (2012). *Anaesthetic and respiratory equipment — Nebulizing systems and components*. Geneva: ISO.

Kwong, W. T. J., Ho, S. L., and Coates, A. L., (2000). Comparison of nebulized particle size distribution with Malvern laser diffraction analyzer versus Andersen cascade impactor and low-flow Marple personal cascade impactor. *J. Aerosol Med.* 13, 303–314. doi: 10.1089/jam.2000.13.303

Longest, P. W., and Hindle, M. (2012). Condensational growth of combination drug-excipient submicrometer particles: Comparison of CFD predictions with experimental results. *Pharm. Res.* 29, 707–721.

Marple, V. A., Olson, B. A., Santhanakrishnan, K., Mitchell, J. P., Murray, S. C., and Hudson-Curtis, B. L. (2003). Next Generation Pharmaceutical Impactor (A New Impactor for Pharmaceutical Inhaler Testing). Part II: Archival Calibration. *J. Aerosol Med.* 16, 301–324.

Martin, A. R., and Finlay, W. H. (2005). The effect of humidity on the size of particles delivered from metered-dose inhalers. *Aerosol Sci. Technol.* 39, 283–289.

Martin, A. R., Kwok, D. Y., and Finlay, W. H. (2005). Investigating the evaporation of metered-dose inhaler formulations in humid air: single droplet experiments. *J. Aerosol Med.* 18, 218–224.

Martin, G. P., Bell, A. E., and Marriott, C. (1988). An in vitro method for assessing particle deposition from metered pressurized aerosols and dry powder inhalers. *Int. J. Pharm.* 44, 57–63.

Nerbrink, O. L., Pagels, J., Pieron, C. A., and Dennis, J. H. (2003). Effect of humidity on constant output and breath enhanced nebulizer designs when tested in the EN13544-1 EC Standard. *Aerosol Sci. Technol.* 37, 282–292.

Newman, S. P. (2003). Drug delivery to the lungs from dry powder inhalers. *Curr. Opin. Pulm. Med.* 9, S17–S20.

Newman, S. P., Steed, K. P., Reader, S. J., Hooper, G., and Zierenberg, B. (1996). Efficient delivery to the lungs of flunisolide aerosol from a new portable hand-held multidose nebulizer. *J. Pharm. Sci.* 85, 960–964.

O'Doherty, I. J., and Miller, R. F. (1993). Aerosols for therapy and diagnosis. *Eur. J. Nucl. Med.* 20, 1201–1213.

Prokop, R. M., Finlay, W. H., Stapleton, K. W., and Zuberbuhler, P. (1995). The effect of ambient relative humidity on regional dosages delivered by a jet nebulizer. *J. Aerosol Med.* 8, 363–372.

Rao, N., Kadrichu, N., and Ament, B. (2010). Application of a droplet evaporation model to aerodynamic size measurement of drug aerosols generated by a vibrating mesh nebulizer. *J. Aerosol Med. Pulm. Drug Deliv.* 23, 295–302.

Sagalla, R. B., and Smaldone, G. C. (2014). Capturing the efficiency of vibrating mesh nebulizers: minimizing upper airway deposition. *J. Aerosol Med. Pulm. Drug Deliv.* 27, 341–348.

Samuel, J., and Smaldone, G. C. (2020). Maximizing Deep Lung Deposition in Healthy and Fibrotic Subjects During Jet Nebulization. *J. Aerosol Med. Pulm. Drug Deliv.* 33, 108–115.

Sangwan, S., Condos, R., and Smaldone, G. C. (2003). Lung deposition and respirable mass during wet nebulization. *J. Aerosol Med.* 16, 379–386.

Solomita, M., and Smaldone, G. C. (2009). Reconciliation of Cascade Impaction during Wet Nebulization. *J. Aerosol Med. Pulm. Drug Deliv.* 22, 11–18.

Spence, B. M., Longest, W., Wei, X., Dhapare, S., and Hindle, M. (2019). Development of a High Flow Nasal Cannula and Pharmaceutical Aerosol Combination Device. *J. Aerosol Med. Pulm. Drug Deliv.* 32, 224–241.

Stapleton, K. W., and Finlay, W. H. (1998). Errors in characterizing particle size distributions with cascade impactors. *J. Aerosol Med.* 11, S80–S83.

Telko, M. J., and Hickey, A. J. (2005). Dry powder inhaler formulation. *Respir. Care.* 50, 1209–1227.

USP 28-Nf 23. (2005). *Chapter 601 - Physical tests and determinations: Aerosols.*Rockville, MD: United States Pharmacopeia. 2359–2377.

Van Oort, M., Downey, B., and Roberts, W. (1996). Verification of operating the Andersen Cascade Impactor at different flow rates. *Pharmacopeia Forum* 22, 2211–2215.

Vecellio None, L., Grimbert, D., Becquemin, M. H., Boissinot, E., Le Pape, A., Lemarié, E., et al. (2001). Validation of laser diffraction method as a substitute for cascade impaction in the European Project for a Nebulizer Standard. *J. Aerosol Med.* 14, 107–114.

Willeke, K., and Baron, P. A. (1993). *Aerosol Measurement: Principles, Techniques, and Applications.* New York: Van Nostrand Reinhold.

Zhang, Z., Kleinstreuer, C., and Kim, C. S. (2006). Water vapor transport and its effects on the deposition of hygroscopic droplets in a human upper airway model. *Aerosol Sci. Technol.* 40, 1–16.

Zhou, Y., Ahuja, A., Irvin, C. M., Kracko, D. A., McDonald, J. D., and Cheng, Y. S. (2005a). Medical nebulizer performance: effects of cascade impactor temperature. *Respir. Care.* 50, 1077–1082.

Zhou, Y., Ahuja, A., Irvin, C. M., Kracko, D., McDonald, J. D., and Cheng, Y. S. (2005b). Evaluation of nebulizer performance under various humidity conditions. *J. Aerosol Med.* 18, 283–293.

12

Glycated Albumin Triggers an Inflammatory Response in the Human Airway Epithelium and Causes an Increase in Ciliary Beat Frequency

Moira L. Aitken[1], Ranjani Somayaji[1], Thomas R. Hinds[2], Maricela Pier[1], Karla Droguett[3], Mariana Rios[3], Shawn J. Skerrett[1,3] and Manuel Villalon[3]*

[1] *Department of Medicine, School of Medicine, University of Washington, Seattle, WA, United States,* [2] *Department of Pharmacy, School of Medicine, University of Washington, Seattle, WA, United States,* [3] *Department of Physiology, Faculty of Biological Sciences, Pontificia Universidad Católica de Chile, Santiago, Chile*

***Correspondence:**
Moira L. Aitken
moira@uw.edu

The role of inflammation in airway epithelial cells and its regulation are important in several respiratory diseases. When disease is present, the barrier between the pulmonary circulation and the airway epithelium is damaged, allowing serum proteins to enter the airways. We identified that human glycated albumin (GA) is a molecule in human serum that triggers an inflammatory response in human airway epithelial cultures. We observed that single-donor human serum induced IL-8 secretion from primary human airway epithelial cells and from a cystic fibrosis airway cell line (CF1-16) in a dose-dependent manner. IL-8 secretion from airway epithelial cells was time dependent and rapidly increased in the first 4 h of incubation. Stimulation with GA promoted epithelial cells to secrete IL-8, and this increase was blocked by the anti-GA antibody. The IL-8 secretion induced by serum GA was 10–50-fold more potent than TNF_{α} or LPS stimulation. GA also has a functional effect on airway epithelial cells *in vitro*, increasing ciliary beat frequency. Our results demonstrate that the serum molecule GA is pro-inflammatory and triggers host defense responses including increases in IL-8 secretion and ciliary beat frequency in the human airway epithelium. Although the binding site of GA has not yet been described, it is possible that GA could bind to the receptor for advanced glycated end products (RAGE), known to be expressed in the airway epithelium; however, further experiments are needed to identify the mechanism involved. We highlight a possible role for GA in airway inflammation.

Keywords: airways, airway disease, glycated albumin, inflammation, cytokine, human, ciliary beat frequency

---

Abbreviations: BAL, Bronchial alveolar lavage; COPD, Chronic obstructive pulmonary disease; CBF, Ciliary beat frequency; CF, Cystic fibrosis; GA, Glycated albumin; HBSS, Hank's balanced salt solution; HRP, Horseradish peroxidase; IL-8, Interleukin 8; IEF, Isoelectric focusing; KSFM, Keratinocyte serum-free medium; PMNs, Polymorphonuclear granulocytes; PVDF, Polyvinylidene difluoride; SEM, Standard error of the mean; TCA, Trichloroacetic acid; UP, Unknown protein.

INTRODUCTION

Airway epithelial cells participate in host defense by generating a wide variety of cytokines and chemokines that initiate or amplify acute and chronic inflammation by mediating the recruitment, activation, and survival of inflammatory cells within the airway (Standiford et al., 1990; Marini et al., 1992; Levine, 1995). Interleukin 8 (IL-8) is a pro-inflammatory molecule that is found in high concentration in the bronchial alveolar lavage (BAL) of patients with airway inflammatory diseases like cystic fibrosis (CF) (Konstan et al., 1994; O'Sullivan and Fredman, 2009), asthma (Lamblin et al., 1998), and chronic obstructive pulmonary disease (COPD) (Keatings et al., 1996; Hollander et al., 2007) and in the nasal mucosa of patients with allergic rhinitis (Cui et al., 2015). Respiratory epithelial cells (or cell lines) produce IL-8 in response to stimulation with IL-1α or TNFα or with other stimuli including neutrophil elastase, viruses, bacteria, and bacterial products (Standiford et al., 1990; Nakamura et al., 1992; Kwon et al., 1994; Levine, 1995). IL-8 is thought to play a major regulatory role in the airways as a potent chemo-attractant of polymorphonuclear granulocytes (PMNs) (Nakamura et al., 1991).

In airway diseases such as CF, asthma, and respiratory infections including viral infections notably SARS-CoV-2, the epithelial barrier is injured causing increased permeability and markedly greater plasma and serum protein movement across this barrier (McElvaney et al., 1992), a possible mechanism leading to a worse outcome in COVID-19 patients. Macromolecules of very different size and charge (i.e., 60-kDa albumin and the 700-kDa α_2-macroglobulin) have been demonstrated to move equally across all barriers that exist between the venular compartment and the mucosal surface of airways (Svenson et al., 1995). The airway epithelium also participates in host defense through mucociliary clearance (MCC) which is designed to remove bacteria and contaminant particles from entering the lung parenchyma (Knowles and Boucher, 2002). MCC is determined by the frequency of ciliated cells and the rheological properties of the mucus released by secretory cells (van der Baan, 2000). The efficiency of MCC is affected by airway inflammation, which in turn induces the release of local pro-inflammatory molecules resulting in mucus hypersecretion or ciliary dysfunction (Seybold et al., 1990; Cowley et al., 1997; Waugh and Wilson, 2008; Schmid et al., 2010; Koblizek et al., 2011).

Limited understanding exists regarding the precise roles of serum molecules in the inflammatory response of the airway epithelium affecting MCC. We conducted the study herein to identify the protein in serum leading to this pro-inflammatory effect. We hypothesized that this protein induces increased airway inflammation and will cause functional effects such as on ciliary function, which plays an important role in chronic airway diseases.

MATERIALS AND METHODS

Human Airway Epithelial Cells

We obtained nasal mucosa samples of 22 non-CF patients (mean age 47 years, range: 19–71 years); bronchial mucosa sample from one CF patient (33 years, cystic fibrosis genotype F508del homozygous); and adenoid tissue from non-CF patients (mean age 7 years, range: 3–12 years) who had undergone surgery for adenoid hypertrophy.

We also used an immortalized cell line from CF nasal polyp airway epithelial cells (CF 1-16 cells) with a homozygous F508del genotype, a gift from Dr. Christine Halbert, Fred Hutchinson Cancer Research Center, Seattle, WA, United States (Halbert et al., 1996). Tissue acquisition was approved by the ethic committee of the Pontificia Universidad Católica de Chile and the Human Subjects Review Committee of the University of Washington.

Nasal and Bronchial Mucosa Samples

Nasal epithelial cells were isolated from the mucosa by methodologies previously described (Standiford et al., 1990; Nakamura et al., 1991; McElvaney et al., 1992; Levine, 1995). Primary cultures from adenoid explant epithelial cells were prepared in Rose chambers as previously described (Gonzalez et al., 2013).

Human epithelial cells were isolated from the mucosa by methodologies previously described (Nakamura et al., 1991; McElvaney et al., 1992; Aitken et al., 1993, 1995; Levine, 1995; Gras et al., 2010; Gonzalez et al., 2013). Briefly, cells were rinsed and plated onto Vitrogen (Collagen Biomedical, Palo Alto, CA, United States)-coated 12-well plates (Costar, Cambridge, MA, United States) and cultured in 3.0 mL keratinocyte serum-free medium (KSFM) (Gibco BRL, Grand Island, NY, United States) with 5% fetal calf serum (FCS) (HyClone, Logan, UT, United States). After 12–24 h, the medium was changed to KSFM with 5 ng/mL epidermal growth factor (Gibco BRL, Grand Island, NY, United States) and 50 μg/mL bovine pituitary extract (Gibco BRL) until confluent (4–14 days). Experiments were performed on confluent cells. The monolayers were rinsed three times with either Hank's balanced salt solution (HBSS) (H9269, Sigma, St Louis, MO, United States) or KSFM and incubated with KSFM under various experimental conditions.

Adenoid Tissue

Primary cultures were prepared to obtain explants of epithelial cells in Rose chambers as previously described (Gonzalez et al., 2013). Briefly, small pieces of adenoid tissue (2–4 mm) were washed with HBSS and rinsed in NHS media (137 mM NaCl, 5.09 mM KCl, 1.14 mM Na_2HPO_4, × 2 H_2O, 0.18 mM KH_2PO_4, 0.923 mM $MgCl_2$ × $6H_2O$, 0.91 mM $CaCl_2$ × $2H_2O$, 4.07 mM $NaHCO_3$, 21.5 mM glucose, pH 7.4) supplemented with 1% vitamins, 1% essential amino acids, 1% non-essential amino acids, and 1% pyruvate and antibiotics (neomycin 0.2 mg/mL and penicillin 0.12 mg/mL) (all these reagents: Invitrogen Corp, NY, United States). Small pieces of epithelium were placed on a cover glass pretreated with 0.1% gelatin (G9391, VWR Scientific, Radnor, PA, United States) and then placed in Rose chambers. Explants were covered with a sterile dialysis membrane pretreated with the NHS culture medium. The Rose chambers were filled with 2 mL of NHS medium, which contain 10% of horse inactivated serum (Biological Industries, Israel) (pH 7.2–7.4), and the explants were incubated at 37°C. The culture media within the Rose chambers were renewed every 48 h.

After approximately 7 days, patches of epithelial cells with synchronized activity were obtained.

Stimulation of Human Airway Epithelial Cells

Nasal human epithelial cell cultures were incubated in KSFM supplemented with commercial pooled serum (AB-Human Serum from Life Technologies, Biocompare, South San Francisco, CA, United States), single-donor serum, or plasma-derived serum, at concentrations ranging from 0.1 to 50%. In the stimulation experiments, after specified time intervals, supernatants were harvested and stored at -70°C. In some experiments, cells were incubated with single-donor serum in the presence of a neutralizing human monoclonal antibody against GA (A717, Exocell, Inc., Philadelphia, PA, United States. RRID:AB_2225805) at a concentration of 10 pg/mL.

The different serums were prepared as follows: single-donor serum was prepared from blood from a healthy subject. Blood was allowed to clot at room temperature, spun at 1,000 × g for 15 min, and subsequently the serum fraction was stored at −70°C. For plasma-derived serum, whole blood (50 mL) from a single donor was collected into a chilled syringe (4°C) containing 5 mL of 3.8% sodium citrate. The citrated blood was then centrifuged at 30,000 × g for 20 min at 4°C. The plasma was removed and mixed with 1.0 M $CaCl_2$ (1:50) and then incubated at 37°C for 2 h and centrifuged at 25,000 × g for 20 min at room temperature. Serum was collected and stored at −70°C.

IL-8 ELISA in the Monolayer Cells

Measurement of IL-8 was performed using "sandwich" enzyme-linked immunosorbent assay (ELISA). A 96-well plate was coated overnight with 100 μL of monoclonal antibody against human IL-8 (I2519, Sigma, RRID:AB_260157) at a concentration of 0.5 μg/mL, rinsed with PBS-Tween 20, and blocked with 2% BSA. The samples were then diluted, run in triplicate, and allowed to incubate at room temperature for 2 h. The plates were washed three times with PBS-Tween 20. A polyclonal antibody conjugated to horseradish peroxidase (HRP) was added to the plate, incubated, and washed. The chromogenic substrate 3,3′,5,5′-tetramethylbenzidine was added, and the absorbance was read at 450 nm. Unknowns were compared to serial dilution standards (0–2,000 pg/mL). IL-8 measurements are expressed in ng/mL considering 1×10^6 cells per culture well.

IL-8 ELISA in Rose Chamber Adenoid Cells

IL-8 production was measured from supernatants which were stored at −20°C until used. We used ELISA KIT Quantikine® (minimum detectable dose: 3.5 pg/mL, D8000C, R&D Systems, Minneapolis, MN, United States). IL-8 measurements are expressed in ng/mL/mg of total protein with approximately 3×10^6 cells per culture/mL.

Identification of the Serum Factor (Glycated Albumin) That Increased IL-8 Secretion

Chromatography of Human Serum on DEAE Cellulose, pH 7: Ion exchange chromatography of human serum was performed on a 12-mL DEAE cellulose column (Whatman Specialty Products, Fairfield, NJ, United States) equilibrated in 50 mM NaCl, 10 mM phosphate, pH 7.5. Three milliliter of human serum dialyzed in equilibration buffer was added to the column, washed with seven column volumes of buffer, and collected in four equal fractions (zero absorbance in fourth fraction). A linear 50-mL salt gradient of 50–1,000 mM NaCl (in 10 mM phosphate, pH 7.5) was used to elute proteins from the column, and 0.6-mL fractions were collected. The salt concentration was monitored with an osmometer. The protein concentration was measured at 280 nm with a Beckman DU/64 spectrophotometer with a micro cuvette. Between 85 and 90 percent of the IL-8 secretory activity of primary non-CF nasal epithelial cells was found in the pre-gradient wash buffer fractions; these fractions were pooled and concentrated.

Protein G Column

Immunoglobulins were removed from the pooled active fractions with a protein G Sepharose column (P3296, Sigma). A 5.0-mL column was washed in buffer containing 137 mM NaCl, 10 mM phosphate, pH 6.5. Serum or DEAE flow-through was dialyzed against the column buffer and applied to the column. The flow-through was collected along with 10 column volumes of wash buffer. Bound IgG was eluted with 100 mM of glycine, pH 2.5, and immediately neutralized with 0.5 N NaOH to pH 6.5. The flow-through and the eluted immunoglobulins were concentrated to their original volume with Millipore Ultrafree-15 centrifugal filters and dialyzed against 137 mM NaCl, 10 mM phosphate buffer, pH 7.5 (PBS). The majority of the IL-8 secretory activity of primary non-CF nasal epithelial cells was found in the flow-through and wash buffer fraction. No IL-8 secretion was found associated with the eluted immunoglobulin.

Gel Filtration

The molecular size of the active protein from the previous steps was determined with a 12-mL S-200 Sephacryl gel column (GE17-0584-10, Sigma). The column was run with PBS. Two hundred microliters of concentrated protein was layered onto the gel, and 150-μL fractions were collected. The protein concentration was measured at 280 nm with a Beckman DU/64 spectrophotometer with a micro cuvette.

Sequencing of IL-8-Stimulating Protein

The identity of the unknown protein (UP) was determined by sequencing. The most active protein fraction in stimulating IL-8 secretion (fraction 38, **Figure 1B**) was electrophoresed on a native 7.5% acrylamide gel. Following electrophoresis, the gel was equilibrated for 5 min in a blotting buffer consisting of 100 mL of 10 mM CAPS buffer and 10% methanol, pH 11.0. The gel and a polyvinylidene difluoride (PVDF) membrane (Millipore, Bedford, MA, United States) were sandwiched and blotted for

45 min at 4°C. The membrane was washed and stained with Coomassie Blue R-250 for 5 min. Then, the membrane was destained in 50% methanol until the bands were clearly visible. The blotted membrane was rinsed in water and stored wet in a saran wrap at -20°C. The protein band of interest was sequenced from a trypsin digest of protein excised out of the PVDF and chromatographed by HPLC on a C18 column. Three peptides were separated out and sequenced using mass spectroscopy. The sequences obtained were used in a BLAST (RRID:SCR_004870)[1] search of human proteins as a means to identify the protein.

IEF (Isoelectric Focusing) Gel Electrophoresis

To further compare the UP with commercial human albumin (A1887, Sigma) and commercial glycated human albumin (A8301, Sigma), the iso-electro point of the three proteins was determined (**Figure 1C**). Equal amounts (6.9 μg) of the three proteins were run along with standards on a precast Bio-Rad IEF gel pH 3–10 (Bio-Rad, Hercules, CA, United States). The IEF standards were soybean trypsin inhibitor, 4.6 pI (10109886001, Sigma), and bovine milk β-lactoglobulin A, 5.1 pI (L3908, Sigma). The protein bands of interest were flanked on both sides by the standards in the gel. The gel was run for 3 h at various voltages; 1 h at 100 V, 1 h at 250 V, and 30 min at 500 V. The gel was fixed in 10% trichloroacetic acid (TCA) for 10 min. Excess ampholytes were removed by an additional overnight 1% TCA soak. To detect the protein bands, the gel was washed in water three times and stained with GELCODE Blue Stain Reagent (Pierce, Rockville, IL, United States).

Western Blot With the Anti-GA Antibody

Human albumin (HA, A3782, Sigma), GA, and the UP were electrophoresed on a 4–20% native gradient gel (**Figure 1D**). Each lane contained 20 μg of protein. After electrophoresis, the proteins were transferred onto polyvinylidene difluoride (PVDF) membranes (Millipore, Bedford, MA, United States) and blocked with 2% gelatin in PBS pH 7.4 overnight. The blot was probed with a human monoclonal antibody against GA (A717, Exocell, Inc., Philadelphia, PA, United States. RRID: AB 2225805) diluted 1:500. It was then incubated with a secondary polyclonal antibody rabbit anti-mouse conjugated to HRP diluted 1:2,000 and visualized with ECL substrate (Amersham Biosciences Corp, Piscataway, NY, United States).

Stimulation of CF1-16 Cells With GA, TNFα, and LPS

The levels of production measured through ligand stimulation with GA, TNFα, and LPS on epithelial cells were determined. CF1-16 cells were cultured with increasing concentrations of TNFα (0.2–20 ng/mL, T6674, Sigma), LPS (1–1,000 ng/mL, L3137 Sigma), and GA (0.2 μg/mL–2.0 mg/mL, A8301, Sigma). After a 5 h incubation at 5% CO_2, 37°C, the supernatants were harvested and stored at -70°C until analyzed for IL-8 secretion by ELISA. Samples were run in triplicate and compared to a standard curve in the same methods described above. To calculate the EC50 and the extrapolated value for Vmax (maximum response), we used a standard model for fitting the data (non-cooperative activity). GraphPad Prism (RRID:SCR_002798)[2].

Ciliary Beat Frequency (CBF) Measurements

CBF was measured by microphotodensitometry as previously described (Hermoso et al., 2001; Barrera et al., 2004). Light fluctuations produced by the ciliary beat were sensed by a photodiode (FDS015, Thorlabs Inc., Newton, NJ, United States) placed on a phase microscope (Nikon 300 Diaphot Inverted Microscope). Signal was processed and displayed by a spectral analyzer (SAI-51C Honeywell, Charlotte, North Caroline, United States). Human adenoid epithelial cells in Rose chambers with spontaneous ciliary activity were washed with HBSS. Cultures were left with 2 mL of HBSS as supernatants. CBF was tested in monolayers of human epithelial cells in Rose Chambers. CBF was measured from 2 to 3 cells in each culture, and a CBF baseline was established for 30 min prior to adding a substrate. CBF was then measured every 15 min for up to 4 h. From each adenoid sample, we obtained around five cultures, each one with four or five explants surrounded by a monolayer of ciliated cells. In this study, we used 34 cultures of ciliated cells, obtained from seven patients. Each time course on CBF effect or Il-8 measurements was performed in 4–5 cultures.

Statistical Analysis

Data were expressed as means ± standard error of the mean (SEM). Correlations between groups were calculated using the Spearman's rank test. We used Student *t*-tests for mean comparisons between experimental groups, and linear regression was conducted to compare trends over time between groups. Dose–response curves on Il-8 secretion for GA, TNFα, and LPS were analyzed by one-way ANOVA followed by Holm–Sidak's multiple-comparison test, using a square-root transformation of the original data. Graphics were performed using GraphPad Prism (see text footnote 2, RRID:SCR_002798). CBF data were analyzed following arcsin transformation. A $p < 0.05$ was considered statistically significant.

RESULTS

Identification of the Serum Component Responsible for Stimulation of IL-8 Secretion

Serum from four healthy donors and commercial pooled AB serum all stimulated IL-8 secretion from primary airway epithelial cells at a range of 0.4–1.3 ng/mL/10^5 cells.

We did not use pooled samples; rather, the individual whose serum had caused consistently the higher IL-8 response (1.7 ng/mL/10^5 cells). Human nasal epithelial cells were incubated for 6 h at concentrations from 0.1 to 50% of the volume, and the level

[1] http://blast.ncbi.nlm.nih.gov/Blast.cgi

[2] http://www.graphpad.com/

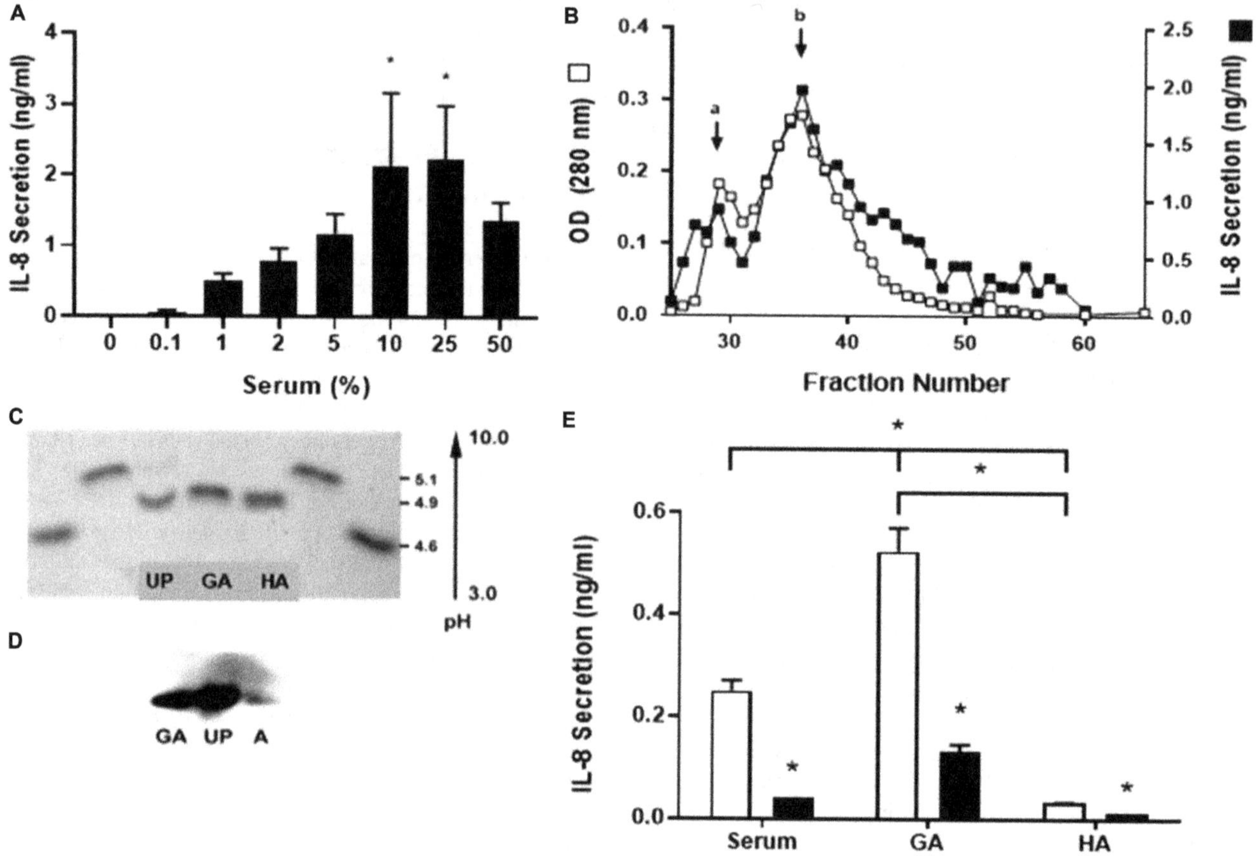

FIGURE 1 | Identification of the serum component responsible for stimulation of IL-8 secretion. Human single-dose serum induced IL-8 secretion in a dose-dependent manner. **(A)** Nasal epithelial cells were incubated for 5 h with a different percentage of human single-dose serum, and IL-8 secretion was measured. Serum induced a dose-dependent IL-8 secretion with a maximum at 25%. * Indicates a statistically significant increase ($p < 0.05$) in IL-8 compared to control. **(B)** Different serum fractions obtained from an S-200 Sephacryl gel column were assayed for IL-8 secretion, and the optical densities at 280 nm were compared. Two peaks were obtained (a and b); the major peak (b) seems to be a dimmer of the active protein. These peptides from a trypsin digest of the peak protein were analyzed by MS and used in a BLAST search of human proteins to identify the unknown protein (UP). **(C)** UP was isoelectric focused with glycated albumin (GA) and human albumin (HA) to determine their isoelectric point (pI). Two standards used soybean trypsin inhibitor (4.6 pI) and bovine β-lactoglobulin A (5.1 pI) loaded at both sides from the bands of interest. UP has the same pI as GA and HA. **(D)** A Western blot with anti-glycated albumin antibody was carried out. GA, UP, and HA were recognized with the same molecular weight. **(E)** IL-8 secretion induced by serum and glycated albumin (GA) in CF1-16 cells was reduced with an anti-human GA antibody. The CF epithelial cell line was incubated for 5 h with commercial pooled human serum (serum), GA (2 mg/mL), or albumin (HA, 2 mg/mL) and an anti-human GA antibody (black bar). Open bars have no antibody. Serum and GA increased IL-8 secretion, which was blocked when cells were coincubated with the GA antibody. * Indicates a statistically significant ($p < 0.05$) reduction in IL-8 secretion in the presence of the antibody in all groups (open vs. black bar) or higher IL-8 secretion in cell cultures incubated with GA compared to serum or HA and serum compared to HA. $n = 3$ for experiments included in **(A,E)**. Experiments for **(B–D)** were repeated three times.

of IL-8 secretion was measured. Serum induced a dose-dependent IL-8 secretion with a maximum of 25% (**Figure 1A**).

To identify the serum component responsible for stimulating IL-8 secretion, an ion exchange chromatography of human serum was performed to identify the unknown protein (UP) (**Figure 1B**). When fractionated, two distinct peaks were identified: a major peak with a molecular weight of about 65 kDa (non-glycated albumin) and a minor peak at approximately 130 kDa (glycated albumin). In subsequent purifications, we noticed that the minor peak quantity was variable. It was postulated that the IL-8 released was associated with both peaks and that the minor peak could be a dimer or aggregate of the active UP. The most active fraction (fraction 38) was sent for sequencing, and the resultant sequence was used in a BLAST search against human proteins as a mean to identify the UP. The BLAST result indicated with a high probability that the UP was human serum albumin which has a molecular weight of ~69 kDa which was similar to the UP weight (**Figure 1C**).

UP was isoelectric focused with glycated albumin (GA) and human albumin (HA) to determine their isoelectric point (pI). Two standards, soybean trypsin inhibitor (4.6 pI) and bovine β-lactoglobulin A (5.1 pI), were loaded at both sides from the bands of interest. UP have the same pI as GA and HA (**Figure 1D**).

A Western blot with equal amounts of anti-glycated albumin antibody was carried out. The results demonstrated that the UP and GA had a strong signal while HA had a very small response as expected, as the monoclonal antibody used targeted GA and thus may not react with non-glycated albumin. Further, all three proteins had equivalent electrophoretic mobility on the 7.7% SDS PAGE gel with a molecular weight of about 67 kDa (**Figure 1E**).

IL-8 secretion induced by serum and glycated albumin (GA) in CF1-16 cells was reduced significantly with an anti-human GA antibody ($p = 0.01$). CF1-16 epithelial cells were incubated for 5 h with commercial pooled human serum, GA (2 mg/mL) or human albumin (HA, 2 mg/mL), and with an anti-human GA antibody. Open bars have no antibody; black bars have an anti-human GA antibody. Serum and GA increased IL-8 secretion, which was blocked when cells were incubated with a GA antibody. HA was unable to increase IL-8 secretion supporting the need for glycation of albumin for this to occur ($p = 0.24$).

Human Upper and Lower Airway Epithelial Cells Had Varying Responses in Il-8 Production With Human Serum Stimulation

We wished to determine if the IL-8 secretion response was similar using the immortalized human CF cell line and the bronchial CF cells (**Figure 2A**). Cells were incubated for 6 h at concentrations from 0.1 to 50%, and the level of IL-8 secretion was measured. A dose response was demonstrated in all three cell types shown in human nasal cells (**Figure 1A**) and immortalized CF1-16 and CF bronchial cells (**Figure 2A**) with a maximal serum concentration of 25% (**Figures 1A, 2A**), and a maximum IL-8 secretion of 22.30 ng/mL in the CF bronchial cells.

Further, we wished to determine if immortalized CF 1-16 cells incubated with 5% of single-donor serum or medium over 4–24 h would show an IL-8 response (**Figure 2B**).

In the three epithelial cell types (human nasal epithelial cells, immortalized CF1-16 cell line, and CF bronchial epithelial cells), the ED_{50} for serum was 5, 5, and 3% with extrapolated maximums of 2.3, 2.8, and 24 ng/mL of IL-8, respectively. The magnitude of the IL-8 response in CF-bronchial cells was 10-fold higher compared to immortalized CF 1–16 airway epithelial cells ($p = 0.02$) (**Figure 2A**). A parallel experiment using plasma-derived serum free of platelet factor contamination demonstrated a similar IL-8 dose–response relationship (to a maximum of 10%) in airway epithelial cells (data not shown).

The time dependence of IL-8 secretion was determined using CF1-16 cell cultures (**Figure 2B**). CF1-16 cells were incubated with 5% of single-donor serum in KSFM, or with KSFM alone, and the supernatants were harvested at 4, 8, 12, 16, 20, and 24 h. By 4 h of incubation, human serum induced a significant increase of IL-8 secretion compared to the control group (**Figure 2B**). No significant changes were observed for IL-8 secretion after a longer incubation period in either group.

IL-8 Secretion Induced by Glycated Albumin Compared to TNFα and LPS

The efficacy of GA to stimulate the airway epithelium to secrete IL-8 was comparatively assessed in CF 1–16 cells with other two pro-inflammatory molecules, TNFα and LPS. The concentrations of TNFα and LPS used were selected based on their pathological concentrations described in the literature (Demling et al., 2005; Kakazu et al., 2011). All induced a dose-dependent IL-8 secretion, with a maximum effect on Il-8 production for LPS and TNF of 0.419 and 0.471 ng/mL, respectively, but GA was over four times more effective, reaching a maximum effect of 2.0 ng/mL. The EC_{50} for LPS was 0.071 and 0.00193 μg/mL for TNF compared to 424 μg/mL for GA (**Figure 3**).

Glycated Albumin Increased IL-8 Secretion and CBF in Human Adenoid Cell Cultures

Next, human primary adenoid epithelial ciliated cell cultures were used to measure IL-8 secretion following 3 h of incubation with culture medium (control), HA, and GA. An elevated level of IL-8 secretion only occurred in the cultures stimulated with GA, while there was no difference between control and HA treated cultures ($p = 0.12$) (**Figure 4A**). When ciliary beat frequency was assessed, a progressive increment was detected in response to GA incubation, compared to control or HA groups ($p < 0.001$ for GA group). Furthermore, the most significant effect upon CBF was observed following 2–4 h of incubation with GA (**Figure 4B**). CBF, expressed as area under the curve (AUC, background was subtracted), was significantly greater in the GA-treated cultures compared to HA and culture medium cultures (GA 139.40 ± 4.54; HA 66.58 ± 1.99; medium 79.67 ± 2.87, $p < 0.05$).

The temporal relationship between the effect of GA and IL-8 secretion on CBF was examined by comparing the time changes in CBF induced by GA (2 mg/mL) and IL-8 (10 nM). GA and IL-8 both induced an increase in CBF in the first 30 min of exposure, but only the increase of CBF induced by GA remained elevated. In contrast, no changes were observed in CBF in cultures incubated with HA (2 mg/mL) or medium alone (**Figures 5A,B**).

DISCUSSION

We purified a human serum factor that increases IL-8 secretion from airway epithelial cells and, using molecular and mass spectrometric methods, identified it as human serum (glycated) albumin. Through comparative assessment, we demonstrated human serum glycated albumin (GA) to be a potent pro-inflammatory molecule with functional effects on the ciliary airway. GA was able to stimulate IL-8 secretion in different epithelial respiratory cell models, including primary cultures of human epithelial nasal cells, adenoid epithelial cells, CF bronchial cells, and an immortalized CF airway epithelial cell line. GA had a greater effect on IL-8 secretion compared with conventional pro-inflammatory molecules of TNF-α and LPS. Furthermore, both GA and IL-8 increased CBF in non-CF human adenoid epithelial cells.

GA is an advanced glycation end product (AGE) considered a pro-inflammatory molecule. AGEs are formed from condensation and oxidation processed between proteins and sugars (Sorci et al., 1833). Clinically, serum GA levels, used to detect early glycemic changes (Hoonhorst et al., 2016), may be twice the normal range in diabetes (Dolhofer and Wieland, 1980;

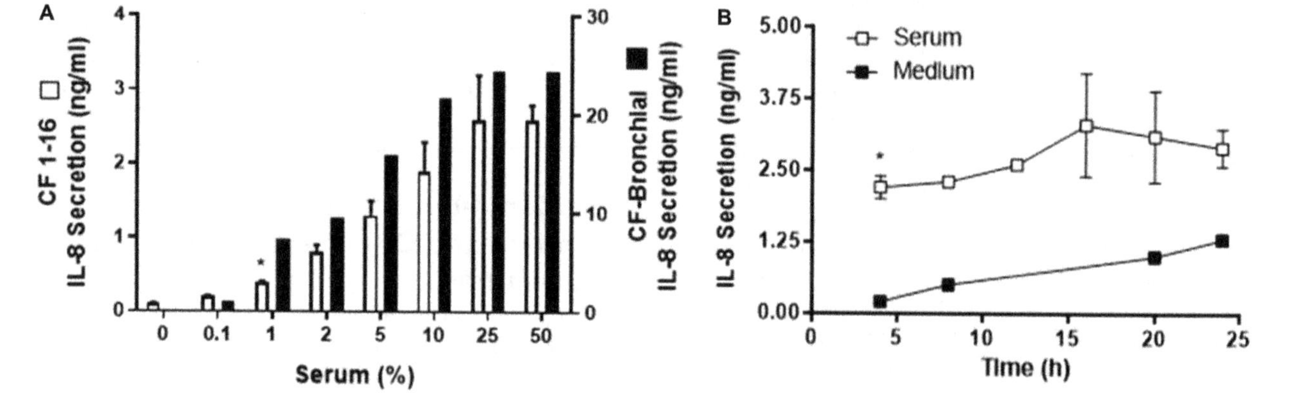

FIGURE 2 | Human serum induced IL-8 secretion from a cystic fibrosis (CF) epithelial cell line. **(A)** Immortalized CF nasal epithelial cell line (CF 1–16) (open bars, $n = 3$) and CF bronchial epithelial cells (black bars, $n = 2$) were incubated for 6 h with increasing percentages of human serum, and IL-8 secretion was measured. Human serum induced a dose-dependent IL-8 secretion in both CF cell line and the CF bronchial cells. **(A)** * indicates the lowest % of serum capable of producing a significant increase in IL-8 production. CF bronchial epithelial cells' response to serum to produce IL-8 secretion is almost one order of magnitude higher compared to the cystic fibrosis epithelial cell line. **(B)** CF 1–16 cells were incubated with 5% of single-donor serum (□, $n = 3$) or medium (■, $n = 2$), and IL-8 secretion ($n = 3$–4) was determined at 4, 8, 12, 16, 20, and 24 h. At 4 h of incubation, human serum induced a significant increase in IL-8 secretion compared to the control group. **(B)** * indicates a statistically significant ($p < 0.05$) increase in IL-8 secretion after 4 h of incubation with serum compared to the control group. No significant changes were observed for IL-8 secretion after longer period of incubation.

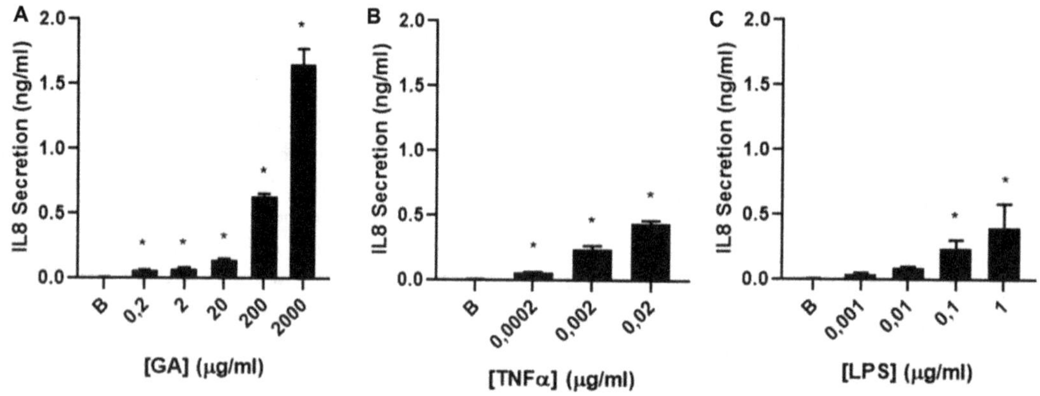

FIGURE 3 | IL-8 secretion by glycated albumin (GA) compared to TNFα and LPS. **(A)** dose–response curve of IL-8 secretion was determined in CF1-16 cells induced by **(A)** GA ($n = 3$), **(B)** TNFα ($n = 3$), and **(C)** LPS ($n = 3$). All induced a dose-dependent IL-8 secretion, with a maximum effect on Il-8 production for TNF and LPS of 477.6 and 424 ng/mL, respectively, but GA was 4–5 times more effective, reaching a max effect of 2.0 ng/mL. The EC_{50} for LPS was 0.071 and 0.00193 μg/mL for TNF compared to 424 μg/mL for GA. * indicates a significant increase ($p < 0.05$) in IL-8 secretion compared to the background **(B)**.

Jones et al., 1983). IL-8 expression is significantly elevated in patients with type II diabetes (Herder et al., 2005). These higher levels of GA are recognized as a major cause of diabetes complications such as atherosclerosis, cardiovascular disorders, nephropathy, and chronic inflammation (Sorci et al., 1833). In addition, GA has been identified as important in the induction of inflammation in retinal epithelial cells and monoclonal antibodies against GA ameliorate diabetic nephropathy in a mouse model (Cohen et al., 1994). In endothelial cells, the presence of GA is deleterious, making cells more procoagulant and promoting inflammatory responses (Rubenstein et al., 2011). Using enzyme-linked immunoassay, GA-treated human retinal pigment epithelial cells secrete levels of IL-8 detectable within 4 h (Bian et al., 1996). In human retinal pigment epithelial cells and in vascular smooth muscle cells, GA induces the expression of IL-8 by a mechanism that involves activation of kinases, including PKC, and transcription factors such as NF-κβ (Chen et al., 2000; Bian et al., 2001; Dahrouj et al., 2015). NF-kβ induces the expression of inflammatory response-related mRNAs, such as TNFα (tumor necrosis factor α) and IL-6 (interleukin-6) (Svenson et al., 1995), inflammatory mediators that have been related with functional changes in cilia activity (Chen et al., 2000; Papathanasiou et al., 2008). Furthermore, kinases like PKC also modify the mechanism associated with cilia activity regulation by ATP (Barrera et al., 2004; Gonzalez et al., 2013).

In human primary airway epithelial ciliated cell cultures, we observed that GA induced an increase in IL-8 and CBF. Previous studies have shown that macromolecules, such as soluble hyaluronic acid, can increase CBF of tracheal ovine epithelial cells through an unknown membrane receptor (Lieb et al., 2000).

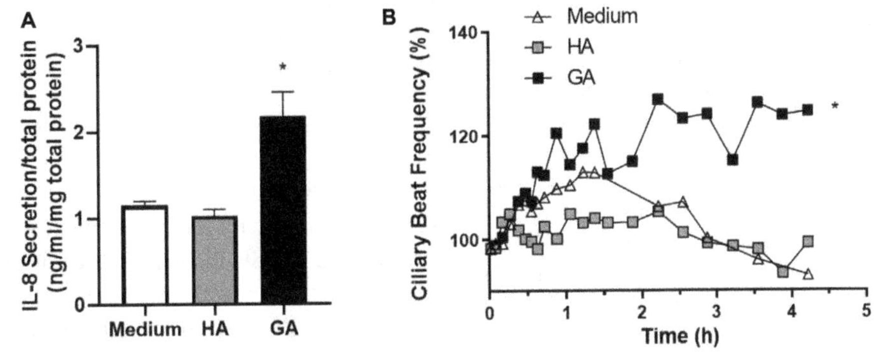

FIGURE 4 | GA increased IL-8 secretion and CBF in human adenoid epithelial cell cultures. **(A)** Human primary adenoid epithelial ciliated cell cultures were incubated with culture medium, HA (2 mg/mL), or GA (2 mg/mL) for 3 h. GA increased the statistical significance of IL-8 secretion with respect to HA and medium. Values are expressed as ng/mL of IL-8 corrected by mg of protein in primary culture. $^{*}p < 0.05$. **(B)** Time-course changes in CBF of non-CF human adenoid ciliated cell culture treated with GA (■, 2 mg/mL), HA (□, 2 mg/mL), and control solution (△, medium). The most significant effect upon CBF was observed after 2–4 h of incubation with GA. $n = 4$–5 cultures were used for each experimental point included in the Il-8 secretion experiments and the time course changes on CBF exposed to medium, HA, and GA.

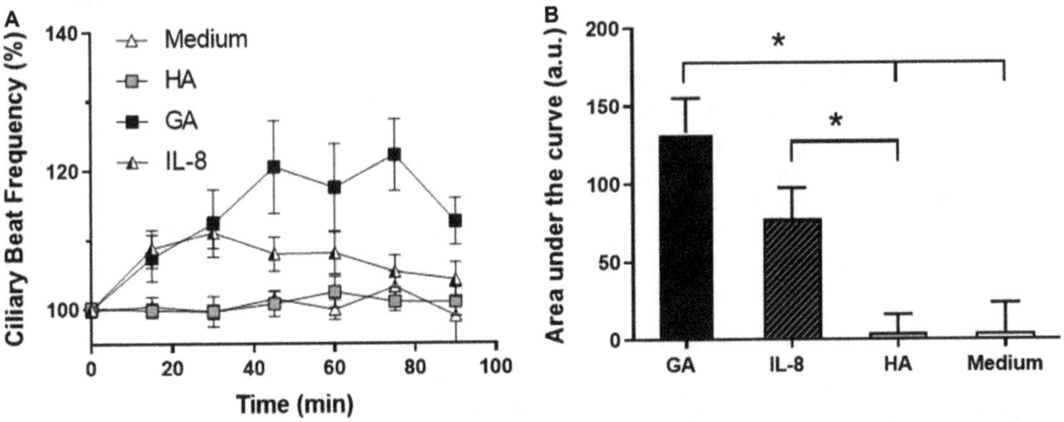

FIGURE 5 | Effect of glycated albumin (GA) and IL-8 in CBF. **(A)** Time-course changes in CBF of human adenoid epithelial ciliated cells cultures treated with GA (■, 2 mg/mL), IL-8 (□, 10 nM), albumin (HA, ○, 2 mg/mL), and culture medium (△). GA and IL-8 induced an increase in CBF in the first 30 min of exposure, but only the increase of CBF induced by GA was sustained. **(B)** Time course of CBF in **(A)** expressed as area under the curve (AUC). GA induced a statistically significant increase in CBF with respect to HA and medium, and IL-8 with respect to HA. $^{*}p < 0.05$. $n = 4$–5 cultures were used for each experimental point included in the time-course changes on CBF exposed to medium, HA, Il-8, and GA.

Non-glycated HA was unable to modify CBF. Although the binding site of GA has not yet been described, it is possible that GA could bind to the receptor for advanced glycated end products (RAGE), known to be expressed in the airway epithelium (Milutinovic et al., 2012). RAGE regulates a number of cellular processes such as inflammation, regulation of cell mass, and cell mobility (Xie et al., 2013; Whitsett and Alenghat, 2014). Studies in retinal pigment epithelial cell cultures indicate that glycated albumin-induced breakdown of RPE function is mediated by RAGE and vascular endothelial growth factor (VEGF) receptor (del Campo et al., 2011). RAGE has been shown to be present in epithelial cells and contribute to allergic airway disease, as it can act as a mediator in one or more pro-inflammatory pathways that eventuate in the altered physiology seen in allergic airways disease (Milutinovic et al., 2012). RAGE knockout mice present a lower production of IL-8 and NF-kβ activation when they are exposed to pulmonary ischemia and reperfusion (Sternberg et al., 2008). In addition to binding AGEs, RAGE also is a signal transduction receptor for amyloid-β (Aβ) and S100/calgranulins, suggesting that RAGE could be involved in the recognition of a variety of macromolecules associated with the respiratory innate immunity response of the airway epithelium (Ma et al., 2007).

The CF 1-16 cell line in the study responded to human serum, increasing IL-8 secretion after 4 h of incubation. CF bronchial epithelial cells also responded to human serum, increasing IL-8 secretion, but CF bronchial cells appeared to be more responsive releasing 10 times more IL-8. Patients with CF suffer from chronic infections and severe inflammation and present high levels of pro-inflammatory molecules such as IL-8, IL-6, TNF_{α}, and arachidonic acid metabolites (Nakamura et al., 1992; Khan et al., 1995; O'Sullivan and Fredman, 2009), indicating a possible pro-inflammatory state of these cells. In addition, CF patients with CF-related diabetes mellitus have a more rapid decline in lung function and an increased mortality rate (Milla et al., 2000). It is possible that increased GA in the airways of these patients enhances the inflammatory response in their lungs.

Previous studies have shown that TNFα induces IL-8 expression in cultured human airway epithelial cells (Kwon et al., 1994). Furthermore, LPS, a TLR4 agonist, increases IL-8 production through phosphorylation of p38 (Mizunoe et al., 2012). When we compared the effectiveness of GA to induce IL-8 secretion with TNFα and LPS, GA was 10 times more effective to induce IL-8 secretion, suggesting a critical role of GA to initiate an inflammatory response.

IL-8 induced an increase in CBF in adenoid epithelial cultures showing a correlation with the effect of GA in the first 30 min. The CXC chemokine receptor (CXCR-1/IL-8) has been found to be expressed in human small airway epithelial cells and to induce the release of IL-6 (Gras et al., 2010). Although the specific mechanism of Il-8 stimulation of CBF has not been identified, it has been reported that Il-8 can increase PLC and intracellular calcium levels, both well-known ciliary beat activators (Barrera et al., 2004). Murine primary sino-nasal cultures treated with the mouse homologue of IL-8 increased basal CBF at 24 and 48 h (Shen et al., 2012). However, IL-8 inhibits beta-agonist ciliary stimulation in bovine bronchial epithelial cells (Allen-Gipson et al., 2004). It is possible that GA and IL-8 affect CBF directly or, alternately, that IL-8 secretion induced by GA enhances CBF (Choi et al., 2010). Furthermore, it is possible that the initial activation of CBF induced by Il-8 could be reverted after longer periods of inflammation, with a deleterious effect upon mucociliary clearance.

Our results suggest that plasma exudation of serum molecules such as GA onto the airway epithelium could induce an inflammatory response, initially producing IL-8 secretion and modifying mucociliary transport by the effect on ciliary activity. A progression of this inflammatory response could involve the release of other chemotactic cytokines, an influx of polymorphonuclear neutrophils, and contribute to airway inflammation observed in chronic airway diseases (Reutershan and Ley, 2004). Future directions may include measurement of GA in several airway diseases, including SARS-CoV-2, and correlate GA levels with patient clinical outcomes. Recent studies have contributed to identifying the location of the receptor of advanced glycation end products (RAGE) in the airways, as a mediator of GA effects on the systemic inflammatory response (Hoonhorst et al., 2016). A study reported by Demling et al. (2005) reported that the RAGE receptor on alveolar epithelial type 1 cells (AT 1) was localized in the basolateral membrane, suggesting a morphological role for the receptor by strengthening the adherence of ATI cells to the alveolar basement membrane. In our study, we used different cellular epithelial cell types, including polarized and non-polarized cells, but we did not identify the specific location of the RAGE receptor. Future studies using double chambers to produce polarized cell cultures will be necessary to identify the RAGE receptor location and activation on the apical or basal membrane by GA inducing an inflammatory response, helping to identify potential blockers to prevent the deleterious effect of AGE, including GA, on the airway epithelium.

In our study, we used different epithelial cell types including polarized and non-polarized cells. However, we did not identify the specific location of the RAGE receptor. Future studies using double chambers to produced polarized cell culture will be necessary to identify the RAGE receptor location and activation on the apical or basal membrane using GA to induce an inflammatory response to assist in identifying potential blockers to prevent the deleterious effects of AGE including GA, on the airway epithelium.

In summary, our results suggest that plasma exudation of serum molecules such as GA onto the airway epithelium can induce an inflammatory response, initially producing IL-8 secretion and modifying mucociliary transport by the effect on ciliary activity. A progression of this inflammatory response could involve the release of other chemotactic cytokines, an influx of polymorphonuclear neutrophils, and contribute to airway inflammation observed in chronic airway diseases. Future directions may include measurement of GA in several airway diseases, including SARS-CoV-2, and correlate GA levels with patient clinical outcomes. Recent studies have contributed to our understanding by identifying the location of the receptor of advanced glycation end products (RAGE) in the airways, as a mediator of GA effects on the inflammatory response (Buckley and Ehrhardt, 2010; Hoonhorst et al., 2016). However, a study by Demling et al. (2005) reported that the RAGE receptor on the alveolar epithelial type I cells (AT I) was localized in the basolateral membrane, suggesting a morphological role for the receptor by strengthening the adherence of AT I cells to the alveolar basal membrane.

CONCLUSION

In conclusion, our findings suggest that a serum protein, GA, may have an important role in the airway inflammatory response.

AUTHOR CONTRIBUTIONS

MA, TH, SS, and MV planned the experimental designs. MA, RS, TH, MP, KD, MR, SS, and MV wrote the manuscript. MA and SS identified a serum factor that induced inflammation. TH and MP identified glycated albumin as the inflammatory protein. MP performed the dose escalation experiments. KD, MR, and MV performed the experiments on CBF. All authors contributed to the revision and final draft of the manuscript.

ACKNOWLEDGMENTS

We thank Dr. Ernest Weymueller from the Department of Otolaryngology, University of Washington, Seattle, WA; Dr. Claudia Gonzalez and Dr. Claudio Callejas, from the Department of Otolaryngology, Faculty of Medicine, Pontificia Universidad Católica de Chile; Carmen Llados and Llilian Arzola PhD from the Department of Physiology, Faculty of Biological Science, Pontificia Universidad Católica de Chile for tissue; Christine Halbert PhD, Research Scientist, Fred Hutchinson Cancer Research Center, Seattle, WA, for the CF cell line; and Marissa Anne Lopez Pier PhD U Arizona and Wen Yu Wong PhD U Arizona for their detailed review of the manuscript.

REFERENCES

Aitken, M., Villalon, M., Pier, M., Verdugo, P., and Nameroff, M. (1995). Characterization of a marker for tracheal basal cells. *Exp. Lung. Res.* 21, 1–16. doi: 10.3109/01902149509031741

Aitken, M., Villalon, M., Pier, M., Verdugo, P., and Nameroff, M. (1993). Characterization of a marker of differentiation for tracheal ciliated cells independent of ciliation. *Am. J. Respir. Cell Mol. Biol.* 9, 26–32. doi: 10.1165/ajrcmb/9.1.26

Allen-Gipson, D., Romberger, D. J., Forget, M. A., May, K. L., Sisson, J. H., and Wyatt, T. A. (2004). IL-8 inhibits isoproterenol-stimulated ciliary beat frequency in bovine bronchial epithelial cells. *J. Aerosol. Med.* 17, 107–115. doi: 10.1089/0894268041457138

Barrera, N., Morales, B., and Villalón, M. (2004). Plasma and intracellular membrane inositol 1, 4, 5-trisphosphate receptors mediate the Ca(2+) increase associated with the ATP-induced increase in ciliary beat frequency. *Am. J. Physiol. Cell Physiol.* 287, C1114–C1124.

Bian, Z., Elner, S. G., Strieter, R. M., Glass, M. B., Lukacs, N. W., Kunkel, S. L., et al. (1996). Glycated serum albumin induces chemokine gene expression in human retinal pigment epithelial cells. *J. Leukoc. Biol.* 60, 405–414. doi: 10.1002/jlb.60.3.405

Bian, Z., Elner, V. M., Yoshida, A., Kunkel, S. L., and Elner, S. G. (2001). Signaling pathways for glycated human serum albumin-induced IL-8 and MCP-1 secretion in human RPE cells. *Invest. Ophthalmol. Vis. Sci.* 42, 1660–1668.

Buckley, S. T., and Ehrhardt, C. (2010). The Receptor for advanced glycation end products (RAGE) and the Lung. *J. Biomed. Biotechnol.* 2010:917108. doi: 10.1155/2010/917108

Chen, J., Takeno, S., Osada, R., Ueda, T., and Yayin, K. (2000). Modulation of ciliary activity by tumor necrosis factor-alpha in cultured sinus epithelial cells. Possible roles of nitric oxide. *Hiroshima J. Med. Sci.* 49, 49–55.

Choi, K., Park, J. W., Kim, H. Y., Kim, Y. H., Kim, S. M., Son, Y. H., et al. (2010). Cellular factors involved in CXCL8 expression induced by glycated serum albumin in vascular smooth muscle cells. *Atherosclerosis* 209, 58–65. doi: 10.1016/j.atherosclerosis.2009.08.030

Cohen, M., Hud, E., and Wu, V. Y. (1994). Amelioration of diabetic nephropathy by treatment with monoclonal antibodies against glycated albumin. *Kidney Int.* 45, 1673–1679. doi: 10.1038/ki.1994.219

Cowley, E., Wang, C. G., Gosselin, D., Radzioch, D., and Eidelman, D. H. (1997). Mucociliary clearance in cystic fibrosis knockout mice infected with *Pseudomonas aeruginosa*. *Eur. Respir. J.* 10, 2312–2318. doi: 10.1183/09031936.97.10102312

Cui, X., Chen, X., Yu, C. J., Yang, J., Lin, Z. P., Yin, M., et al. (2015). Increased expression of toll-like receptors 2 and 4 and related cytokines in persistent allergic rhinitis. *Otolaryngol. Head Neck Surg.* 152, 233–238. doi: 10.1177/0194599814562173

Dahrouj, M., Desjardins, D. M., Liu, Y., Crosson, C. E., and Ablonczy, Z. (2015). Receptor mediated disruption of retinal pigment epithelium function in acute glycated-albumin exposure. *Exp. Eye Res.* 137, 50–56. doi: 10.1016/j.exer.2015.06.004

del Campo, R., Martinez, E., del Fresno, C., Alenda, R., Gómez-Piña, V., Fernández-Ruíz, I., et al. (2011). Translocated LPS might cause endotoxin tolerance in circulating monocytes of cystic fibrosis patients. *PLoS One* 6:e295777. doi: 10.1371/journal.pone.0029577

Demling, N., Ehrhardt, C., Kasper, M., Laue, M., Knels, L., and Rieber, E. P. (2005). Promotion of cell adherence and spreading: a novel function of RAGE, the highly selective differentiation marker of human alveolar epithelial type I cells. *Cell Tissue Res.* 323, 475–488. doi: 10.1007/s00441-005-0069-0

Dolhofer, R., and Wieland, O. H. (1980). Increased glycosylation of serum albumin in diabetes mellitus. *Diabetes* 29, 417–422. doi: 10.2337/diabetes.29.6.417

Gonzalez, C., Espinosa, M., Sanchez, M. T., Droguett, K., Rios, M., Fonseca, X., et al. (2013). Epithelial cell culture from human adenoids: a funcional study model for ciliated and secretory cells. *Biomed. Res. Int.* 2013:478713.

Gras, D., Tiers, L., Vachier, I., de Senneville, L. D., Bourdin, A., Godard, P., et al. (2010). Regulation of CXCR/IL-8 in human airway epithelial cells. *Int. Arch. Allergy Immunol.* 152, 140–150. doi: 10.1159/000265535

Halbert, C., Aitken, M. L., and Miller, A. D. (1996). Retroviral vectors efficiently transduce basal and secretory airway epithelial cells *in vitro* resulting in persistent gene expression in organotypic culture. *Hum. Gene. Ther.* 7, 1871–1881. doi: 10.1089/hum.1996.7.15-1871

Herder, C., Haastert, B., Muller-Scholze, S., Koenig, W., Thorand, B., Holle, R., et al. (2005). Association of systemic chemokine concentrations with impaired glucose tolerance and type 2 diabetes: results from the Cooperative Health Research in the Region of Augsburg Survey S4 (KORA S4). *Diabetes* 54, S11–S17.

Hermoso, M., Barrera, N., Morales, B., Perez, S., and Villalon, M. (2001). Platelet activating factor increases ciliary activity in the hamster oviduct through epithelial production of prostaglandin E2. *Pflugers Arch.* 442, 336–345. doi: 10.1007/s004240100550

Hollander, C., Sitkauskiene, B., Sakalauskas, R., Westin, U., and Janciauskiene, S. M. (2007). Serum and bronchial lavage fluid concentrations of IL-8, SLPI, sCD14 and sICAM-1 in patients with COPD and asthma. *Respir. Med.* 101, 1947–1953. doi: 10.1016/j.rmed.2007.04.010

Hoonhorst, S. J. M., Lo Tam Loi, A. T., Pouwels, S. D., Faiz, A., Telenga, E. D., van den Burge, M., et al. (2016). Advanced glycation endproducts and their receptor in different body compartments in COPD. *Respir. Res.* 17:46. doi: 10.1186/s12931-016-0363-2

Jones, I., Owens, D. R., Williams, S., Ryder, R. E., Birtwell, A. J., Jones, M. K., et al. (1983). Glycosylated serum albumin: an intermediate index of diabetic control. *Diabetes Care* 6, 501–503. doi: 10.2337/diacare.6.5.501

Kakazu, E., Ueno, Y., Kondo, Y., Inoue, J., Ninomiya, M., Kimura, O., et al. (2011). Plasma L-Cystine/L-Glutamate imbalance increases tumor necrosis factor-Alpha from CD14+ circulating monocytes in patients with advanced cirrhosis. *PLoS One* 6:e23402. doi: 10.1371/journal.pone.0023402

Keatings, V., Collins, P. D., Scott, D. M., and Barnes, P. J. (1996). Differences in interleukin-8 and tumor necrosis factor-alpha in induced sputum from patients with chronic obstructive pulmonary disease or asthma. *Am. J. Respir. Crit. Care Med.* 153, 530–534. doi: 10.1164/ajrccm.153.2.8564092

Khan, T., Wagener, J. S., Bost, T., Martinez, J., Accurso, F. J., and Riches, D. W. (1995). Early pulmonary inflammation in infants with cystic fibrosis. *Am. J. Respir. Crit. Care Med.* 151, 1075–1082.

Knowles, M. R., and Boucher, R. C. (2002). Mucus clearance as a primary innate defense mechanism for mammalian airways. *J. Clin. Invest.* 109, 571–577. doi: 10.1172/jci0215217

Koblizek, V., Tomsova, M., Cermakova, E., Papousek, P., Pracharova, S., Mandalia, R. A., et al. (2011). Impairment of nasal mucociliary clearance in former smokers with stable chronic obstructive pulmonary disease relates to the presence of a chronic bronchitis phenotype. *Rhinology* 49, 397–406.

Konstan, M., Hilliard, K. A., Norvell, T. M., and Berger, M. (1994). Bronchoalveolar lavage findings in cystic fibrosis patients with stable, clinically mild lung disease suggest ongoing infection and inflammation. *Am. J. Respir. Crit. Care Med.* 150, 448–454. doi: 10.1164/ajrccm.150.2.8049828

Kwon, O., Au, B. T., Collins, P. D., Adcock, I. M., Mak, J. C., Robbins, R. R., et al. (1994). Tumor necrosis factor-induced interleukin-8 expression in cultured human airway epithelial cells. *Am. J. Physiol.* 267, L398–L405.

Lamblin, C., Gosset, P., Tillie-Leblond, I., Saulnier, F., Marquette, C. H., Wallaert, B., et al. (1998). Bronchial neutrophilia in patients with noninfectious status asthmaticus. *Am. J. Respir. Crit. Care Med.* 157, 394–402. doi: 10.1164/ajrccm.157.2.97-02099

Levine, S. (1995). Bronchial epithelial cell-cytokine interactions in airway inflammation. *J. Invest. Med.* 43, 241–249.

Lieb, T., Forteza, R., and Salathe, M. (2000). Hyaluronic acid in cultures ovine tracheal cells and its effect on ciliary beat frequency *in vitro*. *J. Aerosol. Med.* 13, 231–237. doi: 10.1089/jam.2000.13.231

Ma, W., Lee, S. E., Guo, J., Qu, W., Hudson, B. I., Schmidt, A. M., et al. (2007). RAGE ligand upregulation of VEGF secretion in ARPE-19 cells. *Invest. Ophthalmol. Vis. Sci.* 48, 1355–1361. doi: 10.1167/iovs.06-0738

Marini, M., Vittori, E., Hollemborg, J., and Mattoli, S. (1992). Expression of the potent inflammatory cytokines, granulocyte-macrophage-colony-stimulating factor and interleukin-6 and interleukin-8, in bronchial epithelial cells of patients with asthma. *J. Allergy Clin. Immunol.* 89, 1001–1009. doi: 10.1016/0091-6749(92)90223-o

McElvaney, N., Nakamura, H., Birrer, P., Hébert, C. A., Wong, W. L., Alphonso, M., et al. (1992). Modulation of airway inflammation in cystic fibrosis. In vivo suppression of interleukin-8 levels on the respiratory epithelial surface by aerosolization of recombinant secretory leukoprotease inhibitor. *J. Clin. Invest.* 90, 1296–1301. doi: 10.1172/jci115994

Milla, C., Warwick, W. J., and Moran, A. (2000). Trends in pulmonary function in patients with cystic fibrosis correlate with the degree of glucose intolerance at baseline. *Am. J. Respir. Crit. Care Med.* 162, 891–895. doi: 10.1164/ajrccm.162.3.9904075

Milutinovic, P., Alcorn, J. F., Englert, J. M., Crum, L. T., and Oury, T. D. (2012). The receptor for advanced glycation end products is a central mediator of asthma. *Am. J. Pathol.* 181, 1215–1225. doi: 10.1016/j.ajpath.2012.06.031

Mizunoe, S., Shuto, T., Suzuki, S., Matsumoto, C., Watanabe, K., Ueno-Shuto, K., et al. (2012). Synergism between interleukin (IL)-17 and Toll-like receptor 2 and 4 signals to induce IL-8 expression in cystic fibrosis airway epithelial cell. *J. Pharmacol. Sci.* 118, 512–520. doi: 10.1254/jphs.11240fp

Nakamura, H., Yoshimura, K., Jaffe, H. A., and Crystal, R. G. (1991). Interleukin-8 gene expression in human bronchial epithelial cells. *J. Biol. Chem.* 266, 19611–19617. doi: 10.1016/s0021-9258(18)55037-7

Nakamura, H., Yoshimura, K., McElvaney, N. G., and Crystal, R. G. (1992). Neutrophil elastase in respiratory epithelial lining fluid of individuals with cystic fibrosis induces interleukin-8 gene expression in a human bronchial epithelial cell line. *J. Clin. Invest.* 89, 1478–1484. doi: 10.1172/jci115738

O'Sullivan, B., and Fredman, S. D. (2009). Cystic fibrosis. *Lancet* 373, 1891–1904.

Papathanasiou, A., Djahanbakhch, O., Saridogan, E., and Lyons, R. A. (2008). The effect of interleukin-6 on ciliary beat frequency in the human fallopian tube. *Fertil Steril* 90, 391–394. doi: 10.1016/j.fertnstert.2007.07.1379

Reutershan, J., and Ley, K. (2004). Bench-to-bedside review: acute respiratory distress syndrome - how neutrophils migrate into the lung. *Crit. Care* 8, 453–461.

Rubenstein, D., Maria, Z., and Yin, W. (2011). Glycated albumin modulates endothelial cell thrombogenic and inflammatory responses. *J. Diabetes Sci. Technol.* 5, 703–713. doi: 10.1177/193229681100500325

Schmid, A., Sutto, Z., Schmid, N., Novak, L., Ivonnet, P., Horvath, G., et al. (2010). Decreased soluble adenylyl cyclase activity in cystic fibrosis is related to defective apical bicarbonate exchange and affects ciliary beat frequency regulation. *J. Biol. Chem.* 285, 29998–30007. doi: 10.1074/jbc.m110.113621

Seybold, Z., Mariassy, A. T., Stroh, D., Kim, C. S., Gazeroglu, H., and Wanner, A. (1990). Mucociliary interaction *in vitro*: effects of physiological and inflammatory stimuli. *J. Appl. Physiol.* 68, 1421–1426. doi: 10.1152/jappl.1990.68.4.1421

Shen, J., Chen, B., and Cohen, N. A. (2012). Keratinocyte chemoattractant (interleukin-8) regulation of sinonasal cilia function in a murine model. *Int. Forum. Allergy Rhinol.* 2, 75–79. doi: 10.1002/alr.20087

Sorci, G., Riuzzi, F., Giambanco, I., and Donato, R. (1833). RAGE in tissue homeostasis, repair and regeneration. *Biochim. Biophys. Acta* 10:2013.

Standiford, T., Kunkel, S. L., Basha, M. A., Chensue, S. W., Lynch, J. P., Toews, G. B., et al. (1990). Interleukin-8 gene expression by a pulmonary epithelial cell line. A model for cytokine networks in the lung. *J. Clin. Invest.* 86, 1945–1953. doi: 10.1172/jci114928

Sternberg, D., Gowda, R., Mehra, D., Qu, W., Weinberg, A., Twaddell, W., et al. (2008). Blockade of receptor for advanced glycation end product attenuates pulmonary reperfusion injury in mice. *J. Thorac. Cardiovasc. Surg.* 136, 1576–1585. doi: 10.1016/j.jtcvs.2008.05.032

Svenson, C., Gronneberg, R., Andersson, M., Alkner, U., Andersson, O., Billing, B., et al. (1995). Allergen challenge-induced entry of alpha-2-macroglobulin and trystase into human nasal and bronhial airways. *J. Allergy Clin. Immunol.* 96, 239–246. doi: 10.1016/s0091-6749(95)70013-7

van der Baan, B. (2000). Ciliary function. *Acta Otorhinolaryngol. Belg.* 54, 293–298.

Waugh, D. J. J., and Wilson, C. (2008). The interleukin-8 pathway in cancer. *Clin. Cancer Res.* 14, 6735–6741. doi: 10.1158/1078-0432.ccr-07-4843

Whitsett, J., and Alenghat, T. (2014). Respiratory epithelial cells orchestrate pulmonary innate immunity. *Nat. Immunol.* 16, 27–37. doi: 10.1038/ni.3045

Xie, J., Méndez, J. D., Méndez-Valenzuela, V., and Aguilar-Hernández, M. M. (2013). Cellular signaling of the receptor for advanced glycation end products (RAGE). *Cell. Signal.* 25, 2185–2197. doi: 10.1016/j.cellsig.2013.06.013

13

An Inflamed Human Alveolar Model for Testing the Efficiency of Anti-Inflammatory Drugs *in vitro*

Barbara Drasler[1], Bedia Begum Karakocak[1], Esma Bahar Tankus[1], Hana Barosova[1], Jun Abe[2], Mauro Sousa de Almeida[1], Alke Petri-Fink[1,3] and Barbara Rothen-Rutishauser[1]*

[1] Institut Adolphe Merkle, Faculté des Sciences et de Médecine, Université de Fribourg, Fribourg, Switzerland, [2] Department of Oncology, Microbiology and Immunology, Faculty of Science and Medicine, University of Fribourg, Fribourg, Switzerland, [3] Département de Chimie, Faculté des Sciences et de Médecine, Université de Fribourg, Fribourg, Switzerland

***Correspondence:**
Barbara Rothen-Rutishauser
barbara.rothen@unifr.ch

A large number of prevalent lung diseases is associated with tissue inflammation. Clinically, corticosteroid therapies are applied systemically or via inhalation for the treatment of lung inflammation, and a number of novel therapies are being developed that require preclinical testing. In alveoli, macrophages and dendritic cells play a key role in initiating and diminishing pro-inflammatory reactions and, in particular, macrophage plasticity (M1 and M2 phenotypes shifts) has been reported to play a significant role in these reactions. Thus far, no studies with *in vitro* lung epithelial models have tested the comparison between systemic and direct pulmonary drug delivery. Therefore, the aim of this study was to develop an inflamed human alveolar epithelium model and to test the resolution of LPS-induced inflammation *in vitro* with a corticosteroid, methylprednisolone (MP). A specific focus of the study was the macrophage phenotype shifts in response to these stimuli. First, human monocyte-derived macrophages were examined for phenotype shifts upon exposure to lipopolysaccharide (LPS), followed by treatment with MP. A multicellular human alveolar model, composed of macrophages, dendritic cells, and epithelial cells, was then employed for the development of inflamed models. The models were used to test the anti-inflammatory potency of MP by monitoring the secretion of pro-inflammatory mediators (interleukin [IL]-8, tumor necrosis factor-α [TNF-α], and IL-1β) through four different approaches, mimicking clinical scenarios of inflammation and treatment. In macrophage monocultures, LPS stimulation shifted the phenotype towards M1, as demonstrated by increased release of IL-8 and TNF-α and altered expression of phenotype-associated surface markers (CD86, CD206). MP treatment of inflamed macrophages reversed the phenotype towards M2. In multicellular models, increased pro-inflammatory reactions after LPS exposure were observed, as demonstrated by protein secretion and gene expression measurements. In all scenarios, among the tested mediators the most pronounced anti-inflammatory effect of MP was observed for IL-8. Our findings demonstrate that our inflamed multicellular human lung model is a promising tool for the evaluation of anti-inflammatory potency of drug candidates *in vitro*. With the presented setup, our model allows a meaningful comparison of the systemic vs. inhalation administration routes for the evaluation of the efficacy of a drug *in vitro*.

Keywords: inflammation, lung, *in vitro*, multicellular models, macrophage phenotype, anti-inflammatory drugs, corticosteroids

INTRODUCTION

Lung inflammation plays an important role in the pathogenesis of a number of respiratory diseases, such as pneumonia, acute respiratory distress syndrome, or chronic inflammatory disorders such as asthma and chronic obstructive pulmonary disease (Johnson and Matthay, 2010; Roth, 2014). As the lung is the vital organ for gas exchange, excessive inflammation in the lung tissue can be life-threatening (Moldoveanu et al., 2009). Lung tissue inflammation, as well as the anti-inflammatory reactions, involve complex interactions between and among the immune cells and the structural lung cells (Nicod, 2005; Holt et al., 2008). The airways and the lung parenchyma contain dense networks of immune cells, e.g., dendritic cells and alveolar macrophages, which play a key role in regulating the body's immune responses (Holt et al., 2008). Dendritic cells are professional antigen-presenting cells (APCs) linking innate and adaptive immunity (Banchereau and Steinman, 1998; Cook and MacDonald, 2016). Another type of APCs, macrophages, are located in the apical part of the epithelium, and their main role is professional phagocytosis (Brain, 1988; Lehnert, 1992; Hussell and Bell, 2014). Macrophages and dendritic cells are capable of triggering rapid pro-inflammatory reactions in response to inhaled foreign materials, as well as bacterial, viral, and fungal infections through the release of pro-inflammatory mediators, such as tumor necrosis factor α (TNF-α), interleukin (IL)-1β, and IL-8, along with the increased release of reactive oxygen and nitrogen species (Condon et al., 2011; Laskin et al., 2011). In particular, macrophages also play a pivotal role in the resolution of alveolar inflammation (Frankenberger et al., 2005; Moldoveanu et al., 2009; Tu et al., 2017; Lu et al., 2018). The biological activity of macrophages is mediated by their phenotypically distinct subpopulations, i.e., the M1 and M2 phenotypes, which develop and shift in response to the mediators in their microenvironment. According to the basic dichotomic macrophage polarization classification, M1 macrophage polarization, the pro-inflammatory phenotype is stimulated by specific pathogens (Atri et al., 2018). The M1 phenotype is associated with the release of pro-inflammatory mediators, with the expression of toll-like receptors (TLR-2 and TLR-4) and co-stimulatory molecules, such as cluster of differentiation (CD) 86 (Martinez and Gordon, 2014). The activity of M1 macrophages is balanced by those with M2 phenotypes through the secretion of anti-inflammatory mediators (Martinez and Gordon, 2014). The M2 subset is stimulated with anti-inflammatory agents, such as steroids (Laskin et al., 2011; Wang et al., 2014; Jaroch et al., 2018; Desgeorges et al., 2019). The M2 phenotype is associated with expression of the mannose receptor-1 (CD206) as well as macrophage scavenger receptors (CD204 and CD163) (Gordon, 2003).

Due to the distinctive roles of macrophages in the lung, they have been proposed as the main cellular targets in the treatment of lung-inflammation-related disorders (Laskin et al., 2011). Clinically, immunosuppressant drugs, such as corticosteroids, among them methylprednisolone (MP), play an integral role in anti-inflammatory treatments of pulmonary diseases, particularly in asthma, acute lung injury, and acute respiratory distress syndrome (Silva et al., 2009; Barnes, 2011; Marik et al., 2011; Liu et al., 2013). The efficacy of corticosteroids in suppressing lung inflammation has been confirmed by both systemic administration and inhalation (Sethi and Singhal, 2008; Higham et al., 2015). MP has been shown to attenuate acute lung injury, induced with bacterial endotoxin lipopolysaccharide (LPS), via promoting macrophage polarization into the M2 subset (Tu et al., 2017). Although corticosteroids are widely used agents for the treatment of lung inflammation, strong systemic side effects such as respiratory tract infections, allergies, wound healing impairment, and bronchitis have been reported (Liu et al., 2013; Waljee et al., 2017). As a result, alternative anti-inflammatory therapies are currently being investigated (da Silva et al., 2017).

The role of macrophage phenotypes in lung inflammation and its resolution has been investigated extensively in murine models *in vivo* (Leite-Junior et al., 2008; Katsura et al., 2015; Florentin et al., 2018; Lu et al., 2018). The anti-inflammatory activity of corticosteroids in murine lung epithelia has also been investigated *in vivo*, both for the treatment of allergic asthma (Klaßen et al., 2017) and in order to determine their contribution to fetal lung maturation (Habermehl et al., 2011). On the other hand, based on the findings of clinical studies, it has been proposed that distinctive macrophage phenotype populations play an important role in anti-inflammatory treatment, e.g., in that of chronic obstructive pulmonary disease with poor response to corticosteroids (Barnes, 2011; Chana et al., 2014). Nevertheless, it should be noted that dendritic cells and the alveolar epithelium also contribute significantly to glucocorticoid-mediated immunosuppressive effects (Zach et al., 1993; Piemonti et al., 1999; Rozkova et al., 2006; Klaßen et al., 2017).

With respect to human lung models, mono- and multicellular models, primary or cell line-derived, have been developed to mimic human airway epithelia and the alveolar epithelial-endothelial tissue barrier (Hermanns et al., 2004; Steimer et al., 2005; Bur and Lehr, 2008; Haghi et al., 2015; Hittinger et al., 2016; Yonker et al., 2017; Costa et al., 2019; Artzy-Schnirman et al., 2020). These models have been employed in investigations of lung inflammation to study various lung diseases and disorders, such as cystic fibrosis (Castellani et al., 2018), chronic obstructive pulmonary disorder (Haghi et al., 2015; Zhou et al., 2019), and acute respiratory distress syndrome (Viola et al., 2019). Also, these models have been employed to investigate the safety and efficacy of aerosolized and dry powder formulations for pulmonary drug delivery (Hittinger et al., 2016), including that of steroid drugs (Bur and Lehr, 2008; Haghi et al., 2015). Finally, an *in vitro* human airway model differentiated from primary human bronchial cells has been proposed for pharmacokinetics studies (Rivera-Burgos et al., 2016). LPS is a major component of the outer membrane of Gram-negative bacteria, such as *Haemophilus influenzae*, which are considered one of the main causes of infectious lung diseases (King, 2012). For induction of inflammation, LPS is often used as a stimulus to investigate lung inflammation *in vitro*, to study the efficacy of drugs or vaccinations, or to elucidate the mechanisms of the pulmonary response to bacterial ligands (Knapp, 2009; Bisig et al., 2019;

Nova et al., 2019). To date, however, there have been no studies demonstrating a comparison of drug delivery approaches, i.e., systemic vs. direct pulmonary delivery of anti-inflammatory drugs, using 3D multicellular systems of human lung epithelial tissue *in vitro*.

Given this paucity and the high potential utility of such a comparative study, this study was aimed at the development of an inflamed, immunocompetent, multicellular human lung model, including macrophages and dendritic cells. The simultaneous presence of both immune cell types is important in the cellular interplay in response to exposure to an inflammatory mediator, such as the endotoxin LPS (Bisig et al., 2019; Nova et al., 2019). As a model cell type for human alveolar pneumocytes, the epithelial A549 cell line, isolated from a pulmonary adenocarcinoma, was used. A549 cells possess characteristics of squamous type II epithelial cells of the alveolar region; these cells carry lamellar bodies containing densely packed phospholipids, the constituents of the pulmonary surfactant (Shapiro et al., 1978), and release the surfactant upon exposure to air-liquid interface (ALI) (Blank et al., 2006). In this study, a widely used anti-inflammatory drug, the corticosteroid MP, was initially tested for its ability to induce macrophage phenotype shifts in primary human monocyte-derived macrophages (MDMs) from the pro-inflammatory (M1) towards the anti-inflammatory (M2) subset, and vice-versa. Then, a 3D multicellular human lung epithelial tissue barrier model composed of the same macrophage type along with an alveolar epithelial cell layer, and monocyte-derived dendritic cells (MDDCs) (Rothen-Rutishauser et al., 2005), was stimulated with LPS from either the basal or apical side, mimicking systemic or alveolar lumen-derived inflammation, respectively. These inflamed lung models were further treated with MP in the co-presence of the pro-inflammatory stimulus (LPS) applied from the opposite side of the human lung model, simulating either intravenous drug administration or aerosolized drug administration via inhalation. In the last step, the LPS was removed prior to the anti-inflammatory treatment, mimicking a lower degree of inflammation in the tissue, and the steroid therapy was applied via the respiratory route, i.e., onto the apical side of the tissue. We employed the adverse outcome pathway (AOP) concept for pulmonary fibrosis as it involves a strong inflammatory component. As a result, the focus herein is on so-called key event two (KE2), which is the release of pro-inflammatory cytokines (e.g., tumor necrosis factor-alpha [TNF-α], interleukin [IL]-1β, and IL-8) and the loss of alveolar barrier integrity (Labib et al., 2016; Vietti et al., 2016; Villeneuve et al., 2018).

Herein, we provide experimental evidence for suppression of pro-inflammatory reactions *in vitro* using a widely used anti-inflammatory drug, a corticosteroid MP. We discuss these reactions with respect to the macrophage phenotype shifts towards pro- and anti-inflammatory subsets. We demonstrate the responsiveness of our 3D human lung model to pro- and anti-inflammatory agents, both at the pro-inflammatory protein secretion and gene expression levels. The presented model may serve as a diseased human lung model for *in vitro* pre-clinical testing of the safety, potency, and efficacy of newly developed anti-inflammatory formulations and also can serve as a diseased model to assess occupational exposures to all types of aerosols.

MATERIALS AND METHODS

Chemicals, Reagents, and Laboratory Conditions

All the chemical reagents were purchased from Sigma-Aldrich (Switzerland), while all cell culture reagents were purchased from Gibco and Thermo Fisher Scientific (Switzerland) unless stated otherwise. MilliQ water (ultrapure water of 18.2 MΩ.cm) was used in all the experiments. Methylprednisolone (MP; Cayman Chemical, Ann Arbor, MI, United States) powder was dissolved in absolute ethanol to 5 mg/mL. At every step during cell culture and exposure, cells were kept in an incubator under controlled conditions (humidified atmosphere, 37°C, 5% CO_2). Cell numbers were determined using an EVE^{TM} bench-top automated cell counter (Witec AG, Switzerland) with the trypan blue exclusion method (0.4% trypan blue solution in phosphate buffer saline [PBS]).

Isolation and Differentiation of Primary Human Peripheral Blood-Derived Immune Cells

Human MDMs and MDDCs were prepared from monocytes isolated from buffy coats provided by the Swiss Transfusion Center (Bern, Switzerland), as described previously (Barosova et al., 2020). In brief, isolated blood monocytes were cultured in 6-well tissue culture plates (Corning, FALCON®, United States) for six days at a density of 10^6 cells/mL in 3 mL Roswell Park Memorial Institute (RPMI)-1640 cell culture medium supplemented with 10% (v/v) fetal bovine serum (42G1189K), 2 mM L-glutamine, and penicillin-streptomycin (100 units/mL and 100 μg/mL, respectively), referred to as the complete cell culture medium (cRPMI). For MDM differentiation, 10 ng/mL of macrophage colony-stimulating factor (M-CSF) was added to cRPMI. MDDC differentiation was performed in the presence of 10 ng/mL of recombinant human interleukin 4 (IL-4) and 10 ng/mL of granulocyte-macrophage colony-stimulating factor (GM-CSF; all the factors were obtained from Milteny Biotec, Germany). Experiments involving primary monocyte isolation from human blood were approved by the committee of the Federal Office for Public Health Switzerland (reference number: 611-1, Meldung A110635/2) for the Adolphe Merkle Institute.

Macrophage Phenotype Shifts: Monoculture Experiments

Macrophage Challenge With Pro- and Anti-inflammatory Agents

After six days of MDMs differentiation, cRPMI containing the growth factor was aspirated and replaced with either 2.5 mL fresh cRPMI or cRPMI containing lipopolysaccharide (LPS; 1 μg/mL; isolated from *E. coli*, strain O55:B5, Sigma-Aldrich, Switzerland). After 24 h, cRPMI containing MP or vehicle was added to the cells (the summary of the treatments is presented in **Table 1**).

TABLE 1 | Treatments of the differentiated MDMs.

Sample Description	0 to 24 h	24 to 48 h
Untreated cells	cRPMI (3 mL)	cRPMI not changed
Negative control	cRPMI (2.5 mL)	Vehicle (0.5 mL)
LPS	cRPMI (2.5 mL) with LPS (1 μg/mL)	Vehicle (0.5 mL)
LPS + MP10	cRPMI (2.5 mL) with LPS (1 μg/mL)	MP (0.5 mL of 0.06 mM stock in cRPMI). Final concentration 0.01 mM
MP control	cRPMI (2.5 mL)	MP (0.5 mL of 0.06 mM stock in cRPMI). Final concentration 0.01 mM
IL-4+IL-13 (M2 control)	cRPMI with IL-4 and IL-13 (20 ng/mL)	Treatment not changed
Triton X-100 (positive control for LDH)	cRPMI (3 mL)	Triton X-100 (0.3 mL). Final concentration 0.2% (v/v)

Vehicle is a solution of absolute ethanol (0.005% in cRPMI; v/v).

Flow Cytometry

Immunostaining for cell surface protein markers

After stimulation of MDMs, supernatant and non-adherent cells were removed, centrifuged (500 RCF, 5 min), and kept at 4°C or −80°C until being subjected to a cell viability assay or enzyme-linked immunosorbent assay (ELISA), respectively. Adherent cells were gently washed with PBS and detached from the wells using a cell scraper (SARSTEDT, United States) in fresh PBS. Cells from two identically treated wells in a 6-well plate were pooled in flow cytometry tubes (FALCON® 5 mL Polystyrene Round-Bottom Tube, Corning, Switzerland), counted, centrifuged (5702R, Eppendorf; 500 RCF, 5 min), and resuspended in cold flow cytometry buffer (PBS with 1% BSA, 0.1% NaN3, 1 mM ethylenediaminetetraacetic acid [EDTA] at pH 7.4). Before antibody labeling, cells were incubated with Fc-receptor-blocking reagent (Miltenyi Biotec, Germany) according to the supplier's protocol. After incubation for 10 min, the suspensions were split into two separate flow cytometry tubes at a density of 1×10^6 cells/mL for staining or as unstained controls.

Cells were stained with Alexa Fluor 488 conjugated anti-human CD86 (B7-2) monoclonal antibody (clone IT2.2; at 1.25 μg/mL), and APC conjugated anti-human CD206 (MMR) monoclonal antibody (clone 19.2; at 3 μg/mL), as M1 and M2 macrophage markers, respectively, in cold flow cytometry buffer containing 2 μM 4,6-diamidino-2-phenylindole (DAPI; Sigma Aldrich, Switzerland) for dead cell exclusion. Both antibodies were obtained from eBioscience™ (Thermo Fisher Scientific, Switzerland). Additional untreated samples were prepared for fluorescence minus one control staining using OneComp™ ebeads compensation beads (Thermo Fisher Scientific, Switzerland) to set up the cytometer. After antibody labeling for 30 min at 4°C in the dark, the cells were washed with flow cytometry buffer (3 mL) and centrifuged (500 RCF, 5 min, 4°C). The cell pellet was resuspended with cold flow cytometry buffer and stored at 4°C until data acquisition (up to 2 h). Data were acquired using LSRFortessa (BD Biosciences, Switzerland) and analyzed using FlowJo software (Version 10.6.1, TreeStar, United States).

Cytokine Secretion

The amount of released pro-inflammatory mediators (IL-8, IL-1β, and TNF-α) was quantified using a DuoSet ELISA Development Kit (R&D Systems, Switzerland) according to the supplier's protocol. For IL-8, all the samples were diluted 1:4 (v/v) in reagent diluent for the measured values to remain within the detection limit of the instrument. TNF-α and IL-1β were measured in polystyrene high-binding surface 96-well plates (Corning®, Switzerland) without dilution. Standards and samples were run in triplicate. The concentrations of the cytokines released in the cell culture medium were calculated based on the standard curves and fitted with a four-parameter logistic (4PL) approach using GraphPad Prism 8 software (GraphPad Software Inc., San Diego, CA, United States).

Cell Viability/Membrane Rupture

Cell viability was evaluated by the lactate dehydrogenase (LDH; cytosolic enzyme) released in cRPMI, analyzed in triplicate using LDH cytotoxicity detection kit (Roche Applied Science, Mannheim, Germany) according to the manufacturer's protocol. The absorbance of the colorimetric product was determined spectrophotometrically (Benchmark Microplate reader, BioRad, Switzerland) at 490 nm with a reference wavelength of 630 nm with 30-s intervals for 10 measurements. The values were expressed as fold increase of slopes (0–5 min reaction) of the treated samples relative to those of untreated samples of the multicellular models.

MULTICELLULAR HUMAN LUNG MODEL ASSEMBLY

The multicellular models of human alveolar epithelial type II cell line A549, MDMs, and MDDCs were prepared as previously described (Barosova et al., 2020). In brief, A549 cells were maintained in cRPMI (passage number 5 to 25). A549 cells were seeded on transparent cell culture inserts (surface area of 4.2 cm^2, 3.0 μm pore diameter, high pore density, polyethylene terephthalate [PET] membranes for 6-well plates; Falcon, BD Biosciences, Switzerland) at a cell density of 28.0×10^4 cells/cm^2 in 2 mL of cRPMI at 58×10^4 cells/mL. The membrane inserts with cells were placed in tissue culture plates (6-well plates; Falcon, BD Biosciences, Switzerland) containing 3 mL of cRPMI and cultured for four days to form a confluent monolayer. For the multicellular model composition, membrane inserts with A549 cells were removed from the 6-well plates and placed in a sterile glass petri dish turned upside down. Cells that had grown through the pores on the basal side of the inserts were gently abraded with a cell scraper. MDDCs were pipetted onto the bottom side of the inserts: 300 μL of cell suspension in cRPMI at 98.0×10^4 cells/mL

(29.4×10^4 cells/insert, corresponding to a seeded cell density of 7×10^4 cells/cm^2) and incubated for 70 min at 37°C and 5% CO_2. Membrane inserts were placed back into 6-well plates containing 3 mL of pre-heated fresh cRPMI. Then, 2 mL of a MDM suspension at concentration 2.95×10^4 cells/mL in cRPMI was gently added on the top of the A549 cells on inserts (5.9×10^4 cells/insert, corresponding to 1.4×10^4 cells/cm^2). The assembled multicellular models were exposed for 24 h to air at the ALI to allow for surfactant production by the A549 cells. MDDCs and MDMs prepared from one buffy coat donor and A549 cells from an individual passage were used for each independent experiment. The A549 cell line was purchased from the American Tissue Type Culture Collection (ATCC®CCL-185™) and was authenticated using short tandem repeat (STR) profiling. Cells were regularly tested for the absence of mycoplasma.

Inflamed Model: Induction and Assessment of Pro-inflammatory Reactions

The assembled multicellular model was challenged with 1 μg/mL LPS for 48 h, from either apical or basal compartments. LPS stock (1 mg/mL in water) was diluted in cRPMI. Old cRPMI was aspirated from the bottom compartments in all samples. Then, either cRPMI (3 mL) with LPS was applied to the basal compartment, and nothing to the apical (approach 1), or fresh cRPMI was added to the basal compartment and 0.2 mL of cRPMI with LPS to the apical side, referred to as pseudo-ALI conditions (Endes et al., 2014) (approach 2).

Inflammatory Reactions

Secretion of pro-inflammatory mediators

After the LPS challenge, the concentration of IL-8, IL-1β, and TNF-α released in the cell culture medium in the basal compartment was quantified by ELISA, as described for the monoculture experiments.

Response at Gene Expression Levels

Upon collection of supernatants in the basal compartment, models were washed with PBS, and inserts with cells were cut out of the plastic holders. Half of each insert was incubated in RNA protection buffer (Qiagen, Germany). The cells were removed from the membranes by extensive vortexing and kept at 4°C for up to seven days (the other half was fixed for immunofluorescence staining). Then, RNA isolation was performed using ReliaPrep™ RNA Miniprep Systems (Promega, Switzerland) according to the manufacturer's protocol. RNA concentrations in samples were analyzed with a NanoDrop 2000 spectrophotometer (Thermo Scientific, United States) and stored at −20°C. Complementary DNA (cDNA) was synthesized with the Omniscript RT system (Qiagen, Germany), Oligo dT (Microsynth, Switzerland), and RNasin Inhibitor (Promega, Switzerland). Reverse transcriptase reactions were performed in 10 μL volumes with an RNA concentration of 25 ng/μL (Omniscript RT, Qiagen) and Oligo dT primers (Qiagen). RNase inhibitor (0.25 μL; RNasin Plus RNase Inhibitor, Promega) was added to the reverse transcriptase reactions. A total of 2 μL of the tenfold diluted cDNA was used for real-time PCR in reaction volumes of 10 μL with SYBR Green as reporter dye (Fast SYBR Green master mix, 7500 fast real-time PCR system, Applied Biosystems, United States). The mRNA levels were calculated using the double delta of cycle threshold (ΔΔCt) method, calculated based on the expression of a standard gene (glyceraldehyde-3-phosphate dehydrogenase; GAPDH) and the respective gene expressions in untreated cells. Primer sequences and database accession numbers are listed in the **Supplementary Material (Supplementary Table S1)**.

Suppression of LPS-Induced Pro-inflammatory Reactions

To prepare inflamed cell-culture models, LPS was added either from the basal compartment or from the apical compartments and left to stand for 24 h, following the procedure described above. After the first 24 h, MP was added and left to stand for an additional 24 h while LPS was still present. In approach 1, the MP stock (13 mM in absolute ethanol) was diluted in PBS to the final concentrations of 10 and 100 μM, and 200 μL was applied directly to the apical side of the models. In approach 2, MP stock was diluted in the existing cRPMI in the basolateral compartment to the same final concentrations and left to stand for 24 h. For negative control samples, the vehicle, absolute ethanol, was added at a final concentration of 0.07% or 0.7% to gauge potential biological effects of the solvent alone for comparison with entirely untreated samples. LPS-treated samples were considered as the positive controls for the pro-inflammatory scenario. In parallel, the effects of MP treatments on non-inflamed models were tested following the same procedure as described in approaches 1 and 2, but without LPS in cRPMI. After treatment, the biological responses of the models were assessed by ELISA, real-time RT-qPCR, and confocal microscopy.

Suppression of Pro-inflammatory Reactions Upon LPS Removal

In approaches 3 and 4, inflamed models were established by a 24-h pre-challenge with LPS from the apical side at the pseudo-ALI (**Figure 1**). After 24 h, the apical sides were gently rinsed with PBS, and MP was added to the apical side at the pseudo-ALI for an additional 24 h. In approach 3, the basal cell culture medium was not changed before the MP treatment. In approach 4, the models were washed with PBS from both sides, and cRPMI in the basal compartment was refreshed. Positive controls ("LPS") and "MP only" controls were treated with the vehicle at the pseudo-ALI. Upon completion of the treatment, the biological response was assessed as described above.

Multicellular Model Visualization

Tissue morphology of both LPS-challenged and MP-treated models, immuno-fluorescently stained, was visualized via confocal laser scanning fluorescence microscopy (LSM).

Immunofluorescent Staining

Upon completion of the exposures, the models were washed with PBS, and half of the membrane inserts (the remaining half which was not used for real-time RT-qPCR) were fixed in 4%

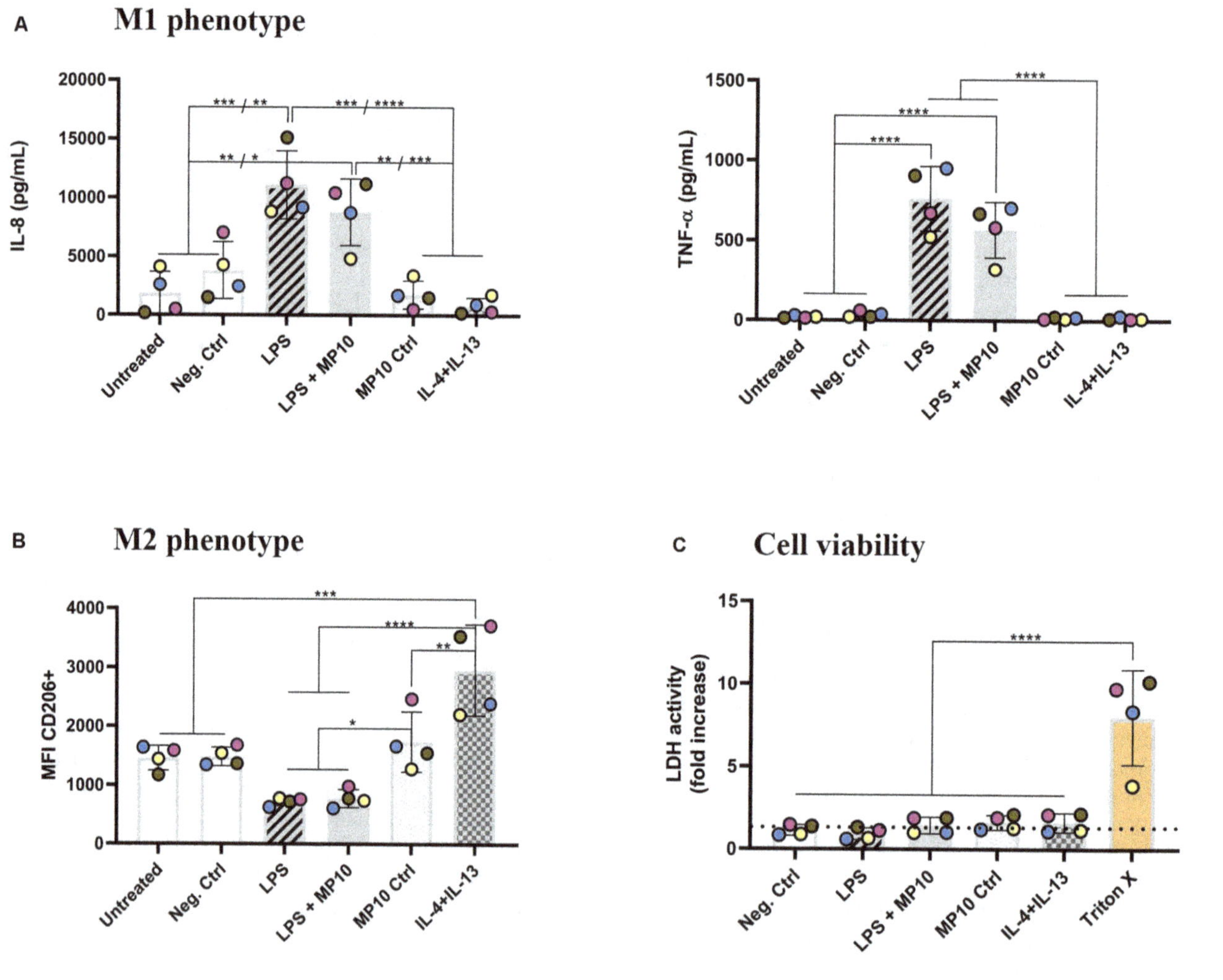

FIGURE 1 | Phenotype shift in macrophage monocultures upon exposure to pro- and anti-inflammatory stimuli. **(A)** Secretion of pro-inflammatory mediators (IL-8 and TNF-α; in pg/mL) in cell-culture medium in the basal compartment, assessed via ELISA. **(B)** Expression of CD206 surface marker (median fluorescence intensity), denoting M2 phenotype, assessed via flow cytometry analysis. The CD206 intensity histogram is shown in **Supplementary Figure S2**. **(C)** Cell viability of MDMs after all of the treatments, assessed via membrane rupture (LDH assay), presented as fold increase over untreated cells (the dotted line). The data is presented as the mean of the four biological repetitions ± standard deviation, whereas individual values from biological repetitions are presented as circles, color-coded for the data from the same biological repetitions (donors). Statistically significant differences among the groups (One-way ANOVA, Tukey's *post hoc*; $\alpha = 0.05$): $^{*}p \leq 0.05$; $^{**}p \leq 0.01$; $^{***}p \leq 0.001$, $^{****}p \leq 0.0001$. Abbreviations: IL-8, interleukin 8; TNF-α, tumor necrosis factor α; MFI, median fluorescence intensity; CD206, cluster of differentiation 206, mannose receptor; IL-4+IL-13, interleukins 4 and 13 (both applied at 20 ng/mL for 48 h); LDH, lactate dehydrogenase; Pos. ctrl Triton X, positive control for LDH assay, i.e., cells exposed to 0.2% Triton X-100 (v/v; 24 h).

paraformaldehyde (in PBS, v/v) for 15 min, washed three-times with PBS and stored at 4°C until the staining procedure. Then, cells were permeabilized with 0.2% Triton X-100 (in PBS, v/v) for 15 min and washed (three-times with 0.1% w/v BSA in PBS). The models were immersed in a mixture of primary antibodies for 2 h: mouse mature macrophage marker monoclonal antibody (clone eBio25F9; eBioscience™; Thermo Fisher Scientific, Germany) at 5 μg/mL and rabbit anti-CD83 antibody (clone EPR22405, Abcam, Switzerland) at 10 μg/mL in 0.1% BSA in PBS. After washing (three-times with 0.1% BSA in PBS), the models were incubated for 2 h in a mixture of secondary antibodies: 20 μg/mL of goat anti-mouse polyclonal secondary antibody, Alexa 647 conjugated (ab150115, Abcam, United Kingdom), 9 μg/mL goat anti-rabbit DY 488 conjugated (AS09 633; Agisera, Sweden) and 0.66 μM rhodamine-phalloidin (Thermo Fisher Scientific, Switzerland) in 0.1% BSA in PBS. After washing (three-times with 0.1% BSA in PBS), the inserts were incubated for an additional 10 min with 1 μg/mL DAPI (Sigma Aldrich, Switzerland) in 0.1% BSA in PBS. All the staining steps were performed in the dark at room temperature. After staining, the cells were washed with PBS, and half of the membranes were cut with a scalpel into two pieces. For optical analysis, both pieces of each sample were mounted in glycergel (DAKO Schweiz AG, Switzerland) to visualize both sides of the model.

Confocal Laser Scanning Microscopy

Visualization of the models was conducted with an inverted LSM Zeiss 710 microscope (Carl Zeiss, Switzerland) equipped with a

40x objective lens (EC Plan-Neofluar 40x/1.30 Oil DIC M27). Representative images (z-stacks) of both apical and basal sides were collected and were further processed using the ImageJ-based software Fiji [ImageJ, NIH, US (Schindelin et al., 2012)].

Barrier Integrity

The barrier integrity of the multicellular models was assessed via a permeability assay using fluorescein isothiocyanate-dextran solution (70 kDa; FITC-dextran). FITC-dextran (stock at 25 mg/mL in water) and EDTA (stock at 0.5 M in water) solutions were prepared in Hank's Balanced Salt Solution (HBSS) without Mg and Ca salts at 2 mg/mL and 10 mM, respectively. After exposure, the models were washed with HBSS and placed in 6-well plates containing 2 mL of HBSS in the basal compartment. First, 1 mL of HBSS buffer was added to the apical compartment of untreated, LPS-, and MP-exposed models, whereas 1 mL of 10 mM EDTA solution was added for positive control samples for barrier integrity disruption. Then, 1 mL of a 2 mg/mL FITC-dextran solution was added to the apical compartments of all the samples and incubated for 60 min (dark, 37°C). In parallel, a blank insert without cells but with HBSS and FITC-dextran was prepared as described above. After incubation, membrane inserts were immediately removed from the cell-culture plates. The supernatants of HBSS containing FITC-dextran were collected from the basal compartments with precise collected volumes noted for each sample. Samples were kept in the dark until the measurements. Fluorescence intensity was measured in triplicate in black 96-well plates using a microplate reader (Tristar LB 941, Berthold Technologies; using the following filters setup: $\lambda ex/\lambda em$: 485/535 nm). Results were corrected with the supernatant volumes (i.e., fluorescence intensity per mL) and expressed as relative to the average fluorescence measured in blank samples.

Cell Viability/Membrane Rupture

Lactate dehydrogenase activity was measured in the basal cell culture medium of exposed models and analyzed in triplicate using the LDH cytotoxicity detection kit, as described for the monoculture experiments. Apical application of 0.2 mL Triton-X (0.2% in sterile-filtered ultrapure water) for 24 h served as a positive control. LDH values are presented as fold increase values relative to untreated cells.

Statistical Analysis

Statistical analysis was performed using GraphPad Prism 8 software (GraphPad Software Inc., San Diego, CA, United States). Parametric one-way analysis of variance (ANOVA; $\alpha = 0.05$) with *post hoc* Tukey's multiple comparison test was used to compare values among the different treatments. Statistically significant values among the treatments are shown as: $^{*}p \leq 0.05$; $^{**}p \leq 0.01$; $^{***}p \leq 0.001$, $^{****}p \leq 0.0001$.

RESULTS

The anti-inflammatory effects of MP were first tested on MDM monocultures with respect to the drug's priming potential to shift macrophage phenotypes towards the anti-inflammatory subset. In the multicellular human alveolar model, LPS-induced inflammation, triggered from apical and basal sides of the model, is demonstrated, followed by four experimental approaches of pro-inflammation induction and its suppression, mimicking various scenarios of lung inflammation and treatment in clinics.

Macrophage Phenotype Plasticity Upon Pro- and Anti-inflammatory Treatments

Alveolar macrophages play a pivotal role in both pro- and anti-inflammatory reactions in the lung. Therefore, in this study, a known phenomenon of macrophage phenotype plasticity, i.e., the shift from M1 (pro-inflammatory) to M2 (anti-inflammatory) and vice-versa, in response to their microenvironment was initially tested. MDMs were treated with LPS for the first 24 h, and MP was added for an additional 24 h while LPS was left in the system (**Table 1**). After the exposure, the secretion of pro-inflammatory cytokines was assessed via ELISA and expression of surface markers via flow cytometry. LPS stimulation induced statistically significant secretion of IL-8 and TNF-α (**Figure 1A** and **Table 2**), demonstrating that MDMs exhibit responsiveness to LPS stimulation. In contrast, the expression of the M1 marker CD86 remained unchanged (**Supplementary Figure S2**). LPS exposure resulted in lower CD206 expression than untreated cells, while a combined IL-4 + IL-13 treatment, which is known to induce M2 polarization, induced its significant upregulation (**Figure 1B**). Next, we tested whether treatment with MP during the latter half of LPS stimulation mitigates manifestation of M1 polarization. Treatment of inflamed MDMs with MP or vehicle alone did not induce secretion of pro-inflammatory cytokines, nor did it cause a phenotypic shift. In contrast, MP treatment of LPS-stimulated MDMs for 24 h resulted in decreased secretion of IL-8 and TNF-α (**Figure 1A**), while leaving the expression of CD86 and CD206 unchanged (**Figure 1B** and **Supplementary Figure S2**). Thus, MP inhibited the secretion of the tested pro-inflammatory markers (IL-8, TNF-α) but did not reprogram the MDM phenotype. None of the treatments used affected the viability of MDMs (**Figure 1C** and **Supplementary Figure S2a**). There are four individual repetitions representing the four blood donors. The gating strategy is presented in the **Supplementary Material** (**Supplementary Figure S1**).

LPS-Induced Inflamed Multicellular Human Lung Model

As the next step, we adapted a more complex lung model to investigate the orchestrated immune cell responses upon exposure to LPS with or without the presence of MP: multicellular models, composed of alveolar epithelial cells (A549) and immune cells (MDDCs and MDMs on basal and apical sides, respectively). The models were challenged with LPS for 48 h from either basal (approach 1) or apical (approach 2) sides. As inflammation in an epithelial tissue often leads to impaired epithelial barrier integrity, the permeability of the model to labeled dextran (70 kDa) was first assessed. LPS challenge from the basal side resulted in increased tissue permeability, demonstrated by the absence of significant differences compared

TABLE 2 | A summary of the pro-inflammatory reactions in monocultures and multicellular human lung models.

		MDMs			*LPS or MP application / in vivo significance*	*Approach 1*			*Approach 2*			*Approach 3*			*Approach 4*		
	Treatment	**MP10 Ctrl**	**LPS**	**LPS + MP10**	**LPS**	**Basal / blood-derived inflammation**			**Apical / inflammation from the airways**			**Apical / inflammation from the airways**			**Basal and apical / strong tissue inflammation**		
Surface marker expression	**CD86**	0	+	0	**MP**	*Apical / pulmonary drug delivery*			*Basal /systemic drug administration*			*Apical / pulmonary drug delivery*			*Apical / pulmonary drug delivery*		
Pro-inflammatory mediators secretion	**IL-8**	0	+++	++		–	++	+	–	+	+	*NA*	++	+	*NA*	+	–
	TNF-α	0	+++	++		–	+	+	–	++	+		+	+		+	+
	IL-1β	*NA*	*NA*	*NA*		–	+	+	–	+	+		+	+		+	+
			Pro-inflammatory gene expression		***CXCL8***	–	++	–	–	++	–		++	–		++	–
					TNF	–	–	++	–	–	+		+	–		++	–
					IL1B	–	0	0	–	++	+		++	0		+	–

to the positive control (EDTA-treated) models, indicating a disruption of barrier integrity (approach 1). In contrast, apical LPS application (approach 2) did not alter the permeability compared to untreated cells but there was statistical significance observed compared to the positive control models (**Figure 2A**). Neither of the treatments induced membrane rupture as assessed by LDH release in the basal cRPMI (**Figure 2B**). The morphology of the epithelial layer on the apical side of the insert was impaired in approach 1 and also slightly after the apical LPS challenge in approach 2. In contrast, the morphology of the basal sides of the inserts, i.e., at the side of MDDCs, was comparable with untreated cells for both approaches (**Figure 2C**).

LPS stimulation significantly increased the expression of pro-inflammatory mediators at protein and gene expression levels, irrespective of the approach used. In both approaches, LPS induced the secretion of IL-8, TNF-α, and IL-1β (the IL-1β secretion was statistically significant only in approach 2; **Figure 3A**). Accordingly, in both approaches, increased mRNA levels were observed compared to untreated cells, with the lowest difference observed for *IL1B* in approach 2 (**Figure 3B**). LPS-induced oxidative stress was evidenced with the onset of mitochondrial antioxidant superoxide dismutase-2 (*SOD2*) mRNA levels in both approaches (**Figure 3C**). The absence of pro-apoptotic reactions was evidenced by unaltered *FAS* mRNA expression levels in both the approaches after 48-h LPS treatments (**Figure 3D**).

Corticosteroids Suppress Pro-inflammatory Reactions in the Inflamed Model

Next, we examined whether the MP treatment of LPS-stimulated multicellular model leads to decreased production of pro-inflammatory factors IL-1 β, IL-8, and TNF-α, following four approaches of LPS and MP application. In approaches 1 and 2, MP treatment of inflamed models was performed in the presence of LPS. LPS and MP were applied either in the basal or the apical compartments (approach 1) or vice-versa (approach 2), respectively (**Figure 4**; left panel). Alternatively, in approaches 3 and 4, LPS was removed from the system before the application of MP. In approach 3, inflamed models were treated with MP while being in contact with LPS-conditioned medium, whereas the basal compartment was refilled with fresh medium in approach 4 (**Figure 4**; right panel). At the protein level, there was an overall trend of slightly reduced secretion of pro-inflammatory mediators (**Figure 5A**). Interestingly, however, the mRNA levels of all three factors were found to have dropped significantly 24 h after the addition of MP in approach 1, which generally induced higher expression of mRNA of the pro-inflammatory factors. A similar trend was observed when we treated the multicellular model using approach 2 (**Figure 5B**). The trends in pro-inflammatory mediator secretion were also observed in approaches 3 and 4 (**Figure 6A**), where LPS was removed before the apical application of MP (**Figure 4**; right panel). Reduced mRNA levels of pro-inflammatory mediators were observed upon

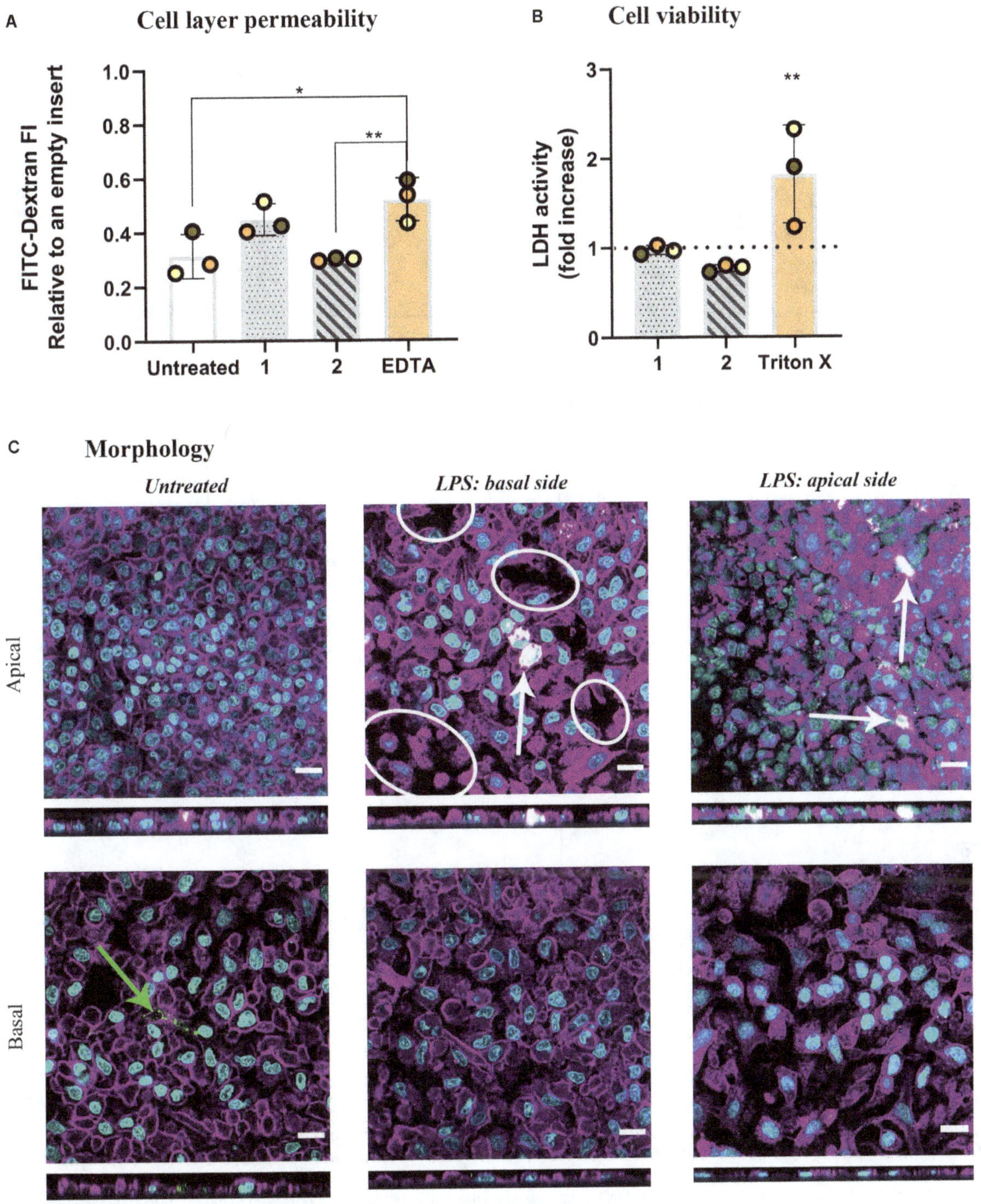

FIGURE 2 | The results of barrier permeability, viability, and morphology assessment of inflamed multicellular models after LPS challenge (1 μg/mL, 48 h) from either basal (approach 1) or apical compartment (approach 2). **(A)** Barrier permeability assessed via FITC-Dextran (70 kDa) permeability assay. The data is presented as fluorescence intensity of FITC-Dextran, measured in the basal compartment, normalized to the values of empty inserts, as the mean of three biological repetitions ± standard deviation. Individual values from biological repetitions are presented as circles, color-coded to represent the data from the same biological repetitions. EDTA (5 mM, 60 min) was used as a positive control for the barrier disruption analysis. **(B)** Cell viability assessed via a membrane rupture assay based on the LDH enzyme released in the cell culture medium of the basal compartment presented as fold increase over untreated cells (the dotted line). Positive control cells were apically exposed to Triton X-100 (0.2%; 24 h). Statistically significant differences among the groups (One-way ANOVA, Tukey's *post hoc*; $\alpha = 0.05$) or to untreated cells (LDH assay): $^{*}p \leq 0.05$; $^{**}p \leq 0.01$. **(C)** Morphology, visualized via confocal laser scanning microscopy of apical and basal sides of the inserts, shown as XY and XZ projections. Immuno-fluorescence labeling: nuclei (cyan), cytoskeleton (magenta), MDMs (mature macrophage marker 25F9; white), MDDCs (CD 83; green). White ellipsoids point out the regions with epithelial barrier disruption. The white arrow denotes MDMs, whereas the green arrow denotes MDDCs. Scale bars are 20 μm.

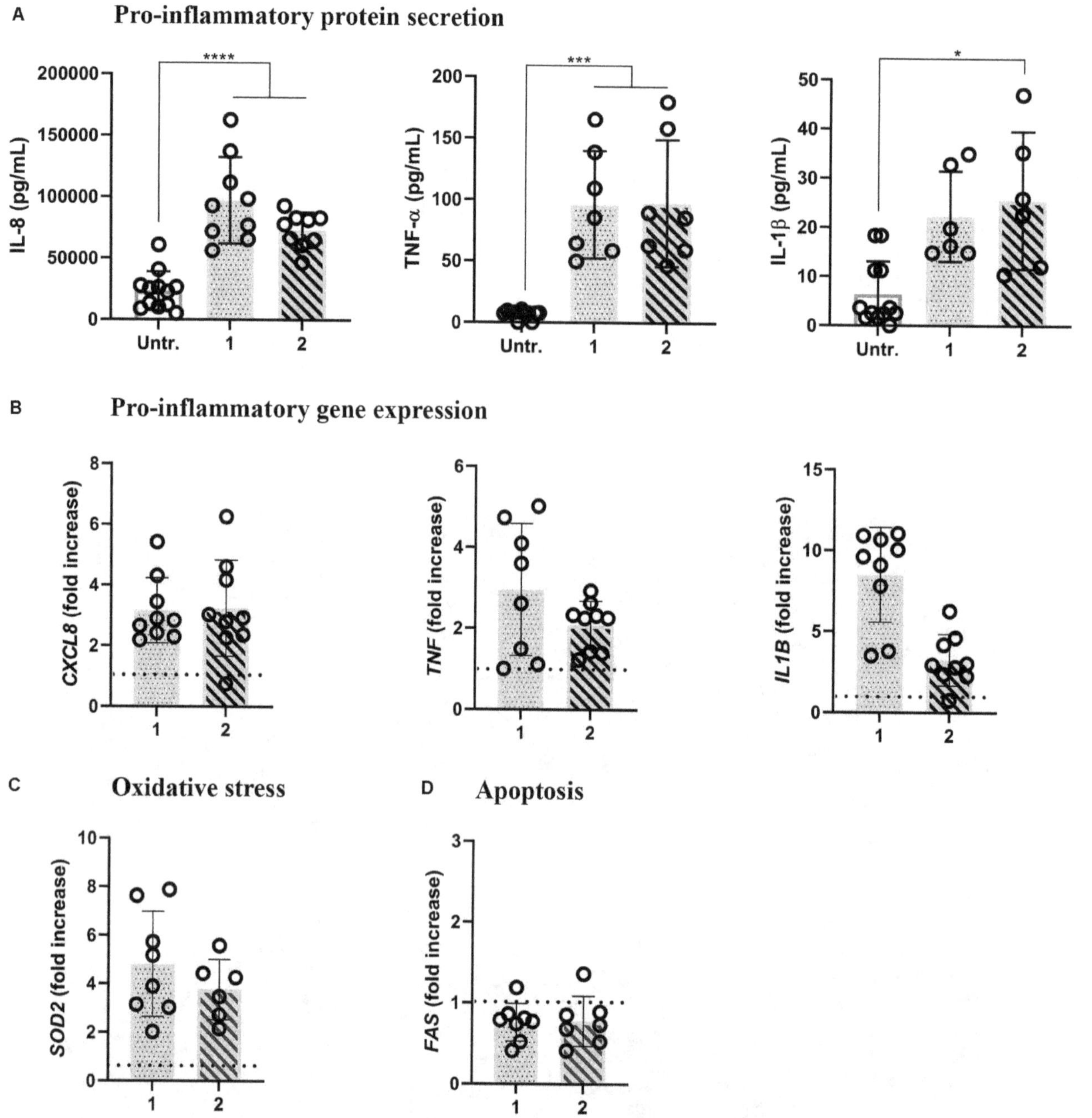

FIGURE 3 | Pro-inflammatory, oxidative stress, and apoptotic reactions in inflamed multicellular models upon LPS challenge (1 μg/mL, 48 h) from either basal (approach 1) or apical compartment (approach 2). **(A)** Secretion of pro-inflammatory mediators IL-8, TNF-α, and IL-1β (upper panel) and **(B)** the respective gene expressions (lower panel). The data for protein secretion are shown in pg/mL, measured in the basal compartment via ELISA. The data on gene expression, assessed via real-time RT-qPCR, is shown as a fold increase of mRNA calculated via the ΔΔCt method, i.e., normalized to the expression of the housekeeping gene GAPDH and the expression of the gene of interest in the untreated samples. The dotted lines denote the mean values of the untreated cells. **(C)** Oxidative stress and **(D)** apoptotic gene expression levels, assessed via real-time RT-qPCR. Statistical analysis for ELISA was performed on pg/mL values using One-way ANOVA (Tukey's *post hoc*; $\alpha = 0.05$). For gene expression, statistically significant differences compared to the untreated cells are shown. $^{*}p \leq 0.05$; $^{**}p \leq 0.01$; $^{***}p \leq 0.001$, $^{****}p \leq 0.0001$. Abbreviations: Untr., untreated models; IL-8, *CXCL8*, interleukin 8; TNF-α, *TNF*, tumor necrosis factor α; IL-1β, *IL1B*, interleukin1β; *SOD2*, superoxide dismutase; *FAS*, Fas cell surface death receptor.

exposure to MP for 24 h compared to positive controls ("LPS"; **Figure 4**), yet this was statistically significant for *CXCL8* in both approaches 3 and 4, *TNF* in approach 4 and *IL1B* in approach 3 (**Figure 6B**). Of the three mediators, MP treatment decreased the IL-8 level the most. A summary of results regarding pro-inflammatory mediator secretion and mRNA levels, along with the monoculture phenotype-associated endpoints, are presented in **Table 2**.

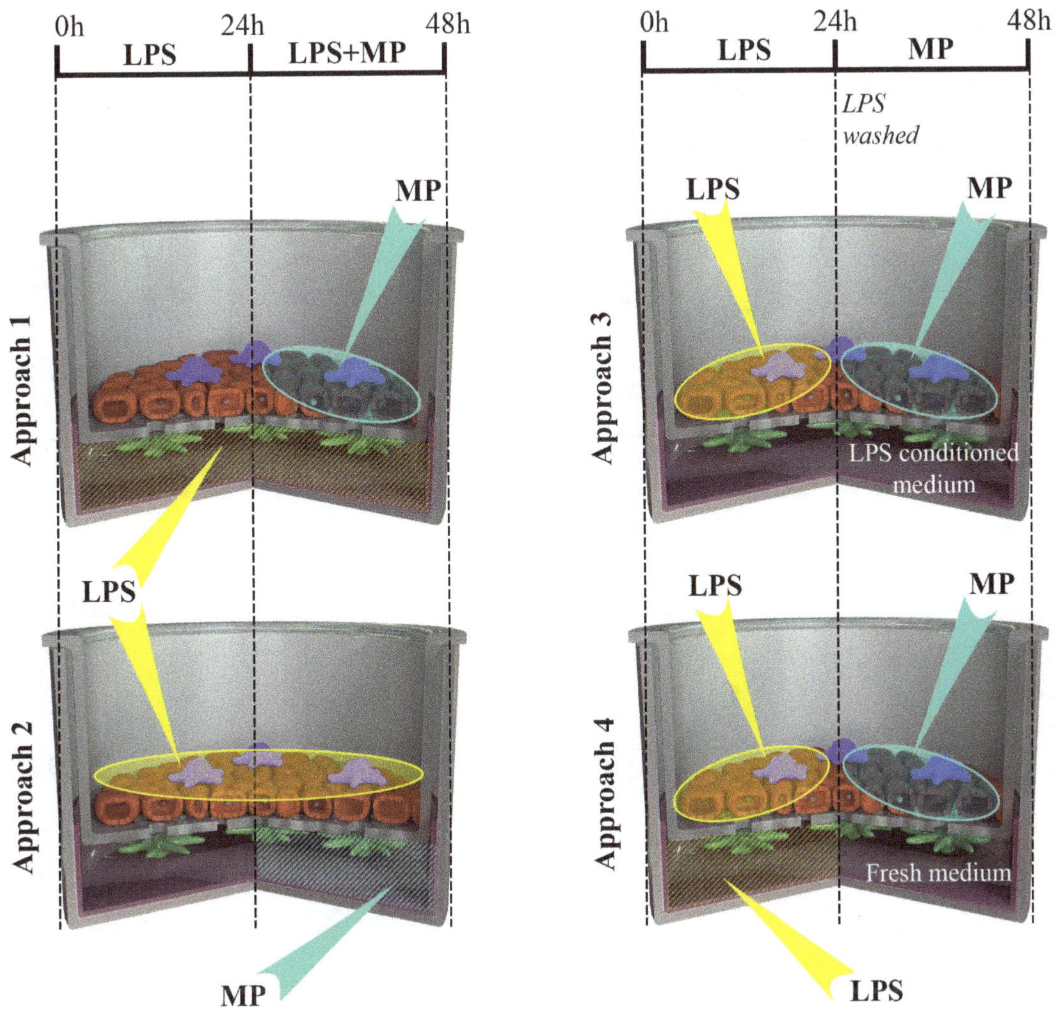

FIGURE 4 | Schematic representation of the four scenarios (approaches 1 to 4) of LPS and MP applications to the multicellular models. Multicellular human lung models, composed of alveolar epithelial cells (A549; red) and human monocyte-derived macrophages (MDMs; blue) and dendritic cells (MDDCs; green), were cultivated at the air-liquid interface conditions (ALI) for 24 h. Subsequently, the models were challenged with LPS (at time 0 h), followed by treatment with MP following four distinct approaches. **Approach 1**: LPS was applied in the basal compartment (1 μg/mL in 3 ml cRPMI), and after the first 24 h, MP was added to the apical side as a thin layer of liquid (i.e., at pseudo-ALI) at 10 or 100 μM, for an additional 24 h. **Approach 2**: LPS was added to the apical compartment at the pseudo-ALI for the first 24 h, and then MP was added in co-exposure from the basal compartment for the next 24 h. **Approach 3**: LPS, applied apically at the pseudo-ALI, was removed after 24 h, and the models were then exposed to the pre-conditioned medium during the MP treatment for an additional 24 h. **Approach 4**: Multicellular models were challenged with LPS both from the apical and basal compartment for 24 h. Then, LPS was removed from both the compartments, the model was washed, and a fresh cell-culture medium was applied during the MP treatment. Abbreviations: LPS, lipopolysaccharide; MP, methylprednisolone.

In all four approaches, the resolution of LPS-induced oxidative stress that had occurred in inflamed models (**Supplementary Figure S3**) was observed, as evidenced by increased levels of the mitochondrial antioxidant superoxide dismutase-2 (*SOD2*) compared to the positive control models ("LPS"; **Figure 4**). These trends were more pronounced in multicellular models treated through approaches 1 and 2, where LPS was applied for 48 h (**Supplementary Figure S3**). None of the treatments exerted notable effects on apoptotic gene expression levels (*FAS* mRNA levels; **Supplementary Figure S3b**). Morphology of the apical epithelial layer remained mostly unaffected after all of the treatments (**Figure 7**), similar to what was observed for untreated cells (**Figure 2C**); only in approaches 1 and 2 did the cell layer integrities appear to be slightly disrupted (**Figure 7A**). The morphological appearance remained unaltered after the apical or basal application of MP alone (**Figure 7D**) relative to the untreated counterparts (**Figure 2C**). These healthy models (in the absence of LPS) treated with MP alone served as a control to rule out the potential effects of MP alone. Exposure to MP at 100 μM both apically and basally did not induce changes in barrier integrity and cell viability (**Supplementary Figures S4a,b**). Levels of secreted IL-8, TNF-α, and IL-1β were lower than in the untreated cells, although the differences were not statistically significant. Similarly, the mRNA content

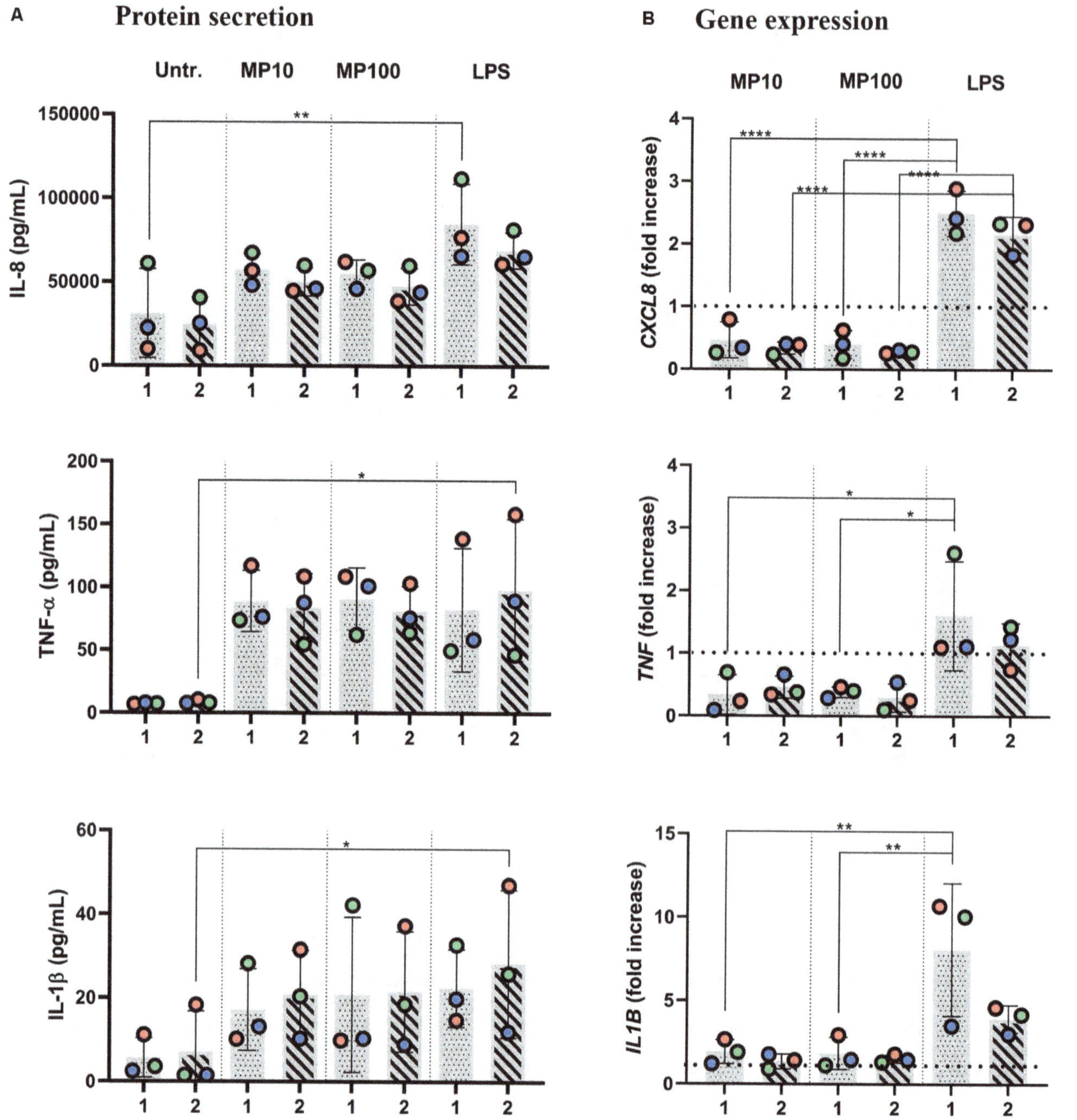

FIGURE 5 | Anti-inflammatory reactions after the addition of MP to inflamed multicellular models in the co-presence of LPS. The *x*-axis represents the number of the approach applied: approaches 1 and 2. Inflamed models were triggered with LPS from either basal (approach 1) or apical (approach 2) compartments for 24 h; then, MP was applied to the opposite compartment for an additional 24 h at 10 or 100 μM. **(A)** Secretion of pro-inflammatory mediators IL-8, TNF-α, and IL-1β and **(B)** the respective gene expressions. The data of protein secretion is shown in pg/mL, measured in the basal compartment via ELISA. The data on gene expression, assessed via real-time RT-qPCR, is shown as fold increase of mRNA calculated via the ΔΔCt method, i.e., normalized to the expression of the housekeeping gene *GAPDH* and the expression of the gene of interest in the untreated samples. Dotted lines denote the mean value of untreated cells. Statistical analysis for ELISA was performed on pg/mL values using One-way ANOVA (Tukey's *post hoc*; $\alpha = 0.05$). For gene expression, statistically significant differences to untreated cells are shown. *$p \leq 0.05$; **$p \leq 0.01$; ***$p \leq 0.001$, ****$p \leq 0.0001$. Abbreviations: Untr.: untreated models; MP10 and MP100: models treated with LPS (24 h) followed by methylprednisolone at 10 or 100 μM for an additional 24 h; LPS: positive control models, i.e., treated with LPS for 48 h.

was slightly reduced in all MP-treated samples, with the most pronounced effect observed for *CXCL8* (**Supplementary Figure S4c**). MP treatment resulted in a slight reduction in *SOD2* mRNA levels in approaches 1 and 2 (**Supplementary Figure S4d**) while leading to a modest increase in the mRNA level of the apoptotic gene *FAS* (**Supplementary Figure S4e**). Given the small

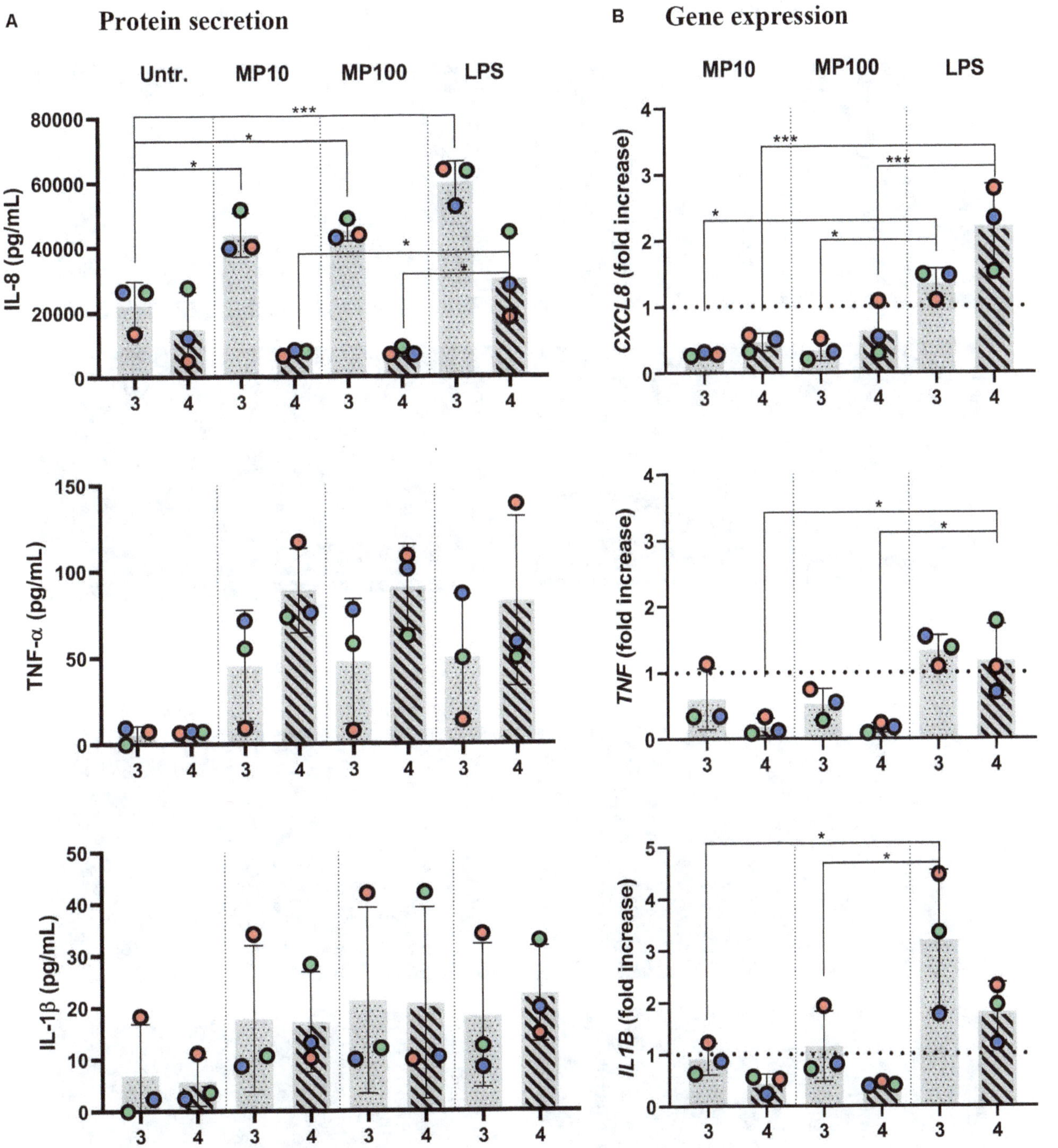

FIGURE 6 | Anti-inflammatory reactions after addition of MP to inflamed multicellular models upon removal of LPS. The *x*-axis represents the number of the approach applied: approaches 3 and 4. Inflamed models were triggered with LPS from the basal compartment (approach 3) or both sides (approach 4) for 24 h. Then, either LPS was removed from the apical side with the cRPMI left in during the apical MP treatment (approach 3) or cRPMI was removed, and inserts were thoroughly washed before MP application (approach 4) for an additional 24 h, at 10 or 100 μM MP. **(A)** Secretion of pro-inflammatory mediators IL-8, TNF-α, and IL-1β and **(B)** the respective gene expressions. The data of protein secretion is shown in pg/mL, measured in the basal compartment via ELISA. The data on gene expression, assessed via real-time RT-qPCR, is shown as fold increase of mRNA calculated via the ΔΔCt method, i.e., normalized to the expression of the housekeeping gene *GAPDH* and the expression of the gene of interest in the untreated samples. The dotted lines denote the mean value of untreated cells. Statistical analysis for ELISA was performed on pg/mL values using One-way ANOVA (Tukey's *post hoc*; $\alpha = 0.05$). For gene expression, statistically significant differences to untreated cells are shown. *$p \leq 0.05$; **$p \leq 0.01$; ***$p \leq 0.001$. Abbreviations: Untr., untreated models; MP10 and MP100, models treated with LPS (24 h) followed by methylprednisolone at 10 or 100 μM for additional 24 h; LPS, positive control models, i.e., treated with LPS for 24 h, then washed accordingly and treated with the vehicle instead of MP.

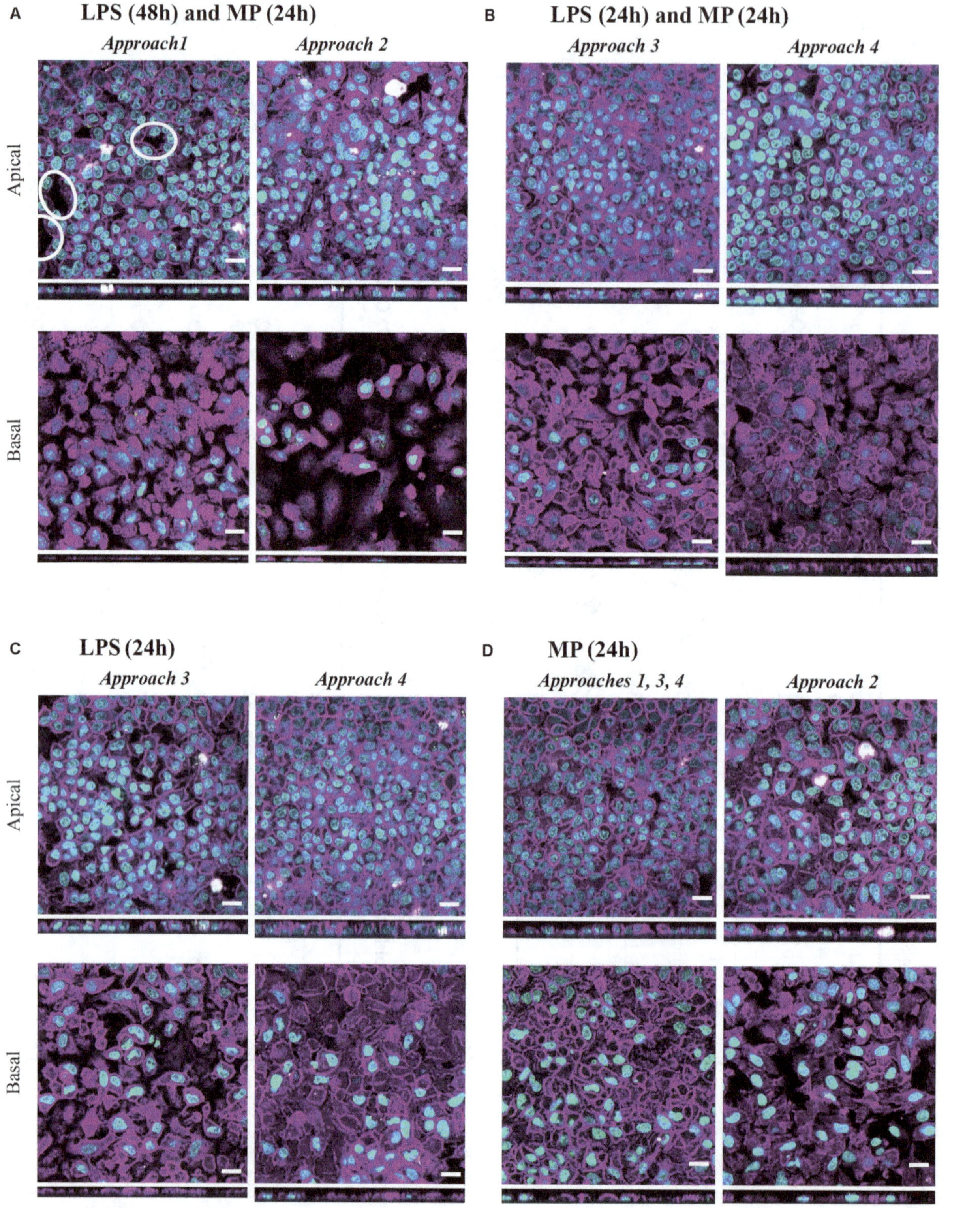

FIGURE 7 | Confocal microscopy images representing the tissue morphology upon exposures to LPS+MP, and LPS or MP alone for 24 h. Multicellular models were treated with **(A)** LPS (24 h + 24 h) and MP at 100 μM from either apical (approach 1) or basal (approach 2) compartments, with **(B)** LPS (24 h) and MP at 100 μM (24 h) corresponding to approaches 3 and 4, respectively **(C)** LPS (24 h) corresponds to the positive controls in approaches 3 and 4. **(D)** MP control tissues, treated only with MP at 100 μM (24 h) from either apical (approaches 1, 3, 4) or basal (approach 2) compartments. Confocal laser scanning microscopy of apical and basal sides of the inserts, shown as XY and XZ projections. Immuno-fluorescence labeling: nuclei (cyan), cytoskeleton (magenta), MDMs (mature macrophage marker 25F9; white), MDDCs (CD 83; green). White ellipsoids point out the regions with epithelial barrier disruption. Scale bars are 20 μm.

degree of differences, however, we considered these effects as biologically insignificant.

DISCUSSION

In this study, we present a multicellular human lung model and the resolution of LPS-induced inflammation *in vitro* using a corticosteroid drug, MP. Four experimental approaches to pro-inflammation induction and its suppression are presented, mimicking various scenarios of lung inflammation and treatment in clinics. As alveolar macrophages are the main actors in the induction and resolution of pro-inflammatory reactions in the tissue, we discuss the anti-inflammatory effects of MP considering its priming potential to shift macrophage phenotypes towards the anti-inflammatory subset and with the potential to reduce pro-inflammatory reactions *in vitro* (**Table 2**).

Pro-inflammatory Reactions and Impaired Alveolar Barrier Integrity in Inflamed Models

Initially, we used a previously established multicellular model of the human alveolar epithelium (Bisig et al., 2019; Barosova et al., 2020) to induce an inflammatory model via a 48-h challenge with LPS. The LPS was applied either from the basal side of the models simulating a systemically derived alveolar inflammation or from the apical side mimicking the source of the tissue inflammation derived from inhaled stimulants. Microbial products such as LPS are a widely used pro-inflammatory stimulus in *in vitro* assays because of their prominent activity to stimulate innate immune responses (Rosadini and Kagan, 2017). The primary mechanism of LPS-induced response begins through its action towards the toll-like receptor 4 (TLR-4), which is present on both of the immune cell types within the model, i.e., macrophages and dendritic cells (Visintin et al., 2001; Fekete et al., 2012). Upon activation of TLR-4, the onset of the nuclear factor kappa B (NF-kB) signaling pathway results in an increase in the secretion of pro-inflammatory cytokines and chemokines, such as the main actor of central inflammation, TNF-α, and interleukins, e.g., IL-1 (Beutler, 2000; Nova et al., 2019). As LPS-induced macrophage phenotype shifts towards M1 have been observed (Wang et al., 2014; Lu et al., 2018; Orecchioni et al., 2019), we employed LPS as the pro-inflammatory stimulus in both the macrophage monocultures and multicellular experiments.

The onset of pro-inflammatory reactions of both the mono- and multicellular models upon LPS challenge can be explained by the high expression of TLR-4 in mononuclear cells (Beutler and Rietschel, 2003; Lawrence and Natoli, 2011), i.e., MDMs and MDDCs. Additionally, the CD14 receptor present in these cells is also involved in the extracellular binding of LPS, which contributes to the initiation of the NF-kB signaling cascade (Beutler, 2000; Lu et al., 2008). Stimulation of MDM monocultures with LPS induced secretion of pro-inflammatory mediators (IL-8, TNF-α) depleted the mannose receptor (CD206) expression (**Figure 1**) and slightly increased CD86 expression, which are established markers of M2 and M1 activation, respectively (Lawrence and Natoli, 2011; Smith et al., 2016). It is important to note that the classical division into distinctive macrophage phenotypes has been questioned in multiple studies, which have proposed that cells adopt a mixed phenotype depending on the stimuli present in their microenvironment, rather than polarization into two distinctive phenotypes (Smith et al., 2016; Atri et al., 2018; Orecchioni et al., 2019). M-CSF, used for monocytes differentiation into macrophages, is also very effective in polarizing macrophages towards the M2 phenotype (Fleetwood et al., 2007; Orecchioni et al., 2019). In fact, by the time we removed the M-CSF from the MDM differentiation culture, the cells were already skewed towards the M2 phenotype, and the addition of LPS might not have been a strong enough stimulus to trigger surface marker expression alterations. The addition of interferon-γ to LPS likely has a synergistic effect of facilitating skewing towards the M1 phenotype along with LPS, as was observed in parallel experiments (data not shown) and in previous reports (Müller et al., 2017; Orecchioni et al., 2019). In this study, however, we focused on LPS-challenged MDMs to compare the onset and suppression of pro-inflammatory reactions between a 2D monoculture setting and more realistic exposures in 3D models.

It should be noted that in *in vivo* settings, macrophages and dendritic cells both respond to microbial danger signals by secretion of inflammatory cytokines and interact with the alveolar epithelial cells as well as one another (Banchereau and Steinman, 1998; Beutler and Rietschel, 2003; Gordon, 2003; Fekete et al., 2012; Cook and MacDonald, 2016). Therefore, *in vitro* multicellular models simulate *in vivo* settings more faithfully than do 2D monocultures (Fitzgerald et al., 2015), as they enable an interplay between the three relevant cell types of alveolar epithelial tissue to take place *in vitro* (Rothen-Rutishauser et al., 2005; Blank et al., 2007). In addition to the immune cells in the model, epithelial cells themselves are also responsive to a pro-inflammatory stimulus, such as LPS (Guillot et al., 2004). LPS stimulation of monocultures of A549 cells results in increased pro-inflammatory marker secretion (IL-8, TNF-α) and the respective gene expression (CXCL8 and TNFA). However, the pro-inflammatory response is significantly lower as compared to that in the co-culture model including immune cells (Bisig et al., 2019; Barosova et al., 2020). Indeed, we observed more pronounced pro-inflammatory reactions in the inflamed multicellular alveolar models, regardless of the side of LPS application, relative to their untreated counterparts (**Figure 3**). However, it is important to note that stressor-induced inflammation in a tissue is a highly complex process involving a combination of events. According to the recently proposed adverse outcome pathway (AOP) framework (Villeneuve et al., 2018), the pro-inflammatory reactions observed in our experiments can be classified as part of the second general key event (KE2): increased pro-inflammatory mediators and a loss of the alveolar barrier integrity (Villeneuve et al., 2018) due to tight junction disruption (Chignard and Balloy, 2000; Eutamene et al., 2005). The latter was observed in the multicellular model upon 48 h of basal LPS exposure (approach 1; **Figure 2A**). Reduced barrier integrity upon basal LPS challenge (approach 1) was also confirmed by the change in the morphological appearance of the multicellular models.

In essence, distinctive patches of ruptured tissue were observed on the apical side of the inserts, whereas the confluency of the apical cell layer in approach 2 was comparable to untreated cells (**Figure 2C**). As we have shown earlier that tight junctions in A549 appear irregularly (Hilton et al., 2019) we did not perform a tight junction staining but assessed the barrier integrity by a permeability assay using FITC-dextran. This suggests that the cytokines released by the MDDCs, present on the basal side of the multicellular model, may affect tight junctions in the epithelial barrier via the release of pro-inflammatory cytokines (Prakash et al., 2014; Agrawal, 2017) and it seems that MDMs are more effective at resolving the inflammation. Consequently, the epithelial permeability is enhanced, which, in *in vivo* settings, allows for infiltration of immune cells at the site of infection/inflammation (Martin et al., 1997). Our observations thus suggest that our inflamed multicellular model can mimic a combination of inflammation-distinctive features in the human lung tissue.

Oxidative and apoptotic reactions are other hallmarks of LPS-induced tissue inflammation (Mukhopadhyay et al., 2006; Ma et al., 2010; Nova et al., 2019). Expression of an oxidative stress-related gene, a mitochondrial antioxidant, manganese-dependent superoxide dismutase (MnSOD) SOD2 was upregulated in the LPS-challenged multicellular models as compared to untreated cells (**Figure 2C**). This result is in line with observations of LPS-challenged monocytes, macrophage cell lines, and primary cells *in vitro*, where *SOD2* upregulation is associated with the NF-kB pathway activation (Sharif et al., 2007; Widdrington et al., 2018). Another reason for the increased SOD2 expression can be attributed to MDDCs (Jin et al., 2010). In our untreated multicellular models, MDDCs induced by GM-CSF and IL-4 remain in their immature state, with the ability to take up and process antigen (Fekete et al., 2012). When the models are stimulated with LPS, MDDCs undergo their maturation process, which is accompanied by a 28-fold upregulation of *SOD2* in 24 h (Jin et al., 2010). Activation of the Fas-mediated apoptosis pathway has been reported to play a key role in inflammation-induced damage of the alveolar epithelium (Ma et al., 2010). In our study, we did not observe a statistically significant upregulation of *FAS* mRNA levels, nor was there any increase in cell membrane rupture as a measure of cell viability in either multicellular models or monoculture (**Figures 1C, 2B**, and **Supplementary Figure S2a**). This was nevertheless expected, as we had chosen a sub-cytotoxic LPS concentration based on our previous studies (Bisig et al., 2019).

Anti-inflammatory Reactions Induced With Corticosteroids

In the next step of the study, we treated the inflamed monocultures and multicellular models with a known anti-inflammatory therapy, corticosteroids. Corticosteroids exert anti-inflammatory activity through their binding to corticosteroid hormone receptors, and this process operates via several molecular mechanisms (Barnes, 2011). When corticosteroids bind to glucocorticoid receptors (GR), which are expressed in almost all cell types, the resulting GR-glucocorticoid complex can take either of two paths: (i) the activated GR complex upregulates the expression of anti-inflammatory proteins the nucleus or (ii) the GR complex represses the expression of pro-inflammatory cytokines and chemokines, or their mRNA degradation (Barnes, 2011).

In the monoculture experiments, we investigated the effect of MP on the priming of inflamed MDMs towards the anti-inflammatory M2 phenotype, as has been reported for MP and other corticosteroids in ex vivo and *in vitro* human and *in vivo* animal studies (Frankenberger et al., 2005; Tu et al., 2017; Desgeorges et al., 2019; Xie et al., 2019). We observed decreased IL-8 and TNF-α secretions and CD86 expression, together with increased CD206 expression, relative to that of LPS-treated cells, albeit without statistical significance among the two groups (**Figure 1** and **Supplementary Figure S2; Table 2**). Thus, these findings suggest that MP inhibits the secretion of pro-inflammatory mediators but does not appear to reprogram the MDM phenotype. A possible reason for the absence of more pronounced differences in cellular phenotypes upon MP treatment in our study is that LPS was not removed from the medium before the MP treatment in order to make the environment comparable with approaches 1 and 2 of the multicellular system. However, as discussed above, the M1/M2 paradigm should not be perceived as two distinctive sub-populations, but rather as a continuum of macrophage polarization states (Edholm et al., 2017; Tu et al., 2017). Therefore, our findings on the increased percentage of M2-associated surface markers accompanied by decreased M1 markers present a valid observation, and suggest that MP helped to balance the macrophage population by shifting them towards the anti-inflammatory phenotype.

Furthermore, in multicellular models, the efficiency of MP in dampening pro-inflammatory reactions was confirmed in models in all of the four different experimental settings applied herein. Overall, the reduction of inflammation compared to the positive controls ("LPS") was comparable among the four approaches (summarized in **Table 2**). Consistent trends were observed in the resolution of LPS-induced inflammation by MP (**Figure 5**). Analogous to the monoculture data (**Figures 1A,B**), the absence of a potent anti-inflammatory effect can be attributed to the simultaneous presence of LPS during the anti-inflammatory treatment. Our findings suggest that the multicellular model recapitulated the effect of MP treatment observed in the monocellular culture of MDMs (summarized in **Table 2**), but potentially with delayed kinetics. In fact, the *in vivo* immunosuppressive properties of corticosteroids, including MP, are primarily associated with their influence on macrophages and T lymphocytes (Coutinho and Chapman, 2011), yet their immunosuppressive effect on dendritic cells and alveolar epithelial cells should not be neglected (Zach et al., 1993; Piemonti et al., 1999; Rozkova et al., 2006; Klaßen et al., 2017). Therefore, it is vital to use an immunocompetent multicellular lung model, i.e., one including immune cells along with epithelial cells, to achieve a realistic assessment of the anti-inflammatory and immunosuppressive actions of corticosteroids. Namely, by applying LPS in the basal compartment and the drug at the apical side (approach 1), we mimicked a systemic inflammation caused by blood-derived danger signals and an anti-inflammatory treatment via inhalation. Vice versa, in approach 2, alveolar inflammation was mimicked by applying LPS apically and MP in the basal compartment, simulating an intravenous steroid therapy (**Figure 4**). Our findings of reduced pro-inflammation in approaches 1 and 2 suggest that MP can be used as an anti-inflammatory drug to model corticosteroid therapy of severe alveolar inflammation in the absence of other treatments that facilitate the resolution of inflammation (such as an antibiotic-based bacteria elimination).

Having demonstrated that a reduction of pro-inflammatory reactions can be assessed *in vitro* in the presence of the stimulus, we developed this test system further by reducing the inflammation. With these *in vitro* conditions, we simulated *in vivo* settings involving pre- or concurrent therapy with agents other than corticosteroids (approaches 3 and 4; **Figure 4**). Similar trends in the reduction of secretion of the pro-inflammatory mediators and their respective mRNA levels (**Figure 6**) were observed as in the MP treatments following the previous two approaches (**Figure 5** and **Table 2**). The mildly disrupted cell layer integrities in approaches 1 and 2 (**Figure 7A**) can be attributed to the extended LPS challenge (48 vs. 24 h), as similar disintegration of the apical cell layer was observed for the positive control models, i.e., those treated with LPS for 48 h (**Figure 2C**), and less disintegration was observed after 24 h (**Figure 7B**). Overall, inflamed models treated with MP presented higher cell-layer integrity than positive control samples (LPS), especially those following approach 3 (**Figures 2C**, **7**). This was expected, however, as MP has been demonstrated to lead to complete resolution of *in vivo* and *in vitro* mechanical and histological lung alterations in mice (Silva et al., 2009). Furthermore, a minimal reduction of pro-inflammatory reactions in healthy tissues was observed upon treatment with MP for all the pro-inflammatory mediators (**Supplementary Figure S4c**). A possible explanation for this is that the assembly of the immunocompetent multicellular human lung model itself triggers a certain amount of pro-inflammatory response, which can then be further reduced with an anti-inflammatory drug. This is indeed consistent with the common side effects of steroid drugs, which can also affect untargeted, healthy cells and tissues (Waljee et al., 2017).

We observed high variations, especially in the cytokine secretion data upon treatment with MP (**Figures 5A**, **6A**, **Supplementary Figure S4c**). This can be explained by biological variations of the immune cell source. First, for each experiment, i.e., for each biological replicate, human blood-derived monocytes were isolated from a different blood donor. Second, the medical history of blood donors cannot be revealed due to ethical reasons; thus, it was unknown whether the patient had an ongoing inflammation and/or treatment at the time of blood sampling. Therefore, we consider that the high variations in our results reflect the variability in donors and not the poor robustness of our model.

The anti-inflammatory activity of MP appeared to be independent of the doses tested. In approaches 1, 3, and 4, MP was applied at the pseudo-ALI in concentrations of 10 and 100 μM, whereas in approach 2, MP was diluted with 1.2 mL of cRPMI, with the same final concentrations of 10 and 100 μM. We set two main criteria for the development of our *in vitro* system: (i) the pro-inflammatory reactions fall within a comparable range irrespective of the side of LPS application (as explained under inflamed model) (Bisig et al., 2019; Barosova et al., 2020), and (ii) MP is applied at a clinically relevant dose (Vichyanond et al., 1989) which is high enough to promote anti-inflammatory reactions in an *in vitro* system without causing adverse effects on the tissues. Overall, the concentrations tested in the study (10 or 100 μM) are in the range of MP concentrations evaluated in human bronchioalveolar fluid upon intravenous drug administration, i.e., 2000 ng/mL [corresponding to 5.2 μM (Vichyanond et al., 1989)] and are in line with the doses tested in the *in vivo* and *in vitro* study of the effects of MP on mice macrophage polarization (Tu et al., 2017).

Clinical Significance

In a clinical setting, MP is predominantly administered intravenously or orally (Kinoshita et al., 2017; Meduri et al., 2018), while other corticosteroid drugs, such as budesonide and formoterol, have proven clinical benefits when inhaled (Barnes, 2011). However, the aim of this study was not to evaluate the action of MP by itself but rather to show the responsiveness of the model to corticosteroid treatment *in vitro*. The purpose of this study was to develop a versatile *in vitro* system to test newly developed drugs, including nanoparticle-based candidates, for the treatment of lung inflammation.

In all of the tested approaches to LPS and MP applications, an efficient reduction of pro-inflammatory reactions was observed at both the protein secretion and gene expression levels (**Table 2**). The authors recommend assessment of the suppression of pro-inflammatory reactions at the gene expression level for inclusion in the endpoint assessment because the decrease in these reactions was more evident than the changes in the secretion of pro-inflammatory factors. In particular, IL-8 (*CXCL8*) yielded the most significant differences among the tested markers (**Table 2**). Our model provides a flexible choice of the scenarios to test novel drug candidates, depending on the research question. For example, if testing the efficiency of a systemically administered drug is the aim, approach 2 can be employed (**Figure 4**). This approach also showed the most pronounced reduction of pro-inflammatory reactions at both protein secretion and gene expression levels (**Table 2**). In contrast, to test candidates for pulmonary drug delivery, approaches 1, 3, and 4 can be followed. Furthermore, a decrease in barrier integrity was observed for the basal application of LPS for 48 h (approach 1). Therefore, where the AOP framework for inflammation and fibrosis (Villeneuve et al., 2018; Halappanavar et al., 2020) is applied, the use of approach 1 is recommended. When a newly developed therapy is envisaged in a combined treatment with, for example, antibiotics, approach 3 or 4 can be employed to test the anti-inflammatory activities of the candidate when the source of inflammation (bacteria) is removed from the microenvironment. Another advantage of the multiple approaches adopted in our study is that the action of the tested drug in respiratory and systemic delivery models can be compared using approaches 1 and 2, respectively. The advantage of creating such a model is that the interplay between the representative cell types is now in an *in vitro* human lung setting, which successfully mimics several key aspects of an *in vivo* setting.

Depending on the stimulus of interest and the research question, additional cell types can also be added to the model, or part of the model elements can be replaced with a relevant type. For the purpose of this study to showcase the responsiveness of the model, A549 have been selected as the epithelial cell type as they are the most widely used cell lines in human respiratory research. An important feature of A549-based model is that surfactant is secreted at the apical surface when cultivated at the air-liquid interface, a key feature to recapitulate *in vivo* conditions in the model. The A549 cell model also has been used to assess the biokinetic distribution of apically administered liposomal Ciclosporin A, and the data was in agreement with the clinically observed pharmacokinetics profile (Schmid et al., 2017). Thus, this model offers a reliable and relevant *in vitro* platform to study the effects of aerosolized substances. Furthermore, depending on the research question and availability of cells the epithelial cells can be replaced for instance with bronchial cells such as the bronchial cell line 16HBE14o-, or with primary alveolar type I-like cells (Lehmann et al., 2011). Importantly, the choice of immune cells is also versatile. Epithelial cells can be co-cultured with other immune cells, such as natural killer cells (Roth et al., 2017). Immune cells such as macrophages can be replaced with differentiated macrophage-like cells (THP-1), and mast cells and/or endothelial cells can be included in similar models (Klein et al., 2013). Additionally, inclusion of polymorphonuclear cells, such as neutrophils, is foreseen, which would, for instance, enable exploration of neutrophil transepithelial migration. However, the importance of other barriers and immune cells needs to be explored in future studies.

An interesting future application of the presented model could be to compare the responsiveness of the model triggered with LPS with the reactions upon stimulation with other inflammatory agents derived from organic dust, such as mold spores (mold antigens). The latter model resembles, for example, a specific respiratory syndrome such as hypersensitivity pneumonitis or extrinsic allergic alveolitis (Riario Sforza and Marinou, 2017) where MP has been used as one of the main treatment drugs (Buchvald et al., 2011).

In conclusion, we have established an *in vitro* human 3D multicellular alveolar epithelial model that is responsive to both pro-inflammatory stimulation and anti-inflammatory treatment. Responses of the model correlated well with phenotypic shifts of macrophages, highlighting their importance in the faithful reproduction of *in vivo* settings. Supported by the use of permeable membranes, our new model also enables the assessment of the permeability of agents through the barrier. Further development is aimed at coupling our multicellular human lung models with an aerosolization system to assess the efficiency of nebulized compounds. Given that a large number of researchers are currently exploring novel anti-inflammatory formulations, and in particular nanoparticle-based candidates intended for administration via inhalation, we anticipate that our "inflammable" human lung model will serve as a versatile and realistic toolkit for efficient evaluation of the efficiency and safety of various drug candidates.

AUTHOR CONTRIBUTIONS

BD designed and planned the study, carried out majority of the experiments, analyzed and interpreted the data, and finally drafted the manuscript. BK and ET supported the planning and execution of the tissue culture experiments, and BK also supported the writing process of the main text. HB assisted with monocyte isolation and multicellular model experiments. JA provided expert knowledge on flow cytometry. MS provided lab support with the real-time RT-PCR experiments. AP-F and BR-R were involved in the planning and technical advisory of the study and critically revised the manuscript draft for important intellectual content and approved publication of the content. All authors contributed to the article and approved the submitted version.

ACKNOWLEDGMENTS

The authors would like to thank Dr. Miguel Spuch-Calvar for the multicellular human lung model scheme in **Figure 4**.

REFERENCES

Agrawal, A. (2017). Dendritic cell-airway epithelial cell cross-talk changes with age and contributes to chronic lung inflammatory diseases in the elderly. *Int. J. Mol. Sci.* 18:1206. doi: 10.3390/ijms18061206

Artzy-Schnirman, A., Lehr, C.-M., and Sznitman, J. (2020). Advancing human in vitro pulmonary disease models in preclinical research: opportunities for lung-on-chips. *Expert Opin. Drug Deliv.* 17, 621–625. doi: 10.1080/17425247.2020.1738380

Atri, C., Guerfali, F. Z., and Laouini, D. (2018). Role of human macrophage polarization in inflammation during infectious diseases. *Int. J. Mol. Sci.* 19:1801. doi: 10.3390/ijms19061801

Banchereau, J., and Steinman, R. M. (1998). Dendritic cells and the control of immunity. *Nature* 392, 245–252. doi: 10.1038/32588

Barnes, P. J. (2011). Glucocorticosteroids: current and future directions. *Br. J. Pharmacol.* 163, 29–43. doi: 10.1111/j.1476-5381.2010.01199.x

Barosova, H., Drasler, B., Petri-Fink, A., and Rothen-Rutishauser, B. (2020). Multicellular human alveolar model composed of epithelial cells and primary immune cells for hazard assessment. *J. Vis. Exp.* 6:e61090. doi: 10.3791/61090

Beutler, B. (2000). Tlr4: central component of the sole mammalian LPS sensor. *Curr. Opin. Immunol.* 12, 20–26. doi: 10.1016/S0952-7915(99)00046-1

Beutler, B., and Rietschel, E. T. (2003). Innate immune sensing and its roots: the story of endotoxin. *Nat. Rev. Immunol.* 3, 169–176. doi: 10.1038/nri1004

Bisig, C., Voss, C., Petri-Fink, A., and Rothen-Rutishauser, B. (2019). The crux of positive controls - Pro-inflammatory responses in lung cell models. *Toxicol. Vitro* 54, 189–193. doi: 10.1016/j.tiv.2018.09.021

Blank, F., Rothen-Rutishauser, B., and Gehr, P. (2007). Dendritic cells and macrophages form a transepithelial network against foreign particulate antigens. *Am. J. Respir. Cell Mol. Biol.* 36, 669–677. doi: 10.1165/rcmb.2006-0234OC

Blank, F., Rothen-Rutishauser, B. M., Schurch, S., and Gehr, P. (2006). An optimized *in vitro* model of the respiratory tract wall to study particle cell interactions. *J. Aerosol. Med.* 19, 392–405. doi: 10.1089/jam.2006.19.392

Brain, J. D. (1988). Lung macrophages: how many kinds are there? What do they do? *Am. Rev. Respir. Dis.* 137, 507–509. doi: 10.1164/ajrccm/137.3.507

Buchvald, F., Petersen, B. L., Damgaard, K., Deterding, R., Langston, C., Fan, L. L., et al. (2011). Frequency, treatment, and functional outcome in children with hypersensitivity pneumonitis. *Pediatr. Pulmonol.* 46, 1098–1107. doi: 10.1002/ppul.21479

Bur, M., and Lehr, C. M. (2008). Pulmonary cell culture models to study the safety and efficacy of innovative aerosol medicines. *Expert Opin. Drug Deliv.* 5, 641–652. doi: 10.1517/17425247.5.6.641

Castellani, S., Di Gioia, S., di Toma, L., and Conese, M. (2018). Human cellular models for the investigation of lung inflammation and mucus production in cystic fibrosis. *Anal. Cell. Pathol.* 2018:3839803. doi: 10.1155/2018/3839803

Chana, K. K., Fenwick, P. S., Nicholson, A. G., Barnes, P. J., and Donnelly, L. E. (2014). Identification of a distinct glucocorticosteroid-insensitive pulmonary macrophage phenotype in patients with chronic obstructive pulmonary disease. *J. Allergy Clin. Immunol.* 133, 207.e1–e11–216.e1–e11. doi: 10.1016/j.jaci.2013.08.044

Chignard, M., and Balloy, V. (2000). Neutrophil recruitment and increased permeability during acute lung injury induced by lipopolysaccharide. *Am. J. Physiol. Lung. Cell Mol. Physiol.* 279, L1083–L1090. doi: 10.1152/ajplung.2000.279.6.L1083

Condon, T. V., Sawyer, R. T., Fenton, M. J., and Riches, D. W. H. (2011). Lung dendritic cells at the innate-adaptive immune interface. *J. Leukoc. Biol.* 90, 883–895. doi: 10.1189/jlb.0311134

Cook, P. C., and MacDonald, A. S. (2016). Dendritic cells in lung immunopathology. *Semin. Immunopathol.* 38, 449–460. doi: 10.1007/s00281-016-0571-3

Costa, A., de Souza Carvalho-Wodarz, C., Seabra, V., Sarmento, B., and Lehr, C. M. (2019). Triple co-culture of human alveolar epithelium, endothelium and macrophages for studying the interaction of nanocarriers with the air-blood barrier. *Acta Biomater.* 91, 235–247. doi: 10.1016/j.actbio.2019.04.037

Coutinho, A. E., and Chapman, K. E. (2011). The anti-inflammatory and immunosuppressive effects of glucocorticoids, recent developments and mechanistic insights. *Mol. Cell. Endocrinol.* 335, 2–13. doi: 10.1016/j.mce.2010.04.005

da Silva, A. L., Cruz, F. F., Rocco, P. R. M., and Morales, M. M. (2017). New perspectives in nanotherapeutics for chronic respiratory diseases. *Biophys. Rev.* 9, 793–803. doi: 10.1007/s12551-017-0319-x

Desgeorges, T., Caratti, G., Mounier, R., Tuckermann, J., and Chazaud, B. (2019). Glucocorticoids shape macrophage phenotype for tissue repair. *Front. Immunol.* 10:1591. doi: 10.3389/fimmu.2019.01591

Edholm, E.-S., Rhoo, K. H., and Robert, J. (2017). Evolutionary aspects of macrophages polarization. *Results Probl. Cell Differ.* 62, 3–22. doi: 10.1007/978-3-319-54090-0_1

Endes, C., Schmid, O., Kinnear, C., Mueller, S., Camarero-Espinosa, S., Vanhecke, D., et al. (2014). An in vitro testing strategy towards mimicking the inhalation of high aspect ratio nanoparticles. *Part. Fibre Toxicol.* 11:40. doi: 10.1186/s12989-014-0040-x

Eutamene, H., Theodorou, V., Schmidlin, F., Tondereau, V., Garcia-Villar, R., Salvador-Cartier, C., et al. (2005). LPS-induced lung inflammation is linked to increased epithelial permeability: role of MLCK. *Eur. Respir. J.* 25, 789–796. doi: 10.1183/09031936.05.00064704

Fekete, T., Szabo, A., Beltrame, L., Vivar, N., Pivarcsi, A., Lanyi, A., et al. (2012). Constraints for monocyte-derived dendritic cell functions under inflammatory conditions. *Eur. J. Immunol.* 42, 458–469. doi: 10.1002/eji.201141924

Fitzgerald, K. A., Malhotra, M., Curtin, C. M., Brien, F. J. O., and O'Driscoll, C. M. (2015). Life in 3D is never flat: 3D models to optimise drug delivery. *J. Control. Release* 215, 39–54. doi: 10.1016/j.jconrel.2015.07.020

Fleetwood, A. J., Lawrence, T., Hamilton, J. A., and Cook, A. D. (2007). Granulocyte-macrophage colony-stimulating factor (CSF) and macrophage CSF-Dependent macrophage phenotypes display differences in cytokine profiles and transcription factor activities: implications for CSF blockade in inflammation. *J. Immunol.* 178, 5245–5252. doi: 10.4049/jimmunol.178.8.5245

Florentin, J., Coppin, E., Vasamsetti, S. B., Zhao, J., Tai, Y.-Y., Tang, Y., et al. (2018). Inflammatory macrophage expansion in pulmonary hypertension depends upon mobilization of blood-borne monocytes. *J. Immunol.* 200, 3612–3625. doi: 10.4049/jimmunol.1701287

Frankenberger, M., Haussinger, K., and Ziegler-Heitbrock, L. (2005). Liposomal methylprednisolone differentially regulates the expression of TNF and IL-10 in human alveolar macrophages. *Int. Immunopharmacol.* 5, 289–299. doi: 10.1016/j.intimp.2004.09.033

Gordon, S. (2003). Alternative activation of macrophages. *Nat. Rev. Immunol.* 3, 23–35. doi: 10.1038/nri978

Guillot, L., Medjane, S., Le-Barillec, K., Balloy, V., Danel, C., Chignard, M., et al. (2004). Response of human pulmonary epithelial cells to lipopolysaccharide involves Toll-like receptor 4 (TLR4) dependent signaling pathways: evidence for an intracellular compartmentalization of TLR4. *J. Biol. Chem.* 279, 2712–2718. doi: 10.1074/jbc.M305790200

Habermehl, D., Parkitna, J. R., Kaden, S., Brügger, B., Wieland, F., Gröne, H. J., et al. (2011). Glucocorticoid activity during lung maturation is essential in mesenchymal and less in alveolar epithelial cells. *Mol. Endocrinol.* 25, 1280–1288. doi: 10.1210/me.2009-0380

Haghi, M., Hittinger, M., Zeng, Q., Oliver, B., Traini, D., Young, P. M., et al. (2015). Mono- and cocultures of bronchial and alveolar epithelial cells respond differently to proinflammatory stimuli and their modulation by salbutamol and budesonide. *Mol. Pharm.* 12, 2625–2632. doi: 10.1021/acs.molpharmaceut.5b00124

Halappanavar, S., van den Brule, S., Nymark, P., Gaté, L., Seidel, C., Valentino, S., et al. (2020). Adverse outcome pathways as a tool for the design of testing strategies to support the safety assessment of emerging advanced materials at the nanoscale. *Part. Fibre Toxicol.* 17:16. doi: 10.1186/s12989-020-00344-4

Hermanns, M. I., Unger, R. E., Kehe, K., Peters, K., and Kirkpatrick, C. J. (2004). Lung epithelial cell lines in coculture with human pulmonary microvascular endothelial cells: development of an alveolo-capillary barrier in vitro. *Lab. Invest.* 84, 736–752. doi: 10.1038/labinvest.3700081

Higham, A., Booth, G., Lea, S., Southworth, T., Plumb, J., and Singh, D. (2015). The effects of corticosteroids on COPD lung macrophages: a pooled analysis. *Respir. Res.* 16:98. doi: 10.1186/s12931-015-0260-0

Hilton, G., Barosova, H., Petri-Fink, A., Rothen-Rutishauser, B., and Bereman, M. (2019). Leveraging proteomics to compare submerged versus air-liquid interface carbon nanotube exposure to a 3D lung cell model. *Toxicol. In Vitro* 54, 58–66. doi: 10.1016/j.tiv.2018.09.010

Hittinger, M., Mell, N. A., Huwer, H., Loretz, B., Schneider-Daum, N., and Lehr, C.-M. (2016). Autologous Co-culture of primary human alveolar macrophages and epithelial cells for investigating aerosol medicines. Part II: evaluation of IL-10-loaded microparticles for the treatment of lung inflammation. *Altern. Lab. Anim.* 44, 349–360. doi: 10.1177/026119291604400405

Holt, P. G., Strickland, D. H., Wikstrom, M. E., and Jahnsen, F. L. (2008). Regulation of immunological homeostasis in the respiratory tract. *Nat. Rev. Immunol.* 8, 142–152. doi: 10.1038/nri2236

Hussell, T., and Bell, T. J. (2014). Alveolar macrophages: plasticity in a tissue-specific context. *Nat. Rev. Immunol.* 14, 81–93. doi: 10.1038/nri3600

Jaroch, K., Jaroch, A., and Bojko, B. (2018). Cell cultures in drug discovery and development: the need of reliable in vitro-in vivo extrapolation for pharmacodynamics and pharmacokinetics assessment. *J. Pharm. Biomed. Anal.* 147, 297–312. doi: 10.1016/j.jpba.2017.07.023

Jin, P., Han, T. H., Ren, J., Saunders, S., Wang, E., Marincola, F. M., et al. (2010). Molecular signatures of maturing dendritic cells: implications for testing the quality of dendritic cell therapies. *J. Transl. Med.* 8:4. doi: 10.1186/1479-5876-8-4

Johnson, E. R., and Matthay, M. A. (2010). Acute lung injury: epidemiology, pathogenesis, and treatment. *J. Aerosol Med. Pulm. Drug Deliv.* 23, 243–252. doi: 10.1089/jamp.2009.0775

Katsura, Y., Harada, N., Harada, S., Ishimori, A., Makino, F., Ito, J., et al. (2015). Characteristics of alveolar macrophages from murine models of OVA-induced allergic airway inflammation and LPS-induced acute airway inflammation. *Exp. Lung Res.* 41, 370–382. doi: 10.3109/01902148.2015.1044137

King, P. (2012). *Haemophilus influenzae* and the lung (*Haemophilus* and the lung). *Clin. Transl. Med.* 1:10. doi: 10.1186/2001-1326-1-10

Kinoshita, Y., Ishii, H., Kushima, H., Watanabe, K., and Fujita, M. (2017). High-dose steroid therapy for acute respiratory distress syndrome lacking common risk factors: predictors of outcome. *Acute Med. Surg.* 5, 146–153. doi: 10.1002/ams2.321

Klaßen, C., Karabinskaya, A., Dejager, L., Vettorazzi, S., Van Moorleghem,

J., Lühder, F., et al. (2017). Airway epithelial cells are crucial targets of glucocorticoids in a mouse model of allergic asthma. *J. Immunol.* 199, 48–61. doi: 10.4049/jimmunol.1601691

Klein, S. G., Serchi, T., Hoffmann, L., Blömeke, B., and Gutleb, A. C. (2013). An improved 3D tetraculture system mimicking the cellular organisation at the alveolar barrier to study the potential toxic effects of particles on the lung. *Part. Fibre Toxicol.* 10:31. doi: 10.1186/1743-8977-10-31

Knapp, S. (2009). LPS and bacterial lung inflammation models. *Drug Discov. TodayDis. Models* 6, 113–118. doi: 10.1016/j.ddmod.2009.08.003

Labib, S., Williams, A., Yauk, C. L., Nikota, J. K., Wallin, H., Vogel, U., et al. (2016). Nano-risk Science: application of toxicogenomics in an adverse outcome pathway framework for risk assessment of multi-walled carbon nanotubes. *Part Fibre Toxicol.* 13:15. doi: 10.1186/s12989-016-0125-9

Laskin, D. L., Sunil, V. R., Gardner, C. R., and Laskin, J. D. (2011). Macrophages and tissue injury: agents of defense or destruction? *Annu. Rev. Pharmacol. Toxicol.* 51, 267–288. doi: 10.1146/annurev.pharmtox.010909.105812

Lawrence, T., and Natoli, G. (2011). Transcriptional regulation of macrophage polarization: enabling diversity with identity. *Nat. Rev. Immunol.* 11, 750–761. doi: 10.1038/nri3088

Lehmann, A. D., Daum, N., Bur, M., Lehr, C. M., Gehr, P., and Rothen-Rutishauser, B. M. (2011). An in vitro triple cell co-culture model with primary cells mimicking the human alveolar epithelial barrier. *Eur. J. Pharm. Biopharm.* 77, 398–406. doi: 10.1016/j.ejpb.2010.10.014

Lehnert, B. E. (1992). Pulmonary and thoracic macrophage subpopulations and clearance of particles from the lung. *Environ. Health Perspect.* 97, 17–46. doi: 10.1289/ehp.929717

Leite-Junior, J. H., Garcia, C. S., Souza-Fernandes, A. B., Silva, P. L., Ornellas, D. S., Larangeira, A. P., et al. (2008). Methylprednisolone improves lung mechanics and reduces the inflammatory response in pulmonary but not in extrapulmonary mild acute lung injury in mice. *Crit. Care Med.* 36, 2621–2628. doi: 10.1097/CCM.0b013e3181847b43

Liu, D., Ahmet, A., Ward, L., Krishnamoorthy, P., Mandelcorn, E. D., Leigh, R., et al. (2013). A practical guide to the monitoring and management of the complications of systemic corticosteroid therapy. *AllergyAsthmaClin. Immunol.* 9:30. doi: 10.1186/1710-1492-9-30

Lu, H. L., Huang, X. Y., Luo, Y. F., Tan, W. P., Chen, P. F., and Guo, Y. B. (2018). Activation of M1 macrophages plays a critical role in the initiation of acute lung injury. *Biosci. Rep.* 38:BSR20171555. doi: 10.1042/bsr20171555

Lu, Y.-C., Yeh, W.-C., and Ohashi, P. S. (2008). LPS/TLR4 signal transduction pathway. *Cytokine* 42, 145–151. doi: 10.1016/j.cyto.2008.01.006

Ma, X., Xu, D., Ai, Y., Ming, G., and Zhao, S. (2010). Fas inhibition attenuates lipopolysaccharide-induced apoptosis and cytokine release of rat type II alveolar epithelial cells. *Mol. Biol. Rep.* 37, 3051–3056. doi: 10.1007/s11033-009-9876-9

Marik, P. E., Meduri, G. U., Rocco, P. R. M., and Annane, D. (2011). Glucocorticoid treatment in acute lung injury and acute respiratory distress syndrome. *Crit. Care Clin.* 27, 589–607. doi: 10.1016/j.ccc.2011.05.007

Martin, L. D., Rochelle, L. G., Fischer, B. M., Krunkosky, T. M., and Adler, K. B. (1997). Airway epithelium as an effector of inflammation: molecular regulation of secondary mediators. *Eur. Respir. J.* 10, 2139–2146. doi: 10.1183/09031936.97.10092139

Martinez, F. O., and Gordon, S. (2014). The M1 and M2 paradigm of macrophage activation: time for reassessment. *F1000Prime Rep.* 6:13. doi: 10.12703/p6-13

Meduri, G. U., Siemieniuk, R. A. C., Ness, R. A., and Seyler, S. J. (2018). Prolonged low-dose methylprednisolone treatment is highly effective in reducing duration of mechanical ventilation and mortality in patients with ARDS. *J. Intensive Care* 6:53. doi: 10.1186/s40560-018-0321-9

Moldoveanu, B., Otmishi, P., Jani, P., Walker, J., Sarmiento, X., Guardiola, J., et al. (2009). Inflammatory mechanisms in the lung. *J. Inflammation Res.* 2, 1–11.

Mukhopadhyay, S., Hoidal, J. R., and Mukherjee, T. K. (2006). Role of TNFα in pulmonary pathophysiology. *Respir. Res.* 7:125. doi: 10.1186/1465-9921-7-125

Müller, E., Christopoulos, P. F., Halder, S., Lunde, A., Beraki, K., Speth, M., et al. (2017). Toll-Like receptor ligands and Interferon-γ synergize for induction of antitumor M1 macrophages. *Front. Immunol.* 8:1383. doi: 10.3389/fimmu.2017.01383

Nicod, L. P. (2005). Lung defences: an overview. *Eur. Respi. Rev.* 14, 45–50. doi: 10.1183/09059180.05.00009501

Nova, Z., Skovierova, H., and Calkovska, A. (2019). Alveolar-capillary membrane-related pulmonary cells as a target in endotoxin-induced acute lung injury. *Int. J. Mol. Sci.* 20:831. doi: 10.3390/ijms20040831

Orecchioni, M., Ghosheh, Y., Pramod, A. B., and Ley, K. (2019). Macrophage polarization: different gene signatures in M1(LPS+) vs. Classically and M2(LPS-) vs. alternatively activated macrophages. *Front. Immunol.* 10:1084. doi: 10.3389/fimmu.2019.01084

Piemonti, L., Monti, P., Allavena, P., Sironi, M., Soldini, L., Leone, B. E., et al. (1999). Glucocorticoids affect human dendritic cell differentiation and maturation. *J. Immunol.* 162, 6473–6481.

Prakash, S., Agrawal, S., Vahed, H., Ngyuen, M., BenMohamed, L., Gupta, S., et al. (2014). Dendritic cells from aged subjects contribute to chronic airway inflammation by activating bronchial epithelial cells under steady state. *Mucosal Immunol.* 7, 1386–1394. doi: 10.1038/mi.2014.28

Riario Sforza, G. G., and Marinou, A. (2017). Hypersensitivity pneumonitis: a complex lung disease. *Clin. Mol. Allergy* 15:6. doi: 10.1186/s12948-017-0062-7

Rivera-Burgos, D., Sarkar, U., Lever, A. R., Avram, M. J., Coppeta, J. R., Wishnok, J. S., et al. (2016). Glucocorticoid clearance and metabolite profiling in an in vitro human airway epithelium lung model. *DrugMetab. Dispos.* 44, 220–226. doi: 10.1124/dmd.115.066365

Rosadini, C. V., and Kagan, J. C. (2017). Early innate immune responses to bacterial LPS. *Curr. Opin. Immunol.* 44, 14–19. doi: 10.1016/j.coi.2016.10.005

Roth, M. (2014). [Fundamentals of chronic inflammatory lung diseases (asthma. COPD, fibrosis)]. *Ther. Umsch.* 71, 258–261. doi: 10.1024/0040-5930/a000510

Roth, M., Usemann, J., Bisig, C., Comte, P., Czerwinski, J., Mayer, A. C. R., et al. (2017). Effects of gasoline and ethanol-gasoline exhaust exposure on human bronchial epithelial and natural killer cells in vitro. *Toxicol. In Vitro* 45(Pt 1), 101–110. doi: 10.1016/j.tiv.2017.08.016

Rothen-Rutishauser, B. M., Kiama, S. G., and Gehr, P. (2005). A three-dimensional cellular model of the human respiratory tract to study the interaction with particles. *Am. J. Respir. Cell Mol. Biol.* 32, 281–289. doi: 10.1165/rcmb.2004-0187OC

Rozkova, D., Horvath, R., Bartunkova, J., and Spisek, R. (2006). Glucocorticoids severely impair differentiation and antigen presenting function of dendritic cells despite upregulation of Toll-like receptors. *Clin. Immunol.* 120, 260–271. doi: 10.1016/j.clim.2006.04.567

Schindelin, J., Arganda-Carreras, I., Frise, E., Kaynig, V., Longair, M., Pietzsch, T., et al. (2012). Fiji: an open-source platform for biological-image analysis. *Nat. Methods* 9, 676–682. doi: 10.1038/Nmeth.2019

Schmid, O., Jud, C., Umehara, Y., Mueller, D., Bucholski, A., Gruber, F., et al. (2017). Biokinetics of aerosolized liposomal ciclosporin a in human lung cells in vitro using an air-liquid cell interface exposure system. *J. Aerosol Med. Pulm. Drug Deliv.* 30, 411–424. doi: 10.1089/jamp.2016.1361

Sethi, G. R., and Singhal, K. K. (2008). Pulmonary diseases and corticosteroids. *Indian J. Pediatr.* 75, 1045–1056. doi: 10.1007/s12098-008-0209-0

Shapiro, D. L., Nardone, L. L., Rooney, S. A., Motoyama, E. K., and Munoz, J. L. (1978). Phospholipid biosynthesis and secretion by a cell line (A549) which resembles type II alveolar epithelial cells. *Biochim. Biophys. Acta Lipids Lipid Metab.* 530, 197–207. doi: 10.1016/0005-2760(78)90005-X

Sharif, O., Bolshakov, V. N., Raines, S., Newham, P., and Perkins, N. D. (2007). Transcriptional profiling of the LPS induced NF-κB response in macrophages. *BMC Immunol.* 8:1. doi: 10.1186/1471-2172-8-1

Silva, P. L., Garcia, C. S. N. B., Maronas, P. A., Cagido, V. R., Negri, E. M., Damaceno-Rodrigues, N. R., et al. (2009). Early short-term versus prolonged low-dose methylprednisolone therapy in acute lung injury. *Eur. Respir. J.* 33, 634–645. doi: 10.1183/09031936.00052408

Smith, T. D., Tse, M. J., Read, E. L., and Liu, W. F. (2016). Regulation of macrophage polarization and plasticity by complex activation signals. *Integrat. Biol.* 8, 946–955. doi: 10.1039/c6ib00105j

Steimer, A., Haltner, E., and Lehr, C. M. (2005). Cell culture models of the respiratory tract relevant to pulmonary drug delivery. *J. Aerosol Med. Depos. Clear. Effects Lung* 18, 137–182. doi: 10.1089/jam.2005.18.137

Tu, G. W., Shi, Y., Zheng, Y. J., Ju, M. J., He, H. Y., Ma, G. G., et al. (2017). Glucocorticoid attenuates acute lung injury through induction of type 2 macrophage. *J. Transl. Med.* 15:181. doi: 10.1186/s12967-017-1284-7

Vichyanond, P., Irvin, C. G., Larsen, G. L., Szefler, S. J., and Hill, M. R. (1989). Penetration of corticosteroids into the lung - evidence for a difference between methylprednisolone and prednisolone. *J. Allergy Clin. Immunol.* 84, 867–873. doi: 10.1016/0091-6749(89)90381-3

Vietti, G., Lison, D., and van den Brule, S. (2016). Mechanisms of lung fibrosis induced by carbon nanotubes: towards an adverse outcome pathway (AOP). *Part. Fibre Toxicol.* 13:11. doi: 10.1186/s12989-016-0123-y

Villeneuve, D. L., Landesmann, B., Allavena, P., Ashley, N., Bal-Price, A., Corsini, E., et al. (2018). Representing the process of inflammation as key events in adverse outcome pathways. *Toxicol. Sci.* 163, 346–352. doi: 10.1093/toxsci/kfy047

Viola, H., Chang, J., Grunwell, J. R., Hecker, L., Tirouvanziam, R., Grotberg, J. B., et al. (2019). Microphysiological systems modeling acute respiratory distress syndrome that capture mechanical force-induced injury-inflammation-repair. *Apl. Bioengin.* 3:41503. doi: 10.1063/1.5111549

Visintin, A., Mazzoni, A., Spitzer, J. H., Wyllie, D. H., Dower, S. K., and Segal, D. M. (2001). Regulation of toll-like receptors in human monocytes and dendritic cells. *J. Immunol.* 166, 249–255. doi: 10.4049/jimmunol.166.1.249

Waljee, A. K., Rogers, M. A. M., Lin, P., Singal, A. G., Stein, J. D., Marks, R. M., et al. (2017). Short term use of oral corticosteroids and related harms among adults in the United States: population based cohort study. *BMJ* 357:j1415. doi: 10.1136/bmj.j1415

Wang, N., Liang, H., and Zen, K. (2014). Molecular mechanisms that influence the macrophage m1-m2 polarization balance. *Front. Immunol.* 5:614. doi: 10.3389/fimmu.2014.00614

Widdrington, J. D., Gomez-Duran, A., Pyle, A., Ruchaud-Sparagano, M.-H., Scott, J., Baudouin, S. V., et al. (2018). Exposure of monocytic cells to lipopolysaccharide induces coordinated endotoxin tolerance. Mitochondrial biogenesis, mitophagy, and antioxidant defenses. *Front. Immunol.* 9:2217. doi: 10.3389/fimmu.2018.02217

Xie, Y., Tolmeijer, S., Oskam, J. M., Tonkens, T., Meijer, A. H., and Schaaf, M. J. M. (2019). Glucocorticoids inhibit macrophage differentiation towards a pro-inflammatory phenotype upon wounding without affecting their migration. *Dis. Models Mech.* 12:dmm037887. doi: 10.1242/dmm.037887

Yonker, L. M., Mou, H., Chu, K. K., Pazos, M. A., Leung, H., Cui, D., et al. (2017). Development of a primary human co-culture model of inflamed airway mucosa. *Sci. Rep.* 7:8182. doi: 10.1038/s41598-017-08567-w

Zach, T. L., Herrman, V. A., Hill, L. D., and Leuschen, M. P. (1993). Effect of steroids on the synthesis of complement C3 in a human alveolar epithelial cell line. *Exp. Lung Res.* 19, 603–616. doi: 10.3109/01902149309031731

Zhou, T., Hu, Y., Wang, Y., Sun, C., Zhong, Y., Liao, J., et al. (2019). Fine particulate matter (PM2.5) aggravates apoptosis of cigarette-inflamed bronchial epithelium in vivo and vitro. *Environ. Pollut.* 248, 1–9. doi: 10.1016/j.envpol.2018.11.054

14

A High-Throughput System for Cyclic Stretching of Precision-Cut Lung Slices during Acute Cigarette Smoke Extract Exposure

*Jarred R. Mondoñedo[1,2], Elizabeth Bartolák-Suki[1], Samer Bou Jawde[1], Kara Nelson[1], Kun Cao[1], Adam Sonnenberg[3], Walter Patrick Obrochta[1], Jasmin Imsirovic[1], Sumati Ram-Mohan[4], Ramaswamy Krishnan[4] and Béla Suki[1]**

[1] Department of Biomedical Engineering, College of Engineering, Boston University, Boston, MA, United States, [2] Boston University School of Medicine, Boston, MA, United States, [3] Department of Systems Engineering, College of Engineering, Boston University, Boston, MA, United States, [4] Department of Emergency Medicine, Beth Israel Deaconess Medical Center, Harvard Medical School, Boston, MA, United States

***Correspondence:**
Béla Suki
bsuki@bu.edu

Rationale: Precision-cut lung slices (PCLSs) are a valuable tool in studying tissue responses to an acute exposure; however, cyclic stretching may be necessary to recapitulate physiologic, tidal breathing conditions.

Objectives: To develop a multi-well stretcher and characterize the PCLS response following acute exposure to cigarette smoke extract (CSE).

Methods: A 12-well stretching device was designed, built, and calibrated. PCLS were obtained from male Sprague-Dawley rats (N = 10) and assigned to one of three groups: 0% (unstretched), 5% peak-to-peak amplitude (low-stretch), and 5% peak-to-peak amplitude superimposed on 10% static stretch (high-stretch). Lung slices were cyclically stretched for 12 h with or without CSE in the media. Levels of Interleukin-1β (IL-1β), matrix metalloproteinase (MMP)-1 and its tissue inhibitor (TIMP1), and membrane type-MMP (MT1-MMP) were assessed via western blot from tissue homogenate.

Results: The stretcher system produced nearly identical normal Lagrangian strains (E_{xx} and E_{yy}, $p > 0.999$) with negligible shear strain ($E_{xy} < 0.0005$) and low intra-well variability 0.127 ± 0.073%. CSE dose response curve was well characterized by a four-parameter logistic model ($R^2 = 0.893$), yielding an IC_{50} value of 0.018 cig/mL. Cyclic stretching for 12 h did not decrease PCLS viability. Two-way ANOVA detected a significant interaction between CSE and stretch pattern for IL-1β ($p = 0.017$), MMP-1, TIMP1, and MT1-MMP ($p < 0.001$).

Conclusion: This platform is capable of high-throughput testing of an acute exposure under tightly-regulated, cyclic stretching conditions. We conclude that the acute mechano-inflammatory response to CSE exhibits complex, stretch-dependence in the PCLS.

Keywords: stretcher, IL-1b, MMP-1, mechanotrasduction, emphysema

INTRODUCTION

Precision-cut lung slices (PCLSs) have emerged as a valuable tool in lung biology (Tepper et al., 2005; Henjakovic et al., 2008; Khan et al., 2010; Lavoie et al., 2012; Schlepütz et al., 2012; Rosner et al., 2014; Hiorns et al., 2016; Van Dijk et al., 2016). A key advantage of this preparation is that the PCLS can be acutely exposed to disease-modifying conditions, such as enzymatic parenchymal digestion in emphysema (Van Dijk et al., 2016), while recording corresponding structural and functional changes in both space and time (Hiorns et al., 2016; Lavoie et al., 2012). PCLSs also benefit by preserving the native extracellular environment (Sanderson, 2011) and retaining nearly all of the resident cell types in the lung. These technical advantages have thus promoted widespread adoption of the PCLS in models of exposure assessment (Langer et al., 2012; Lauenstein et al., 2014; Uhl et al., 2015; Hess et al., 2016; Watson et al., 2016; Neuhaus et al., 2017), pharmacologic therapy (Switalla et al., 2010; van Rijt et al., 2015; Donovan et al., 2016; Kistemaker et al., 2017), and disease modeling, including chronic obstructive pulmonary disease (COPD) (Chronic Obstructive Lung Disease [COLD], 2017).

The overwhelming majority of this prior work has examined the PCLS under static conditions. However, the lung is continuously and rhythmically stretched during tidal breathing *in vivo* and thus, a more accurate recapitulation of native lung responsiveness demands similar dynamic conditions be imposed *ex vivo* (Suki et al., 2013). For example, the absence of stretch has been shown to influence cellular and enzymatic maintenance of tissue properties (Yi et al., 2016; Jesudason et al., 2010) by impacting the biological phenomenon known as mechanotransduction (Ingber, 2006). One of the few models incorporating cyclic stretching of PCLS showed that stretch magnitude in ventilator induced lung injury (VILI) modulated the nuclear translocation of NF-κB and oxidative stress responses in lung slices (Song et al., 2016; Davidovich et al., 2013b). It has been suggested that analogous mechanisms could facilitate emphysema progression in the lung via stretch-dependent secretion of pro-inflammatory cytokines and enzymes accelerating matrix turnover (Suki et al., 2013). Yet, comparable and potentially transformative studies aimed at elucidating the possible role of mechanotransduction in COPD pathogenesis and progression are lacking.

Here, we report the design and implementation of a multi-well equibiaxial device to cyclically stretch PCLSs obtained from excised rat lungs. Its primary advantages include high-throughput, low variance, and the ability to deliver complex, user-defined stretch patterns to the entire slice. To demonstrate the feasibility of this system in studying the mechano-inflammatory response to an acute pharmacologic exposure, we use cigarette smoke extract (CSE) during cyclic stretching to mimic cigarette smoking *in vivo*. We hypothesize the corresponding physiological response is stretch-pattern dependent. To test this, we first confirm tissue viability in this system and then compare the effects of stretch and CSE exposure on biochemical changes in several molecular markers known to play a role in COPD.

MATERIALS AND METHODS

Device Design

The multi-well stretching system pictured in **Figure 1** was built and calibrated based on previous designs (Arold et al., 2009; Imsirovic et al., 2015). Briefly, one or two 6-well plates with deformable elastic membranes are secured in the upper stage of the stretcher. A linear actuating motor (A1 Series: Servo Cylinder, Ultra Motion, Cutchogue, NY, United States) is used to move the stage vertically. As the stage moves down, the elastic membrane in each well is stretched around a fixed, cylindrical indenter post. As the stage moves back up, the elastic membrane relaxes to its initial configuration. Cyclic stretching is achieved by repeating this process at a prescribed rate and displacement depth, which corresponds to the area strain translated to the elastic membrane. Ball bearings (McMaster-Carr, Elhmhurst, IL, United States) affixed to the top of the indenter posts reduce friction, heat generation, and hysteresis. Detailed designs available by request.

A custom software interface (Embarcadero C++ Developer, Austin, TX, United States) was developed to prescribe any simple or complex stretch pattern with parameters including

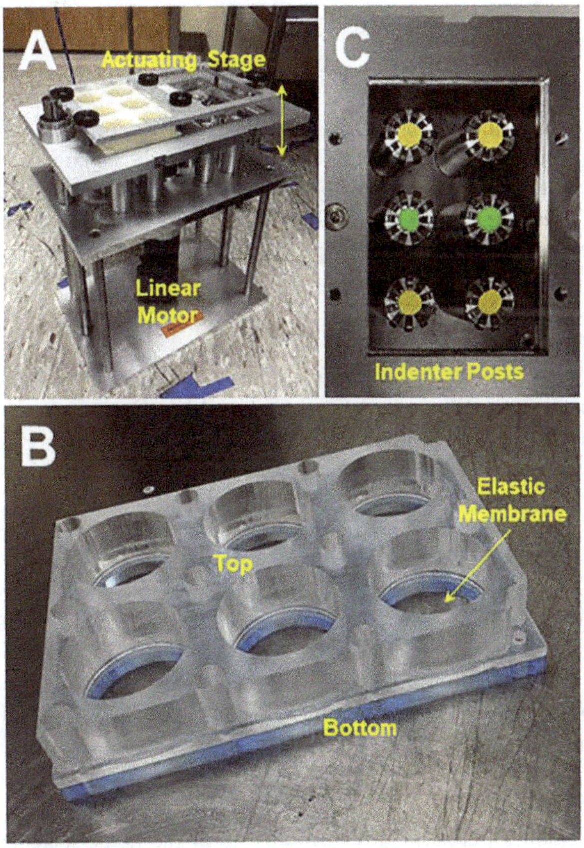

FIGURE 1 | (A) Multi-well device for cyclic stretching of precision-cut lung slices (PCLSs), see text for design details. **(B)** Reusable 6-well flexframe with interchangeable elastic membrane. **(C)** Ball bearings affixed to the indenter posts minimized friction during stretch.

waveform type, frequency, amplitude, and duration. The entire system was constructed from stainless steel and could be moved to a cell culture incubator for stretching under controlled, sterile conditions.

We also designed and fabricated a lightweight, reusable 6-well plate acrylic "flexframe" with an interchangeable elastic, silicone membrane (Specialty Manufacturing, Inc., Saginaw, MI, United States), which we validated by comparison with a commercially available alternative (BioFlex® Culture Plates, Flexcell International Corp., Burlington, NC, United States). The top and bottom components of the flexframe are separable, allowing for replacement of the elastic membrane between experiments.

Device Calibration

To calibrate the relationship between stage displacement and membrane surface area, colored acrylic markers (Pēbēo, Cedex, France) were adhered to the membrane in a circular arrangement and then tracked during quasi-static stretch to compute local radial area change. The corresponding area strain-displacement curve was used to calibrate the stretcher and prescribe area strains for cyclic stretching. Delaunay triangulation and radial displacement of individual beads were used to calculate the Lagrangian strain E_{ij} of the elastic membrane during stretch according to the following relation (Holzapfel, 2000):

$$ds^2 - ds_0^2 = 2E_{ij} da_i da_j$$

where ds and ds_0 are the segment lengths before and after deformation, respectively, of each triangle, while da_i and da_j are the changes in position of the bead vertices. To assess whether repeated stretch induced plastic deformation of the elastic membrane, this calibration procedure was repeated following 12 h of stretch.

Animal Protocol

Protocol #16-025 was reviewed and approved by the Boston University Institutional Animal Care and Use Committee. Male Sprague-Dawley rats (N = 10) with body weight 343.8 ± 60.2 g were sedated via intraperitoneal injection of xylazine (10 mg/kg) and ketamine (90 mg/kg). After ensuring appropriate depth of anesthesia and analgesia, animals were euthanized via abdominal aortic exsanguination. The lungs were excised and insufflated via tracheostomy with 10–12 mL of 1.5% low melt agarose (HyAgarose, ACTGene Inc., Piscataway, NJ, United States) in Hanks' buffered salt solution (HBSS, Sigma) at 37°C, according to previous techniques (Watson et al., 2016). Excised lungs were then placed on ice for 15 min to allow for solidification of the agarose.

Precision-Cut Lung Slices (PCLSs)

Lung lobes were separated, trimmed to fit the tissue stage, and then sliced in cooled HBSS with thickness ~500 μm using a vibratome (752M Vibroslice, Campden Instruments Ltd., United Kingdom). The vibratome tissue stage was modified to include an adjustable, cylindrical sleeve that was filled with agarose to help stabilize the lung lobe during slicing. PCLSs were then "punched" using either a 6 or 10 mm coring tool (Acuderm Inc., Fort Lauderdale, FL, United States) to generate round, symmetric slices. Punching the tissues after slicing the entire lobe was found to yield a greater amount of material compared to coring the lung lobes prior to slicing. PCLSs were then moved to Dulbecco's Modified Eagle's Medium (DMEM, Gibco) supplemented with penicillin, streptomycin, and amphotericin B (Antimycotic-Antibiotic, Gibco). To facilitate removal of residual agarose and other cellular debris, media was changed every 30 min for 0–2 h after slicing, 1 h for 2–4 h, 2 h for 4–8 h, and 24 h thereafter, similar to previous methods (Davidovich et al., 2013a,b; Song et al., 2016). Lung slices were incubated under standard conditions (5% CO_2 at 37°C) and allowed to recover overnight.

MTS Assay

PCLS viability was assessed via MTS assay, which is a colorimetric measure of cell metabolic activity (Berridge et al., 2005). The formazan product yielded by this reaction is proportional to the number of metabolically healthy or active cells and is quantified by measuring the absorbance at 490 nm. The colorimetric MTS assay was used according to manufacturer's specifications. Lung slices (6 mm) were incubated in individual wells with 20 μL of MTS reagent in 200 μL of HBSS for 1.5 h at 37°C. The supernatant was then removed to a 96-well plate for measurement of optical density.

Preparation and Potency of Cigarette Smoke Extract (CSE)

Cigarette smoke extract solutions were prepared fresh by bubbling two cigarettes (Marlboro Red, Philip Morris USA, Richmond, VA, United States) with the filters removed, through 20 mL of DMEM at a rate of 1.0 L/min to yield a stock solution of 0.1 cig/mL. Next, the solutions were sterile filtered using a 0.22 μm pore size membrane vacuum filtration system (Steriflip, EMD Millipore) to remove large tobacco debris and other small particles. To determine the CSE dose response curve, the stock solution was diluted and 6 mm lung slices (N = 93) were incubated in 6-well plates for 12 h with CSE concentrations ranging from 0.001 to 0.050 cig/mL (~3 slices per 3 mL of solution in each well). Following incubation, individual slices were rinsed with warmed HBSS to remove any residual solution containing the CSE-media mix. PCLS were transferred to a 96-well plate for assessment of viability via MTS assay as described above.

Experimental Protocol

Individual lung slices were attached to the center of the elastic membranes in each well using four evenly spaced beads of cyanoacrylate glue along the tissue perimeter. Initial pilot studies confirmed appropriate local tissue stretch with this preparation (**Supplementary Figure S1**). PCLSs were covered with 3 mL of media with or without CSE (0.01 cig/mL) for the treated and control groups, respectively, then sinusoidally stretched for 12 h at 1 Hz under standard incubation conditions. To assess the effect of different stretch patterns, PCLS were randomly assigned to one of the following three stretch amplitude groups: unstretched (US); low-stretch (LS), 5% peak-to-peak amplitude with no static stretch; and high-stretch (HS), 5% peak-to-peak amplitude superimposed on 10% static stretch. These waveforms were arbitrarily selected to simulate regions of lung experiencing different stretch during tidal breathing; a schematic is shown in **Figure 2**. Following cyclic stretch, the PCLSs were collected from each well for biochemical analysis (N = 48). Protease inhibitors EDTA and Halt Protease Inhibitor cocktail (Thermo Scientific) were added to the homogenized tissue samples, then stored at −20°C until further use. PCLSs were also collected to assess tissue viability after stretching (N = 49). Lung slices were trimmed using a 6 mm coring tool to reduce edge effects from slicing and the attachment procedure, then evaluated via MTS as before.

Western Blot

Protein concentrations for the homogenized tissues were determined using the BCA colorimetric protein assay kit (Pierce, Thermo Scientific). The assay was used according to manufacturer's specifications. Equal amounts of protein (~3.7 μg) from each sample were separated via sodium dodecyl sulfate polyacrylamide gel electrophoresis (SDS-PAGE), transferred to a polyvinylidene difluoride (PVDF) membrane, and blocked using 5% bovine serum albumin in phosphate buffered saline containing 0.05% Tween 20 (PBS-T). All groups were run on the same membrane. After blocking for 2 h, the membrane was incubated for 1 h at room temperature with primary antibodies anti-IL-1β (1:250, Abcam), anti-MMP-1 (1:1000, Thermo Fisher Scientific), TIMP1 (1:1000, Abcam), MT1-MMP (1:5000, Abcam), and anti-GAPDH (loading control, 1 μg/ml, Abcam), washed in PBS-T 4 × 15 min, incubated with secondary antibody (anti-mouse, 1:7000, anti-rabbit, 1:10000, Vector Laboratories) for 1 h, and again washed in PBS-T 4 × 15 min. Quantitative densitometry was performed after chemiluminescence detection (SuperSignal West Pico Chemiluminescent Substrate, Pierce) with picomolar sensitivity similar to that of ELISA, with corrections for background and loading control.

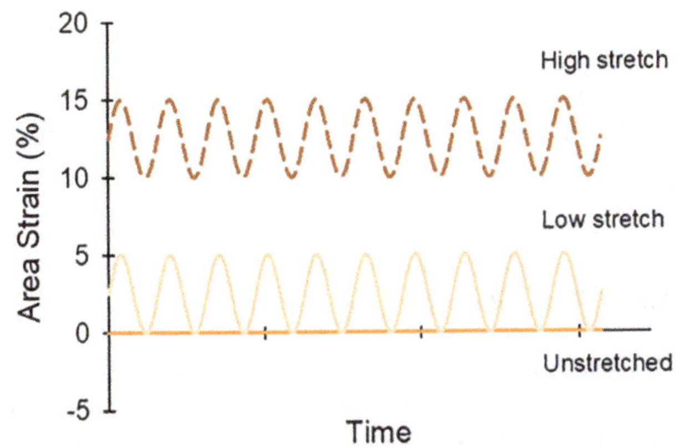

FIGURE 2 | Lung slices were randomly assigned to one of three stretch patterns: unstretched (0%), low stretch (0–5% area strain), or high stretch (10–15% area strain).

Statistical Analysis

Data analysis and fitting were performed using MATLAB (R2016a, MathWorks, Natick, MA, United States) and SigmaPlot (SigmaPlot v12.3, Systat Software, Inc., San Jose, CA, United States). CSE dose response data was fitted using a four-parameter logistic regression as follows:

$$y = a + \frac{b - a}{1 + \left(\frac{x}{c}\right)^d}$$

where y is normalized absorbance; x is CSE concentration a and b are the minimum and maximum values possible, respectively, c is the point of inflection; and d is a coefficient characterizing the slope of the curve. Two-Way analysis of variance (ANOVA) was used to evaluate the influence of stretch and CSE on PCLS viability as well as on IL-1β, MT1-MMP, MMP-1, and TIMP1. Holm-Sidak method was used for *post hoc* comparisons. For all, $p < 0.05$ was considered significant.

RESULTS

Figure 3 presents the calibration and validation of the multi-well stretcher and FlexFrame devices. Vertical displacement of the actuating stage yielded a non-linear relation between area strain and motor position (**Figure 3A**), which was used to prescribe waveforms for cyclic stretching. Note the minimal hysteresis between loading and unloading of the flexframe elastic membrane, 6.34%. Normal Lagrangian strains, E_{xx} and E_{yy}, were nearly identical, $\rho > 0.999$, with negligible shear strain, $E_{xy} < 0.0005$, demonstrating equibiaxial strain of the elastic membrane (**Figure 3B**). Compared to the commercially available BioFlex Culture Plates, our custom fabricated flexframe demonstrated lower intra-well variance for area strain, 0.473 ± 0.717% vs. 0.127 ± 0.073% (Variance Mean ± SD), particularly at larger prescribed strains (**Figure 3C**). Finally, there was no detectable plastic deformation of the membrane due to stretch as there was no difference in measured area strains before and after 12 h of cyclic stretching (slope: 0.998 with R^2 = 0.997; **Figure 3D**).

Figure 4 shows the effects of CSE and cyclic stretch on tissue viability. We first established a sub-toxic concentration mimicking acute cigarette smoke exposure *in vivo* (**Figure 4A**). As expected, PCLS viability decreased with CSE concentration. The corresponding dose response curve was well characterized by a four-parameter logistic model (R^2 = 0.893), yielding an IC_{50} value of 0.018 cig/mL corresponding to the CSE concentration at half-maximal viability. Based on this curve, the CSE concentration was selected to be 0.01 cig/mL for all subsequent experiments. We then confirmed tissue viability following 12 h of cyclic stretching ± CSE (**Figure 4B**). Two-way ANOVA detected no statistical difference in PCLS viability

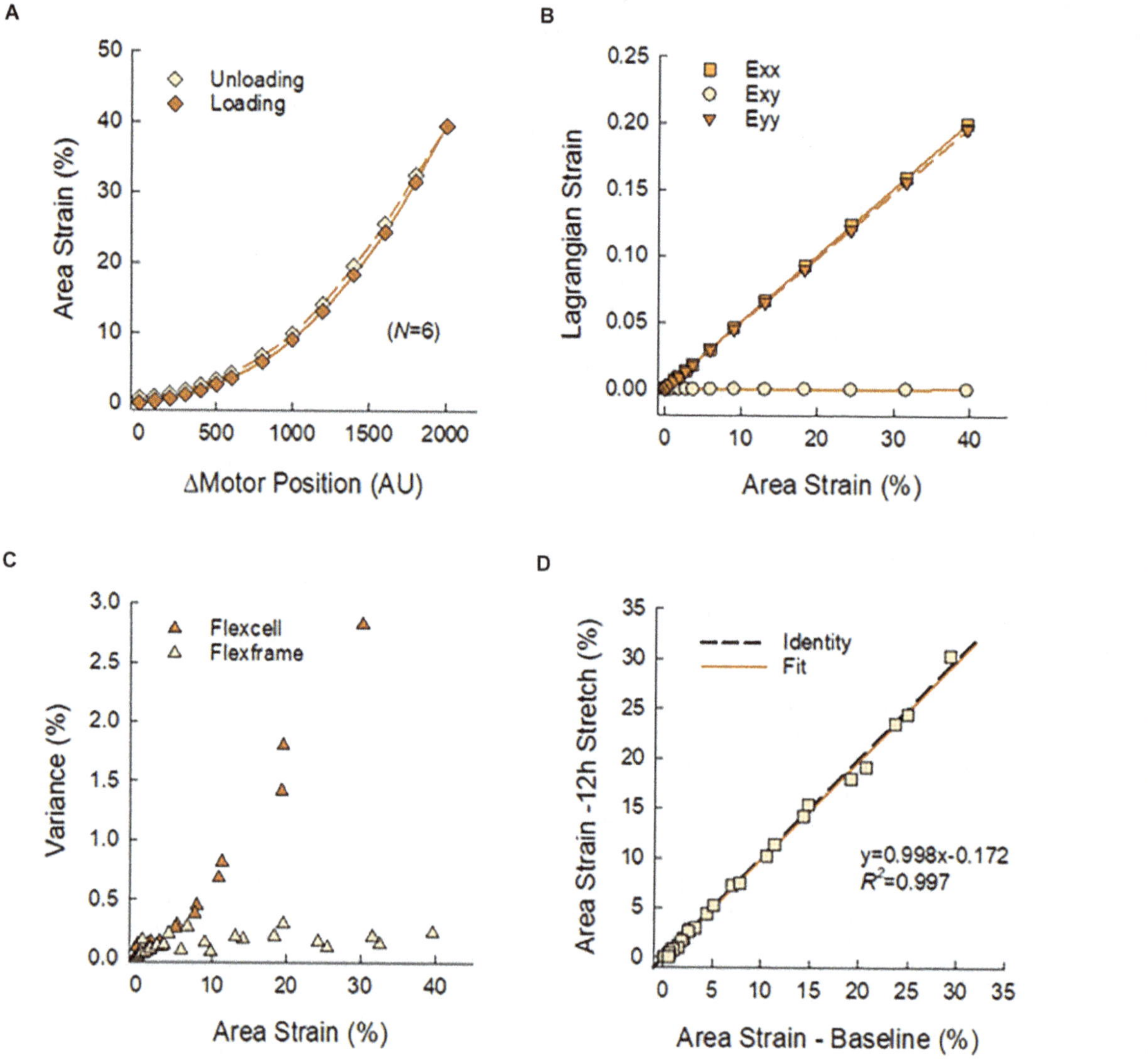

FIGURE 3 | (A) Calibration curve used to prescribe membrane area strain as a function of motor position. Symbols represent means of $N = 6$ wells with standard deviations smaller than symbol sizes. **(B)** Nearly identical normal strains, E_{xx} and E_{yy}, and negligible shear strain, E_{xy}, as estimated by Delaunay triangulation, confirmed equbiaxial strain of the elastic membrane. **(C)** The reusable flexframe exhibited lower variance of area strain in comparison to a commercially available disposable alternative. **(D)** There was no observable mechanical change in the elastic membrane after 12 h of cyclic stretching.

among different stretch patterns ($p = 0.070$), CSE exposure ($p = 0.594$), or their interaction ($p = 0.277$).

As shown in **Figure 5**, Two-Way ANOVA detected a significant interaction between stretch pattern and CSE exposure on the tissue content of all measured molecular markers (IL-1β, $p = 0.017$; MT1-MMP, MMP-1, TIMP1, $p < 0.001$). Each had a unique response to stretch and CSE. We found that IL-1β (**Figure 5A**) exhibited the greatest response to stretching ($p < 0.001$) among the group, and was statistically higher with CSE exposure ($p < 0.001$) for all stretch patterns. CSE also had a significant effect ($p < 0.001$) on MT1-MMP (**Figure 5C**), though regulation directionality depended on stretch pattern ($p < 0.001$). In contrast, stretch pattern had a significant effect on MMP-1 (**Figure 5B**) in the presence of CSE ($p < 0.001$), whereas it only had an effect on TIMP1 (**Figure 5D**) in the absence of CSE ($p < 0.001$). The enzymes MT1-MMP and MMP-1 had the greatest tissue content for LS with CSE exposure, while the tissue content of the inhibitor TIMP1 was the greatest for the same stretch pattern when CSE was absent.

DISCUSSION

In this study, we present the design and implementation of a multi-well stretcher to investigate the mechano-inflammatory response in lung tissue following an acute pharmacologic insult. This is the first report to combine CSE exposure with cyclic PCLS stretching as an *ex vivo* model of the dynamic changes in lung volume that occur during cigarette smoke inhalation *in vivo*. First, we demonstrated this device delivered repeatable,

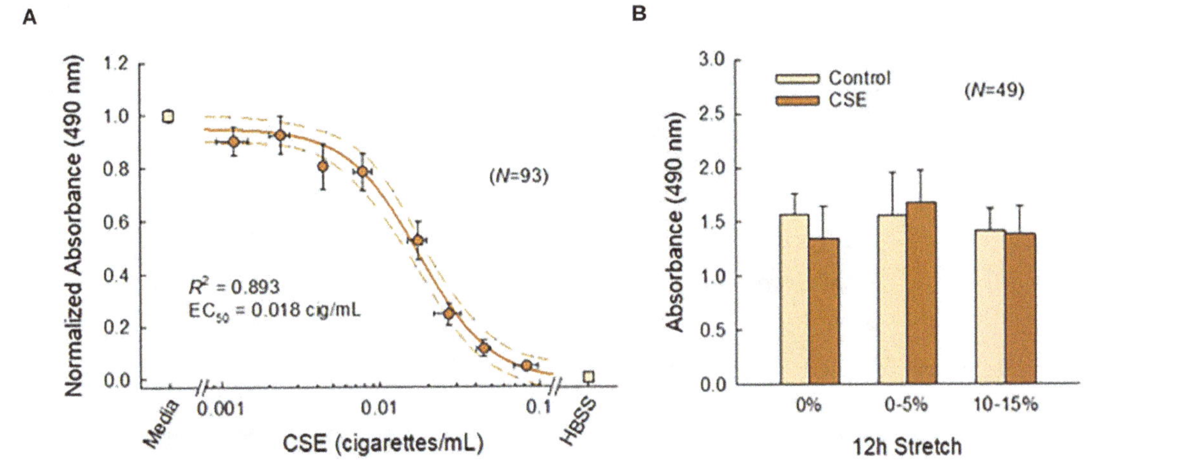

FIGURE 4 | (A) Lung slice (N = 93) viability decreased with CSE concentration and was well characterized (R^2 = 0.893) by a four-parameter logistic curve (solid line) shown with 95% confidence intervals (dashed lines). Binned data across multiple CSE concentrations are shown, vertical and horizontal error bars represent SE and SD, respectively. **(B)** The sub-toxic CSE concentration was selected to be 0.01 cig/mL. Two-way ANOVA detected no effects for stretch and CSE at this concentration, indicating tissue viability was not compromised with this system. Error bars represent SD.

low-variance, equibiaxial stretch. We then characterized the CSE dose response curve in PCLSs and confirmed that cyclic stretching did not compromise tissue viability. Finally, we found the interaction between stretch pattern and CSE exposure had a significant effect on all of the molecular markers, with each exhibiting a unique response pattern. Together, these findings demonstrate the feasibility of using this system to recapitulate tidal breathing-like conditions in PCLS, while identifying specific stretch-dependent molecular responses to acute CSE exposure.

Various approaches have been reported for stretching PCLS. Techniques range from suturing (Davidovich et al., 2013a,b) or clamping (Dassow et al., 2010) the PCLS to a deformable elastic membrane, to compressing it between a polyacrylamide gel and a hollow indenter (Lavoie et al., 2012). While such devices allow for real-time imaging, they can be time consuming, limited to a single lung slice, or constrained to a small area-of-stretch. In contrast, the multi-well device described here provides simultaneous, whole-slice stretching of up to 12 samples with minimal preparation time. A commercially available alternative capable of accommodating multiple lung slices operates by applying a negative pressure vacuum to deform an elastic membrane around a rigid post. However, we found that indenter posts with integrated ball bearings improved hysteresis, stretch homogeneity, and inter-cycle repeatability compared to other designs using grease to reduce friction, which can also cause heat-induced cell damage (Arold et al., 2009). Moreover, the flexframe design introduced here is considerably more economic, easy to build, reusable, and customizable with significantly lower intra-well variance. Although stretcher selection is generally dictated by application and familiarity, our device as described above is ideal for higher throughput testing of acute exposures, either pathologic or therapeutic, under tightly-regulated, physiologic stretching conditions.

This platform is uniquely appropriate for investigating mechano-inflammatory interactions, such as those underlying COPD. Biomechanical forces are known to facilitate emphysema progression (Mishima et al., 1999; Kononov et al., 2001; Yi et al., 2016) along with inflammatory stimuli (*i.e.*, cigarette smoking) that weaken and predispose tissue to failure (Suki et al., 2003). Yet, there is a paucity of data describing their relationship. CSE has been used with *in vitro* (Nana-Sinkam et al., 2007; Stringer et al., 2007; Thaikoottathil et al., 2009; Farid et al., 2013; Ballweg et al., 2014; Chen et al., 2014) and small animal (Chen et al., 2009, 2010; Hanaoka et al., 2011; Lee et al., 2012; He et al., 2015; Chai et al., 2016) models of cigarette smoke exposure given its relatively short incubation time and similarity to pathophysiology *in vivo*. As a proof of concept, we used our system to characterize the PCLS response to acute CSE exposure under various stretch patterns, simulating cigarette smoke inhalation during tidal breathing-like conditions.

IL-1β and MMP-1 expression are often upregulated in patients with COPD (Imai et al., 2001; Ostridge et al., 2016), while MT1-MMP and TIMP1 imbalance can lead to improper lung tissue maintenance (Vandenbroucke et al., 2011; Woode et al., 2015). We observed that the interaction between stretch pattern and CSE exposure had a significant effect on these markers. IL-1β increased with CSE and showed the most robust response to stretch, whereas the enzymes MT1-MMP and MMP-1 and the inhibitor TIMP1 could be either up- or down-regulated by CSE depending on the level of stretch. Interestingly, the low stretch group showed the greatest tissue content of MT1-MMP and MMP-1 when CSE was present, and conversely when it was absent for TIMP1, suggesting this stretch pattern may be most sensitive to an acute exposure. Additional silver staining revealed similar regulatory effects on protein species across a range of molecular weights (**Supplementary Figure S2** and **Supplementary Table S1**). While not a comprehensive model of COPD, the stretch-dependent response to acute CSE exposure observed here suggests a role for mechanotransduction in modulating regional inflammation and enzyme burden on

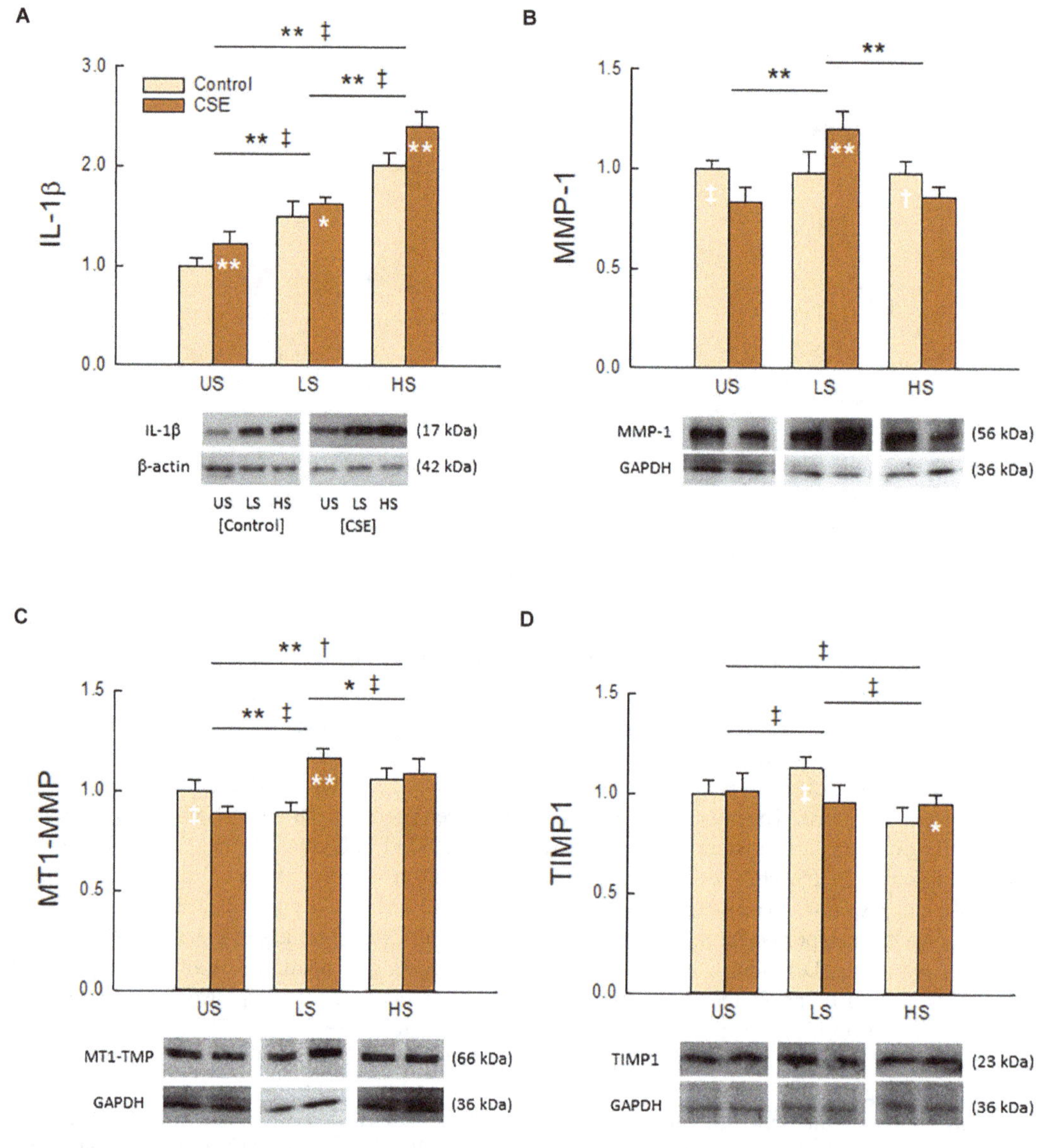

FIGURE 5 | Effects of stretch pattern, CSE, and their interaction on tissue content of IL-1β **(A)**, MMP-1 **(B)**, MT1-MMP **(C)**, and TIMP1 **(D)**. Representative bands with loading controls are also shown. Data (N = 8) are shown as normalized mean and SD ($^{*\dagger}p < 0.05$ and $^{**\ddagger}p < 0.001$ for CSE and Control groups, respectively). For presentation purposes the original images were cut to smaller ones including representative bands in the desired order and, according to standard publication guideless, white spaces were left between them.

the alveoli. One may speculate this could further exacerbate structural disease heterogeneity and emphysema progression, particularly in tissue experiencing abnormal stretch (Mishima et al., 1999; Suki et al., 2003; Bhatt et al., 2016, 2017; Bodduluri et al., 2017; Mondoñedo and Suki, 2017). In any case, these findings show a clear and definitive difference in PCLS response to an acute exposure between cyclically stretched and unstretched conditions, highlighting the need to provide a comparable dynamic environment as experienced by the lung during tidal breathing *in vivo*.

There are some limitations of this study. (1) Bathing the lung slices directly in media simultaneously exposes all cell types to CSE, whereas exposure to inhaled cigarette smoke initially occurs at the airway and alveolar wall interfaces primarily involving epithelial cells. This is an inherent limitation of the PCLS design. Similarly, the MTS analysis does not specify local tissue viability, but could be extended with immunohistochemistry to verify cell origin. (2) The low-melt agarose is likely incompletely removed despite frequent media changes after slicing as in previous studies (Tepper et al., 2005; Sanderson, 2011; Davidovich et al., 2013b), which could affect the apparent stiffness and residual area of the lung slice. Thus, excised lungs were carefully prepared in the same manner each time to minimize disparities between animals. (3) The lack of circulation in the PCLS limits the study of chemotactic factors, including neutrophil recruitment, which participate in the inflammatory response to cigarette smoking (van der Vaart et al., 2004). (4) While this platform does not facilitate real-time imaging, flexframes are easily removed to visualize lung slices immediately after stretching. (5) Although the deformation provided by the equibiaxial stretching is not 3-dimensional uniform expansion, cells experience physiologically appropriate stretch as the aspect ratio is approximately 1 to 16.

In summary, we demonstrated the feasibility of using this device to perform high-throughput testing of an acute exposure under tightly-regulated, cyclic stretching conditions. We showed that pro-inflammatory and enzyme expression-related effects of acute exposure to cigarette smoke extract are stretch-dependent. These findings identify a fundamental difference between static and tidal breathing-like conditions in precision-cut lung slices. Additional studies in PCLS are required to determine whether mechanotransduction could be a key mediator in COPD disease pathogenesis and progression.

AUTHOR CONTRIBUTIONS

JM designed the stretcher and experiments, carried out studies, analyzed the data, and wrote the manuscript. EB-S carried out the biochemical assays and analyzed the data. SB analyzed the data. AS analyzed the data and designed the stretcher. KN, KC, AS, WO, and SR-M carried out the experiments. RK designed the experiments. JI designed the stretcher. BS designed the stretcher and experiments, analyzed the data, and wrote the manuscript.

ACKNOWLEDGMENTS

The authors thank Dr. Niccole Schaible and Ms. Ariana Harvey for their contributions in the early stages of this study.

REFERENCES

Arold, S. P., Bartolák-Suki, E., and Suki, B. (2009). Variable stretch pattern enhances surfactant secretion in alveolar type II cells in culture. *Am. J. Physiol. Lung Cell. Mol. Physiol.* 296, L574–L581. doi: 10.1152/ajplung.90454.2008

Ballweg, K., Mutze, K., Königshoff, M., Eickelberg, O., and Meiners, S. (2014). Cigarette smoke extract affects mitochondrial function in alveolar epithelial cells. *Am. J. Physiol. Lung Cell. Mol. Physiol.* 307, L895–L907. doi: 10.1152/ajplung.00180.2014

Berridge, M. V., Herst, P. M., and Tan, A. S. (2005). Tetrazolium dyes as tools in cell biology: new insights into their cellular reduction. *Biotechnol. Annu. Rev.* 11, 127–152. doi: 10.1016/s1387-2656(05)11004-7

Bhatt, S. P., Bodduluri, S., Hoffman, E. A., Newell, J. D. Jr., Sieren, J. C., Dransfield, M. T., et al. (2017). CT measure of lung at-risk and lung function decline in chronic obstructive pulmonary disease. *Am. J. Respir. Crit. Care Med.* 196, 569–576.

Bhatt, S. P., Bodduluri, S., Newell, J. D., Hoffman, E. A., Sieren, J. C., Han, M. K., et al. (2016). CT-derived biomechanical metrics improve agreement between spirometry and emphysema. *Acad. Radiol.* 23, 1255–1263. doi: 10.1016/j.acra.2016.02.002

Bodduluri, S., Bhatt, S. P., Hoffman, E. A., Newell, JD Jr, Martinez, C. H., Dransfield, M. T., et al. (2017). Biomechanical CT metrics are associated with patient outcomes in COPD. *Thorax* 72, 409–414. doi: 10.1136/thoraxjnl-2016-209544

Chai, X.-M., Li, Y.-L., Chen, H., Guo, S.-L., Shui, L.-L., and Chen, Y.-J. (2016). Cigarette smoke extract alters the cell cycle via the phospholipid transfer protein/transforming growth factor-β1/CyclinD1/CDK4 pathway. *Eur. J. Pharmacol.* 786, 85–93. doi: 10.1016/j.ejphar.2016.05.037

Chen, L., Ge, Q., Tjin, G., Alkhouri, H., Deng, L., Brandsma, C. A., et al. (2014). Effects of cigarette smoke extract on human airway smooth muscle cells in COPD. *Eur. Respir. J.* 44, 634–646. doi: 10.1183/09031936.00171313

Chen, Y., Hanaoka, M., Chen, P., Droma, Y., Voelkel, N. F., and Kubo, K. (2009). Protective effect of beraprost sodium, a stable prostacyclin analog, in the development of cigarette smoke extract-induced emphysema. *Am. J. Physiol. Lung Cell. Mol. Physiol.* 296, L648–L656. doi: 10.1152/ajplung.90270.2008

Chen, Y., Hanaoka, M., Droma, Y., Chen, P., Voelkel, N. F., and Kubo, K. (2010). Endothelin-1 receptor antagonists prevent the development of pulmonary emphysema in rats. *Eur. Respir. J.* 35, 904–912. doi: 10.1183/09031936.00003909

Chronic Obstructive Lung Disease [GOLD] (2017). From the Global Strategy for the Diagnosis, Management and Prevention of COPD, Global Initiative for Chronic Obstructive Lung Disease (GOLD) 2017. Available from: http://goldcopd.org (accessed 5 February, 2017).

Dassow, C., Wiechert, L., Martin, C., Schumann, S., Müller-Newen, G., Pack, O., et al. (2010). Biaxial distension of precision-cut lung slices. *J. Appl. Physiol.* 108, 713–721. doi: 10.1152/japplphysiol.00229.2009

Davidovich, N., Chhour, P., and Margulies, S. S. (2013a). Uses of remnant human lung tissue for mechanical stretch studies. *Cell. Mol. Bioeng.* 6, 175–182. doi: 10.1007/s12195-012-0263-6

Davidovich, N., Huang, J., and Margulies, S. S. (2013b). Reproducible uniform equibiaxial stretch of precision-cut lung slices. *Am. J. Physiol. Lung Cell. Mol. Physiol.* 304, L210–L220. doi: 10.1152/ajplung.00224.2012

Donovan, C., Seow, H. J., Bourke, J. E., and Vlahos, R. (2016). Influenza A virus infection and cigarette smoke impair bronchodilator responsiveness to β-adrenoceptor agonists in mouse lung. *Clin. Sci. (Lond).* 130, 829–837. doi: 10.1042/cs20160093

Farid, M., Kanaji, N., Nakanishi, M., Gunji, Y., Michalski, J., Iwasawa, S., et al. (2013). Smad3 mediates cigarette smoke extract (CSE) induction of VEGF release by human fetal lung fibroblasts. *Toxicol. Lett.* 220, 126–134. doi: 10.1016/j.toxlet.2013.04.011

Hanaoka, M., Droma, Y., Chen, Y., Agatsuma, T., Kitaguchi, Y., Voelkel, N. F., et al. (2011). Carbocisteine protects against emphysema induced by cigarette smoke extract in rats. *Chest* 139, 1101–1108. doi: 10.1378/chest.10-0920

He, Z. H., Chen, P., Chen, Y., He, S. D., Ye, J. R., Zhang, H. L., et al. (2015). Comparison between cigarette smoke-induced emphysema and cigarette smoke extract-induced emphysema. *Tob. Induc. Dis.* 13:6. doi: 10.1186/s12971-015-0033-z

Henjakovic, M., Martin, C., Hoymann, H. G., Sewald, K., Ressmeyer, A. R., Dassow, C., et al. (2008). Ex vivo lung function measurements in precision-cut lung slices (PCLS) from chemical allergen-sensitized mice represent a suitable alternative to in vivo studies. *Toxicol. Sci.* 106, 444–453. doi: 10.1093/toxsci/kfn178

Hess, A., Wang-Lauenstein, L., Braun, A., Kolle, S. N., Landsiedel, R., Liebsch, M., et al. (2016). Prevalidation of the ex-vivo model PCLS for prediction of respiratory toxicity. *Toxicol. In Vitro* 32, 347–361. doi: 10.1016/j.tiv.2016.01.006

Hiorns, J. E., Bidan, C. M., Jensen, O. E., Gosens, R., Kistemaker, L. E., Fredberg,

J. J., et al. (2016). Airway and parenchymal strains during bronchoconstriction in the precision cut lung slice. *Front. Physiol.* 7:309.

Holzapfel, G. A. (2000). *Nonlinear Solid Mechanics: A Continuum Approach for Engineering, New Edition*. Chichester, NY: Wiley.

Imai, K., Dalal, S. S., Chen, E. S., Downey, R., Schulman, L. L., Ginsburg, M., et al. (2001). Human collagenase (matrix metalloproteinase-1) expression in the lungs of patients with emphysema. *Am. J. Respir. Crit. Care Med.* 163(Pt 1), 786–791. doi: 10.1164/ajrccm.163.3.2001073

Imsirovic, J., Wellman, T. J., Mondoñedo, J. R., Bartolák-Suki, E., and Suki, B. (2015). Design of a novel equi-biaxial stretcher for live cellular and subcellular imaging. *PLoS One* 10:e0140283. doi: 10.1371/journal.pone.0140283

Ingber, D. E. (2006). Cellular mechanotransduction: putting all the pieces together again. *FASEB J.* 20, 811–827. doi: 10.1096/fj.05-5424rev

Jesudason, R., Sato, S., Parameswaran, H., Araujo, A. D., Majumdar, A., Allen, P. G., et al. (2010). Mechanical forces regulate elastase activity and binding site availability in lung elastin. *Biophys. J.* 99, 3076–3083. doi: 10.1016/j.bpj.2010.09.018

Khan, M. A., Ellis, R., Inman, M. D., Bates, J. H. T., Sanderson, M. J., and Janssen, L. J. (2010). Influence of airway wall stiffness and parenchymal tethering on the dynamics of bronchoconstriction. *Am. J. Physiol. Lung Cell. Mol. Physiol.* 299, L98–L108. doi: 10.1152/ajplung.00011.2010

Kistemaker, L. E. M., Oenema, T. A., Baarsma, H. A., Bos, I. S. T., Schmidt, M., Facchinetti, F., et al. (2017). The PDE4 inhibitor CHF-6001 and LAMAs inhibit bronchoconstriction-induced remodeling in lung slices. *Am. J. Physiol. Lung Cell. Mol. Physiol.* 313, L507–L515. doi: 10.1152/ajplung.00069.2017

Kononov, S., Brewer, K., Sakai, H., Cavalcante, F. S., Sabayanagam, C. R., Ingenito, E. P., et al. (2001). Roles of mechanical forces and collagen failure in the development of elastase-induced emphysema. *Am. J. Respir. Crit. Care Med.* 164(Pt 1), 1920–1926. doi: 10.1164/ajrccm.164.10.2101083

Langer, M., Duggan, E. S., Booth, J. L., Patel, V. I., Zander, R. A., Silasi-Mansat, R., et al. (2012). Bacillus anthracis lethal toxin reduces human alveolar epithelial barrier function. *Infect. Immun.* 80, 4374–4387. doi: 10.1128/IAI.01011-12

Lauenstein, L., Switalla, S., Prenzler, F., Seehase, S., Pfennig, O., Förster, C., et al. (2014). Assessment of immunotoxicity induced by chemicals in human precision-cut lung slices (PCLS). *Toxicol. In Vitro* 28, 588–599. doi: 10.1016/j.tiv.2013.12.016

Lavoie, T. L., Krishnan, R., Siegel, H. R., Maston, E. D., Fredberg, J. J., Solway, J., et al. (2012). Dilatation of the constricted human airway by tidal expansion of lung parenchyma. *Am. J. Respir. Crit. Care Med.* 186, 225–232. doi: 10.1164/rccm.201202-0368OC

Lee, J. H., Hanaoka, M., Kitaguchi, Y., Kraskauskas, D., Shapiro, L., Voelkel, N. F., et al. (2012). Imbalance of apoptosis and cell proliferation contributes to the development and persistence of emphysema. *Lung* 190, 69–82. doi: 10.1007/s00408-011-9326-z

Mishima, M., Hirai, T., Itoh, H., Nakano, Y., Sakai, H., Muro, S., et al. (1999). Complexity of terminal airspace geometry assessed by lung computed tomography in normal subjects and patients with chronic obstructive pulmonary disease. *Proc. Natl. Acad. Sci. U.S.A.* 96, 8829–8834. doi: 10.1073/pnas.96.16.8829

Mondoñedo, J. R., and Suki, B. (2017). Predicting structure-function relations and survival following surgical and bronchoscopic lung volume reduction treatment of emphysema. *PLoS Comput. Biol.* 13:e1005282. doi: 10.1371/journal.pcbi.1005282

Nana-Sinkam, S. P., Lee, J. D., Sotto-Santiago, S., Stearman, R. S., Keith, R. L., Choudhury, Q., et al. (2007). Prostacyclin prevents pulmonary endothelial cell apoptosis induced by cigarette smoke. *Am. J. Respir. Crit. Care Med.* 175, 676–685. doi: 10.1164/rccm.200605-724oc

Neuhaus, V., Schaudien, D., Golovina, T., Temann, U. A., Thompson, C., Lippmann, T., et al. (2017). Assessment of long-term cultivated human precision-cut lung slices as an ex vivo system for evaluation of chronic cytotoxicity and functionality. *J. Occup. Med. Toxicol.* 12:13. doi: 10.1186/s12995-017-0158-5

Ostridge, K., Williams, N., Kim, V., Bennett, M., Harden, S., Welch, L., et al. (2016). Relationship between pulmonary matrix metalloproteinases and quantitative CT markers of small airways disease and emphysema in COPD. *Thorax* 71, 126–132. doi: 10.1136/thoraxjnl-2015-207428

Rosner, S. R., Ram-Mohan, S., Paez-Cortez, J. R., Lavoie, T. L., Dowell, M. L., Yuan, L., et al. (2014). Airway contractility in the precision-cut lung slice after cryopreservation. *Am. J. Respir. Cell Mol. Biol.* 50, 876–881. doi: 10.1165/rcmb.2013-0166MA

Sanderson, M. J. (2011). Exploring lung physiology in health and disease with lung slices. *Pulm. Pharmacol. Ther.* 24, 452–465. doi: 10.1016/j.pupt.2011.05.001

Schlepütz, M., Rieg, A. D., Seehase, S., Spillner, J., Perez-Bouza, A., Braunschweig, T., et al. (2012). Neurally mediated airway constriction in human and other species: a comparative study using precision-cut lung slices (PCLS). *PLoS One* 7:e47344. doi: 10.1371/journal.pone.0047344

Song, M. J., Davidovich, N., Lawrence, G. G., and Margulies, S. S. (2016). Superoxide mediates tight junction complex dissociation in cyclically stretched lung slices. *J. Biomech.* 49, 1330–1335. doi: 10.1016/j.jbiomech.2015.10.032

Stringer, K. A., Tobias, M., O'Neill, H. C., and Franklin, C. C. (2007). Cigarette smoke extract-induced suppression of caspase-3-like activity impairs human neutrophil phagocytosis. *Am. J. Physiol. Lung Cell. Mol. Physiol.* 292, L1572–L1579.

Suki, B., Lutchen, K. R., and Ingenito, E. P. (2003). On the progressive nature of emphysema: roles of proteases, inflammation, and mechanical forces. *Am. J. Respir. Crit. Care Med.* 168, 516–521. doi: 10.1164/rccm.200208-908pp

Suki, B., Sato, S., Parameswaran, H., Szabari, M. V., Takahashi, A., and Bartolák-Suki, E. (2013). Emphysema and mechanical stress-induced lung remodeling. *Physiology (Bethesda)* 28, 404–413. doi: 10.1152/physiol.00041.2013

Switalla, S., Lauenstein, L., Prenzler, F., Knothe, S., Förster, C., Fieguth, H. G., et al. (2010). Natural innate cytokine response to immunomodulators and adjuvants in human precision-cut lung slices. *Toxicol. Appl. Pharmacol.* 246, 107–115. doi: 10.1016/j.taap.2010.04.010

Tepper, R. S., Ramchandani, R., Argay, E., Zhang, L., Xue, Z., Liu, Y., et al. (2005). Chronic strain alters the passive and contractile properties of rabbit airways. *J. Appl. Physiol.* 98, 1949–1954. doi: 10.1152/japplphysiol.00952.2004

Thaikoottathil, J. V., Martin, R. J., Zdunek, J., Weinberger, A., Rino, J. G., and Chu, H. W. (2009). Cigarette smoke extract reduces VEGF in primary human airway epithelial cells. *Eur. Respir. J.* 33, 835–843. doi: 10.1183/09031936.00080708

Uhl, F. E., Vierkotten, S., Wagner, D. E., Burgstaller, G., Costa, R., Koch, I., et al. (2015). Preclinical validation and imaging of Wnt-induced repair in human 3D lung tissue cultures. *Eur. Respir. J.* 46, 1150–1166. doi: 10.1183/09031936.00183214

van der Vaart, H., Postma, D. S., and Timens, W.. and ten Hacken, N. H. T., (2004). Acute effects of cigarette smoke on inflammation and oxidative stress: a review. *Thorax* 59, 713–721. doi: 10.1136/thx.2003.012468

Van Dijk, E. M., Culha, S., Menzen, M. H., Bidan, C. M., and Gosens, R. (2016). Elastase-induced parenchymal disruption and airway hyper responsiveness in mouse precision cut lung slices: toward anEx vivoCOPD model. *Front. Physiol.* 7:657.

van Rijt, S. H., Bölükbas, D. A., Argyo, C., Datz, S., Lindner, M., Eickelberg, O., et al. (2015). Protease-mediated release of chemotherapeutics from mesoporous silica nanoparticles to ex vivo human and mouse lung tumors. *ACS Nano* 9, 2377–2389. doi: 10.1021/nn5070343

Vandenbroucke, R. E., Dejonckheere, E., and Libert, C. (2011). A therapeutic role for matrix metalloproteinase inhibitors in lung diseases? *Eur. Respir. J.* 38, 1200–1214. doi: 10.1183/09031936.00027411

Watson, C. Y., Damiani, F., Ram-Mohan, S., Rodrigues, S., de Moura Queiroz P, Donaghey, T. C., et al. (2016). Screening for chemical toxicity using cryopreserved precision cut lung slices. *Toxicol. Sci.* 150, 225–233. doi: 10.1093/toxsci/kfv320

Woode, D., Shiomi, T., and D'Armiento, J. (2015). Collagenolytic matrix metalloproteinases in chronic obstructive lung disease and cancer. *Cancers (Basel)* 7, 329–341. doi: 10.3390/cancers7010329

Yi, E., Sato, S., Takahashi, A., Parameswaran, H., Blute, T. A., Bartolák-Suki, E., et al. (2016). Mechanical forces accelerate collagen digestion by bacterial collagenase in lung tissue strips. *Front. Physiol.* 7:287. doi: 10.3389/fphys.2016.00287

15

A Bioinspired *in vitro* Lung Model to Study Particokinetics of Nano-/Microparticles Under Cyclic Stretch and Air-Liquid Interface Conditions

Ali Doryab[1,2], Mehmet Berat Taskin[3], Philipp Stahlhut[3], Andreas Schröppel[1,2], Sezer Orak[1,2], Carola Voss[1,2], Arti Ahluwalia[4,5], Markus Rehberg[1,2], Anne Hilgendorff[1,2,6], Tobias Stöger[1,2], Jürgen Groll[3] and Otmar Schmid[1,2]*

[1] Comprehensive Pneumology Center Munich, Member of the German Center for Lung Research, Munich, Germany, [2] Helmholtz Zentrum München—German Research Center for Environmental Health, Institute of Lung Biology and Disease, Munich, Germany, [3] Department of Functional Materials in Medicine and Dentistry, Bavarian Polymer Institute, University of Würzburg, Würzburg, Germany, [4] Research Center "E. Piaggio", University of Pisa, Pisa, Italy, [5] Department of Information Engineering, University of Pisa, Pisa, Italy, [6] Center for Comprehensive Developmental Care (CDeC^{LMU}), Dr. von Haunersches Children's Hospital University, Hospital of the Ludwig-Maximilians University, Munich, Germany

***Correspondence:**
Otmar Schmid
otmar.schmid@helmholtz-muenchen.de

Evolution has endowed the lung with exceptional design providing a large surface area for gas exchange area (ca. 100 m^2) in a relatively small tissue volume (ca. 6 L). This is possible due to a complex tissue architecture that has resulted in one of the most challenging organs to be recreated in the lab. The need for realistic and robust *in vitro* lung models becomes even more evident as causal therapies, especially for chronic respiratory diseases, are lacking. Here, we describe the **C**yclic ***In VI****tro* **C**ell-stretch (CIVIC) "breathing" lung bioreactor for pulmonary epithelial cells at the air-liquid interface (ALI) experiencing cyclic stretch while monitoring stretch-related parameters (amplitude, frequency, and membrane elastic modulus) under real-time conditions. The previously described biomimetic copolymeric BETA membrane (5 μm thick, bioactive, porous, and elastic) was attempted to be improved for even more biomimetic permeability, elasticity (elastic modulus and stretchability), and bioactivity by changing its chemical composition. This biphasic membrane supports both the initial formation of a tight monolayer of pulmonary epithelial cells (A549 and 16HBE14o$^-$) under submerged conditions and the subsequent cell-stretch experiments at the ALI without preconditioning of the membrane. The newly manufactured versions of the BETA membrane did not improve the characteristics of the previously determined optimum BETA membrane (9.35% PCL and 6.34% gelatin [w/v solvent]). Hence, the optimum BETA membrane was used to investigate quantitatively the role of physiologic cyclic mechanical stretch (10% linear stretch; 0.33 Hz: light exercise conditions) on size-dependent cellular uptake and transepithelial transport of nanoparticles (100 nm) and microparticles (1,000 nm) for alveolar epithelial cells (A549) under ALI conditions. Our results show that physiologic stretch enhances cellular uptake of 100 nm nanoparticles across the epithelial cell barrier, but the barrier becomes permeable for both nano- and micron-sized particles (100 and 1,000 nm). This suggests that currently used static *in vitro* assays may underestimate cellular uptake and transbarrier transport of nanoparticles in the lung.

Keywords: lung cell model, cyclic stretch, ALI culture, bioinspired membrane, particle study

INTRODUCTION

The lung is the largest organ of the human body built to accommodate the extraordinary size of required gas (oxygen-carbon dioxide) exchange surface area (ca. 100 m^2) corresponding to about half the size of a tennis court (Weibel, 1970, 2009) within a relatively small volume (ca. 6 l; <10% of body volume). Direct exposure to airborne particles, such as cigarette smoke particles, urban dust and particles from indoor sources (e.g., cooking and laser printer) jeopardizes the fragile architecture of this organ, causing pulmonary lung diseases, such as asthma and chronic obstructive pulmonary disease (Pope et al., 2009; Hänninen et al., 2010; Schaumann et al., 2014). Out of the wide size range of inhalable particles (up to 10 μm diameter), nanoparticles (NPs) with a diameter between 100 and 300 nm have been shown to undergo epithelial-endothelial translocation, i.e., they can cross the alveolar tissue barrier into the blood circulation and from there to other organs (Kreyling et al., 2013). Moreover, ultrafine NPs (<100 nm in diameter) have received increasing attention due to their enhanced surface area per mass of particles, which has been associated with both acute and chronic lung disease (Peters et al., 1997; Schmid and Stoeger, 2016).

Improvement of the predictive power of pre-clinical *in vitro* models as an alternative to animal experiments according to the 3R principles (replacement, refinement, and reduction) relies on enhancing their biomimetic features. Over the past decades *in vitro* cell culture models of the lung epithelial cells have evolved significantly from technologically simple, non-physiologic, submerged cell culture systems to an advanced level of *in vitro* cell culture models at the air-liquid interface (ALI) (Doryab et al., 2016). In these advanced lung models, epithelial lung cells are seeded on the apical (air) side of a porous/perforated membrane, which is in contact with the cell culture medium located on the basal side. This setup mimics *in vivo* conditions, initiating polarization of cells, and secretion of protective lining fluids (surfactant), which do not occur under submerged conditions where cells are completely covered with cell culture medium (Doryab et al., 2019). Hence, ALI cell cultures provide more physiologic conditions and potentially clinically more relevant results when testing drug/toxin effects on the lung as compared to submerged cultures (Paur et al., 2011).

Moreover, *in vitro* lung models have been developed to exert cyclic mechanical stretch to cells mimicking the breathing-induced cyclic stretch conditions in the alveolar lung tissue in order to include this important stimulus for cell physiology and morphology in the cell culture models (Doryab et al., 2019). Hence, addition of this type of stimulus may prove useful for preclinical drug testing and assessment of toxin- and/or particle-induced toxicity. Most of the studies reported in the literature used commercially available cell-stretch technologies (e.g., Flexcell strain unit; Flexcell International Corp., USA) that are only suitable for submerged culture conditions (Edwards et al., 1999; Vlahakis et al., 1999; Hammerschmidt et al., 2004; Guenat and Berthiaume, 2018; Doryab et al., 2019).

Nevertheless, a variety of *in vitro* models has been developed to combine cyclic cell-stretch and ALI culture conditions for more biomimetic models of the alveolar air-blood barrier. Ideally, these advanced models enable (I) cyclic mechanical activation of the (multi-)cell cultures at the ALI, (II) basal perfusion of the culture medium, mimicking blood circulation, and (III) dose-controlled, aerosolized substance delivery. While the former two items have been implemented in various models, the latter is often missing (Doryab et al., 2019; Artzy-Schnirman et al., 2020). In 2010, the seminal work performed by Ingber et al. at the WYSS Institute of Harvard University introduced a microfluidic lung bioreactor often referred to as "lung-on-a-chip" (Huh et al., 2010). The concept of these systems is comparable to standard (multi-)cell culture models of the lung cultured at the ALI on an elastic, perforated membrane, which can be mechanically activated (stretched) combined with basal medium perfusion on a miniature-scale (shift from milli- to microfluidic system). Nowadays, these microfluidic systems have been evolved from a simple bi-channel structure (Huh et al., 2010; Stucki et al., 2015) to a complex airway network (acini-on-chips) (Artzy-Schnirman et al., 2019). However, wide-spread use of these systems is still hampered by the high degree of complexity associated with operating these systems (Ehrmann et al., 2020). These types of biomimetic alveolar barrier models not only have the potential to predict clinical outcome during early preclinical drug or toxin testing and accurate but also for mimicking drug/particle transport from the lung into the blood. In fact, the latter is part of the clinical testing (phase I of clinical trial) required for regulatory licensing of safety and efficacy of novel drugs.

All of these models and recent developments suffer from a lack of a suitable biomimetic membrane, acting as a cell-substrate. An appropriate membrane should emulate the main characteristics of the supporting extracellular matrix (ECM) of the cells, such as thickness, stiffness, permeability, and bioactivity. Commercially available polycarbonate (PC) and polyethylene terephthalate (PET) membranes are widely used in (static) ALI culture systems that do not mimic the stiffness (or rather "softness") of the ECM in the lung. Silicone-based materials, such as poly(dimethylsiloxane) (PDMS, Sylgard 184) are generally cast for cell-stretch applications due to their suitable mechanoelastic properties (Doryab et al., 2019). Nonetheless, adsorption of proteins/growth factors to and leaching of uncured oligomers from PDMS membranes has been recognized as potential cause of adverse effects on cell physiology (Regehr et al., 2009). Recently, synthetic/natural electrospun scaffolds with a thickness range of ≈20–200 μm have been fabricated with suitable properties for lung cells using co-polymers consisting of poly(ε-caprolactone) (PCL)/star-shaped polyethylene glycols (sPEG) functionalized with biomolecules (Nishiguchi et al., 2017), poly-L-lactic acid (PLLA)/decellularized pig lung ECM (PLECM) (Young et al., 2017), and PCL/gelatin (Higuita-Castro et al., 2017). The stretchability of these scaffolds/membranes has not been determined as they were employed only under static cell culture conditions.

We have recently introduced a novel porous and elastic membrane for *in vitro* cell-stretch models of the lung cultured under ALI conditions (Doryab et al., 2020). This innovative hybrid biphasic membrane, henceforth referred to as **B**iphasic **E**lastic **T**hin for **A**ir-liquid culture conditions (BETA) membrane, was developed to optimize membrane characteristics for the two phases of cell-stretch experiments under ALI conditions, namely the initial cell seeding, attachment and growth phase under submerged cell culture conditions (phase I) followed by an ALI acclimatization and cell-stretch phase at the ALI (phase II). As these phases require distinctly different membrane properties, the BETA membrane has been designed to be biphasic. As the pores are initially filled with a wettable, water-soluble and hence sacrificial material (gelatin), the BETA membrane provides initially a non-porous and wettable enough (WCA ≤ 70°) substrate for initial cell adhesion and growth into a confluent epithelial monolayer on the apical side of the membrane (closed pores avoid inadvertent transmembrane migration of cells) (phase I). Subsequently, dissolution of the sacrificial material results in sufficient porosity, permeability and stretchability for up to 25% reversible linear strain (without plastic deformation), granting suitable ALI cell culture conditions under cyclic mechanical stretch (phase II). In contrast to typically used stretchable poly(dimethylsiloxane) (PDMS) membranes, the BETA membrane is bioactive enough to support the proliferation and formation of a confluent layer of alveolar (A549) and bronchial (16HBE14o$^-$) epithelial cells without pre-coating with ECM proteins (e.g., Matrigel) (Doryab et al., 2020).

Right now, the main limitations of the BETA membrane are the relatively larger thickness (ca. 5 μm) compared to the alveolar-capillary tissue barrier (ca. 1 μm) and higher stiffness [uniaxial Young's modulus: 1.8 ± 0.7 MPa (1D stretch); 0.78 ± 0.24 MPa (3D stretch)], which is similar to or better than other typically used porous membranes for lung cell-stretch cultures (e.g., PDMS), but still about 100-fold lager than the elastic modulus (3–6 kPa) reported for alveolar walls/tissue (Doryab et al., 2020). Moreover, the ideal membrane is as bioactive as possible to provide optimum growth conditions for (primary) cell cultures and perfectly permeable to minimize membrane effects on transbarrier transport measurements.

In the present study, we attempted to improve the previously described limitations of the "optimum" BETA membrane with respect to thickness, permeability, elasticity (elastic modulus and stretchability), and bioactivity by changing its chemical composition. This is supported by newly applied analytical parameters (e.g., 3D porosity and mapping of surface topology of the membrane). Moreover, we provide a detailed technical description of the recently introduced **C**yclic ***In VI**tro* **C**ell-stretch (CIVIC) bioreactor for cell-stretch experiments under ALI conditions (Doryab et al., 2020) with particular attention to refinements over its earlier version (MALI, **M**oving **A**ir-**L**iquid **I**nterface bioreactor) (Cei et al., 2020). Subsequently, the effect of cyclic stretch on the particokinetics of aerosol-delivered nano- (100 nm) and microparticles (1,000 nm) in an alveolar tissue barrier model (A549) cultured under ALI conditions was investigated quantitatively with respect to size-dependent cellular uptake and transepithelial transport of particles.

RESULTS

Advanced *in vitro* Cell-Stretch System (CIVIC)

The **C**yclic ***In VI**tro* **C**ell-stretch (CIVIC) system, which was employed for cell-stretch experiments with the BETA membrane, is a modified version of our previously described MALI system (Cei et al., 2020) mainly with respect to material stability, (BETA) membrane fixation, pressure sealing, and quality control including real-time monitoring of the amplitude and frequency of the cyclically stretched cell-covered membrane. The CIVIC system allows for culturing of lung epithelial cells under ALI, cyclic mechanical stretch, and medium (blood) perfusion conditions in combination with dose-controlled delivery of aerosolized substances to the cells. This *in vitro* scenario resembles closely aerosol deposition onto the air-blood barrier of the lung as encountered during inhalation therapy or breathing of ambient aerosol. The details of the technical aspects of the CIVIC system are presented in **Figures 1A,B** and the Methods and Materials section. A movie of the cyclically stretched membrane in the "breathing" CIVIC system can be found in the **Supplementary Video 1**.

Characterization and Optimization Bioinspired Stretchable Membrane (BETA)

As mentioned above, we recently described an optimized biphasic copolymeric membrane for cell growth inspired by the ECM in the alveolar region of the lung (Doryab et al., 2020). The initially non-porous membrane consists of two polymeric components namely poly(ε-caprolactone) (PCL) and gelatin, tailored to facilitate initial cell adhesion and growth under submerged condition (phase I) (**Figures 1C, 2A**). Upon contact with cell culture medium, the gelatin at the surface of the membrane turns into a hydrogel, which is conducive to cell growth (lowers water contact angle; provides favorable conditions for cell adhesion

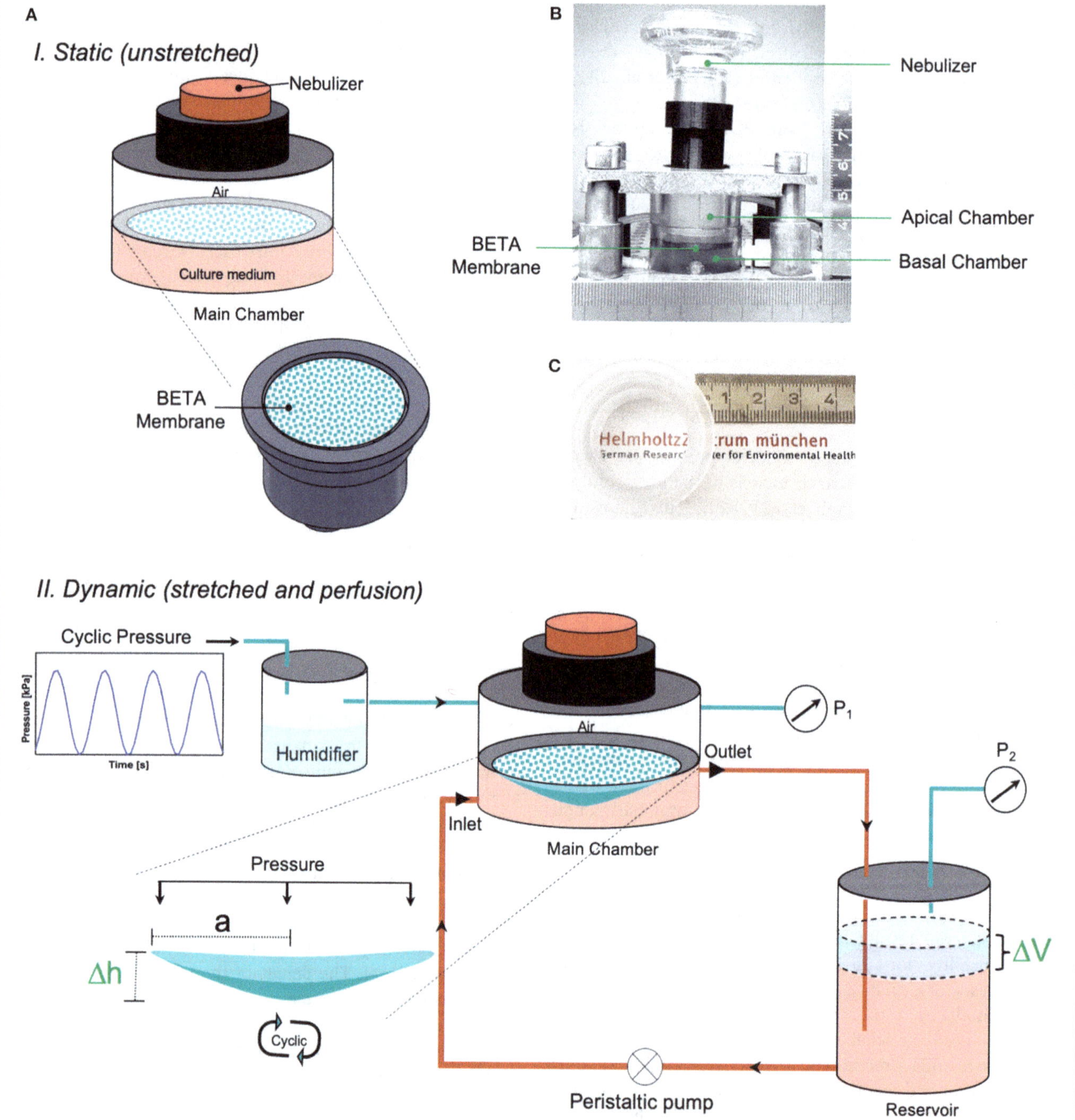

FIGURE 1 | The CIVIC system used in this study. **(A)** Schematic depiction of the CIVIC system under (top) static (unstretched) and (bottom) dynamic (stretched and perfusion) conditions with the pressure-based strain/elasticity monitoring system. A thin, permeable, and stretchable membrane (BETA) placed in the (PDMS-free) main chamber of the bioreactor separates the apical (air) and basal (medium) compartments. Lung cells are grown on the membrane at ALI and perfused with culture medium by circulating the medium in the basal compartment with a perfusion pump to mimic blood flow. Cyclic mechanical stretch is applied to the cells on the membrane by applying cyclic (positive) pressure (P_1) to the apical compartment. The cell/membrane stretch profile can be monitored via a pressure sensor in the air volume of the medium reservoir (P_2), which is connected to the main chamber. The apical compartment of the bioreactor can be connected to a nebulizer to deliver aerosolized particles/drugs to the cells. **(B)** Snapshot of the main chamber of the CIVIC bioreactor system. **(C)** Photograph of the BETA membrane in the PC holder of the CIVIC system, which is transparent, thus favorable for direct cell imaging applications.

and proliferation). Gelatin also serves as "sacrificial" material, i.e., it is gradually dissolved by the medium turning the initially non-porous, stiff membrane into a porous/permeable and more elastic membrane as required for nurturing ALI cell cultures via basolateral medium and during cell-stretch experiments (phase II) (**Figure 2B**). We previously determined the optimum concentrations of PCL and gelatin (9.35% PCL and 6.34% gelatin [w/v solvent]) for membrane fabrication by spin coating with respect to matching the properties of the BETA membrane to the basement membrane of the alveolar tissue using a widely used) optimization approach [design of experiment (DoE)].

Due to remaining limitations of the "optimum" BETA membrane with respect to thickness and stiffness (ca. 100-fold reduction needed to match alveolar basement membrane) (Polio et al., 2018; Doryab et al., 2019; Bou Jawde et al., 2020), we attempted to improve the performance characteristics of the membrane by expanding the previously tested range of PCL/gelatin mixing ratios. For this, new membranes were manufactured with PCL concentration larger than the previously explored upper limit of 10% [w/v solvent], namely 15% PCL mixed with 6, 8, and 10% [w/v] (**Figure 2A**). The characteristics of these three newly generated BETA membranes were compared with previously characterized membranes consisting of 10% PCL mixed with 6, 8, and 10% [w/v] and the optimum BETA membrane (9.35% PCL and 6.34% gelatin [w/v]).

Surface analysis of the optimum BETA membrane (9.35% PCL and 6.34% gelatin [w/v solvent]) using Atomic Force Microscopy (AFM) showed an average roughness height of 1.31 μm (**Figure 2C**). The cross-sectional structure of the membrane was studied using Focused Ion Beam-Scanning Electron Microscopy (FIB-SEM). The data show that gelatin forms spherical "islands" in the PCL membrane (**Figure 2D**, left panel). These gelatin islands also extend deep into the PCL membrane, leaving a favorable interconnected 3D network of pores after dissolution of the gelatin in phase II, as confirmed by Energy Dispersive X-ray Spectroscopy (EDS)-FIB-SEM (**Figure 2D**, right panel).

Analysis of the water contact angle (WCA)—one of the key properties of cell attachment and growth of the three new membranes reveals a range of 70–76° indicating that all of these membranes are wettable (**Figure 2E**). The uniaxial tensile test of the membranes prior to cell seeding (in phase I) revealed that Young's modulus (elastic modulus) varies between 5.33 ± 1.90 and 21.41 ± 4.65 MPa (**Figure 2F**). Moreover, all of the membranes can endure at least 8% linear reversible strain, which is required for physiologic cell stretch conditions in the lung (Doryab et al., 2019), except for PCL 10% gelatin 6% [w/v], which can withstand only 4% linear strain. Another important parameter for culturing of cells under ALI conditions is the porosity of the membrane at the end of phase II (ALI culture), which varies between 1.8 ± 2.5 and 49.7 ± 1.4%, where the highest and lowest porosity corresponds to the membrane consisting of PCL 10% gelatin 10% and PCL 15% gelatin 8% [w/v], respectively (**Figure 2G**). It is noteworthy, that there is excellent agreement between empirically determined porosity and theoretically derived (upper limit of) porosity (volume fraction of gelatin), if the composition-derived theoretical porosity exceeds 40% (here: PCL 10% gelatin 8% and PCL 10% gelatin 10%).

In addition, repeatedly performed WST1 assays showed that the metabolic activity (cell viability) of A549 cells increases with incubation time on the membranes (**Figure 2H**). This indicates that the relatively few initial seeded cells are proliferating and gradually covering the entire membrane as indicated by WST1 values near 100%, representing the WST1 signal obtained for standard Transwell PET inserts. After a 4–6 days growth period (depending on membrane composition), all of the membranes are covered with a confluent monolayer layer of epithelial cells (**Figure 3A**). As an additional measure of cytocompatibility, the release of intracellular lactate dehydrogenase (LDH) from the cytosol due to uncontrolled cell death was measured. The small release of LDH (<0.5% of totally available LDH) indicates that these membranes display low cytotoxicity (**Figure 2I**), which implies that the membranes do not release or leach significant amounts of toxic materials when incubated with the cell culture medium.

In summary, the three new membranes consisting of 15% [w/v] (with 6–10% [w/v] of gelatin) did not improve the key characteristics of a membrane for cell-stretch experiments at the ALI. While their wettability as quantified by WCA was not statistically different from that of the optimum BETA membrane (**Figure 2D**), the membrane with the lowest Young's modulus and hence highest elasticity (prior to removal of gelation) displayed an extremely low porosity of 2% as compared to the 15.32% of the optimum BETA membrane (**Figure 2F**). Such a low porosity value is a knock-out criterion for the membrane since it prevents efficient trans-membrane transport of nutrients (or drugs or nanoparticles) and hence nourishment of cells cultured at the ALI. Hence, the previously determined optimum BETA membrane (9.35% PCL and 6.34% gelatin [w/v solvent]) is superior to all of the 15% PCL membranes and therefore remains the composition of the optimum BETA membrane, which is used for cell experiments described below.

Bioactivity of the BETA Membrane

We also evaluated the bioactivity of the (optimum) BETA membrane using two lung epithelial cell lines namely human lung alveolar epithelial cells (A549) and human bronchial epithelial cells (16HBE14o$^-$). CLSM (confocal laser scanning microscopy) analysis showed that A549 cells grew on the membrane into a confluent cell monolayer resulted in the formation of E-cadherin—a transmembrane adhesion protein—which plays a pivotal role in cell-cell contact and polarization of cells at the ALI. Moreover, F-actin rich regions representing a network of polymeric microfilaments of the cytoskeleton were formed, which is essential for important cellular functions, such as cell motility, cell division, vesicle and organelle movement, cell signaling as well as the establishment and maintenance of cell-cell junctions and cell morphology (**Figure 3A**; images reflect day 6). From the DAPI-stained images (**Figure 3A**) the number of cells (nuclei) per surface area was determined (4.3×10^5 cells cm^{-2}). Since this value is 2.9-fold larger than the seeding density of the cells (1.5×10^5 cells cm^{-2}), this indicates that substantial cell proliferation has occurred during the 6 days of cell growth under submerged culture conditions. For reference, we also compared the bioactivity of the BETA membrane with that of a commercially available standard Transwell® insert (PET) membrane. It is evident that while initial cell growth/metabolic activity (WST1 signal) on the BETA membrane was slower/lower, this difference

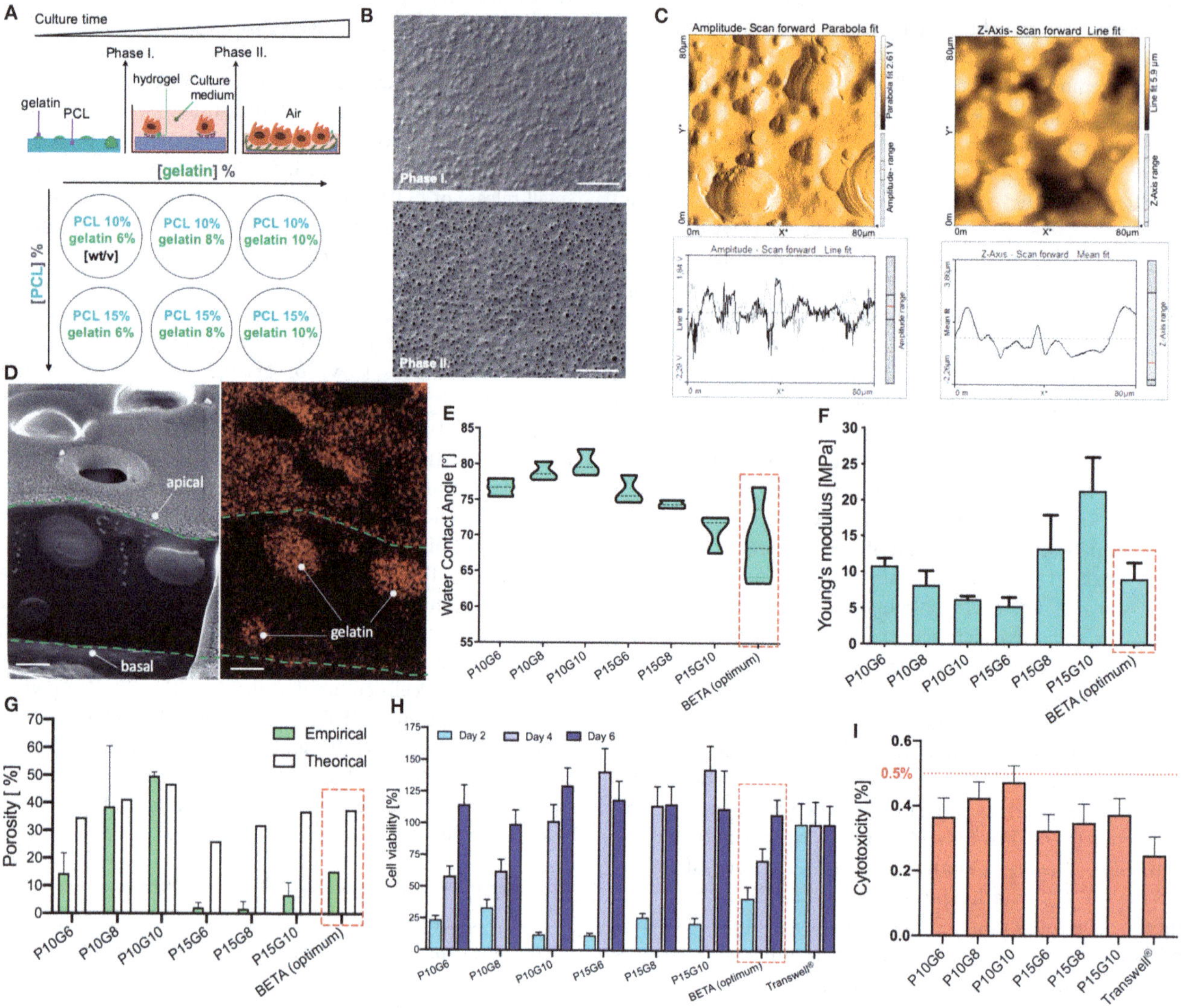

FIGURE 2 | Characterization of the biphasic (BETA) membrane used in this study. **(A)** Schematic depiction of the biphasic membrane concept. (Top) During phase I, gelatin forms a hydrogel due to contact with water (cell culture medium), which serves as adhesion point for epithelial cells of the lung and facilitates subsequent cell proliferation until a confluent epithelial cell layer is formed. After 4 days (phase II), the gelatin has been dissolved in water leaving behind a network of interconnected pores in the PCL membrane, which provides space for further cell spreading and at the same time enhances both membrane permeability and elastic modulus. (Bottom) Different membranes with various combinations of mixing ratio of PCL and gelatin—in the PCL/gelatin solution used for membrane manufacturing—expected to obtain a wide range of physicomechanical properties. **(B)** Top view of the ultrastructure of the "optimum" membrane (9.35% PCL and 6.34% gelatin [w/v of TFE], i.e., P/G = 9.35/6.34), which is also used for the analysis presented in **(C,D)**. The scale bar is 100 μm. **(C)** Surface topography of an 80 × 80 μm^2 section of the membrane analyzed by Atomic Force Microscopy (AFM; left) and its corresponding z-amplitude profile (right) showing an average roughness height of 1.31 μm. **(D)** Cross-sectional analysis of the membrane using Focused Ion Beam-Scanning Electron Microscopy (FIB-SEM, left panel) and Energy Dispersive X-ray Spectroscopy FIB-SEM (EDS-FIB-SEM, right panel), indicating that gelatin is distributed throughout the PCL membrane during the late stage of phase I. The thickness of the membrane thickness ca. 5 μm. The scale bar is 2 μm. The newly manufactured membranes (P15G6, P15G8, and P15G10) are analyzed (and compared to previously reported results (Doryab et al., 2020) with respect to **(E)** Water Contact Angle (WCA), **(F)** Young's modulus (uniaxial, phase I, under dry conditions), **(G)** porosity obtained empirically by the liquid displacement method—and theoretical (maximum) porosity (gelatin volume fraction), **(H)** cell viability analyzed by WST1 assay on days 2, 4, and 6 of culture relative to PET Transwell® cell culture insert **(H)**, and **(I)** cytotoxicity (LDH assay at day 6) of the three newly investigated membranes with different mixing ratios of PCL and gelatin. The LDH release for each membrane was normalized by the maximum possible LDH level (LDH contained in all cells). Typically, LDH < 10% is considered non-cytotoxic. There is no significant difference between the LDH release of Transwell® inserts and the different mixing ratios of BETA membranes. Optimum values for WCA, Young's modulus, empirical porosity, and theoretical (maximum) porosity were 69 ± 5 [°], 9.0 ± 1.9 [MPa], 15.32 [%] and 37.6 [%], respectively. Data are reported as the mean ± SD, $n = 3$.

had disappeared on day 4–6 (**Figure 2H**). The ultrastructural analysis exhibited a flattened cell morphology when cells grew on the BETA membrane (**Figure 3B**). Furthermore, cells showed superior interaction and integration with the BETA membrane as compared to the Transwell® insert (**Figure 3B**).

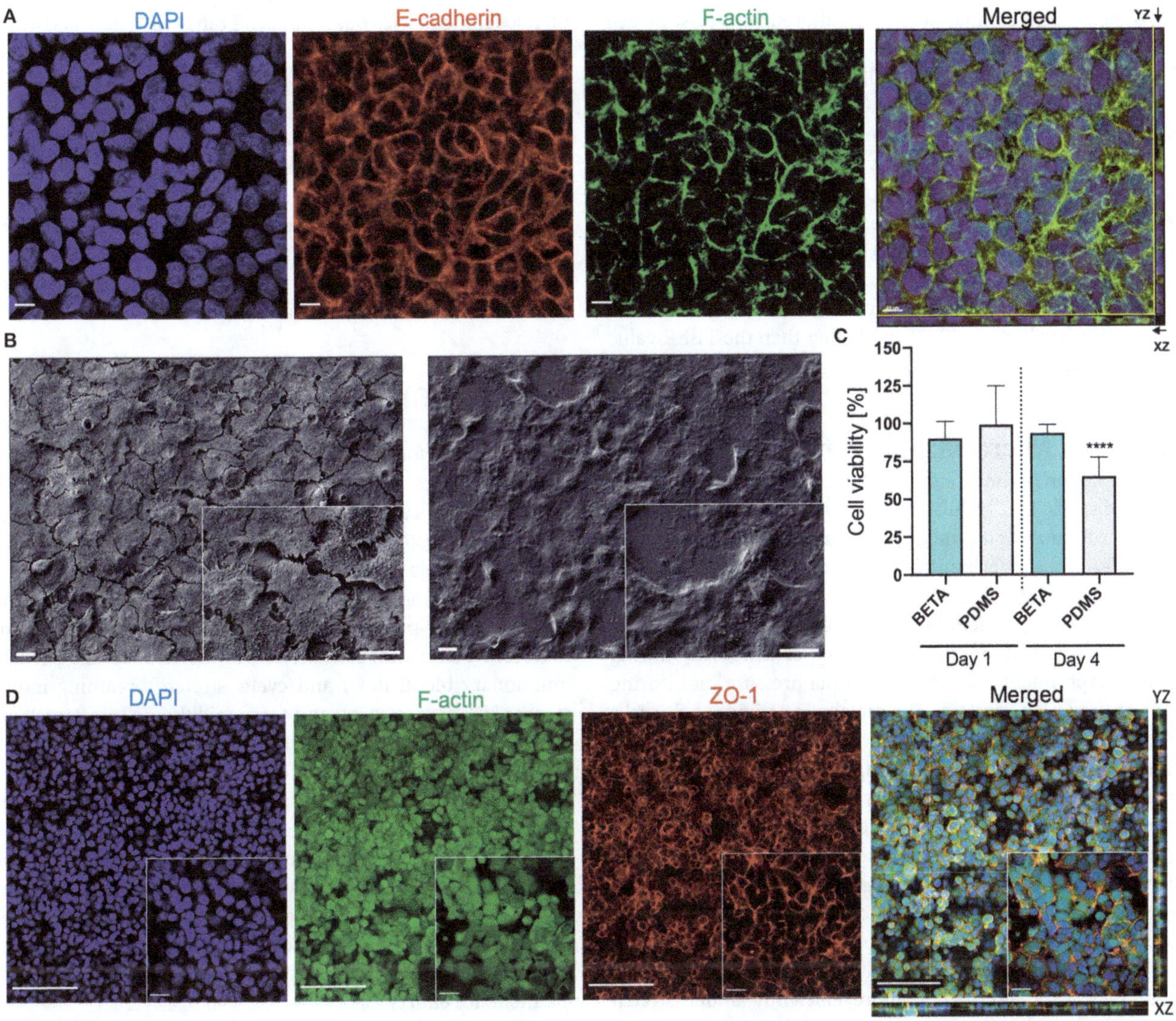

FIGURE 3 | Bioactivity of the BETA membrane (optimum: 9.35% PCL and 6.34% gelatin [w/v of TFE]). **(A)** Z-stack Confocal Laser Scanning Microscopy (CLSM) of human alveolar epithelial cells (A549) on the membrane (under static submerged culture conditions for 6 days) demonstrating the formation of a confluent uniform cell layer. The cell nuclei (DAPI, blue), expression of the cell-cell adhesion protein E-cadherin (red), and formation of F-actin filaments (green). The scale bar is 10 μm. **(B)** SEM image of A549 cells after proliferation on a (left) biphasic membrane and (right) a commercial Transwell® insert (6 days of submerged culture). The scale bar is 10 μm. **(C)** Effect of leaching from BETA and PDMS membrane on cell viability (WST1 assay; A549 cells). BETA and PDMS membranes were incubated for 2 days in cell culture medium and this medium was used to grow A549 cells for 1 and 4 days in a standard 12-well tissue culture well plate. The reduced cell viability for PDMS-conditioned medium after 4 days indicates that some substances (e.g., uncured oligomers) leaching from the PDMS have a cytotoxic effect. This effect is not seen for the BETA membrane. The viability data were normalized that of a standard 12- well cell culture plate with fresh medium. Data are reported as mean ± SD. $n = 8$; $^{****}P < 0.00001$ by one-way ANOVA with Dunnett test. **(D)** Z-stack and orthogonal CLSM view of (XY) with side views of YZ (right) and XZ (bottom) optical projection of the human bronchial epithelial cells (16HBE14o$^-$) on the membrane visualizing a confluent cell monolayer and the formation of tight junctions (culture conditions: 6 days submerged and 24 h ALI culture); cell nucleus (DAPI, blue), F-actin filaments (green); ZO-1 tight junction (red). The scale bars are 100 μm (for the 20× projection view) and 20 μm (for the 63× projection view).

PDMS (Sylgard 184) membranes are commonly used in cell-stretch devices due to their mechano-elastic properties. However, it has been reported that uncured oligomers of PDMS are released into the culture medium during cell culture, which might be toxic for the cells (Regehr et al., 2009; Carter et al., 2020). Hence, we assessed the leaching of unwanted components of the PDMS membrane compared to the (optimum) BETA membrane (**Figure 3C**). Medium incubated for 48 h with PDMS and BETA membranes was used to culture A549 cells under submerged conditions. After 1 day, no significant difference was detected in cell viability for the two materials. However, after 4 days of incubation, a 36% reduction in cell viability was detected for the cells incubated with PDMS-leached medium, while only 6% of viability reduction was observed for the BETA membrane-leached medium as compared to cells cultured with pristine cell culture medium.

We also examined the bioactivity of the BETA membrane using the human bronchial epithelial cell line 16HBE14o$^-$. Cells were grown on the (optimum) BETA membrane for 6 days under submerged and 1 day under ALI conditions. A confluent epithelial barrier with the formation of the F-actin was observed (**Figure 3D**). SEM analysis also confirmed the CLSM findings (**Supplementary Figure 2**). Excellent barrier integrity was also confirmed by a TEER value of 451 $\pm$ 55 Ω cm^2, which is consistent with data reported for 16HBE14o$^-$ cells in the literature (Ehrhardt et al., 2002) and higher than the TEER value for A549 epithelial confluent cell monolayer on the BETA (136 $\pm$ 23 Ω cm^2).

Nano- and Microparticle Kinetics Study

As an application of the *in vitro* cell-stretch lung model (CIVIC), we investigated the cellular uptake by and transepithelial transport of nano- and microparticles of A549 cells under physiologic cyclic mechanical stretch (10% linear, 0.33 Hz) applied for 2 h. The stability of the stretch parameters as well as the stiffness [Young's modulus: 0.78 $\pm$ 0.24 MPa (mean $\pm$ SD, $n = 5$)] of the membrane was monitored continuously during the entire experiment with the differential pressure monitoring system of the CIVIC system. The metabolic activity of the cells did not show any evidence of reduced viability due to aerosol exposure and 2 h of cyclic stretch (**Supplementary Figure 3**).

This study shows that 2 h of cyclic stretch affects cellular uptake and intracellular distribution, but not trans-cellular transport in a size-dependent way. The former is qualitatively evident from CLSM images revealing that cellular uptake of 100 and 1,000 nm particles under unstretched (static) ALI conditions was very limited and cell-associated particles were mostly located close to the air-facing, apical cell surface (**Figure 4B**). In contrast, 100 nm NPs were internalized more efficiently under stretch conditions and co-localized with the F-actin cytoskeleton deeper within the cell (**Figure 4B**). On the other hand, stretch did not enhance cellular uptake of 1,000 nm microparticles and particles were still localized close to the apical cell surface, but positioned preferably between adjacent cells rather than randomly as without stretch (**Figure 4B**). Quantitative fluorescence analysis of the CLSM images revealed a 2.4-fold increase of cellular uptake of 100 nm NPs under stretch, while there was no statistically significant effect of stretch on cellular uptake for 1,000 nm microparticles (**Figure 4C**).

In addition, spectrophotometric analysis of the basal medium revealed the transepithelial transport (translocation) of particles after 2 h under static and stretch-activated conditions of A549 cells on the BETA membrane or on 3 µm pore (static) PET membranes of 6-well Transwell® inserts (**Figure 4D**). For Transwell® inserts, the particles were delivered with a VITROCELL®Cloud 6 system to A549 cells (Lenz et al., 2014) and then cultured under (static) ALI conditions.

After 2 h of incubation time under static conditions, the transport fractions across A549 cells on both Transwell® inserts and BETA membranes for 100 and 1,000 nm particles were below the detection limit, except for the 1.8 $\pm$ 0.4% transport of 1,000 nm particles observed for Transwell® inserts (two-way ANOVA followed by *post-hoc* Tukey's multiple comparison test) (**Figure 4D** and **Table 1**).

For cell-stretch, the transepithelial transport of 100 and 1,000 nm particles across the A549 cell-covered BETA membrane was increased to 30.0 $\pm$ 1.7 and 21.0 $\pm$ 11.3%, respectively, but no statistically significant dependence on size was observed (no stretch can be applied to Transwell® inserts). Hence, cell-stretch significantly increased the translocation of 100 and 1,000 nm particles across the alveolar epithelial barrier independent of particle diameter (see **Table 1** and **Figure 4D**).

DISCUSSION

In the quest for overcoming limitations of traditional *in vitro* models of the lung, the field of bioengineering has witnessed significant efforts toward developing advanced *in vitro* models striving to mimic more closely the human pulmonary environment (de Souza Carvalho et al., 2014). This has led the way from mono-cellular submerged cell lines to primary co-culture cell models at the ALI (air-blood barrier), from static cell culture media and cell layers to medium perfusion (pulmonary blood flow) and cyclic stretch (breathing-induced mechanical tissue strain), and from millifluidic ($\sim$cm^2 cell area, mL of media) into microfluidic systems often referred to as lung/acinar-on-a-chip technologies (Huh et al., 2012, 2013; de Souza Carvalho et al., 2014; Benam et al., 2015; Tenenbaum-Katan et al., 2018; Ainslie et al., 2019; Artzy-Schnirman et al., 2019). While lung-on-a-chip technologies are starting to become commercially available (e.g., Alveolix, Switzerland and Emulate, USA), also millifluidic lung bioreactors are expected to continue to play a role due to their ease-of-handling, a larger amount of cell samples suitable for many standard assay kits, and lower maintenance efforts.

At the core of any cell-stretch lung bioreactor/chip is a porous and elastic membrane on which the cell culture model is cultured. For lung/acinar-on-a-chip systems mainly 3.5–10 µm thick PDMS membranes are used for cell seeding and growth of an alveolar or bronchial tissue barrier (Huh et al., 2010; Stucki et al., 2015). PDMS membranes are widely used for their high mechano-elasticity, with Young's modulus of $\approx$1–3 MPa (Wang et al., 2014). While perforated PDMS membranes are suitable for small-sized lung-on-chip applications ($\sim$mm^2), they are too fragile for larger millifluidic ($\sim$cm^2) devices. Moreover, PDMS membranes have low wettability (WCA $\geq$ 115°) (**Supplementary Figure 1**) and therefore require pre-treatment and/or coating with ECM proteins to facilitate sufficient cell adhesion and proliferation (Wang et al., 2010). Another disadvantage is that uncured oligomers of PDMS can leach into the cell culture medium resulting in changes and cell physiology (Regehr et al., 2009; Carter et al., 2020). Our investigation of a PDMS film has confirmed reports from the literature that cells may experience reduced cell viability due to the leaching of toxins into the cultured in a medium (Regehr et al., 2009). Alternatively, commercial electrospun biocompatible

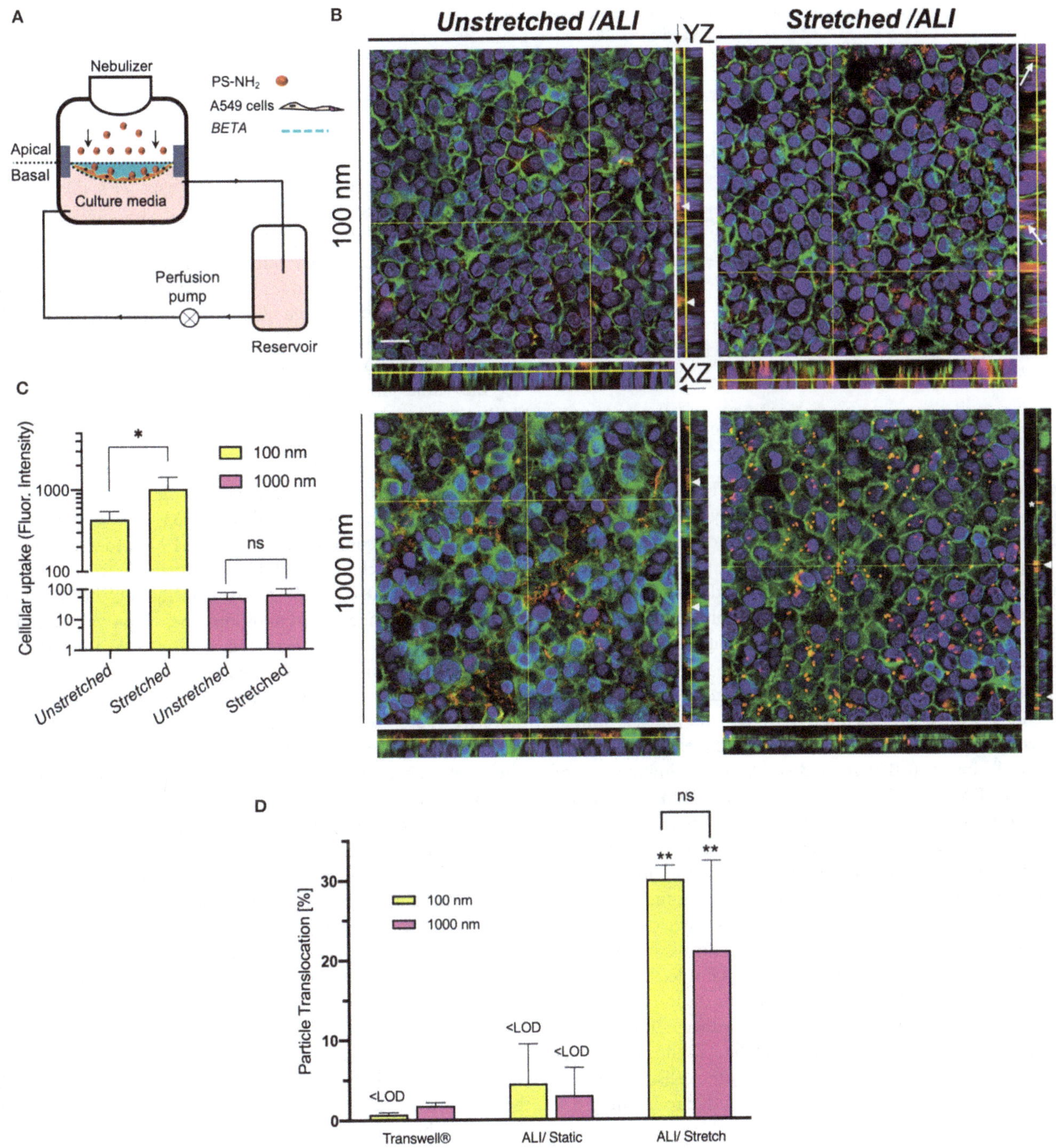

FIGURE 4 | Cellular uptake and membrane-association of aerosolized nano- and microparticles for alveolar epithelial (A549) cells and translocation across the epithelial barrier (2 h incubation). **(A)** Schematic of the CIVIC bioreactor system for particle study. A549 cells were seeded on the BETA membrane (cell density: 2 × 10^5 cells cm^{-2}, 4 days LLC, and 1-day ALI culture). Amine-modified polystyrene ($PS\text{-}NH_2$) nano- and microparticles (100 and 1,000 nm diameter, respectively) are then nebulized onto the cells with the nebulizer of the bioreactor. After 2 h, the cells were fixed and prepared for CLSM analysis. **(B)** 3D reconstruction z-stack of CLSM images presented as orthogonal (XY) and side views (YZ, right) of monolayered, confluent cells on the membrane after nebulization of 100 and 1,000 nm fluorescently labeled, amine-modified polystyrene ($PS\text{-}NH_2$) particles under non-stretched and physiologically stretched (10% linear, 0.33 Hz for 2 h) under ALI conditions. Cell nucleus (DAPI, blue), particles (red) and F-actin filaments of the cytoskeleton (green). Arrows, arrowheads, and asterisk indicate internalized particles, cell-membrane associated (extracellular) particles (on the apical cell surface) and particles located between cells, respectively. (Scale bar: 20 μm). **(C)** Quantitative cellular uptake of particles measured by fluorescence intensity of z-stacks, showing that physiologic cyclic mechanical stretch enhances uptake of 100 nm NPs as compared to static conditions, while there is no effect on 1,000 nm microparticles [Representative images (z-stacks) were recorded at 5 independent fields of view for each sample (n = 4); region of interest: 134.95 × 134.95 μm]. Y-axis is presented fluorescence intensity data in a log scale. Data are reported as the mean ± SD;

(Continued)

FIGURE 4 | *$P < 0.01$ by two-way ANOVA and data were corrected by Sidac for multiple comparison tests. **(D)** Translocation of 100 and 1,000 nm particles across the cell layer grown on unstretched PET Transwell® inserts and on the BETA membrane (under unstretched and stretched conditions) ($n = 3$). ** Show the comparison between stretched with the corresponding experiment under unstretched conditions. Data are reported as the mean ± SD; **$P < 0.001$ by two-way ANOVA and data were corrected by Tukey for multiple comparison tests.

TABLE 1 | Transport of 100 and 1,000 nm particles across A549 cell-layer grown on BETA or PET Transwell® insert membrane (3 μm pores) at ALI within 2 h of particle exposure (mean ± SD; $n = 3$).

Run / Translocation [%]	100 nm	1,000 nm
Transwell®/Unstretched	<LOD*	1.8 ± 0.4
BETA/Unstretched	<LOD	<LOD
BETA/Stretched	30.0 ± 1.7	21.0 ± 11.3

* *<LOD, below limit of detection.*

poly(carbonate)urethane (PCU) membranes (Bionate® II 80A, The Electrospinning Company, UK) have been tested for cell growth in a millifluidic lung bioreactor. They proved inadequate due to their hydrophobic nature (in spite of pre-coating with ECM proteins) and associated poor cell proliferation, their relatively large thickness (ca. 75 μm), and their inability to prevent the formation of multilayered epithelial tissue deep within the membrane rather than at its apical side (Cei et al., 2020).

The BETA membrane, which overcomes some of these limitations (**Figure 5**), has a thickness of ≤5 μm, which is thinner than conventional PET or PC/PET membranes used in static Transwell® inserts (≈10 μm) and similar to the lower range of advanced PDMS membranes (≈3.5–10 μm) (Huh et al., 2010; Stucki et al., 2015). The two polymer components, i.e., gelatin and PCL were chosen for their wettability and mechanical properties, respectively. The presence of gelatin initial non-porous membrane (BETA in phase I) is conducive to cell adhesion/growth without requiring further surface modification and prevents apically seeded epithelial cells from unwanted migration through the membrane to the basal side, fostering the formation of a monolayer of epithelial cells on the apical side. The gradual dissolution of gelatin by cell culture medium induces sufficient porosity for culturing of cells at the ALI and even results in the secretion of innate ECM secreted by the cells. In contrast to PDMS, no adverse effect on cell viability due to leaching has been observed (**Figure 3C**).

As mentioned above, one of the main advantages of the PDMS membranes is their high mechano-elasticity with Young's modulus of ≈1–3 MPa (Wang et al., 2014), which is still ca. 100-fold larger than that of alveolar tissue with 3–6 kPa (Polio et al., 2018; Bou Jawde et al., 2020). Since the previously derived optimized BETA membrane (PCL/gelatin = 9.35%/6.34% [w/v solvent] or P/G = 9.35/6.34) (Doryab et al., 2020) has an initial Young's modulus of 9.0 ± 1.9 MPa (prior dissolution of gelatin), the present study tested the hypothesis that an increased PCL concentration of 15% (rather than 6–10% as tested previously) will result in a more elastic membrane. It became evident, that while a ca. 2-fold lower (uniaxial) Young's modulus (5.3 ± 1.2 MPa for P15G6) could be obtained (**Figure 2F**), the porosity would be prohibitively low (2% for P15G6) for sufficient trans-membrane nutrient transport during ALI culture conditions. Hence, the previously determined optimum BETA membrane (P/G = 9.35/6.34) was used for the cell-stretch cell experiments.

It is important to note that albeit the (optimum) BETA membrane has an initial (uniaxial) Young's modulus of 9.0 ± 1.9 MPa prior to the dissolution of gelatin (prior to phase I), the (uniaxial) Young's modulus reduces to 1.84 ± 0.66 MPa after dissolving sacrificial gelatin (day 6 under submerged conditions; end of phase II) (Doryab et al., 2020). When measured under more realistic, triaxial stretch conditions in the CIVIC (pressure monitoring method), the elastic modulus of the BETA membrane decreased from 1.33 ± 0.14 MPa (day 1; partial gelatin dissolution) to 0.78 ± 0.24 MPa (day 6) (Doryab et al., 2020), which is ca. 2-fold lower than the corresponding uniaxial value (1.84 ± 0.66 MPa). Considering that the latter was measured under dry conditions these two values can be considered equal within expected experimental uncertainties, which indicates that the BETA membrane is quite isotropic.

In the present study, we recognized the limited value of 2D porosity (pore-area fraction at the surface of the membrane), did not correlate well with the gelatin volume fraction of the membrane, for membrane optimization with respect to 3D porosity (through pores) as only an interconnected 3D pore structure allows for sufficient contact between apically located cells and basal medium during ALI cell culturing. The measurement method for 3D porosity described here was in excellent agreement with the theoretically predicted porosity from gelatin volume fraction, if the latter was larger than 41% (**Figure 2G**). This indicates that for gelatin volume factions larger than 41% all of the available gelatin can eventually be reached and hence dissolved by culture medium, i.e., the gelatin-induced 3D pore structure is perfectly interconnected, which is optimum for ALI culture conditions. For gelatin factions below ca. 35%, the 3D porosity falls below 10% implying that increasing "islands" of gelatin are formed, which are completely engulfed by non-soluble PCL (Figure 2B of Doryab et al., 2020). Thus, future efforts for improved membrane composition should focus on gelatin volume fractions near or above 40% to provide sufficient 3D porosity.

In summary, the optimum BETA membrane is relatively thin (≤5 μm) with a suitable permeability (9.9×10^{-6} cm s^{-1} for FITC-dextran 4 kDa and 15.3% 3D porosity), which can provide sufficient contact between ALI cultured cells on the apical and medium on the basal side of the membrane (Weibel, 1970; Doryab et al., 2019). The BETA membrane is also stretchable up to 25% linear strain (during phase

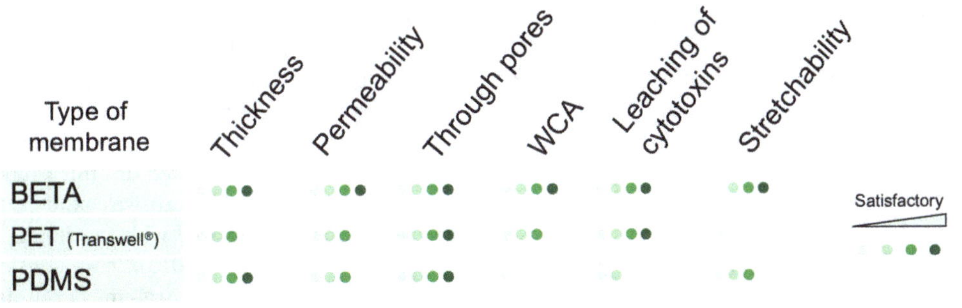

FIGURE 5 | Qualitative comparison between key properties of conventional porous membranes (PET and PDMS) used for static and dynamic (cell-stretch) *in vitro* lung models at the air-liquid interface and the BETA membrane presented here. The scores are based on biomimetic relevance as compared to the alveolar basement membrane. The permeability was measured as apparent permeability (Papp) for FITC-dextran (4 kDa). Stretchability and through pores refer to the elastic modulus and pores connecting the apical and basal sides of the membrane, respectively.

II), which includes the range of physiologic strain (up to 12% linear) and non-physiologic over-stretch conditions as discussed below. While the BETA membrane is more biomimetic than most other membranes currently available due to the low WCA (68°) and 3D interconnectivity of the pores, the BETA membrane still has a ca. 100-fold higher elastic modulus and thickness of the alveolar tissue and basement membrane, respectively (Polio et al., 2018; Doryab et al., 2019; Bou Jawde et al., 2020). The former is expected to alter cell physiology as compared to lung conditions and the latter may result in bias transbarrier transport studies. Future research on membrane technology mimicking the alveolar basement membrane should focus not only on matching the physicochemical properties of the basement membrane but also on its microstructural (network of ECM fibers) and molecular structure.

Thus, further research is needed to close this physiologic gap. Several alternative synthetic scaffolds have presented promising results for lung, such as biofunctionalized or synthetic-peptide-based synthetic scaffold (Nishiguchi et al., 2017). Despite the natural-based scaffold (e.g., collagen type I), synthetic scaffolds can be tailored to have selective tunable properties, mimicking the microenvironment of cells to facilitate cell adherence, proliferation, and differentiation. However, artificial scaffolds, i.e., natural, synthetic, and natural/synthetic introduced until now are unable to concurrently mimic all the physical, mechanical, and biological properties of the natural ECM or basement membrane of the pulmonary cells. The biomimetic biphasic scaffold reported here has excellent structural, mechanical, and biophysical characteristics and can be a suitable alternative for growing epithelial cells not only in the monoculture but also in co-culture and triple co-culture models (Lehmann et al., 2011; Heydarian et al., 2019).

Ultimately, sufficiently biomimetic *in vitro* models of the alveolar tissue should not only focus on the basement membrane but also include more advanced primary alveolar cell models, such as the commercially available primary-derived hAELVi cells (Kuehn et al., 2016) or EpiAlveolar cell model (MatTek, Inc.) (Barosova et al., 2020). The combination of both aspects should lead to even more biomimetic and hence clinically predictive models of the alveolar barrier.

The millifluidic CIVIC bioreactor utilizes positive pressure to mechanically stretch a cell-covered elastic membrane activate stretchable and thus allows for ALI cell culture conditions with medium perfusion, cyclic stretch, and monitoring of the pressures in the apical and basal compartment of the bioreactor is leveraged for real-time monitoring of amplitude and frequency of cyclic stretch and of tri-axial Young's modulus of the cell-covered membrane. This allows for precise selection of stretch conditions and quality control of key experimental conditions during the course of the cell-stretch experiment. Moreover, an aerosol-cell delivery unit using a clinically relevant nebulizer enhances its applicability to drug testing suitable for inhalation therapy.

It is instructive to relate the characteristic stretch and perfusion parameters of the CIVIC equipped with the BETA membrane to clinical conditions. The BETA membrane can sustain linear stretch amplitudes of up to 25% (Doryab et al., 2020). Population-based averages for breathing frequency and tidal volume during heavy exercise are 26 breaths per minute (33 bpm for women) and 1.92 L (1.36 L), respectively (ICRP, 1994). For typical lung inflation of 3.3 L (2.7 L) at functional residual capacity (FRC, at end of exhalation), this tidal volume corresponds to a 58% (50%) increase in lung volume yielding a 17% (15%) linear and 36% (31%) area change (assuming the alveolar sacs are spherical). Analogous, the stretch conditions were chosen here for the particokinetics study (10% linear at 0.33 Hz = 20 bpm) correspond to a tidal volume of 1.09 L (female 0.89 L), which is similar to "light exercise" conditions (male: 1.25 L, 20 bpm; female: 0.99 L, 21 bpm) (ICRP, 1994). Consequently, linear strain larger than 17% (or 35% ΔSA), which may occur for instance during positive pressure ventilation, is considered over-distension or non-physiologic strain, possibly provoking apoptosis and necrosis, increase permeability and release of inflammatory mediators (such as Interleukin-8) in alveolar epithelial cells (Edwards et al., 1999; Vlahakis et al., 1999; Hammerschmidt et al., 2004).

The maximum positive differential pressure applied to the apical side of the cells during a cyclic stretch in the CIVIC

(2.5 kPa) is higher than exerted onto the lung tissue during normal exhalation (0.1–0.5 kPa), but similar to conditions during mechanical ventilation at the intensive care unit of a hospital (normal: 1.5–2.0 kPa, 2.5 kPa acceptable peak value; 3.0 kPa should not be exceeded for an extended period of time) (Hall, 2016). Finally, the medium perfusion rate of 400 μL min^{-1} has to be put into context with the area of gas exchange (membrane area: 5 cm^2) for comparison with the lung. The ratio of area and perfusion rate of the CIVIC is with 1.25 $m^2/(L\ min^{-1})^{-1}$ considerably lower than that of the lung [20 $m^2/(L\ min^{-1})^{-1}$ = 100 $m^{-2}/(5\,L\ min^{-1})$], but the corresponding flow rate of 6.4 L min^{-1} in the CIVIC system technically not be difficult to establish since it would require tubing with much larger diameter enhancing the laboratory footprint unduly.

It is well known that the size of particles plays a key role in cellular uptake and internalization of the particles (Takenaka et al., 2012; Zhu et al., 2013). We found that both 100 and 1,000 nm amine-coated particles could not be internalized by alveolar epithelial cells (A549) under static/unstretched conditions (2 h after aerosolized particle delivery). Moreover, 1,000 nm microparticles were also not taken up by cells under stretched conditions, which can be explained by endocytic uptake (most relevant uptake mechanism for epithelial cells) being limited to ca. 500 nm particles (Winnik and Maysinger, 2013; Zhu et al., 2013; Annika Mareike Gramatke, 2014). In contrast, the relatively efficient cellular uptake of 100 nm NPs is consistent with previous observations that positively charged (amine-coated) NPs tend to interact with the negatively charged cell membrane, which enhances their uptake as compared to neutral or even negatively charged particles of the same size (Rothen-Rutishauser et al., 2006). The observed colocalization of NPs with the F-actin cytoskeleton in A549 cells is conducive for further intracellular trafficking and endocytosis of the NPs within cells (Foroozandeh and Aziz, 2018). For *in vitro* pharmacokinetic testing, ALI culture conditions have several advantages over submerged cell culture settings. In addition to more physiologic and tighter barrier function, burst-like pharmacokinetic profiles as typically seen in patients can only be observed for ALI conditions (Meindl et al., 2015; Schmid et al., 2017) since this resembles rapid depletion of the pulmonary drug reservoir due to drug transport into the blood. Moreover, the cell-delivered dose is often poorly known under submerged conditions due to variable particle-cell transport rates in cell culture medium (Teeguarden et al., 2007; Schmid and Cassee, 2017). In contrast, under ALI conditions, the aerosol dose is delivered immediately directly onto the epithelial barrier mimicking the conditions of inhaled particles in the lung. To date, *in vitro* particokinetic studies are mainly performed under submerged culture conditions, and to the best of our knowledge, no quantitative transbarrier particokinetic (translocation) studies under cell-stretch ALI conditions have been reported, yet.

For sub-100 nm NPs the translocated fraction of particles is inversely proportional to particle size in both static *in vitro* cell and *in vivo* animal models of the lung (Kreyling et al., 2014; Bachler et al., 2015). For A549 cells at ALI and rodent models after NP instillation, the first plateau of particle translocation is achieved within 2 h for 80 nm gold NPs, but it is considerably larger for (static) A549 cells (ca. 2% of the delivered dose) as compared to particle instillation in rats (ca. 0.2%) (Kreyling et al., 2014; Bachler et al., 2015). For A549 cells, receiving doses larger than 0.1 $\mu g\ cm^{-2}$ for gold NPs has resulted in a decrease in the transport rate (Bachler et al., 2015).

The 2 h translocation fraction of 100 nm amine-modified polystyrene particles observed in this study was below the detection limit [ca. 1.0% (Transwell) and ca. 3% BETA], which is in general agreement well with the results from Bachler and colleagues (Bachler et al., 2015), if we consider that the larger than 0.1 $\mu g\ cm^{-2}$ (here 2.1 $\mu g\ cm^{-2}$) cell-delivered dose may have lowered the transport fraction. On the other hand, the 1.8% of translocation fraction for 1,000 nm particles (Transwell inserts) appears relatively large considering that virtually no translocation of microparticles has been reported in *in vivo* biokinetics studies. The absence of 1,000 nm translocation for the BETA membrane (below detection limit of ca. 3%) is consistent with these *in vivo* results. While it may be expected that cyclic stretch affects the transepithelial mobility of particles by, e.g., additional convective particle transport, changes in paracellular barrier integrity, and effects on cellular uptake and transport mechanisms, the relatively large increase to 30 and 20% for 100 and 1,000 nm particles is unexpectedly high. Since these values even agree within experimental uncertainty it is unlikely that this is the result of an active cellular transport process especially since endo-/exocytosis as the most effective cellular uptake and transport mechanism for epithelial cells is limited to sizes below 500 nm. Moreover, substantially enhanced cellular uptake was only observed for 100 nm particles (**Figure 4B**). Therefore, we assume that this large increase in translocation fraction is due to a combination of passive mechanisms, such as rupture of the relatively weak tight junctions of A549 cells yielding intracellular gaps, which allows for enhanced convective transport of particles irrespective of particle size due to leakage of the medium in and out of the apical space where the particles are residing.

CONCLUSION

The "optimum" copolymeric BETA membrane (P/G = 9.35/6.34) applied here is biomimetic in the sense that it is thin ($\leq$5 μm), surface wettable, permeable with proper pore size for cell growth and interconnected 3D pore structure, elastic and bioactive, and somewhat comparable to the ECM in the alveolar region. However, it still is ca. 100-fold too thick and stiff as compared to the basement membrane of the alveolar region. These limitations could not be alleviated by enhancing the poly(ε-)caprolactone (PCL) concentration 15% (w/v). Using the "optimum" we showed that the CIVIC can be utilized for cellular uptake and transepithelial transport studies under physiologic stretch and ALI conditions including aerosolized substance delivery. While the results for static conditions are in general agreement with literature data, unexpectedly high translocation of both 100 and 1,000 nm particles under physiologic stretch (light exercise) was observed for an A549 alveolar lung barrier. This suggests that more appropriate cell (co-)culture models with more pronounced tight junctions and advanced primary cell culture models should be employed for cell-stretch experiments. Studies in the field of respiratory diseases are expected to benefit greatly from the development of more biomimetic and reliable *in vitro* models of the lung as currently available. We believe our system presents a valuable step toward improvement of the predictive value of advanced lung cell models.

MATERIALS AND METHODS

Cell Culture

Human alveolar type-II like epithelial cells (A549) were cultured and maintained in Dulbecco's Modified Eagle Medium: Nutrient Mixture F-12 (DMEM/F12, 1:1 v/v, Gibco) supplemented with 10% FCS (Gibco), 1% (v/v) Pen/Strep (100 U mL^{-1}, Gibco), 1% L-glutamine (2 mM, Gibco), and 2-phospho-L-ascorbic acid (0.1 mM, Sigma). Human bronchial epithelial cells (16HBE14o^{-}) were cultured in MEM/F12 medium (Gibco) supplemented with 10% FCS (Gibco), 1% (v/v) Pen/Strep (100 U mL^{-1}, Gibco) and 1% L-glutamine (2 mM, Gibco).

For longitudinal monitoring of cell viability (WST1), A549 cells were grown on the BETA membranes by seeding cells with a cell density of 1.5×10^5 cells cm^{-2} on a UV sterilized BETA membrane (effective growth area: 1.3 cm^2, depending on application). A PTFE holder was used for keeping the BETA membranes) and on Corning® Costar® Transwell® cell culture inserts (PET, 12-well, 1.1 cm^2; 3 μm pore) (control). Cells were then cultured for 6 days under submerged conditions (basal and apical medium volumes were 1.5 and 0.5 mL, respectively) followed by 24 h under ALI conditions. Similarly, 16HBE14o^{-} cells were also grown on the BETA membrane (cell seeding density: 2×10^5 cells cm^{-2}; effective growth area: 1.3 cm^2) for 6 days under submerged and 24 h under ALI conditions.

Immediately prior to cell-stretch experiments the membrane was placed in the CIVIC and the media volume in the basal and reservoir chamber of the CIVIC were 4 and 12 mL (including 2 mL in the connecting tubing), respectively.

In vitro Cell-Stretch System (CIVIC)

We used the CIVIC system to apply cyclic stretch to cells grown on the BETA membrane under ALI culture conditions (**Figure 1**). The main chamber of the CIVIC bioreactor is separated by the BETA membrane into an apical (humidified air) and a basal (perfused cell culture medium) compartment mimicking the air-blood barrier of the lung including its breathing-related cyclic stretch induced by oscillation of the apical pressure (**Figures 1A,B** and **Supplementary Video 1**). The cell culture medium in the basal compartment is circulated using a peristaltic pump to mimic blood flow (400 μL min^{-1}). Cells grown on the membrane are subjected to a uniform cyclic triaxial strain by applying a cyclic (here: sinusoidal) positive pressure to the apical chamber by cyclic opening of a valve connected to pressurized cleaned house air and a valve connected to ambient air. The entire system is placed in an incubator (37°C) to maintain optimum cell culture conditions. The dry house air is entering the chamber for pressurization via a humidifier and the initially dry air in the apical compartment can be humidified by nebulization of small volume (2 μL) of saline using the nebulizer described below (**Figures 1A,B**). Both amplitude and frequency of stretch can be set by an Arduino integrated development environment (or IDE) software (Arduino IDE 1.0.5 for Windows). For BETA membranes, the CIVIC bioreactor is able to apply physiologic linear strain: (0–17%) and non-physiologic (over-stretch; 17–25%) stretch conditions, as described below.

The CIVIC system is a modified version of the previously described MALI bioreactor system (Cei et al., 2020). The overall setup and geometry of the MALI system have not been changed. However, the following technical improvements were implemented. All of the components in contact with culture medium are now manufactured with PDMS-free material (namely polycarbonate, PC) to prevent potential artifacts due to leaching of toxicants from the PDMS into the cell culture medium. Moreover, an upgraded design of the PC holder more effectively prevents membrane slipping and leakage of culture medium during pressure oscillations required for inducing cyclic cell stretch as described below. The pressure sealing of the main chamber was improved and not only the pressure in the basal compartment (headspace of the medium reservoir, P_2), but also the pressure in the apical compartment was measured continuously (P_1) (**Figure 1A**) using two piezoresistive, monolithic silicon pressure transducers (MPX5050, Freescale Semiconductor, Munich, Germany).

A clinically used vibrating mesh nebulizer (Aeroneb Pro/Lab, Aerogen Inc., Galway, Ireland) is positioned at the top of the apical chamber for delivery of aerosolized substances to the cells on the BETA membrane. This type of nebulizer has liquid output rates and mass median droplet diameters ranging from 0.2 to 0.8 mL min^{-1} and 2.5 to 6 μm, respectively, depending on the specific type of nebulizer (Ding et al., 2020). Nebulization of 10 μL of liquid and subsequent spatially uniform deposition onto the cells cultured on the BETA membrane (5 cm^2) with a deposition efficiency of 52% occurs within 2 min due to cloud settling (Cei et al., 2020). These aerosol delivery parameters are, independent of nebulizer performance in terms of droplet diameter or liquid output rate (Lenz et al., 2014) since cloud settling depends on the fractional aerosol volume in the air only and hence on the nebulized aerosol volume (10 μL) and the volume of the apical compartment of the chamber. Vibrating mesh nebulizers contain a porous membrane for aerosol production, which may be affected by cyclic positive pressure. Since aerosolized substance delivery is short (2 min) relative to typical cell-stretch experiments (>2 h), aerosolized substance application is typically decoupled from cyclic cell stretch, i.e., cell-stretch is not applied during aerosolization. This patented aerosol-cell exposure unit has recently been made commercially available as VITROCELL®Cloud MAX (VITROCELL Systems, Waldkirch, Germany), albeit only for standard transwell inserts, which cannot be subjected to cyclic stretch. When positive pressure is applied apically to the membrane (P_1), the initially relaxed, flat, horizontally oriented membrane is stretched triaxially downwards expanding the volume of the apical compartment by a dome-shaped volume ΔV (**Figures 1A, 4A**). Due to the incompressible nature of water (culture medium), this change in apical volume reduces the air-filled headspace of the medium reservoir by ΔV and the corresponding increase in pressure (P_2) can be directly related to the linear/area amplitude of membrane stretch (**Figure 1A**).

This special feature of the CIVIC bioreactor enables real-time monitoring of the experimental stretch parameters (amplitude, frequency) and Young's modulus of the cell-covered membrane with thickness t during triaxial stretch under wet conditions (contact with culture medium) by continuously monitoring the apical and basal pressures (P_1 and P_2, respectively). While the stretch frequency can be directly derived from the time course of P_1 or P_2, the linear (1D) and area (2D) amplitude as well as Young's modulus (elastic modulus; E, kPa) of the membrane can be determined from the maximal values of P_1 and P_2 according to the Equations (1)–(3) (Flory et al., 2007).

$$\Delta V = \Delta P\left(\frac{V_0}{P_0}\right),\ where\ \Delta P = P_2 - P_0 \tag{1}$$

$$\Delta V = \pi \Delta h\left(\frac{a^2}{2} + \frac{\Delta h^2}{6}\right) \tag{2}$$

$$\Delta P' = (P_1 - P_2) = \frac{4E\left(\frac{\Delta h}{a}\right)t}{3a\left(\left(\frac{\Delta h}{a}\right)^2 + 1\right)}\left(1 - \frac{1}{\left(1 + \left(\frac{\Delta h}{a}\right)^2\right)^3}\right) \tag{3}$$

Initially, the membrane is non-stretched and the pressure in both the apical and basal compartment is at ambient pressure P_0 (on average 98.0 kPa in Munich, Germany) (see **Figure 1A**). Under these conditions, the radius (area) of the membrane a is 1.26 cm (5 cm^2) and the headspace volume in the medium reservoir V_0 is 30 mL (40 mL vessel filled with 10 mL medium). The deflection of the membrane perpendicular to the membrane (Δh) can be obtained from the corresponding change in apical/basal air volume ΔV, which is determined from Equations (1), (2) and the measured pressures P_1 and P_2. Young's modulus (elastic modulus; E, kPa) of the membrane can then be obtained from Equation (3), where t is the thickness of the membrane (ca. 5 μm; calculated by cross-sectional SEM analysis). For dome-shaped geometry (spherical cap), one can find the relative linear and area strain according to Equation (4).

$$\frac{\Delta L}{L} = \frac{\Delta h}{a} \quad or \quad \frac{\Delta S}{S} = \left(\frac{\Delta h}{a}\right)^2 \tag{4}$$

The amplitude of cell stretch can be calculated from Equation (4), where Δh is the membrane deflection ($0 \leq \Delta h \leq 0.11$ cm) (Equations 1–3) and ΔS is membrane change in surface area during the stretch. P_1 and P_2 are 100.5 and 99.5 kPa for physiologic stretch (10% linear strain or 21% ΔS), respectively.

For optimum BETA membrane, the CIVIC bioreactor is able to apply a linear mechanical strain of up to 17% (or 3, which covers both physiologic and non-physiologic (overstretch) conditions. For those conditions, the optimum BETA membrane is resilient to 48 h cyclic stretch with no deformation, rupture, and creep.

Membrane Fabrication

We recently introduced a novel ultra-thin co-polymeric membrane (BETA) transitioning from an initially stiff, hydrophilic, non-porous membrane to an elastic, porous substrate, providing optimum cell culture conditions during the two phases of typical *in vitro* alveolar cell-stretch experiments at the ALI (Doryab et al., 2020). Briefly, we employed a two-component (hybrid) polymeric material consisting of poly(ε-caprolactone) (PCL: Sigma-Aldrich, Mn 80,000) and gelatin (Type A from porcine skin, Sigma) chosen for their mechano-elastic and bioactivity properties, respectively. Different mass ratios of PCL and gelatin were dissolved in TFE [(2,2,2-trifluoroethanol) with >99.8% purity, Carl Roth GmbH, Karlsruhe, Germany] and stirred until the blend became homogenous. The PCL/gelatin mixture was then added to a custom-made spin-coater (2,000 rpm) to produce a thin film which was left to dry under vacuum (**Figure 2A**). The initially non-porous membrane (phase I: initial cell adhesion and growth) becomes gradually permeable (phase II: ALI culture) upon contact with the cell culture medium. The underlying concept of a biphasic membrane for cell-stretch experiments under ALI conditions mimicking the conditions in the alveolar tissue has been described in the introduction. The optimum concentrations of PCL and gelatin was determined previously as 9.35% PCL and 6.34% gelatin [w/v solvent]; solvent: ≥99% TFE (2,2,2-trifluoroethanol) (Doryab et al., 2020). Here, three new membranes with 15% PCL and 6, 8, and 10% of gelatin were manufactured. The membranes were placed in a holder for placement in the CIVIC system during cell-stretch experiments as described below (**Figure 1C**). Membranes were sterilized before cell culture experiments with ethanol and ultraviolet (UV) light exposure. The membrane is optically transparent and hence suitable for modern cell microscopy technologies.

Membrane Characterization

The membranes were characterized in terms of thickness, ultrastructure, pore size, elemental and chemical composition, surface wettability, elastic modulus, 3D porosity, and cell proliferation (viability and cytotoxicity).

Physical, Elemental, and Chemical Characterization

Thickness, ultrastructure, and pore size of the membranes were analyzed by Scanning Electron Microscopy (SEM). The samples were fixed in 6% (v/v) glutaraldehyde (Sigma-Aldrich) and then dehydrated in gradient ethanol solutions followed by HDMS (hexamethyldisilazane, Sigma-Aldrich) for 15 min and subsequently mounted onto aluminum stubs, sputter-coated with platinum using Leica EM ACE600 vacuum coater, and imaged by SEM (Zeiss Crossbeam 340, Carl Zeiss AG, Oberkochen, Germany) with acceleration voltage of 2 kV. We also used Energy Dispersive X-ray Spectroscopy (EDS, X-max^N, Oxford instruments) with an acceleration voltage of 8 kV to study qualitative elemental and the local distributions of certain elements (Carbon and Nitrogen) in the sample. Focused Ion Beam (FIB)/SEM (Zeiss Crossbeam 340, Carl Zeiss AG, Oberkochen, Germany) and FIB/SEM/EDS were employed to investigate the cross-sectional structures of the membranes at high resolution (30 kV; 700 pA and 1.5 nA). Surface roughness was assessed by an Atomic Force Microscope (AFM, Nanosurf Flex-Axiom) at room temperature. A scanning area of 80 μm was chosen. Scan rates of 0.5–0.15 Hz were used during mapping with 512 points per scan.

Surface Wettability (Water Contact Angle)

The surface wettability or Water Contact Angle (WCA) of the membranes was determined with the sessile drop method using an automated contact angle system OCA20 with an image processing system as described previously (Doryab et al., 2020).

Elastic Modulus (Young's Modulus)

Uniaxial (1D) tensile test (BOSE 5500 system, ElectroForce, Eden Prairie, MN, USA) with a load capacity of 22 N at a rate of 0.01 mm/s until rupture was used to calculate Young's modulus of the membrane (in phase I). Young's modulus of the membrane in wet (phase II) condition was measured using our novel pressure-based technique integrated into our CIVIC system described in more detail in **Figure 1A**.

Porosity

We used the liquid displacement method to measure the 3D porosity of the interconnected three-dimensional (3D) pore network of the membranes. Briefly, membranes were submerged in ethanol (EtOH, ≥99% purity) for 24 h. Gravimetric analysis prior to and after soaking the membrane with EtOH revealed the volume of EtOH (V_{EToH}) inside the pores ($V = m/\rho$; m_{EtOH} = difference of mass prior to and after soaking; $\rho_{EtOH} = 0.789$ g cm^{-3}) and the volume of the dry membrane (V_m) [m_m = mass of membrane prior to soaking; ρ_m is the volume-weighted density of PCL (1.145 g cm^{-3}) and gelatin (1.3 g cm^{-3})]. The empirical 3D porosity can then be calculated according to Equation (5).

$$Porosity = \frac{V_{ETоH}}{V_{EToH} + V_m}. \quad (5)$$

To account for EtOH adsorption on and/or microporosity of PCL itself, the apparent porosity of the pure PCL membrane (9.3 ± 1.7%; according to Equation 5) was subtracted from the measured porosity of the PCL/gelatin membranes.

Moreover, one can estimate the upper limit of porosity from the chemical composition of the membrane. Assuming gelatin has been completely dissolved in the culture medium (PCL is insoluble), one finds a theoretical upper limit for porosity from the volume fraction of gelatin based on Equation (6), where V_g and V_{PCL} are the volume fraction of gelatin and PCL in the composite of PCL/gelatin, respectively, and ρ_g and ρ_{PCL} are the density of gelatin and PCL (ρ_g =1.30 g cm^{-3} and ρ_{PCL} =1.45 g cm^{-3}), respectively.

$$Theoretical\ Porosity = \frac{\frac{V_g}{\rho_g}}{\frac{V_g}{\rho_g} + \frac{V_{PCL}}{\rho_{PCL}}} \quad (6)$$

Cell Proliferation, Morphology, and Cell Viability

Cell proliferation was assessed from the known number of cells seeded on the membrane (day 0) and the cells counted based on DAPI-stained (cell nucleus) CLSM images at the end of the submerged cell culture conditions (day 6). Moreover, cell proliferation was monitored indirectly with higher time-resolution by measuring cell viability in terms of a non-destructive metabolic activity assay (WST1, Roche, Mannheim, Germany), provided the metabolic activity of the cells is similar during the 6 days of cell growth. This test was performed on cell covered BETA membranes (1.3 cm^3) and Corning® Costar® Transwell® cell culture inserts (PET, 12-well, 3 μm pore), which was used as a commercial membrane to compare cell viability, cell number and morphology with that of the BETA membrane. Each membrane was incubated with 1 mL diluted WST1 reagent (1:15) at 37°C. After 15 min, 150 μL supernatant was transferred to a 96-well plate (4 times for each membrane) and absorbance was measured in a plate reader (Magellan™ Tecan) at 450 nm. All the results were normalized to the mean value of blank.

Lactate Dehydrogenase (LDH) Release

The cytotoxicity effect of the manufactured membranes was assessed by the detection of the release of lactate dehydrogenase (LDH; Roche Applied Science, Mannheim, Germany) from the cells, which indicates perforation of the cell membrane. According to the manufacturer's protocol, the determination of LDH activity was determined in the basal (and apical) medium by absorbance measurement at a wavelength of 492 nm. The LDH release is presented as the ratio of LDH dose (LDH concentration times medium volume) in the cell culture medium and the high control (cells treated with 2% [w/v] Triton X-100). Transwell inserts were used as a positive control since BETA membranes are more limited in supply than standard Transwell inserts. The LDH release for each membrane was normalized by the maximum possible LDH level (LDH contained in all cells).

PDMS-Leached in Cell Culture Medium

We fabricated PDMS films for studying the leaching of PDMS oligomers into the culture medium. Briefly, the elastomers and crosslinker (1:10, Sylgard 184, Dow Corning) were mixed and degassed under vacuum. After casting, the film was cured in an oven at 60°C overnight. The PDMS film (thickness: 5 μm) was then cut using a standard biopsy punch (size: 5.0 mm; Kai medical, Solingen, Germany). The membranes were washed with PBS (three times) and disinfected using EtOH 80% and UV before immersing in the Dulbecco's Modified Eagle Medium: Nutrient Mixture F-12 (DMEM/F12, 1:1 v/v, Gibco) supplemented with 10% FCS (Gibco), 1% (v/v) Pen/Strep (100 U mL^{-1}, Gibco), 1% L-glutamine (2 mM, Gibco). The PDMS punches and BETA membranes of the same size were soaked in 2 mL of culture medium for 2 days (the ratio of the surface area and the bulk volume of the membrane to the culture medium were 0.1 cm^2 mL^{-1} and 4.9×10^{-5} cm^3 mL^{-1}).

The PDMS- and BETA-incubated media containing leached compounds were used to investigate their effect on cell viability with the WST1 assay. For this, A549 cells (1.5×10^5 cells cm^{-2}) were cultured under submerged conditions in 12-well multiwell plates using PDMS- and BETA membrane-leached media for up to 4 days and repeatedly analyzed for viability (WST1). As a control, A549 cells were seeded on the bottom of the well plate.

Immunofluorescence

Cells were fixed in 4% paraformaldehyde (Sigma-Aldrich), washed with PBS and, permeabilized by 0.3% Triton X-100 (Sigma-Aldrich) in PBS at room temperature. To prevent any unspecific antibody binding, a blocking buffer (5% BSA and 0.1% TritonX-100) was added for 10 min. The cells were then incubated overnight at 4°C with Anti-E-Cadherin (mouse, 1:1,000; Invitrogen) and anti–ZO-1 monoclonal (mouse, 1:100; Invitrogen), in a blocking buffer (5% BSA and 0.1% TritonX-100). Cells were then incubated with secondary antibody Alexa Fluor® 488 goat anti-mouse IgG (1:500; Invitrogen) and Alexa Fluor® 555 goat anti-mouse IgG (1:500; Invitrogen). The F-actin cytoskeleton and cell nuclei were stained with Phalloidin 594 (1:40) and DAPI (1:100), respectively. The cells were then embedded in Glycergel (DAKO Schweiz AG, Baar, Switzerland). All cell images were acquired using a confocal laser scanning microscope (CLSM; LSM710, Carl Zeiss; Oberkochen, Germany) coupled to the Zen2009 software. For intensity quantification of particles, the images were recorded at five independent fields of view (region of interest: $134.95 \times 134.95\,\mu m$) for each sample. The rectangular tool (Fiji) was used to measure the mean fluorescence intensity of background-subtracted images.

TEER Measurement

Trans-epithelial electrical resistance (TEER) measurements of epithelial cells grown on the membrane were measured using the Millicell-ERS system (Millicell ERS-2, Millipore, USA). TEER is calculated by multiplying the cell-specific resistance (Ohm, Ω) and the effective surface area of the membrane (cm^2). The TEER value of the blank BETA membrane was determined as 78 ± 10 ($\Omega\ cm^2$), which was then subtracted from the cell-covered membrane TEER values.

Particokinetic Studies

For particle studies, we chose fluorescent amine-modified polystyrene ($PS\text{-}NH_2$) spheres, fluorescent orange (Sigma-Aldrich, St. Louis, USA), with a mean diameter of 100 and 1,000 nm for particle study (**Figure 4A**) since amine-functionalized surfaces (positively charged particles) are associated with higher cellular uptake and internalization as compared to neutral or negatively charged ones (Rothen-Rutishauser et al., 2006; Zhu et al., 2013). A549 cells were grown on the optimized BETA membrane until confluence (submerged conditions for 6 days) and left for acclimatization at the ALI for 1 day. Particles were then nebulized directly onto the cells [deposited mass dose: 2.1 $\mu g\ cm^{-2}$; surface area dose: 1.2 $cm^2\ cm^{-2}$ (100 nm particles); 0.12 $cm^2\ cm^{-2}$ (1,000 nm)] and incubate with the cells for 2 h under stretched or unstretched conditions.

For the unstretched experiments, the membranes were first put in special holders and placed in a 6-well plate which was then positioned in the aerosol-cell exposure chamber of a VITROCELL®Cloud 6 system (VITROCELL Systems, Waldkirch, Germany; aerosol exposed area: 146 cm^2, deposition factor: 0.97), followed by nebulization of 250 μL of particle suspensions (1.25 mg mL^{-1} in 0.3% NaCl) with subsequent aerosol sedimentation onto the cells with 3 min as described by Lenz and colleagues (Lenz et al., 2014). Corning® Costar® Transwell® cell culture inserts (6-well, PET membrane with 3 μm pores) were also used to compare transepithelial translocation of particles with cells cultured on the BETA membrane under unstretched and stretched conditions. For stretch experiments, particles are delivered to the cells using the nebulizer integrated in the CIVIC as described above (**Figures 1A,B, 4A**) with a known delivery efficiency of 52% (Doryab et al., 2020). Subsequently, a physiologic cyclic mechanical stretch (10% linear at 0.33 Hz) corresponding to respiratory conditions during light exercise was applied to the cells for 2 h.

The fractional particle transport across the epithelial barrier was determined by quantitative fluorescence spectroscopy of the culture media in the basal compartment of both unstretched and stretched treatment using a plate reader (Safire2™, Tecan; excitation: 520 nm, emission: 540 nm). For normalization to the cell-delivered dose a standard curve of the particle suspension in cell culture medium basal medium volume prepared and measured for fluorescence intensity. For the measurement of quantitative cellular uptake of particles with CLSM, the samples were washed with PBS to remove free or weakly adsorbed particles from the apical side of the cell layer. Subsequently, the cells on the membranes were fixed in 4% paraformaldehyde for CLSM analysis. The CLSM images (z-stacks) were then recorded at five randomly selected fields of view for each sample ($n = 4$; region of interest: $134.95 \times 134.95\,\mu m$) and quantified for cumulative fluorescence intensity of z-stacks.

Statistical Analysis

All data were analyzed using GraphPad Prism 8.4 (GraphPad Software, La Jolla, CA, USA). The details of each statistical analysis were presented in the caption of the figures.

AUTHOR CONTRIBUTIONS

AD and OS designed the experiments, analyzed the data, and wrote the manuscript. AD manufactured and characterized the BETA membrane and performed all the cell experiments and particle and particokinetic studies. AD, OS, and AS modified the CIVIC bioreactor systems. AD and PS performed SEM, FIB-SEM, and EDS-SEM. SO assisted AD with particle study of the Transwell® insert under static conditions. JG, MT, TS, AH, CV, AA, and MR provided the input to data interpretation in their respective field of expertise and contributed to the writing of the manuscript. All authors contributed to the article and approved the submitted version.

SUPPLEMENTARY MATERIAL

Supplementary Figure 1 | The Water Contact Angle (WCA) of the PDMS and BETA membranes using an automated contact angle system OCA20 with an image processing system (mean ± SD).

Supplementary Figure 2 | SEM micrograph of bronchial epithelial 16HBE14o^{-} cells grown on the membrane (cultured 6 days submerged and 24 h ALI culture). (Left) Confluent cell layer scale bar of overview and the magnified insert is 25 and 2 μm, respectively. (Right) Pseudocolored cells (using the GNU Image Manipulation Program (GIMP 2.10.8) (http://www.gimp.org/), showing cracks between cells, which were induced due to dehydration of the samples for SEM. The scale bar is 10 μm.

Supplementary Figure 3 | No significant effect of 2 h physiologic stretch and particle exposure (diameter: 100 and 1,000 nm) on cell viability (WST1 assay; A549 cells) was observed. The viability data were normalized by the corresponding value of the Transwell inserts (no stretch) (Data are reported as mean ± SD. $n = 3$; Two-way ANOVA with Sidak test).

Supplementary Video 1 | BETA membrane motion in the CIVIC bioreactor system when a cyclic mechanical stretch (linear strain: 10%; breathing/stretch frequency: 0.33 Hz) is applied to the membrane.

REFERENCES

Ainslie, G. R., Davis, M., Ewart, L., Lieberman, L. A., Rowlands, D. J., Thorley, A. J., et al. (2019). Microphysiological lung models to evaluate the safety of new pharmaceutical modalities: a biopharmaceutical perspective. *Lab Chip* 19, 3152–3161. doi: 10.1039/C9LC00492K

Annika Mareike Gramatke, I. L. H. (2014). Size and cell type dependent uptake of silica nanoparticles. *J. Nanomed. Nanotechnol.* 5:6. doi: 10.4172/2157-7439.1000248

Artzy-Schnirman, A., Lehr, C. M., and Sznitman, J. (2020). Advancing human *in vitro* pulmonary disease models in preclinical research: opportunities for lung-on-chips. *Expert Opin. Drug Deliv.* 17, 621–625. doi: 10.1080/17425247.2020.1738380

Artzy-Schnirman, A., Zidan, H., Elias-Kirma, S., Ben-Porat, L., Tenenbaum-Katan, J., Carius, P., et al. (2019). Capturing the onset of bacterial pulmonary infection in acini-on-chips. *Adv. Biosyst.* 3:1900026. doi: 10.1002/adbi.201900026

Bachler, G., Losert, S., Umehara, Y., von Goetz, N., Rodriguez-Lorenzo, L., Petri-Fink, A., et al. (2015). Translocation of gold nanoparticles across the lung epithelial tissue barrier: combining *in vitro* and *in silico* methods to substitute *in vivo* experiments. *Part. Fibre Toxicol.* 12:18. doi: 10.1186/s12989-015-0090-8

Barosova, H., Maione, A. G., Septiadi, D., Sharma, M., Haeni, L., Balog, S., et al. (2020). Use of EpiAlveolar lung model to predict fibrotic potential of multiwalled carbon nanotubes. *ACS Nano* 14, 3941–3956. doi: 10.1021/acsnano.9b06860

Benam, K. H., Dauth, S., Hassell, B., Herland, A., Jain, A., Jang, K.-J., et al. (2015). Engineered *in vitro* disease models. *Annu. Rev. Pathol. Mech. Dis.* 10, 195–262. doi: 10.1146/annurev-pathol-012414-040418

Bou Jawde, S., Takahashi, A., Bates, J. H. T., and Suki, B. (2020). An analytical model for estimating alveolar wall elastic moduli from lung tissue uniaxial stress-strain curves. *Front. Physiol.* 11:121. doi: 10.3389/fphys.2020.00121

Carter, S. D., Atif, A., Kadekar, S., Lanekoff, I., Engqvist, H., Varghese, O. P., et al. (2020). PDMS leaching and its implications for on-chip studies focusing on bone regeneration applications. *Organs Chip* 2:100004. doi: 10.1016/j.ooc.2020.100004

Cei, D., Doryab, A., Lenz, A., Schröppel, A., Mayer, P., Burgstaller, G., et al. (2020). Development of a dynamic *in vitro* stretch model of the alveolar interface with aerosol delivery. *Biotechnol. Bioeng.* 1–13. doi: 10.1002/bit.27600

de Souza Carvalho, C., Daum, N., and Lehr, C.-M. (2014). Carrier interactions with the biological barriers of the lung: advanced *in vitro* models and challenges for pulmonary drug delivery. *Adv. Drug Deliv. Rev.* 75, 129–140. doi: 10.1016/j.addr.2014.05.014

Ding, Y., Weindl, P., Lenz, A. G., Mayer, P., Krebs, T., and Schmid, O. (2020). Quartz crystal microbalances (QCM) are suitable for real-time dosimetry in nanotoxicological studies using VITROCELL®Cloud cell exposure systems. *Part. Fibre Toxicol.* 17, 1–20. doi: 10.1186/s12989-020-00376-w

Doryab, A., Amoabediny, G., and Salehi-Najafabadi, A. (2016). Advances in pulmonary therapy and drug development: lung tissue engineering to lung-on-a-chip. *Biotechnol. Adv.* 34, 588–596. doi: 10.1016/j.biotechadv.2016.02.006

Doryab, A., Tas, S., Taskin, M. B., Yang, L., Hilgendorff, A., Groll, J., et al. (2019). Evolution of bioengineered lung models: recent advances and challenges in tissue mimicry for studying the role of mechanical forces in cell biology. *Adv. Funct. Mater.* 29:1903114. doi: 10.1002/adfm.201903114

Doryab, A., Taskin, M. B., Stahlhut, P., Schröppel, A., Wagner, D. E., Groll, J., et al. (2020). Stretch experiments with pulmonary epithelial cells at the air-liquid interface. *Adv. Funct. Mater.* 2004707. doi: 10.1002/adfm.202004707

Edwards, Y. S., Sutherland, L. M., Power, J. H., Nicholas, T. E., and Murray, A. W. (1999). Cyclic stretch induces both apoptosis and secretion in rat alveolar type II cells. *FEBS Lett.* 448, 127–130. doi: 10.1016/S0014-5793(99)00357-9

Ehrhardt, C., Kneuer, C., Fiegel, J., Hanes, J., Schaefer, U., Kim, K.-J., et al. (2002). Influence of apical fluid volume on the development of functional intercellular junctions in the human epithelial cell line 16HBE14o^{-}: implications for the use of this cell line as an *in vitro* model for bronchial drug absorption studies. *Cell Tissue Res.* 308, 391–400. doi: 10.1007/s00441-002-0548-5

Ehrmann, S., Schmid, O., Darquenne, C., Rothen-Rutishauser, B., Sznitman, J., Yang, L., et al. (2020). Innovative preclinical models for pulmonary drug delivery research. *Expert Opin. Drug Deliv.* 17, 463–478. doi: 10.1080/17425247.2020.1730807

Flory, A. L., Brass, D. A., and Shull, K. R. (2007). Deformation and adhesive contact of elastomeric membranes. *J. Polym. Sci. B Polym. Phys.* 45, 3361–3374. doi: 10.1002/polb.21322

Foroozandeh, P., and Aziz, A. A. (2018). Insight into cellular uptake and intracellular trafficking of nanoparticles. *Nanoscale Res. Lett.* 13:339. doi: 10.1186/s11671-018-2728-6

Guenat, O. T., and Berthiaume, F. (2018). Incorporating mechanical strain in organs-on-a-chip: lung and skin. *Biomicrofluidics* 12:042207. doi: 10.1063/1.5024895

Hall, J. E. (2016). *Guyton and Hall Textbook of Medical Physiology, 13th Edn.* London: Elsevier.

Hammerschmidt, S., Kuhn, H., Grasenack, T., Gessner, C., and Wirtz, H. (2004). Apoptosis and necrosis induced by cyclic mechanical stretching in alveolar type II cells. *Am. J. Respir. Cell Mol. Biol.* 30, 396–402. doi: 10.1165/rcmb.2003-0136OC

Hänninen, O., Brüske-Hohlfeld, I., Loh, M., Stoeger, T., Kreyling, W., Schmid, O., et al. (2010). Occupational and consumer risk estimates for nanoparticles emitted by laser printers. *J. Nanoparticle Res.* 12, 91–99. doi: 10.1007/s11051-009-9693-z

Heydarian, M., Yang, T., Schweinlin, M., Steinke, M., Walles, H., Rudel, T., et al. (2019). Biomimetic human tissue model for long-term study of neisseria gonorrhoeae infection. *Front. Microbiol.* 10:1740. doi: 10.3389/fmicb.2019.01740

Higuita-Castro, N., Nelson, M. T., Shukla, V., Agudelo-Garcia, P. A., Zhang, W., Duarte-Sanmiguel, S. M., et al. (2017). Using a novel microfabricated model of the alveolar-capillary barrier to investigate the effect of matrix structure on atelectrauma. *Sci. Rep.* 7:11623. doi: 10.1038/s41598-017-12044-9

Huh, D., Kim, H. J., Fraser, J. P., Shea, D. E., Khan, M., Bahinski, A., et al. (2013). Microfabrication of human organs-on-chips. *Nat. Protoc.* 8, 2135–2157. doi: 10.1038/nprot.2013.137

Huh, D., Matthews, B. D., Mammoto, A., Montoya-Zavala, M., Hsin, H. Y., and Ingber, D. E. (2010). Reconstituting organ-level lung functions on a chip. *Science* 328, 1662–1668. doi: 10.1126/science.1188302

Huh, D., Torisawa, Y., Hamilton, G. a., Kim, H. J., and Ingber, D. E. (2012). Microengineered physiological biomimicry: organs-on-chips. *Lab Chip* 12:2156. doi: 10.1039/c2lc40089h

ICRP (1994). Human respiratory tract model for radiological protection. A report of a Task Group of the International Commission on Radiological Protection. *Ann. ICRP* 24, 1–482.

Kreyling, W. G., Hirn, S., Möller, W., Schleh, C., Wenk, A., Celik, G., et al. (2014). Air-blood barrier translocation of tracheally instilled gold nanoparticles inversely depends on particle size. *ACS Nano* 8, 222–233.

doi: 10.1021/nn403256v

Kreyling, W. G., Semmler-Behnke, M., Takenaka, S., and Möller, W. (2013). Differences in the biokinetics of inhaled nano- versus micrometer-sized particles. *Acc. Chem. Res.* 46, 714–722. doi: 10.1021/ar300043r

Kuehn, A., Kletting, S., de Souza Carvalho-Wodarz, C., Repnik, U., Griffiths, G., Fischer, U., et al. (2016). Human alveolar epithelial cells expressing tight junctions to model the air-blood barrier. *ALTEX* 33, 1–20. doi: 10.14573/altex.1511131

Lehmann, A. D., Daum, N., Bur, M., Lehr, C. M., Gehr, P., and Rothen-Rutishauser, B. M. (2011). An *in vitro* triple cell co-culture model with primary cells mimicking the human alveolar epithelial barrier. *Eur. J. Pharm. Biopharm.* 77, 398–406. doi: 10.1016/j.ejpb.2010.10.014

Lenz, A. G., Stoeger, T., Cei, D., Schmidmeir, M., Semren, N., Burgstaller, G., et al. (2014). Efficient bioactive delivery of aerosolized drugs to human pulmonary epithelial cells cultured in air–liquid interface conditions. *Am. J. Respir. Cell Mol. Biol.* 51, 526–535. doi: 10.1165/rcmb.2013-0479OC

Meindl, C., Stranzinger, S., Dzidic, N., Salar-Behzadi, S., Mohr, S., Zimmer, A., et al. (2015). Permeation of therapeutic drugs in different formulations across the airway epithelium *in vitro*. *PLoS ONE* 10:e0135690. doi: 10.1371/journal.pone.0135690

Nishiguchi, A., Singh, S., Wessling, M., Kirkpatrick, C. J., and Möller, M. (2017). Basement membrane mimics of biofunctionalized nanofibers for a bipolar-cultured human primary alveolar-capillary barrier model. *Biomacromolecules* 18, 719–727. doi: 10.1021/acs.biomac.6b01509

Paur, H.-R., Cassee, F. R., Teeguarden, J., Fissan, H., Diabate, S., Aufderheide, M., et al. (2011). *In-vitro* cell exposure studies for the assessment of nanoparticle toxicity in the lung—a dialog between aerosol science and biology. *J. Aerosol Sci.* 42, 668–692. doi: 10.1016/j.jaerosci.2011.06.005

Peters, A., Wichmann, H. E., Tuch, T., Heinrich, J., and Heyder, J. (1997). Respiratory effects are associated with the number of ultrafine particles. *Am. J. Respir. Crit. Care Med.* 155, 1376–1383. doi: 10.1164/ajrccm.155.4.9105082

Polio, S. R., Kundu, A. N., Dougan, C. E., Birch, N. P., Aurian-Blajeni, D. E., Schiffman, J. D., et al. (2018). Cross-platform mechanical characterization of lung tissue. *PLoS ONE* 13:e0204765. doi: 10.1371/journal.pone.0204765

Pope, C. A., Ezzati, M., and Dockery, D. W. (2009). Fine-particulate air pollution and life expectancy in the United States. *N. Engl. J. Med.* 360, 376–386. doi: 10.1056/NEJMsa0805646

Regehr, K. J., Domenech, M., Koepsel, J. T., Carver, K. C., Ellison-Zelski, S. J., Murphy, W. L., et al. (2009). Biological implications of polydimethylsiloxane-based microfluidic cell culture. *Lab Chip* 9:2132. doi: 10.1039/b903043c

Rothen-Rutishauser, B. M., Schürch, S., Haenni, B., Kapp, N., and Gehr, P. (2006). Interaction of fine particles and nanoparticles with red blood cells visualized with advanced microscopic techniques. *Environ. Sci. Technol.* 40, 4353–4359. doi: 10.1021/es0522635

Schaumann, F., Frömke, C., Dijkstra, D., Alessandrini, F., Windt, H., Karg, E., et al. (2014). Effects of ultrafine particles on the allergic inflammation in the lung of asthmatics: results of a double-blinded randomized cross-over clinical pilot study. *Part. Fibre Toxicol.* 11:39. doi: 10.1186/s12989-014-0039-3

Schmid, O., and Cassee, F. R. (2017). On the pivotal role of dose for particle toxicology and risk assessment: exposure is a poor surrogate for delivered dose. *Part. Fibre Toxicol.* 14:52. doi: 10.1186/s12989-017-0233-1

Schmid, O., Jud, C., Umehara, Y., Mueller, D., Bucholski, A., Gruber, F., et al. (2017). Biokinetics of aerosolized liposomal ciclosporin a in human lung cells *in vitro* using an air-liquid cell interface exposure system. *J. Aerosol Med. Pulm. Drug Deliv.* 30, 411–424. doi: 10.1089/jamp.2016.1361

Schmid, O., and Stoeger, T. (2016). Surface area is the biologically most effective dose metric for acute nanoparticle toxicity in the lung. *J. Aerosol Sci.* 99, 133–143. doi: 10.1016/j.jaerosci.2015.12.006

Stucki, A. O., Stucki, J. D., Hall, S. R. R., Felder, M., Mermoud, Y., Schmid, R. A., et al. (2015). A lung-on-a-chip array with an integrated bio-inspired respiration mechanism. *Lab Chip* 15, 1302–1310. doi: 10.1039/C4LC01252F

Takenaka, S., Möller, W., Semmler-Behnke, M., Karg, E., Wenk, A., Schmid, O., et al. (2012). Efficient internalization and intracellular translocation of inhaled gold nanoparticles in rat alveolar macrophages. *Nanomedicine* 7, 855–865. doi: 10.2217/nnm.11.152

Teeguarden, J. G., Hinderliter, P. M., Orr, G., Thrall, B. D., and Pounds, J. G. (2007). Particokinetics *in vitro*: dosimetry considerations for *in vitro* nanoparticle toxicity assessments. *Toxicol. Sci.* 95, 300–312. doi: 10.1093/toxsci/kfl165

Tenenbaum-Katan, J., Artzy-Schnirman, A., Fishler, R., Korin, N., and Sznitman, J. (2018). Biomimetics of the pulmonary environment *in vitro*: a microfluidics perspective. *Biomicrofluidics* 12:042209. doi: 10.1063/1.5023034

Vlahakis, N. E., Schroeder, M. A., Limper, A. H., and Hubmayr, R. D. (1999). Stretch induces cytokine release by alveolar epithelial cells *in vitro*. *Am. J. Physiol. Cell. Mol. Physiol.* 277, L167–L173. doi: 10.1152/ajplung.1999.277.1.L167

Wang, L., Sun, B., Ziemer, K. S., Barabino, G. A., and Carrier, R. L. (2010). Chemical and physical modifications to poly(dimethylsiloxane) surfaces affect adhesion of Caco-2 cells. *J. Biomed. Mater. Res. A* 93, 1260–1271. doi: 10.1002/jbm.a.32621

Wang, Z., Volinsky, A. A., and Gallant, N. D. (2014). Crosslinking effect on polydimethylsiloxane elastic modulus measured by custom-built compression instrument. *J. Appl. Polym. Sci.* 131:41050. doi: 10.1002/app.41050

Weibel, E. R. (1970). Morphometric estimation of pulmonary diffusion capacity. *Respir. Physiol.* 11, 54–75. doi: 10.1016/0034-5687(70)90102-7

Weibel, E. R. (2009). What makes a good lung? *Swiss Med. Wkly.* 139, 375–86. doi: 10.4414/smw.2009.12270

Winnik, F. M., and Maysinger, D. (2013). Quantum dot cytotoxicity and ways to reduce it. *Acc. Chem. Res.* 46, 672–680. doi: 10.1021/ar3000585

Young, B. M., Shankar, K., Allen, B. P., Pouliot, R. A., Schneck, M. B., Mikhaiel, N. S., et al. (2017). Electrospun decellularized lung matrix scaffold for airway smooth muscle culture. *ACS Biomater. Sci. Eng.* 3, 3480–3492. doi: 10.1021/acsbiomaterials.7b00384

Zhu, M., Nie, G., Meng, H., Xia, T., Nel, A., and Zhao, Y. (2013). Physicochemical properties determine nanomaterial cellular uptake, transport, and fate. *Acc. Chem. Res.* 46, 622–631. doi: 10.1021/ar300031y

16

A Novel Fibroblast Reporter Cell Line for *in vitro* Studies of Pulmonary Fibrosis

Julia Nemeth[1†], Annika Schundner[1†], Karsten Quast[2], Veronika E. Winkelmann[1] and Manfred Frick[1]*

[1] Institute of General Physiology, Ulm University, Ulm, Germany, [2] Boehringer Ingelheim Pharma GmbH & Co. KG, Biberach, Germany

***Correspondence:**
Manfred Frick
manfred.frick@uni-ulm.de
orcid.org/0000-0002-4763-1104

† These authors have contributed equally to this work

Idiopathic pulmonary fibrosis (IPF) is a fatal disease of the lower respiratory tract with restricted therapeutic options. Repetitive injury of the bronchoalveolar epithelium leads to activation of pulmonary fibroblasts, differentiation into myofibroblasts and excessive extracellular matrix (ECM) deposition resulting in aberrant wound repair. However, detailed molecular and cellular mechanisms underlying initiation and progression of fibrotic changes are still elusive. Here, we report the generation of a representative fibroblast reporter cell line (10-4A^{BFP}) to study pathophysiological mechanisms of IPF in high throughput or high resolution *in vitro* live cell assays. To this end, we immortalized primary fibroblasts isolated from the distal lung of Sprague-Dawley rats. Molecular and transcriptomic characterization identified clone 10-4A as a matrix fibroblast subpopulation. Mechanical or chemical stimulation induced a reversible fibrotic state comparable to effects observed in primary isolated fibroblasts. Finally, we generated a reporter cell line (10-4A^{BFP}) to express nuclear blue fluorescent protein (BFP) under the promotor of the myofibroblast marker alpha smooth muscle actin (*Acta2*) using CRISPR/Cas9 technology. We evaluated the suitability of 10-4A^{BFP} as reporter tool in plate reader assays. In summary, the 10-4A^{BFP} cell line provides a novel tool to study fibrotic processes *in vitro* to gain new insights into the cellular and molecular processes involved in fibrosis formation and propagation.

Keywords: idiopathic pulmonary fibrosis, lung, myofibroblast, TGF-β, extracellular matrix, alpha smooth muscle actin

INTRODUCTION

Idiopathic pulmonary fibrosis (IPF) is a progressive, irreversible and usually fatal lung disease with poor prognosis. IPF is characterized by subpleural fibrosis, subepithelial fibroblast foci, and microscopic honeycombing (Raghu et al., 2011; Wuyts et al., 2013; Lederer and Martinez, 2018; Sgalla et al., 2018). Various risk factors, including air pollution and smoking, have been associated with the development of IPF (Selman and Pardo, 2001; Kage and Borok, 2012; Liang et al., 2016; Kasper and Barth, 2017; Richeldi et al., 2017). In recent years, it has become clear that IPF is also strongly associated with genetic aberrations (Armanios et al., 2007; Seibold et al., 2011; Ryu et al., 2014; Stuart et al., 2015; Evans et al., 2016). Hence, an approach in understanding IPF pathogenesis is to consider it as a three-stage process: predisposition, initiation, and progression.

The conceptual model for the pathogenesis of IPF postulates that recurrent micro-injuries to the bronchoalveolar epithelium, superimposed on accelerated epithelial aging, result in aberrant wound repair. The reduced renewal capacity of bronchoalveolar stem cells, including alveolar type II cells, leads to reduced alveolar-epithelial cell proliferation, and secretion of profibrotic mediators (Selman and Pardo, 2001; Plantier et al., 2011; Kage and Borok, 2012; Ryu et al., 2014; Chambers and Mercer, 2015; Liang et al., 2016; Xu et al., 2016; Kasper and Barth, 2017; Richeldi et al., 2017; Lederer and Martinez, 2018). The main and most studied profibrotic cytokine is transforming growth factor beta 1 (TGF-β1). Several other cytokines play a major role in immune and inflammation responses for fibrosis formation, including interleukins (IL) like IL-13 (Zhu et al., 1999; Kolodsick et al., 2004; O'Reilly, 2013), IL-33 (Yanaba et al., 2011; Luzina et al., 2012, 2013) and IL-4 (Huaux et al., 2003; Saito et al., 2003), tumor necrosis factor alpha (TNFα) (Sime et al., 1998; Oikonomou et al., 2006; Epstein Shochet et al., 2017) as well as thymic stromal lymphopoietin (TSLP) (Datta et al., 2013; Lee et al., 2017). Profibrotic cytokines promote fibroblast activation and proliferation (Sime et al., 1997; Hinz, 2009; Luzina et al., 2015).

Fibroblast activation results in altered and increased ECM production, deposition, and accumulation (Liu et al., 2010; Bagnato and Harari, 2015). This causes remodeling processes of the pulmonary interstitium, forming scar tissue and modifying its mechanical properties (Booth et al., 2012; Parker et al., 2014). Scarring is accompanied by a strong increase in the tissue stiffness and an overall thickening of the alveolar septae (Horowitz and Thannickal, 2006; Hinz, 2009; Richeldi et al., 2017). During this progression phase, the matrix stiffness can increase from $\sim$ 0.5 to 15 kPa in healthy lung tissue to up to 100 kPa in fibrotic tissue depending on the measured lung compartment (Liu et al., 2010; Booth et al., 2012). The pathologically stiff matrix further propagates remodeling independent of epithelial cell dysfunction. In a feed-forward loop, increased matrix stiffness promotes additional differentiation of fibroblasts to myofibroblasts and matrix deposition (Hinz, 2009; Enomoto et al., 2013; Burgess et al., 2016; Tschumperlin et al., 2018). Overall, these processes result in the destruction of the overall alveolar architecture, leading to a strong impairment of lung function and eventually resulting in the death of the patient (Wuyts et al., 2013).

Studies regarding the onset and progress of IPF are mainly conducted in animal models by the application of fibrosis inducing agents like bleomycin (Gabazza et al., 2004; Xiao et al., 2006; Löfdahl et al., 2018). However, animal models of IPF do not fully recapitulate human pathophysiology (Lederer and Martinez, 2018). These models only partially mimic the events hallmarking IPF but it's challenging to gain a deep insight into cellular and molecular processes. Hence, studies investigating molecular alterations of affected cell populations in response to pro-fibrotic stimuli are essential to get a more in-depth understanding of key processes responsible for development and progression of IPF. In this context, *in vitro* studies mimicking the *in vivo* situation hold great promise to elucidate molecular mechanisms underlying IPF initiation and progression. Sophisticated "lung on a chip" approaches recapitulating the alveolar microenvironment were developed and optimized by different groups (Huh, 2015; Stucki et al., 2018; Felder et al., 2019). These enable co-culture of differentiated alveolar epithelial and mesenchymal cells at air-liquid conditions whilst mimicking breathing motion and blood flow. However, the impact of these *in vitro* models depends on the use of cells representative of the *in vivo* situation.

In order to promote *in vitro* models for studying fibrotic processes, we generated an immortalized pulmonary fibroblast reporter cell line (10-4A^{BFP}) using CRISPR/Cas9 gene-editing. 10-4A^{BFP} cells express nuclear blue fluorescent protein (BFP) under the promotor of the myofibroblast marker alpha smooth muscle actin (*Acta2*). To this end, we isolated primary cells from the distal lung of Sprague-Dawley rats and immortalized them using a recently described technology (Kuehn et al., 2016). We characterized several clones and validated selected clones for suitability in fibrosis studies, directly comparing responsiveness to either mechanical or chemical stimuli to responses observed in primary isolated fibroblasts. We identified clone 10-4A as a matrix fibroblast subpopulation that can be (reversibly) induced to a fibrotic state comparable to primary isolated fibroblasts. The 10-4A clone was then used for generation of a reporter cell line (10-4A^{BFP}) expressing nuclear BFP under the promotor of the myofibroblast marker alpha smooth muscle actin (*Acta2*) using CRISPR/Cas9 technology. Finally, we evaluated the use of 10-4A^{BFP} cells as screening tool in plate reader assays. In summary, the 10-4A^{BFP} cell line provides a novel tool to study fibrotic processes in an *in vitro* co-culture system at high resolution and/or high throughput and thereby enables new insights into the cellular and molecular processes involved in fibrosis formation and propagation.

MATERIALS AND METHODS

Chemicals and Antibodies

Human TGF-β1 was obtained from Proteintech (cat. # HZ-1011, Manchester, United Kingdom), rat IL-13 (cat. # 1945-RL-025) and rat TNF-α (cat. # 510 RT) from R&D Systems (Minneapolis, MN, United States), rat IL-33 (cat. # ab200250) from Abcam (Cambridge, United Kingdom) and rat IL-1β (cat. # 80023-RNAE) from Sino Biological (Vienna, Austria). All other chemicals were obtained from Sigma-Aldrich GmbH (Steinheim, Germany) if not stated otherwise. The following primary and secondary antibodies were used for immunofluorescence staining: αSMA (1:200, cat. # ab5694; Abcam; RRID:AB_2223021), vimentin (1:500, cat. # ab73159; Abcam; RRID:AB_1271458), EpCAM (1:200, cat. # ab71916; Abcam, RRID:AB_1603782), ABCa3 (1:500, cat. # ab24751; Abcam, RRID:AB_448287), Aqp5 (1:200, cat. # ab92320; Abcam, RRID:AB_2049171), caveolin 1 (1:200, cat. # ab2910, Abcam, RRID:AB_303405), CD45 (1:500, cat. # 12-0461-80, Thermo Fisher Scientific, Bonn, Germany, RRID:AB_2572560).

Alexa Fluor® 488 goat anti-chicken (1:300, cat. # A11039; Thermo Fisher Scientific, RRID:AB_142924); Alexa Fluor® 568 goat anti-rabbit (1:300, cat. # A11011; Thermo Fisher Scientific, RRID:AB_143157) Alexa Fluor® 488 goat anti-mouse (1:300, cat. # A11029; Thermo Fisher Scientific, RRID:AB_138404).

Cell Isolation and Cultivation

All lung cells were isolated from 12 to 14-week-old male Sprague-Dawley rats.

Primary alveolar type II (ATII) cells were isolated according to a modified protocol described by Jansing et al. (2018) In short, rats were anesthetized with ketamine (10%) and xylazil (2%) and injected with heparin (400 IU/kg). Lungs were perfused, removed, washed with BSS-A supplemented with EGTA, BSS-A w/o EGTA and BSS-B solution. The tissue was incubated with 0.5 mg/ml elastase (Elastin Products Co., Owensville, MO, United States) for 20 min. Then, 2 mg/ml DNase were added and the tissue was minced with sharp scissors into bits of about 1 mm^3. The enzymatic reaction was stopped by adding FCS (GIBCO® life technologies, Carlsbad, CA, United States) (37°C, 2 min). The digested tissue was filtered through gauze and nylon meshes (mesh sizes: 100, 40, and 10 μm) and the cell filtrate was centrifuged for 8 min at 130 rcf. For further cell separation, density gradient centrifugation was applied by mixing the cells in OptiPrep™ Density Gradient medium (1.077 g/mL) diluted in BSS-B. The cells were centrifuged for 20 min at 200 rcf. The layer containing ATII cells was collected and supplemented with BSS-B to a total volume of 40 ml. Cells were centrifuged at 130 rcf for 8 min, resuspended in MucilAir™ cell culture medium and 1×10^6 cells/cm^2 were seeded apically on 0.4 μm transparent Transwell® filter inserts (Sarstedt, Nümbrecht, Germany). Purity of the ATII cells (>90%) was determined by staining with 0.4 μM Lyso Tracker Red DND 99 for 10 min (Thermo Fisher Scientific, Waltham, MA, United States) and more specifically with an ABCa3 staining. The amount of LTR positive cells was determined using a Countess II FL Automated Cell Counter (Thermo Fisher Scientific, Waltham, MA, United States).

Primary lung fibroblasts and distal lung cells were isolated according to the method of Dobbs et al. (1986) with minor modifications as previously described (Miklavc et al., 2010).

For primary isolated fibroblasts further modifications were applied:

Anesthesia, lung perfusion and removal followed the protocol described for isolation of AT2 cells. The tissue was then incubated with 0.5 mg/ml elastase (Elastin Products Co., Owensville, MO, United States) and 0.05 mg/ml trypsin at 37°C for 30 min. 2 mg/ml DNase were added, the enzymatic reaction was stopped by FCS and the digested tissue was filtered through gauze and nylon meshes (mesh sizes: 100, 70, and 40 μm). For purification of primary fibroblasts, cell suspensions were depleted of leukocytes using anti-CD45 MicroBeads (Miltenyi Biotec, Bergisch Gladbach, Germany) before fibroblasts were isolated using anti- CD90.1 MicroBeads (Miltenyi Biotec, Bergisch Gladbach, Germany) according to manufacturer's instructions. Cells were seeded on polydimethylsiloxane (PDMS) gels or plastic substrate in MucilAir™ culture medium containing 25.6 μg/ml Gentamicin ± 5 ng/mL TGF-β1 at a density of 1 to 5×10^5 cells/cm^2. Cells were cultured at 37°C, 5% CO_2 and 95% humidity for up to 14 days. Culture media were changed every 2 days, with TGF-β1 being added freshly to the medium in corresponding experiments.

Generation of Immortalized Cell Lines

Immortalization was performed by InSCREENeX (Braunschweig, Germany) as previously described (Lipps et al., 2018). In short: Immortalization genes were incorporated with third generation self-inactivating lentiviral vectors. Gene expression is controlled by an internal SV 40 promoter. Integration of the transgenes was verified by PCR and subsequent gel electrophoresis.

Overall, 15 immortalized cell clones were generated, all displaying characteristics of different cell populations of the distal lung. The incorporated genes used for the immortalization process for the cell line 10-4A are TAg, ID2, ID3, Rex, Nanog, and E7.

10-4A cells were maintained in the chemically defined, standardized, cell culture medium MucilAir™ (Epithelix, Genève, Switzerland) containing 25.6 μg/ml Gentamicin (Thermo Fisher Scientific) at 37°C, 5% CO_2 and 95% humidity. Cells were detached upon reaching 80% confluence using TrypLE (Thermo Fisher Scientific), centrifuged, resuspended in cell culture medium ± 5 ng/mL TGF-β1 and seeded on PDMS gels or plastic dishes at a density of 0.5×10^3 to 40×10^3 cells/cm^2. Culture media were changed every 2 days, with TGF-β1 being added freshly to the medium in corresponding experiments. Cells from passage 11 to 25 were used for all experiments.

PDMS Gel Preparation and Coating of Cell Culture Dishes

PDMS gels were prepared with the Sylgard 527 Silicon Dielectric Gel Kit (Dow Europe GmbH, Wiesbaden, Germany) as previously described (Palchesko et al., 2012) with minor modifications. In brief, component A and B were thoroughly mixed in a 1:1 ratio and added to 24 Well Culture Plates (Sarstedt, Nümbrecht, Germany) or ibiTreat μSlide 8 well (ibidi GmbH, Gräfelfing, Germany), respectively. Culture containers were kept under vacuum for 2 h to remove potential air inclusions and then incubated at room temperature for 48 h for polymerization. Fully polymerized PDMS gels were sterilized in a UV Crosslinker (GE Healthcare Europe GmbH, Freiburg im Breisgau, Germany) for 30 min and then coated with a 0.01% w/v polydopamine solution [50 mM Tris–HCl, pH = 8.5, 0.01% (w/v) Dopamine Hydrochloride] for 1 h and a 38 μg/ml rat tail collagen I solution (Advanced BioMatrix Inc., San Diego, CA, United States), diluted in Dulbecco PBS (Biochrom, Berlin, Germany; pH 7.4) over night at 37°C, respectively.

Identical coating conditions were used for culture plastic dishes w/o PDMS to ensure comparability.

RNA Isolation, cDNA Synthesis and qPCR

Total RNA was isolated using the my-Budget RNA Mini Kit (Bio-Budget Technologies GmbH, Krefeld, Germany) with an additional DNA removal step using the RNase free DNase Set (QIAGEN GmbH, Hilden, Germany). cDNA synthesis was performed using the SuperScript® VILO^{TM} cDNA Synthesis Kit (Thermo Fisher Scientific) and cDNA was diluted in a 1:3 ratio with DEPC treated H_2O (Carl Roth, Karlsruhe, Germany) prior qPCR.

Amplification was performed on a StepOnePlus qPCR cycle (Applied Biosystems, Foster City, CA, United States) using EvaGreen QPCR Mix II (Bio-Budget Technologies). The following QuantiTect® Primer assays (QIAGEN GmbH, Hilden Germany) were used: Rn_Plin2_2_SG (QT01624329), Rn_Acta2_1_SG (QT01615901), Rn_Col1a1_1_SG (QT01081059), Rn_Sftpc_1_SG (QT00179368), Rn_ABCa3_1_SG (QT01587936), Rn_Vim_1_SG (QT00178724), Rn_HOPX_1_SG (QT00182693), Rn_Cav1_1_SG (QT00398181), and Rn_Hmbs_1_SG (QT00179123). The relative quantification of mRNA expression was performed according to the method of Pfaffl (2001).

Illumina Library Preparation and Sequencing

The Sequencing library preparation has been done using 200 ng of total RNA input with the TruSeq RNA Sample Prep Kit v2-Set B (RS-122-2002, Illumina Inc., San Diego, CA, United States) producing a 275 bp fragment including adapters in average size. In the final step before sequencing, eight individual libraries were normalized and pooled together using the adapter indices supplied by the manufacturer. Pooled libraries have then been clustered on the cBot Instrument from Illumina using the TruSeq SR Cluster Kit v3 - cBot - HS (GD-401-3001, Illumina Inc., San Diego, CA, United States) sequencing was then performed as 50 bp, single reads and 7 bases index read on an Illumina HiSeq2000 instrument using the TruSeq SBS Kit HS- v3 (50-cycle) (FC-401-3002, Illumina Inc., San Diego, CA, United States).

mRNA-Seq Bioinformatics Pipeline

RNA-Seq reads were aligned to the rat genome using the STAR Aligner v2.5.2a (Dobin et al., 2013) with the Ensembl 84 reference genome[1]. Sequenced read quality was checked with FastQC v0.11.2[2] and alignment quality metrics were calculated using the RNASeQC v1.18 (Deluca et al., 2012). Following read alignment, duplication rates of the RNA-Seq samples were computed with bamUtil v1.0.11 to mark duplicate reads and the dupRadar v1.4 Bioconductor R package for assessment (Sayols et al., 2016). The gene expression profiles were quantified using Cufflinks software version 2.2.1 (Trapnell et al., 2013) to get the Reads Per Kilobase of transcript per Million mapped reads (RPKM) as well as read counts from the feature counts software package (Liao et al., 2014). The matrix of read counts and the design file were imported to R, normalization factors calculated using trimmed mean of M-values (TMM) and subsequently voom normalized, before subjected to downstream descriptive statistics analysis.

[1]http://www.ensembl.org

[2]http://www.bioinformatics.babraham.ac.uk/projects/fastqc/

Western Blot

Cells were washed twice with PBS, collected with RIPA Buffer (Sigma-Aldrich) and sonicated (Sonifier 250, Branson Ultrasonics Corporation, Danbury, CT, United States) prior loading on gels. The protein concentration was determined by Pierce BCA Protein Assay (Thermo Fisher Scientific). Protein Loading Buffer and NuPAGE reducing agent (Thermo Fisher Scientific) were added in a 1:5 and 1:10 ratio, respectively. Samples were incubated at 70°C for 10 min, separated by SDS-PAGE and blotted on a nitrocellulose membrane. Immunodetection of αSMA and HSP90 was performed using Anti-alpha smooth muscle actin (1:200, cat # ab5694; Abcam, RRID:AB_2223021) and HSP90 α/β antibodies (F-8) (1:500, cat. # sc-13119; Santa Cruz Biotechnology, Dallas, TX, United States, RRID:AB_675659) in combination with fluorescent labeled secondary antibodies [1:20,000; IRDye® 800CW Donkey anti-Rabbit (cat. # 926-32213, RRID:AB_621848), IRDye® 680RD Donkey anti-Mouse (cat. # 926-68072, RRID:AB_10953628)] diluted in Intercept® Blocking Buffer (cat. # 927-60001) (all from LI-COR Biosciences, Lincoln, NE, United States). Primary antibodies were incubated over night at 4°C, secondary antibodies for 1 h at RT, respectively. Membranes were analyzed with the Odyssey Fc Imaging System (LI-COR Biosciences).

Immunofluorescence

For immunofluorescence staining, cells were washed with DPBS (Biochrom, Berlin, Germany; pH 7.4) and fixed in a 4% paraformaldehyde solution (dissolved in DPBS) for 10 min followed by a 1 min incubation in ice-cold 99.8% MeOH. Cells were permeabilized in a 0.2% w/v saponin solution (dissolved in DPBS) containing 10% FBS (Thermo Fisher Scientific) and 50 mM HEPES. Subsequently, cells were stained for 1 h with primary antibodies, washed twice with DPBS and stained with secondary antibodies diluted in saponin solution for 1 h. Images were taken on an iMIC digital microscope (FEI Munich GmbH, Gräfelfing, Germany) with an Olympus UApo/340 40x/1.35 Oil Iris, Infinity/0.17 lens (Olympus Europa SE & Co. KG, Hamburg, Germany) and the corresponding software (Live Aquisition v2.6.0.14).

Generation of the *Acta2*-BFP Reporter Cell Line

CRISPR/Cas9 dependent gene editing of 10-4A cells was performed according to the method described in Ran et al. (2013).

A 20 bp single guide RNA (sgRNA) (AAACAGGAGT ATGACGAAGC), binding at the end of the coding region of the *Acta2* gene was designed by using the R&D Benchling software[3]. The sgRNA was cloned into SpCas9(BB)-2A-GFP (Addgene plasmid ID: 48138). A donor vector was designed to allow for in-frame fusion of a T2A-BFP-NLS (BFP from Evrogen, Heidelberg, Germany) cassette at the 3′ end of the *Acta2* gene. Primers used were listed in **Table 1**. DNA sequences flanking the sgRNA cutting site at the 5′and 3′ end were amplified from genomic DNA isolated from 10-4A cells (isolated with DNeasy Blood ans Tissue Kit, QIAGEN GmbH), and

[3]https://www.benchling.com

TABLE 1 | Primers used for cloning of T2A-BFP-NLS and homology arms into donor vector pGEX-6P-1.

Primer Name	Sequence 5′ → 3′
pGEX-6P-1_fwd	tgtggaattgtgagcggataac
pGEX-6P-1_rev	cattatacgcgatgattaattg
T2A-BFP-NLS_fwd	tcggctcgtataatggagggcagaggaag tctgct
T2A-BFP-NLS_rev	gctcacaattccacattatacctttctcttcttt tttgga
*Acta2*_right_homologous_right_arm_fwd	tcggctcgtataatgccctctgtgttgggcag
*Acta2*_right_homologous_right_arm_rev	acttcctctgccctcccacatctgctgga aggtaga
*Acta2*_left_homologous_right_arm_fwd	caggaaacagtattcgtcacgcccccaccct
*Acta2*_left_homologous_right_arm_rev	aacttccagatccgatgtaaacacatgtata attgtttttacttatccggtcac
pGEX-6P-1_T2A-BFP-NLS_right_arm_rev	cattatacgcgatgattaattgtcaacag
pGEX-6P-1_T2A-BFP-NLS_right_arm_fw	gagggcagaggaagtctgctaac
pGEX-6P-1_T2A-BFP-NLS_left_arm_fw	tcggatctggaagttctgttccagg
pGEX-6P-1_T2A-BFP-NLS_left_arm_rev	gaatactgtttcctgtgtgaaattgttatccg

subcloned into the targeting pGEX-6P-1 Vector (GE Healthcare, 28-9546-48) using the In-Fusion kit (Clontech, Mountain View, CA, United States). 10-4A cells were co-transfected with the sgRNA/SpCas9(BB)-2A-GFP plasmid and the pGEX-6P-1 donor plasmid in a ratio of 2:1 using Lipofectamine LTX (Ratio: LTX Reagent: PLUS™ Reagent, 1:1) (Thermo Fisher Scientific). The efficiency of sgRNA/Cas9-mediated integration of the BFP was evaluated after addition of 5 ng/ml TGF-β1 via fluorescence microscopy. 72 h after transfection, isolation of clonal cells was achieved by fluorescent activated cell sorting (FACS). Cells were selected for GFP and BFP expression using the BD FACSAria™ III (Becton Dickinson GmbH) with the corresponding BD FACSDiva™ v6.1.3 software. Single cells were seeded in 96-well plates containing cell culture medium.

Functional Testing of BFP Integration

The DNA of the cell clones was extracted as described above. The region of interest was amplified by PCR and the respective products (WT: 1000 bp, with BFP insert: 1880 bp) were verified by Sanger Sequencing (Eurofins).

Additionally, in order to verify the functionality of the *Acta2* coupled BFP reporter system, cells were seeded in plastic or 5 kPa PDMS coated ibiTreat μSlide 8 well at a density of 25000/cm^2 in MucilAir ± 5 ng/ml TGF-β1. Pictures were taken with an iMIC Digital Microscope (FEI Munich GmbH). All images were obtained using an Olympus Objective UApo/340 40x/1.35 Oil ∞/0.17 and a 405 nm excitation filter for BFP.

Microplate Reader Assay

Cells were seeded in PDMS coated 96-well plates (Sarstedt, Nümbrecht, Germany). Respective growth factors were added 24 h post-seeding and the BFP signal was measured at indicated time points. For fluorescence measurements, cells were trypsinized, transferred to a collagen (Advanced BioMatrix Inc.) coated black 96-well plate (Sarstedt) and let adhere for 3 h. Cells were stained with Calcein AM (Thermo Fisher Scientific) for 30 min in bath solution (in mM: 140 NaCl, 5 KCl, 1 MgCl2, 2 CaCl2, 5 glucose, and 10 HEPES; pH 7.4), washed twice with PBS w/o Ca^{2+}/Mg^{2+} and maintained in 200 μl bath solution during analysis of BFP signal with the plate reader (Tecan, Salzburg, Austria). Excitation wavelength were 385 nm and 485 nm and BFP and Calcein emissions were collected at 445 nm and 535 nm, respectively. BFP and Calcein signals were background subtracted and the BFP signal was normalized to the Calcein signal to adjust for cell number.

Statistical Analysis

GraphPad Prims7 software (GraphPad, La Jolla, CA, United States) was used for statistical analysis, curve fitting and data representation. Respective tests are given within the figure legend. Data are represented as means ± SEM unless stated otherwise. Statistical significance was determined using the non-parametric Mann–Whitney-*U* test for comparison of two independent samples at the same time point. The number of experiments (N) indicates individual animals for primary fibroblasts and cells from varying passages for immortalized fibroblasts. Data was considered significant if the p value was < 0.05 and is indicated with an asterisk. Statistical significance is indicated in the graphs as follows: p-values < 0.05: *, p-values < 0.01: **, p-values < 0.001: ***.

RESULTS

10-4A Cells Resemble Matrix Fibroblasts but Not Myo-/Lipofibroblasts

Isolation and immortalization of primary cells from the distal lung yielded 15 individual cell clones (**Figure 1A**). Subsequently, cell clones were analyzed for phenotypic expression patterns resembling primary epithelial and mesenchymal cells. Expression of marker genes for alveolar type II (ATII) [*Abca3*, *Sftpc* (Beers et al., 2017)], alveolar type I (ATI) [*Hopx*, *Aqp5*, *Cav1* (McElroy and Kasper, 2004; Beers et al., 2017)], pan-epithelial [*Epcam* (Hasegawa et al., 2017)], leukocyte [*CD45* (Barletta et al., 2012)], and mesenchymal [*Vim* (Cheng et al., 2016)] cells was analyzed on the gene and protein level. Both, semi-quantitative RT-PCR and immunofluorescence data identified the presence of mesenchymal and absence of epithelial and leukocyte cell markers in several clones (**Figures 1B,C**). Taking into consideration that *Cav1* is also expressed in lung fibroblasts (Xiao et al., 2006) the data indicate a fibroblast phenotype of all investigated cell clones.

Based on gene expression analysis and protein localization, clone 10-4A was selected for further analysis. In-depth characterization was performed by transcriptomic analysis. Gene expression in 10-4A cells was also compared to expression in healthy primary distal lung fibroblasts and primary ATII cells. The 10-4A cell line exhibits high expression of matrix fibroblast marker genes, in particular *Col1a1* and *Vim*, and low expression of myofibroblast marker genes. Lipofibroblast marker gene expression was low in 10-4A cells when compared to primary fibroblasts (**Figure 2**). Expression of specific pan- and alveolar

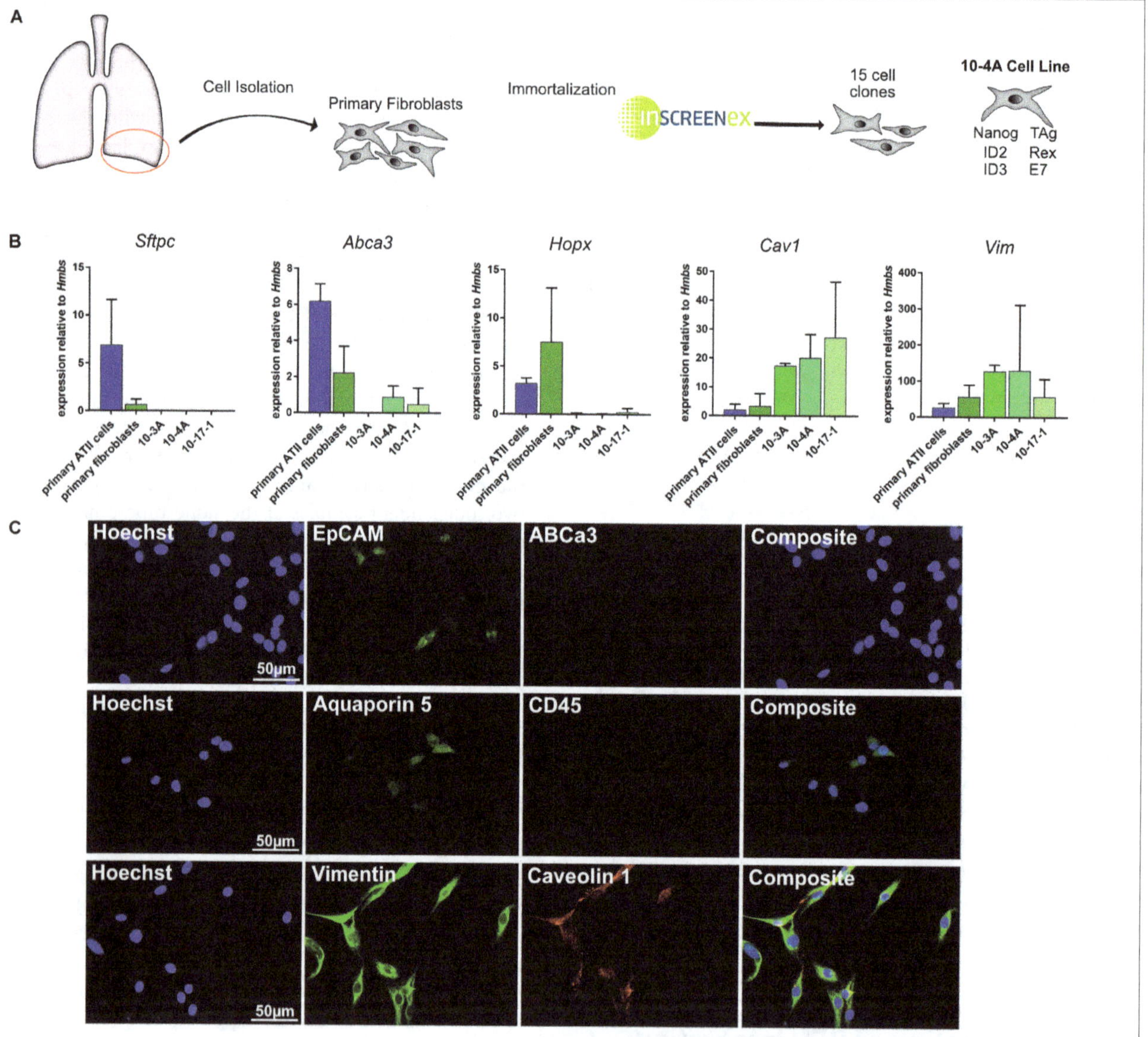

FIGURE 1 | Gene and protein expression pattern of the immortalized cell lines. **(A)** Schematic representation of the immortalization process. *Right:* Genes incorporated in 10-4A cells for immortalization **(B)** Semi-quantitative RT-PCR of ATII cell (*Sftpc*, *Abca3*), ATI cell (*Hopx*, *Cav1*), and mesenchymal cell (*Vim*) marker genes. $N = 5$ **(C)** Immunofluorescent staining of 10-4A cells for expression of epithelial cell (EpCAM), alveolar type II cell (ABCa3), alveolar type I cell (aquaporin 5, caveolin 1), leukocyte (CD45), and mesenchymal cell (vimentin) marker expression. 10-4A cells predominantly express mesenchymal marker vimentin and caveolin-1, that is also expressed in lung fibroblasts. Scale bar = 50 µm.

epithelial marker genes was very low. Together these data suggest that 10-4A cells exhibit a matrix fibroblast phenotype (Zepp et al., 2017; Xie et al., 2018).

Interestingly, 10-4A exhibited high expression of *Pdgfrα*, which is associated with the capability of myofibroblast differentiation (Li et al., 2018).

Increased Substrate Stiffness Exhibits of Myofibroblast Characteristics in 10-4A Cells

The high expression of *Pdgfrα* suggested that these cells may constitute a model to study activation/differentiation of fibroblast cells observed in pulmonary fibrosis. To test whether 10-4A cells resemble a suitable surrogate cell model for *in vitro* fibrosis studies, we first investigated the responsiveness of 10-4A cells to mechanical stimuli (Hinz, 2009). We analyzed expression of myofibroblast marker genes in response to changes in substrate stiffness. Results in 10-4A cells were compared to effects on freshly isolated primary fibroblasts.

Expression of myofibroblast marker *Acta2* and ECM component *Col1a1* were unchanged over a 14 days period in 10-4A and primary fibroblasts when maintained on soft PDMS gels with physiological stiffness (Young's Modulus of 5 kPa) (Palchesko et al., 2012). In line, with maintenance of a quiescent phenotype, *Plin2*, a marker for lipofibroblasts, did not

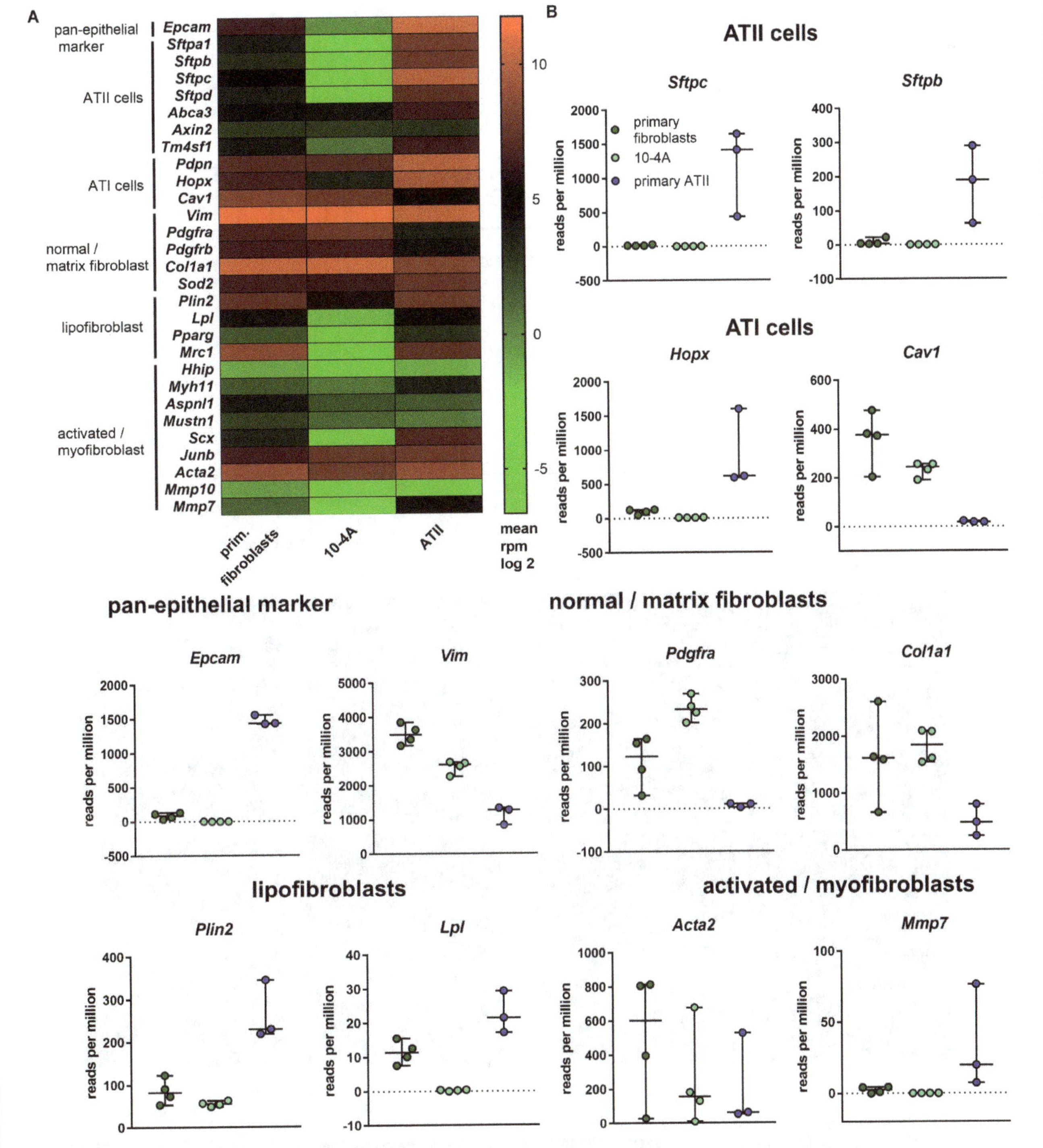

FIGURE 2 | Transcriptomic profile of 10-4A compared to freshly isolated rat fibroblasts and ATII cells. **(A)** Heat map of selected pan-epithelial, ATII, ATI and different fibroblast subtype marker genes. Values are given as log2-fold change of the mean reads per million base pairs. 10-4A and primary fibroblasts, $N = 4$, primary ATII cells, $N = 3$. **(B)** Detailed presentation of rpm values obtained for selected marker genes.

significantly change (**Figures 3A–C**). In some cases, a faint alpha smooth muscle actin (αSMA) signal (the product of *Acta2*) was detected in Western Blots at day 0 in 10-4A.

In contrast, culture on rigid plastic substrate resulted in significantly increased *Acta2* expression in 10-4A (day 4, $p = 0.008$; day 7, $p = 0.03$; day 14, $p = 0.008$) and primary fibroblasts (day 4, $p = 0.007$; day 7, $p = 0.053$; day 14, $p = 0.03$) (**Figure 3A**). Consistently, αSMA stress fiber formation was detected from day 7 onward, in immunofluorescence experiments and was confirmed by Western Blot (**Figures 3D,E**).

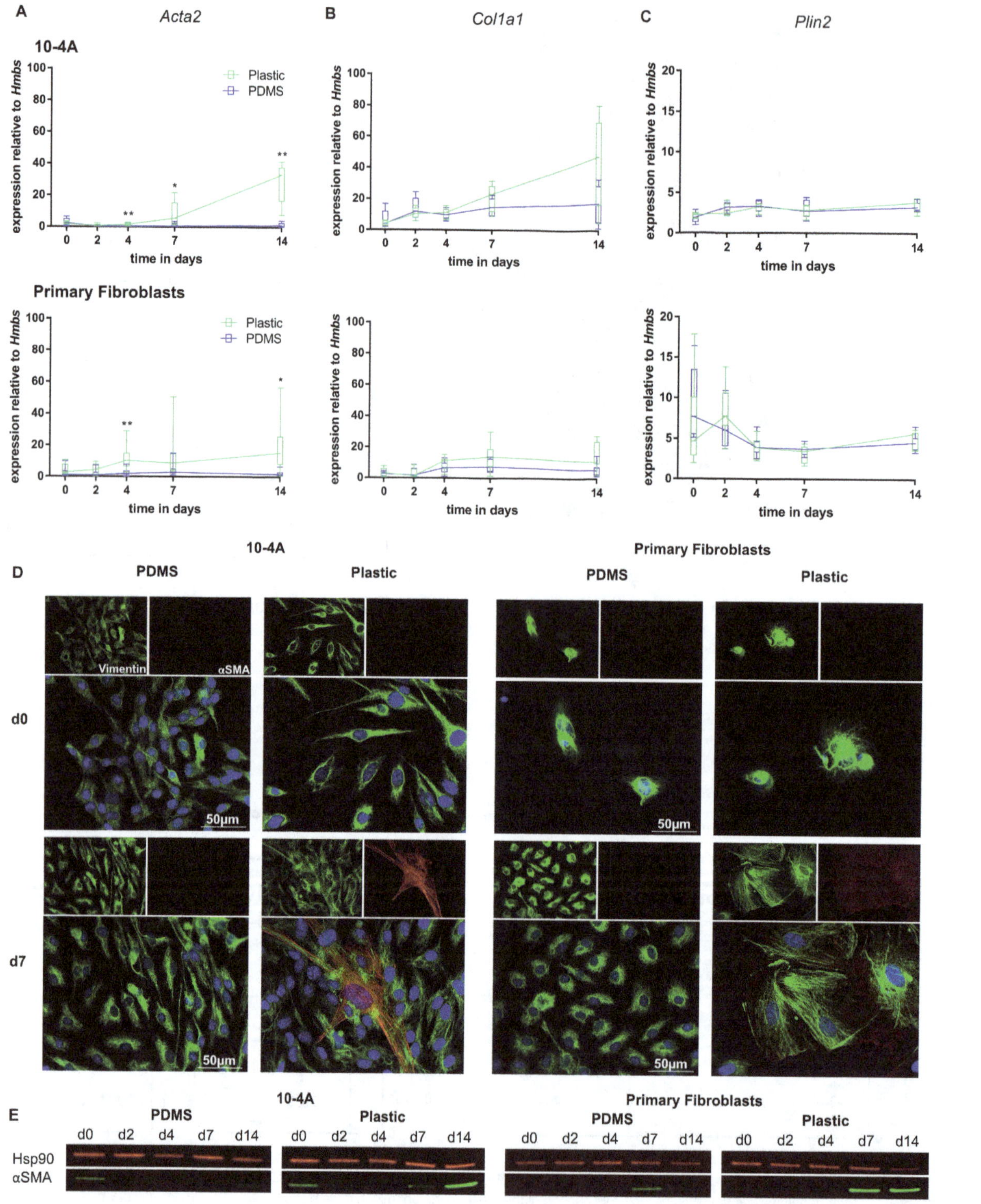

FIGURE 3 | Mechanical stimulation of 10-4A cells and primary fibroblasts. Semi-quantitative RT-PCR analysis of *Acta2* **(A)**, *Col1a1* **(B)**, and *Plin2* **(C)** expression in 10-4A cells **(top graph)** and primary fibroblasts **(bottom graph)** maintained on soft PDMS or stiff plastic substrate, respectively. Data are expressed as fold expression of the housekeeping gene hydroxymethylbilane synthase (*Hmbs*). Primary fibroblast data were obtained from seven different animals, 10-4A data from five different passages. Statistical significance for the respective time points was tested with the non-parametric Mann–Whitney-*U*-Test. Statistical significance is indicated as follows: p-values < 0.05: *, p-values < 0.01: **. Box plots show data as median values, the boxes represent percentiles, the whiskers indicate the minimum/maximum. **(D)** Immunofluorescence staining of 10-4A cells **(left)** or primary fibroblasts either seeded on PDMS or plastic directly after adherence (d0) or 7 days post-seeding. Cells were stained for the mesenchymal marker vimentin (green) and the pro-fibrotic protein αSMA (red). Scale bar = 50 μm. **(E)** Western Blot for αSMA in 10-4A cells and primary fibroblasts cultured over 14 days on soft (PDMS) and stiff (Plastic) matrices, respectively. HSP90 was used as loading control.

This likely originates from αSMA expressed during cell culture in plastic culture flasks that had not been degraded by the time samples were collected (approx. 6 h after seeding on PDMs substrate). Expression of *Col1a1* and *Plin2* were not affected by stiff substrate within the 14 days culture period, suggesting that the time course might not be sufficiently long enough for full differentiation and activation of fibroblasts. A weak αSMA signal was detected in Western blots for day 0 samples from 10-4A cells.

TGF-β1 Induces a Transient Myofibroblast Phenotype in 10-4A Cells

To further characterize the response of 10-4A cells to fibrotic stimuli, we stimulated the cells with the potent profibrotic cytokine TGF-β1.

Transforming growth factor beta 1 (5 ng/ml) treatment resulted in significantly increased *Acta2* gene expression after 2 days in 10-4A cells (day 2, $p = 0.008$; day 4, $p = 0.008$; day 7, $p = 0.057$; day 14, $p = 0.03$) and after 4 days in primary fibroblasts (day 4, $p = 0.003$; day 7, $p = 0.003$; day 14, $p = 0.003$) (**Figure 4A**). In line, αSMA stress fiber formation was more prominent from day 2 post-seeding onward in 10-4A cells as well as primary fibroblasts (**Figures 4D,E**). Interestingly, the TGF-β1-induced increase in *Acta2* expression followed a transient course in the 10-4A cells, peaking at day 2 after TGF-β1 addition and returning to baseline at day 4–5. A similar trend was noticeable in primary fibroblast post day 7. In contrast to mechanical stimulation, TGF-β1 administration also resulted in significantly increased *Col1a1* (day 2, $p = 0.008$, day 7, $p = 0.03$, day 14, $p = 0.03$) and a reduced *Plin2* (day 2, $p = 0.008$, day 4, $p = 0.02$) gene expression in 10-4A cells (**Figures 4B,C**) and primary fibroblasts (*Col1a1* day 4, $p = 0.003$, *Plin2*, day 4, $p = 0.003$). Together these data suggest that TGF-β1 administration triggers changes observed in fibrosis in 10-4A cells and primary fibroblasts, respectively. However, the effect was not sustained over a 14-day time course, despite constant exposure to TGF-β1.

Combination of Stiff Matrix and TGF-β1 Stimulation Leads to Strong and Persistent Expression of Myofibroblast Markers in 10-4A Cells

In pulmonary fibrosis mechanical and chemical cues act simultaneously. Therefore, we investigated the combination of mechanical and chemical stimulation seeding cells on plastic substrate and stimulated them with TGF-β1.

The combination of mechanical and chemical stimulation resulted in significantly increased *Acta2* gene expression in 10-4A cells from day 2 onward (day 2, $p = 0.008$, day 4, $p = 0.008$, day 7, $p = 0.008$, day 14, $p = 0.008$) and 4 days onward in primary fibroblasts (day 4, $p = 0.003$, day 7, $p = 0.003$, day 14, $p = 0.003$) (**Figure 5A**). This was also observed on the protein level (**Figures 5D,E**). Similar changes were observed for *Col1a1* (**Figure 5B**) (10-4A: day 2, $p = 0.008$, day 4, $p = 0.008$, day 7, $p = 0.008$, day 14, $p = 0.008$; primary fibroblasts: day 4, $p = 0.05$, day 7, $p = 0.003$, day 14, $p = 0.003$). In line, *Plin2* expression (**Figure 5C**) was decreased in both cell types after 4 and 2 days, respectively (10-4A: day 2, $p = 0.008$, day 4, $p = 0.02$, day 14, $p = 0.03$; primary fibroblasts: day 4, $p = 0.005$, day 14, $p = 0.003$).

Overall, the combination of mechanical and chemical stimulation induced a robust and persistent expression of myofibroblast markers in 10-4A cells and primary fibroblasts. Interestingly the transient effect observed by TGF-β1 treatment alone was counteracted by increased substrate stiffness.

Generation of a 10-4A Reporter Cell Line to Monitor Fibroblast to Myofibroblast Differentiation in Live Cell *in vitro* Assays

In order to track fibroblast to myofibroblast differentiation within living cells, we designed a reporter system targeting the *Acta2* gene locus in 10-4A cells by generating a BFP-reporter of *Acta2* expression. We inserted a T2A-BFP-NLS sequence at the end of the *Acta2* CDS in 10-4A cells (10-4A^{BFP}). The correct integration of the BFP sequence was verified via PCR and Sanger sequencing. Induction of myofibroblast differentiation (TGF-β1) resulted in a nuclear BFP signal in 10-4A^{BFP} cells (**Figures 6A,B**).

To exclude changes in *Acta2* gene expression arising from genetic modifications, we compared the 10-4A^{BFP} cell line to wildtype 10-4A cells during quiescence (on PDMS, soft matrix) and after TGF-β1 stimulation, respectively. 10-4A^{BFP} cells showed similar responses to PDMS and TGF-β1 stimulation as 10-4A cells when analyzing *Acta2*, *Col1a1*, and *Plin2* gene expression (**Figures 6C–E**), indicating no adverse effects of T2A-BFP-NLS cassette integration.

Next, we tested on the protein level, whether the BFP signal correlated with αSMA expression. TGF-β1 treatment resulted in double-positive cells, whereas cells cultured on soft substrate without TGF-β1 were negative for BFP and αSMA (**Figure 6F**). Correlating the αSMA and BFP signal within individual cells, confirmed a linear correlation between BFP intensity and αSMA expression ($R^2 = 0.82, p < 0.0001$) (**Figure 6G**).

For a high throughput evaluation of fibrotic signals, a fluorescence-based 96-well assay was established. First, a linear correlation between BFP signal and cell count was verified under different culture conditions.

For a more thorough characterization and verification of the 10-4A^{BFP} cells, cytokines elevated during pulmonary fibrosis (TGF-β1, IL-33, IL-4, and TSLP) were screened to establish dose- and time-response curves (**Figure 7**). EC_{50} values following a 2-day incubation post-seeding were 1.45 ng/ml for TGF-β1, 400 pg/ml for TSLP, 12 ng/ml for IL-4, and 22 pg/ml for IL-33. Time course analysis of BFP signal expression revealed that the BFP signal was transiently increasing following TGF-β1 and IL-33, respectively, similar to what was observed for wildtype 10-4A cells (**Figure 4**). In contrast, TSLP and IL-4 show an increase in BFP expression until day 2 and afterward a stable BFP expression up to day 7.

In summary, the 10-4A^{BFP} cell line resembles a valuable tool for high throughput analysis of factors driving fibroblast to myofibroblast differentiation in pulmonary fibrosis, enabling screening with limited sample preparation and processing.

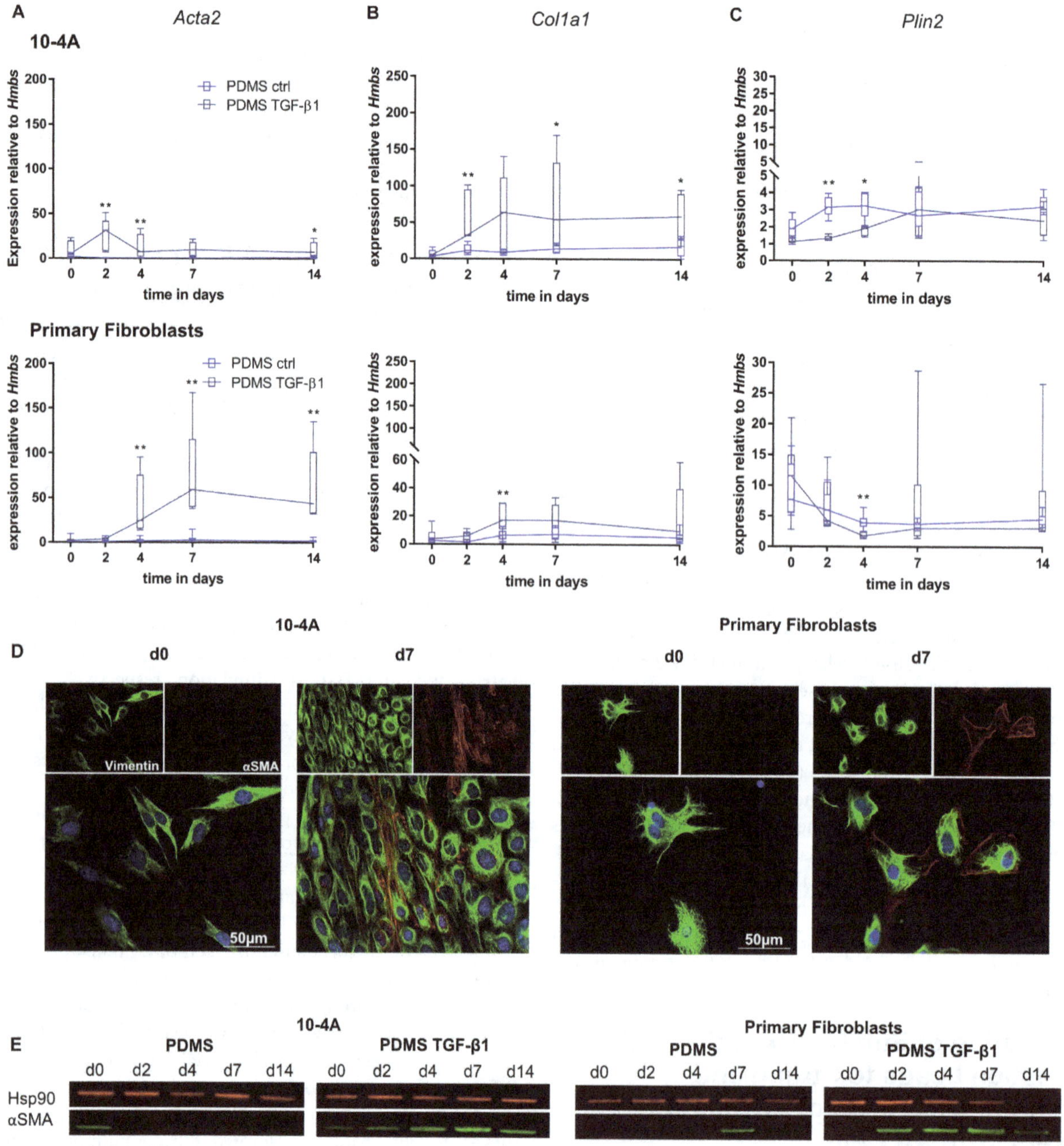

FIGURE 4 | Chemical stimulation of 10-4A cells and primary fibroblasts with TGF-β1 on a physiological substrate. Semi-quantitative RT-PCR of *Acta2* **(A)**, *Col1a1* **(B)**, and *Plin2* **(C)** expression in 10-4A cells **(top graph)** and primary fibroblasts **(bottom graph)** cultured in the presence or absence of 5 ng/ml TGF-β1 on a soft PDMS substrate, respectively. Data are expressed as fold expression of housekeeping gene *Hmbs*. Primary fibroblast data were obtained from 5 different animals, 10-4A data from five independent passages. The respective time points were tested with the non-parametric Mann–Whitney-*U*-Test. Statistical significance is indicated as follows: *p*-values < 0.05: *, *p*-values < 0.01: **. Box plots show data as median values, the boxes represent percentiles, the whiskers indicate the minimum/maximum. **(D)** Immunofluorescence staining of 10-4A cells **(left)** or primary fibroblasts seeded on PDMS with administration of 5 ng/ml TGF-β1 directly after adherence (d0) or 7 days post-seeding. Cells were stained for the mesenchymal marker vimentin (green) and the pro-fibrotic protein αSMA (red). Scale bar = 50 μm. **(E)** Western Blot for αSMA in 10-4A cells and primary fibroblasts cultured over 14 days on PDMS substrate in the presence or absence of TGF-β1, respectively. HSP90 was used as loading control.

DISCUSSION

Frequently, when studying molecular and cellular mechanisms in pulmonary fibrosis, primary fibroblasts are used for *in vitro* experiments (Pierce et al., 2007; Huang et al., 2012; Pardo and Selman, 2016). However, use of primary cells is often limited by availability, restricted propagation, ethical hurdles, the cost and difficulty of repetitive cell isolations and often

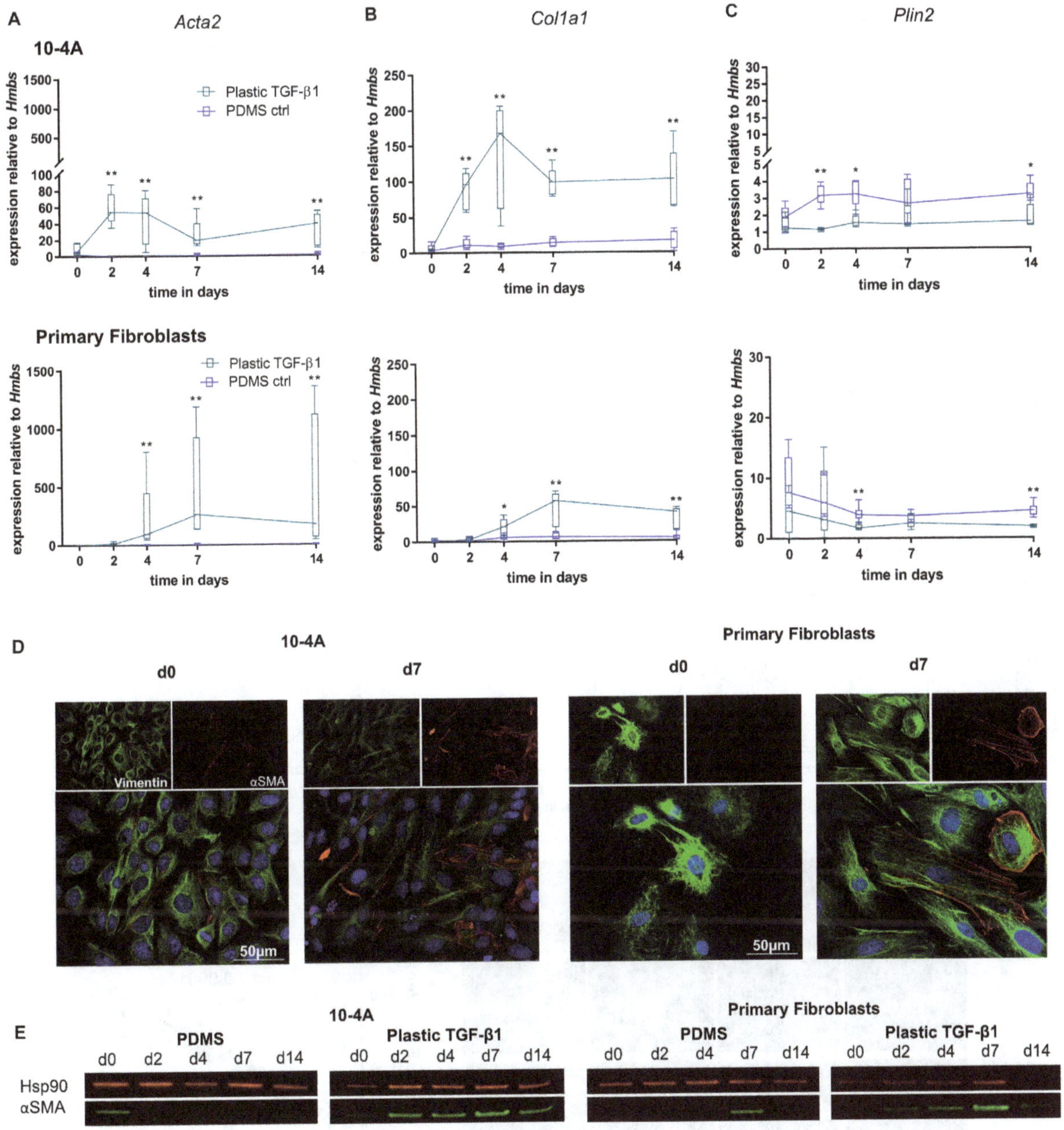

FIGURE 5 | Combination of chemical and mechanical stimulation of 10-4A cells and primary fibroblasts with TGF-β1 on a physiological substrate. Semi-quantitative RT-PCR of *Acta2* **(A)**, *Col1a1* **(B)**, and *Plin2* **(C)** expression in 10-4A cells (top graph) and primary fibroblasts (bottom graph) cultured on either soft substrate (PDMS) or in the presence of 5 ng/ml TGF-β1 stiff substrate (Plastic), respectively. Data are expressed as fold expression of housekeeping gene *Hmbs*. Primary fibroblast data were obtained from five different animals, 10-4A data from five independent cell culture experiments. The respective time points were tested with the non-parametric Mann–Whitney-*U*-Test. Statistical significance is indicated as follows: p-values < 0.05: *, p-values < 0.01: **. Box plots show data as median values, the boxes represent percentiles, the whiskers indicate the minimum/maximum. **(D)** Immunofluorescence staining of 10-4A cells (left) or primary fibroblasts seeded on PDMS with administration of 5 ng/ml TGF-β1 directly after adherence (d0) or 7 days post-seeding. Cells were stained for the mesenchymal marker Vimentin (green) and the pro-fibrotic protein αSMA (red). Scale bar = 50 μm. **(E)** Western Blot for αSMA in 10-4A cells and primary fibroblasts cultured over 14 days on PDMS substrate or on Plastic in the presence of TGF-β1, respectively. HSP90 was used as loading control.

a heterogeneity of isolated cells within or between isolations from different donors (Kaur and Dufour, 2012). Thus, well-characterized, representative cell lines provide a useful alternative for high-throughput, live-cell assays and can be used for *in vitro* disease modeling. Genetic modifications are easily introduced to study specific signaling pathways. In addition, they offer the opportunity for long-term studies replicating diseases progression *in vitro*. The aim of our work was to generate a representative cell line to be used for *in vitro* fibrosis research. To this end, we immortalized primary rat lung cells, screened them

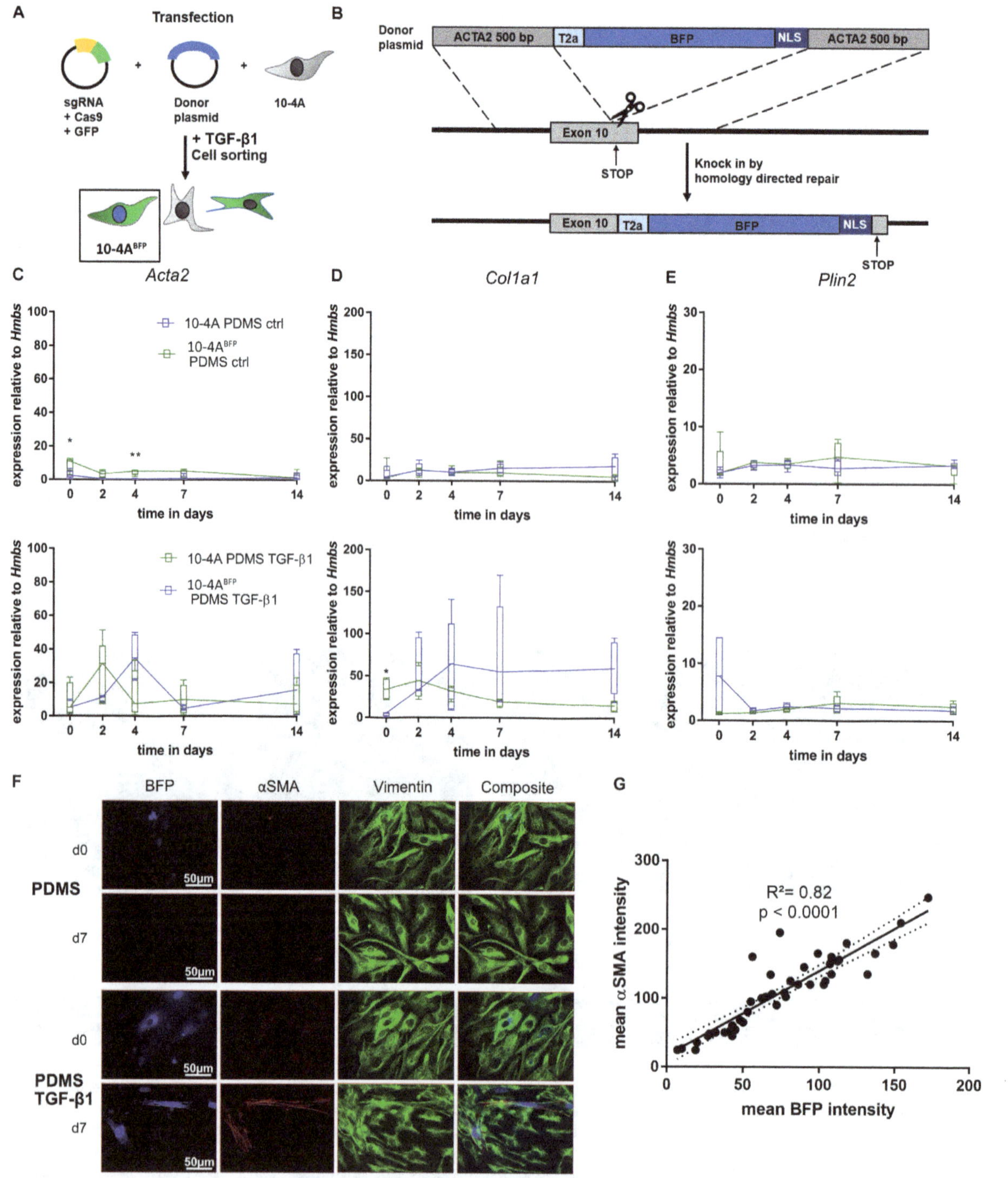

FIGURE 6 | Generation and verification of an *Acta2* coupled BFP reporter cell line. **(A,B)** Schematic representation of 10-4A cell transfection. Cells were transfected with a plasmid containing Cas9 and the sgRNA binding at the desired gene (exon 10) and a donor plasmid. The donor plasmid contained a BFP flanked by a self-cleaving T2A cassette, a nuclear localization sequence and two 500 bp homologous arms of the sgRNA cutting site. After cell transfection, *Acta2* gene expression was induced by addition of 5 ng/ml TGF- β1 and cells were FACS sorted for BFP. Semi-quantitative RT-PCR analysis of *Acta2* **(C)**, *Col1a1* **(D)**, and *Plin2* **(E)** expression in 10-4A and 10-4A^{BFP} cells with and without administration of 5 ng/ml TGF-β1 on a soft PDMS substrate, respectively. Values are means from five individual culture experiments. The respective time points were tested with the non-parametric Mann–Whitney-*U*-Test. Statistical significance is indicated as follows: *p*-values < 0.05: *, *p*-values < 0.01: **. Box plots show data as median values, the boxes represent percentiles, the whiskers indicate the minimum/maximum. **(F)** Immunofluorescence staining of 10-4A^{BFP} cells seeded on PDMS with and without administration of 5 ng/ml TGF-β1 directly after adherence (d0) or 7 days post-seeding. Cells were monitored for BFP and stained for the mesenchymal marker vimentin (green) and the pro-fibrotic protein αSMA (red). Scale bar = 50 μm. **(G)** Correlation of the BFP and αSMA signal intensity within individual cells 7 days post seeding. *N* = 48 cells. A linear regression line and the corresponding indicator *R* and *p*-value show the linear dependency of BFP and αSMA signal.

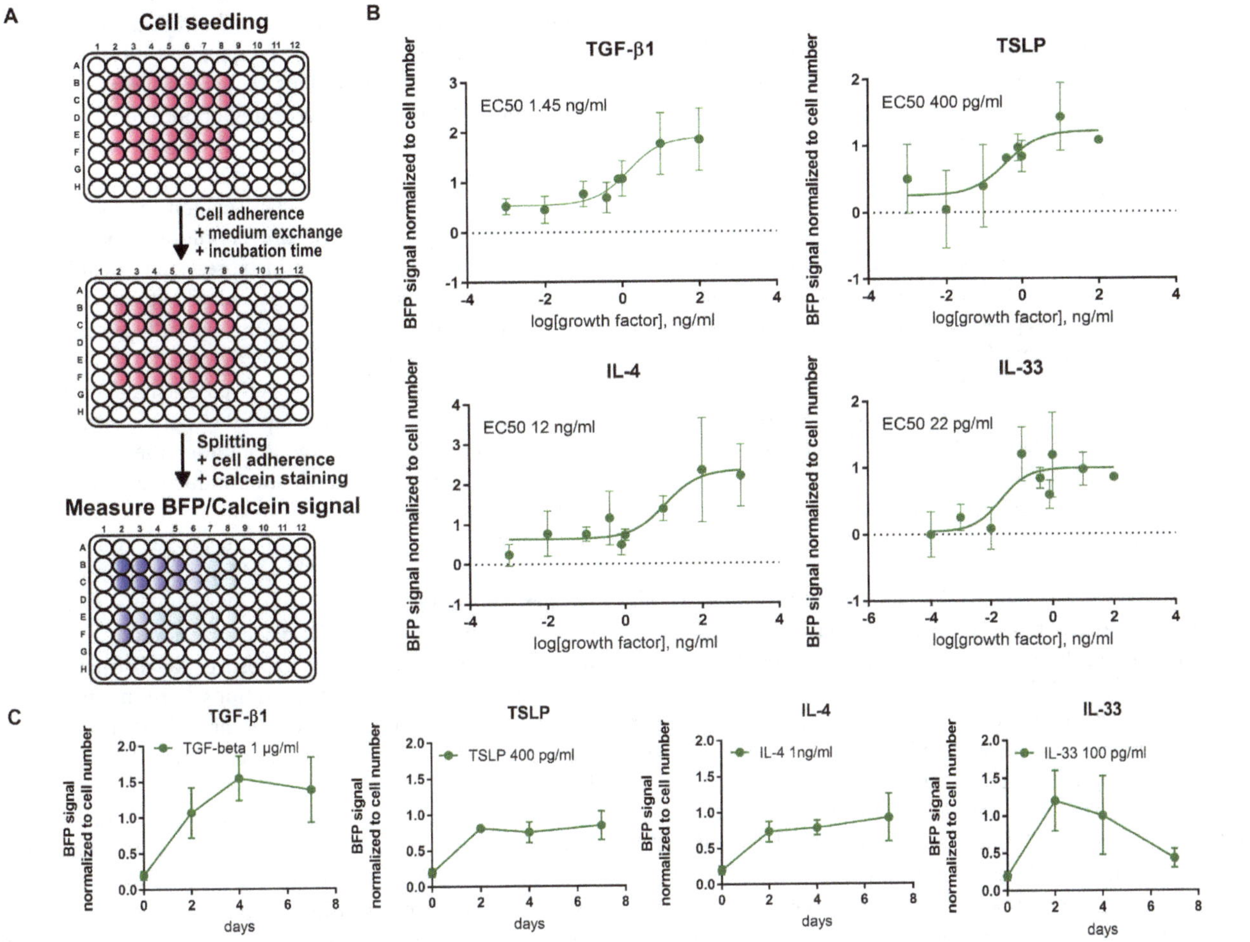

FIGURE 7 | High-throughput screening using the 10-4A^{BFP} cell line. **(A)** Schematic of plate reader assay to study the fibrotic response of 10-4A^{BFP} to cytokine treatment in live cell assays. For normalization to the cell number, cells were stained with Calcein AM. **(B)** Dose-response curves of BFP expression in 10-4A^{BFP} cells in response to 2 days exposure with increasing doses of TGF-β1, TSLP, IL-4, and IL-33. **(C)** Time-response curve of 10-4A^{BFP} cells to continuous exposure to TGF-β1, TSLP, IL-4, and IL-33.

for fibroblast characteristics and tested the induction of fibrosis after mechanical as well as chemical stimulation.

Within recent years, various cell and, in particular, fibroblast subpopulations were reported for the distal lung. Diverse roles in development, lung homeostasis, aging and injury repair were attributed to distinct populations, raising the complexity for modeling pulmonary fibrosis (Zepp et al., 2017; Xie et al., 2018). Interestingly, some myo-and lipofibroblast marker genes like *Mmp7*, *Mmp10* or *Plin2* (Adams et al., 2019; Reyfman et al., 2019; Strunz et al., 2019) were also expressed in ATII cells, emphasizing the importance to look in detail at a combination of distinct marker genes in order to assign cells to a cellular group. The presence of *Epcam* in the RNA sequencing data from primary fibroblasts likely indicates small impurities of epithelial cells, whereas the presence of *Vim* indicates minor impurities in the epithelial cell in the primary cell isolates. The presence of small fractions of other cell types after the isolation of primary lung cells is also described by other groups (Dobbs et al., 1986; Driscoll et al., 2012; Lee et al., 2018).

Regarding the fibroblast subpopulations stated by Xie et al. (2018), our 10-4A cell line neither exhibits a classical myofibroblast nor a lipofibroblast phenotype, but rather a matrix fibroblast phenotype with unexpected high expression of *Pdgfrα*. On a molecular level, the 10-4A cells could also be clearly differentiated from alveolar epithelial cells. The ATI-related genes *Cav1* as well as *Pdpn*, often used to discriminate ATI and ATII cells, are both also highly expressed in lung fibroblasts (Xiao et al., 2006; Quintanilla et al., 2019). Considering lineage-tracing and CRISPR/Cas9 *knock-in* experiments, *Pdgfrα* positive cells have been shown to give rise to either myofibroblasts or lipofibroblasts during development and to be able to differentiate into myofibroblasts in the adult lung (Ntokou et al., 2015; Zepp et al., 2017; Li et al., 2018). This directed differentiation of fibroblasts into myofibroblasts, as described for *Pdgfrα* positive cells, is one of the major requirements when studying pulmonary fibrosis. Thus, the gene and protein expression pattern of the 10-4A cell line indicates their suitability to study the mechanisms involved in the initiation and progression of pulmonary fibrosis.

Congruent with previous findings, we were also able to verify that myofibroblast differentiation can be induced mechanically (Wipff et al., 2007; Huang et al., 2012; Asano et al., 2017) and/or chemically (Chambers et al., 2003; Thannickal et al., 2003; Goffin et al., 2006; Blaauboer et al., 2011; Shi et al., 2013; El Agha et al., 2017) in 10-4A cells. Moreover, our data confirmed that fibroblasts grown on a substrate with physiological stiffness (Huang et al., 2012; Asano et al., 2017) and serum free medium (Baranyi et al., 2019) stay in a quiescent state over a time-course of 14 days. Since it is well established that fetal bovine serum exerts a heterogeneous influence on cellular behavior in cell culture due to batch-dependent variations and variable growth factor levels (Krämer et al., 2005; Mannello and Tonti, 2009; Baranyi et al., 2019), we decided to use a chemically defined, standardized, serum-free culture medium. Thereby, we were able to exclude potential variations in cellular responses due to heterogeneity of our culture conditions.

With regards to mechanical activation of the 10-4A cell line, the increase in gene and protein expression of αSMA was comparable to what has been described for primary fibroblasts as well as cell lines (Wipff et al., 2007; Huang et al., 2012; Asano et al., 2017). In line, a recent report from Tschumperlin et al., has shown that *Col1a1* mRNA levels were stable above a substrate stiffness of 0.1 kPa (Liu et al., 2010).

Transforming growth factor beta 1 in combination with a soft substrate resulted in an increase of *Acta2*, *Col1a1* and decrease of *Plin2* gene expression as well as an increase of αSMA on the protein level. These observations are in accordance to already published data in several studies of human (Chambers et al., 2003; Thannickal et al., 2003; Blaauboer et al., 2011; El Agha et al., 2017) and rodent lung fibroblasts (Goffin et al., 2006; Shi et al., 2013; El Agha et al., 2017). Interestingly, continuous stimulation with TGF-β1 induced an early but transient increase in profibrotic marker gene expression. *Acta2* expression was downregulated after 4 days in 10-4A cells continuously treated with TGF-β1. This effect was also observed in primary fibroblasts from two out of five animals after 7 days. In accordance, *Col1a1* and *Plin2* expression also adopt to control conditions for the primary fibroblasts. This indicates, that TGF-β1 stimulation alone, is not sufficient to maintain a myofibroblast phenotype and that changes in substrate stiffness are essential to induce a robust, persistent fibrotic response. The dependence of TGF-β1 on mechanical activation was already described by Shi et al. (2013). However, due to the lack of long-term studies examining the TGF-β1 effect beyond >4 days, comparable data are not available. Likewise, it has been reported, that TGF-β1 requires mechanical induction to be able to regulate myofibroblast differentiation (Hinz, 2009). This is again in accordance with our data, that the combination of chemical and mechanical stimulation is necessary to fully resemble the aspects of myofibroblast differentiation. This is also more likely to reflect the *in vivo* situation where fibrosis might be triggered by chemical stimuli but shifts to a self-perpetuating state with increasing stiffening of the lung tissue (spreading from fibrotic foci). We limited the observation time to 14 days as cellular overgrowth under fibrotic conditions, due to increased proliferation rates, resulted in inconsistent findings at observation periods beyond 14 days.

In order to accelerate and facilitate the read-out of fibroblast differentiation in a live cell, high-throughput setting, we generated an *Acta2*-BFP coupled reporter system using CRISPR/Cas9 technology. This reporter system is intended for use in live-cell, long-term screening applications. CRISPR/Cas9 can lead to off-target mutations. Therefore, we have verified correct insertion of BFP-NLS by Sanger sequencing and that 10-4A^{BFP} and 10-4A cells exhibit a similar behavior under physiological cell culture conditions and after fibrotic stimulation. Minor differences in expression of *Acta2* and *Col1a1* at day 0 might indicate a slightly delayed RNA turnover in 10-4A^{BFP} during adjustment to non-fibrotic culture conditions after transfer from culture flasks (Kitsera et al., 2007). On the protein level, αSMA signal and the respective BFP signal correlated very well, confirming appropriate reporter characteristics. Similarly, the regulation of BFP expression under the αSMA promoter could be confirmed by the targeted induction of the BFP signal after TGF-β1 administration.

Finally, in order to confirm the proper functionality and the suitability to use 10-4A^{BFP} cells in high throughput assays, we performed plate-reader based experiments to analyze the dose- and time-response of *Acta2* expression (i.e., myofibroblast induction) in response to exposure to distinct profibrotic cytokines. The effective concentrations were in agreement with previous reports for induction of fibrosis (Saito et al., 2003; Yanaba et al., 2011; Datta et al., 2013; Lee et al., 2017; Jones et al., 2019).

One potential limitation of the presented reporter cell line is its origin from rat rather than human. Several human pulmonary fibroblast cell lines are already available. However, in contrast to the cell line presented here, none of the currently available human cell lines has been characterized in detail with regards to the representation of a specific mesenchymal cell sub-population (Adams et al., 2019; Reyfman et al., 2019; Valenzi et al., 2019; Habermann et al., 2020; Liu et al., 2020; Travaglini et al., 2020). This might not only affect cellular responses to pro-fibrotic mechanical and chemical cues, but also affect epithelial-mesenchymal crosstalk and fibrotic remodeling when used in complex co-culture *in vitro* models (e.g., lung-on-a-chip). It is also accepted that *in vivo* animal models do not fully recapitulate all features of IPF pathogenesis (Moore et al., 2013). The reasons are not fully understood. The human lung contains structural and cellular differences to the rodent lung, however, the alveolus is one of the most conserved regions between rodents and human lungs and whether the mesenchymal and epithelial cells believed to be central to development of IPF are different is still a matter of debate. Even lipofibroblasts, a cell that's presence has been found in rodents but has long been controversial in the human lung (Tahedl et al., 2014), has recently been identified in human lung (Liu et al., 2020; Travaglini et al., 2020). Therefore, we believe that the cell line reported here provides a valuable tool for fibrosis research, offering the opportunity to investigate molecular and cellular responses of a representative mesenchymal cell to mechanical and/or chemical stimuli with high resolution and in high throughput formats.

In summary, our data clearly demonstrate that the 10-4A cell line can be used as a valuable, novel tool for studying the onset and progression of fibrotic changes observed in pulmonary fibrosis. Additionally, the deviated 10-4A^{BFP} reporter cell line is a useful tool for high-throughput live cell, *in vitro* assays to directly monitor fibrotic changes over time.

AUTHOR CONTRIBUTIONS

JN, AS, and MF conceived and designed the study, interpreted results of the experiments, and edited and revised the manuscript. JN, AS, and VW performed the experiments. JN, KQ, and AS analyzed the data. JN and AS prepared the figures. JN, AS, KQ, and MF drafted the manuscript. All authors approved final version of manuscript.

ACKNOWLEDGMENTS

We thank Achim Riecker and Tatiana Felder for help with primary cell isolation, Susan Tavakoli and Kay Gottschalk for advice with PDMS gel preparation and handling, and Prof. Dr. C. Buske and the Core Facility Cytometry Ulm University for performance of cell sorting. We also want to thank Coralie Viollet, Head of the Genomics Lab at Boehringer Ingelheim, Biberach, for the Illumina library preparation.

REFERENCES

Adams, T., Schupp, J., Poli, S., Ayaub, E., Neumark, N., Ahangari, F., et al. (2019). Single Cell RNA-seq reveals ectopic and aberrant lung resident cell populations in idiopathic pulmonary fibrosis. *bioRxiv* [preprint]. doi: 10.1101/759902

Armanios, M. Y., Chen, J. J. L., Cogan, J. D., Alder, J. K., Ingersoll, R. G., Markin, C., et al. (2007). Telomerase mutations in families with idiopathic pulmonary fibrosis. *N. Engl. J. Med.* 356, 1317–1326. doi: 10.1056/NEJMoa066157

Asano, S., Ito, S., Takahashi, K., Furuya, K., Kondo, M., Sokabe, M., et al. (2017). Matrix stiffness regulates migration of human lung fibroblasts. *Physiol. Rep.* 5, 1–11. doi: 10.14814/phy2.13281

Bagnato, G., and Harari, S. (2015). Cellular interactions in the pathogenesis of interstitial lung diseases. *Eur. Respir. Rev.* 24, 102–114. doi: 10.1183/09059180.00003214

Baranyi, U., Winter, B., Gugerell, A., Hegedus, B., Brostjan, C., Laufer, G., et al. (2019). Primary human fibroblasts in culture switch to a myofibroblast-like phenotype independently of TGF Beta. *Cells* 8:721. doi: 10.3390/cells8070721

Barletta, K. E., Cagnina, R. E., Wallace, K. L., Ramos, S. I., Mehrad, B., and Linden, J. (2012). Leukocyte compartments in the mouse lung: distinguishing between marginated, interstitial, and alveolar cells in response to injury. *J. Immunol. Methods* 375, 100–110. doi: 10.1016/j.jim.2011.09.013

Beers, M. F., Moodley, Y., Stem, R., and Hall, E. J. S. (2017). When is an alveolar Type 2 cell an alveolar Type 2 Cell? A conundrum for lung stem cell biology and regenerative medicine. *Am. J. Respir. Cell Mol. Biol.* 57, 1–31. doi: 10.1165/rcmb.2016-0426PS

Blaauboer, M. E., Smit, T. H., Hanemaaijer, R., Stoop, R., and Everts, V. (2011). Cyclic mechanical stretch reduces myofibroblast differentiation of primary lung fibroblasts. *Biochem. Biophys. Res. Commun.* 404, 23–27. doi: 10.1016/j.bbrc.2010.11.033

Booth, A. J., Hadley, R., Cornett, A. M., Dreffs, A. A., Matthes, S. A., Tsui, J. L., et al. (2012). Acellular normal and fibrotic human lung matrices as a culture system for in vitro investigation. *Am. J. Respir. Crit. Care Med.* 186, 866–876. doi: 10.1164/rccm.201204-0754OC

Burgess, J. K., Mauad, T., Tjin, G., Karlsson, J. C., and Westergren-Thorsson, G. (2016). The extracellular matrix - the under-recognized element in lung disease? *J. Pathol.* 240, 397–409. doi: 10.1002/path.4808

Chambers, R. C., Leoni, P., Kaminski, N., Laurent, G. J., and Heller, R. A. (2003). Global expression profiling of fibroblast responses to transforming growth factor-β1 reveals the induction of inhibitor of differentiation-1 and provides evidence of smooth muscle cell phenotypic switching. *Am. J. Pathol.* 162, 533–546. doi: 10.1016/S0002-9440(10)63847-3

Chambers, R. C., and Mercer, P. F. (2015). Mechanisms of alveolar epithelial injury, repair, and fibrosis. *Ann. Am. Thoracic Soc.* 12, S16–S20. doi: 10.1513/AnnalsATS.201410-448MG

Cheng, F., Shen, Y., Mohanasundaram, P., Lindström, M., Ivaska, J., Ny, T., et al. (2016). Vimentin coordinates fibroblast proliferation and keratinocyte differentiation in wound healing via TGF-β-Slug signaling. *Proc. Natl. Acad. Sci. U.S.A.* 113, E4320–E4327. doi: 10.1073/pnas.1519197113

Datta, A., Alexander, R., Sulikowski, M. G., Nicholson, A. G., Maher, T. M., Scotton, C. J., et al. (2013). Evidence for a functional thymic stromal lymphopoietin signaling axis in fibrotic lung disease. *J. Immunol.* 191, 4867–4879. doi: 10.4049/jimmunol.1300588

Deluca, D. S., Levin, J. Z., Sivachenko, A., Fennell, T., Nazaire, M. D., Williams, C., et al. (2012). RNA-SeQC: RNA-seq metrics for quality control and process optimization. *Bioinformatics* 28, 1530–1532. doi: 10.1093/bioinformatics/bts196

Dobbs, L. G., Gonzalez, R., and Williams, M. C. (1986). An improved method for isolating type II cells in high yield and purity. *Am. Rev. Respir. Dis.* 134, 141–145. doi: 10.1164/arrd.1986.134.1.141

Dobin, A., Davis, C. A., Schlesinger, F., Drenkow, J., Zaleski, C., Jha, S., et al. (2013). STAR: ultrafast universal RNA-seq aligner. *Bioinformatics* 29, 15–21. doi: 10.1093/bioinformatics/bts635

Driscoll, B., Kikuchi, A., Lau, A. N., Lee, J., Reddy, R., Jesudason, E., et al. (2012). Isolation and characterization of distal lung progenitor cells. *Methods Mol. Biol.* 879, 109–122. doi: 10.1007/978-1-61779-815-3_7

El Agha, E., Moiseenko, A., Kheirollahi, V., De Langhe, S., Crnkovic, S., Kwapiszewska, G., et al. (2017). Two-way conversion between lipogenic and myogenic fibroblastic phenotypes marks the progression and resolution of lung fibrosis. *Cell Stem Cell* 20, 261.e3–273.e3. doi: 10.1016/j.stem.2016.10.004

Enomoto, N., Suda, T., Kono, M., Kaida, Y., Hashimoto, D., Fujisawa, T., et al. (2013). Amount of elastic fibers predicts prognosis of idiopathic pulmonary fibrosis. *Respir. Med.* 107, 1608–1616. doi: 10.1016/j.rmed.2013.08.008

Epstein Shochet, G., Brook, E., Israeli-Shani, L., Edelstein, E., and Shitrit, D. (2017). Fibroblast paracrine TNF-α signaling elevates integrin A5 expression in idiopathic pulmonary fibrosis (IPF). *Respir. Res.* 18:122. doi: 10.1186/s12931-017-0606-x

Evans, C. M., Fingerlin, T. E., Schwarz, M. I., Lynch, D., Kurche, J., Warg, L., et al. (2016). Idiopathic pulmonary fibrosis: a genetic disease that involves mucociliary dysfunction of the peripheral airways. *Physiol. Rev.* 96, 1567–1591. doi: 10.1152/physrev.00004.2016

Felder, M., Trueeb, B., Stucki, A. O., Borcard, S., Stucki, J. D., Schnyder, B., et al. (2019). Impaired wound healing of alveolar lung epithelial cells in a breathing lung-on-a-chip. *Front. Bioeng. Biotechnol.* 7:3. doi: 10.3389/fbioe.2019.00003

Gabazza, E. C., Kasper, M., Ohta, K., Keane, M., D'Alessandro-Gabazza, C., Fujimoto, H., et al. (2004). Decreased expression of aquaporin-5 in bleomycin-induced lung fibrosis in the mouse. *Pathol. Int.* 54, 774–780. doi: 10.1111/j.1440-1827.2004.01754.x

Goffin, J. M., Pittet, P., Csucs, G., Lussi, J. W., Meister, J. J., and Hinz, B. (2006). Focal adhesion size controls tension-dependent recruitment of α-smooth muscle actin to stress fibers. *J. Cell Biol.* 172, 259–268. doi: 10.1083/jcb.200506179

Habermann, A. C., Gutierrez, A. J., Bui, L. T., Yahn, S. L., Winters, N. I., Carla, L., et al. (2020). Single-cell RNA-sequencing reveals profibrotic roles of distinct epithelial and mesenchymal lineages in pulmonary fibrosis. *Sci. Adv.* 6. doi: 10.1101/753806

Hasegawa, K., Sato, A., Tanimura, K., Uemasu, K., Hamakawa, Y., Fuseya, Y., et al. (2017). Fraction of MHCII and EpCAM expression characterizes distal lung epithelial cells for alveolar type 2 cell isolation. *Respir. Res.* 18, 1–13. doi: 10.1186/s12931-017-0635-5

Hinz, B. (2009). Tissue stiffness, latent TGF-β1 activation, and mechanical signal transduction: implications for the pathogenesis and treatment of fibrosis. *Curr. Rheumatol. Rep.* 11, 120–126. doi: 10.1007/s11926-009-0017-1

Horowitz, J. C., and Thannickal, V. J. (2006). Epithelial-mesenchymal interactions in pulmonary fibrosis. *Semin. Respir. Crit. Care Med.* 27, 600–612. doi: 10.1055/s-2006-957332

Huang, X., Yang, N., Fiore, V. F., Barker, T. H., Sun, Y., Morris, S. W., et al. (2012). Matrix stiffness-induced myofibroblast differentiation is mediated by intrinsic mechanotransduction. *Am. J. Respir. Cell Mol. Biol.* 47, 340–348. doi: 10.1165/rcmb.2012-0050OC

Huaux, F., Liu, T., McGarry, B., Ullenbruch, M., and Phan, S. H. (2003). Dual Roles of IL-4 in lung injury and fibrosis. *J. Immunol.* 170, 2083–2092. doi: 10.4049/jimmunol.170.4.2083

Huh, D. (2015). A human breathing lung-on-a-chip. *Ann. Am. Thoracic Soc.* 12, 42–44. doi: 10.1513/AnnalsATS.201410-442MG

Jansing, N. L., McClendon, J., Kage, H., Sunohara, M., Alvarez, J. R., Borok, Z., et al. (2018). Isolation of rat and mouse alveolar type II epithelial cells. *Methods Mol. Biol.* 1809, 69–82. doi: 10.1007/978-1-4939-8570-8_6

Jones, D. L., Haak, A. J., Caporarello, N., Choi, K. M., Ye, Z., Yan, H., et al. (2019). TGFβ-induced fibroblast activation requires persistent and targeted HDAC-mediated gene repression. *J. Cell Sci.* 132:jcs233486. doi: 10.1242/jcs.233486

Kage, H., and Borok, Z. (2012). EMT and interstitial lung disease: a mysterious relationship. *Curr. Opin. Pulm. Med.* 18, 517–523. doi: 10.1097/MCP.0b013e3283566721

Kasper, M., and Barth, K. (2017). Potential contribution of alveolar epithelial type I cells to pulmonary fibrosis. *Biosci. Rep.* 37:BSR20171301. doi: 10.1042/bsr20171301

Kaur, G., and Dufour, J. (2012). Cell lines: valuable tools or useless artifacts. *Spermatogenesis* 2, 1–5. doi: 10.4161/spmg.19885

Kitsera, N., Khobta, A., and Epe, B. (2007). Destabilized green fluorescent protein detects rapid removal of transcription blocks after genotoxic exposure. *BioTechniques* 43, 222–227. doi: 10.2144/000112479

Kolodsick, J. E., Toews, G. B., Jakubzick, C., Hogaboam, C., Moore, T. A., McKenzie, A., et al. (2004). Protection from fluorescein isothiocyanate-induced Fibrosis in IL-13-Deficient, but Not IL-4-Deficient, mice results from impaired collagen synthesis by fibroblasts. *J. Immunol.* 172, 4068–4076. doi: 10.4049/jimmunol.172.7.4068

Krämer, D. K., Bouzakri, K., Holmqvist, O., Al-Khalili, L., and Krook, A. (2005). Effect of serum replacement with Plysate on cell growth and metabolismin primary cultures of human skeletal muscle. *Cytotechnology* 48, 89–95. doi: 10.1007/s10616-005-4074-7

Kuehn, A., Kletting, S., De Souza Carvalho-Wodarz, C., Repnik, U., Griffiths, G., Fischer, U., et al. (2016). Human alveolar epithelial cells expressing tight junctions to model the air-blood barrier. *Altex* 33, 251–260. doi: 10.14573/altex.1511131

Lederer, D. J., and Martinez, F. J. (2018). Idiopathic pulmonary fibrosis. *N. Engl. J. Med.* 378, 1811–1823. doi: 10.1056/NEJMra1705751

Lee, D. F., Salguero, F. J., Grainger, D., Francis, R. J., MacLellan-Gibson, K., and Chambers, M. A. (2018). Isolation and characterisation of alveolar type II pneumocytes from adult bovine lung. *Sci. Rep.* 8:11927.

Lee, J. U., Chang, H. S., Lee, H. J., Jung, C. A., Bae, D. J., Song, H. J., et al. (2017). Upregulation of interleukin-33 and thymic stromal lymphopoietin levels in the lungs of idiopathic pulmonary fibrosis. *BMC Pulm. Med.* 17:39. doi: 10.1186/s12890-017-0380-z

Li, R., Bernau, K., Sandbo, N., Gu, J., Preissl, S., and Sun, X. (2018). Pdgfra marks a cellular lineage with distinct contributions to myofibroblasts in lung maturation and injury response. *eLife* 7, 1–20. doi: 10.7554/eLife.36865

Liang, J., Zhang, Y., Xie, T., Liu, N., Chen, H., Geng, Y., et al. (2016). Hyaluronan and TLR4 promote surfactant-protein-C-positive alveolar progenitor cell renewal and prevent severe pulmonary fibrosis in mice. *Na. Med.* 22, 1285–1293. doi: 10.1038/nm.4192

Liao, Y., Smyth, G. K., and Shi, W. (2014). FeatureCounts: an efficient general purpose program for assigning sequence reads to genomic features. *Bioinformatics* 30, 923–930. doi: 10.1093/bioinformatics/btt656

Lipps, C., Klein, F., Wahlicht, T., Seiffert, V., Butueva, M., Zauers, J., et al. (2018). Expansion of functional personalized cells with specific transgene combinations. *Nat. Commun.* 9:994. doi: 10.1038/s41467-018-03408-4

Liu, F., Mih, J. D., Shea, B. S., Kho, A. T., Sharif, A. S., Tager, A. M., et al. (2010). Feedback amplification of fibrosis through matrix stiffening and COX-2 suppression. *J. Cell Biol.* 190, 693–706. doi: 10.1083/jcb.201004082

Liu, X., Rowan, S. C., Liang, J., Yao, C., Huang, G., Deng, N., et al. (2020). Definition and signatures of lung fibroblast populations in development and fibrosis in mice and men. *bioRxiv* [preprint]. doi: 10.1101/2020.07.15.203141

Löfdahl, A., Rydell-Törmänen, K., Larsson-Callerfelt, A. K., Wenglén, C., and Westergren-Thorsson, G. (2018). Pulmonary fibrosis in vivo displays increased p21 expression reduced by 5-HT2B receptor antagonists in vitro - A potential pathway affecting proliferation. *Sci. Rep.* 8:1927. doi: 10.1038/s41598-018-20430-0

Luzina, I. G., Kopach, P., Lockatell, V., Kang, P. H., Nagarsekar, A., Burke, A. P., et al. (2013). Interleukin-33 potentiates Bleomycin-induced lung injury. *Am. J. Respir. Cell Mol. Biol.* 49, 999–1008. doi: 10.1165/rcmb.2013-0093OC

Luzina, I. G., Pickering, E. M., Kopach, P., Kang, P. H., Lockatell, V., Todd, N. W., et al. (2012). Full-Length IL-33 promotes inflammation but not Th2 response in vivo in an ST2-Independent fashion. *J. Immunol.* 189, 403–410. doi: 10.4049/jimmunol.1200259

Luzina, I. G., Todd, N. W., Sundararajan, S., and Atamas, S. P. (2015). The cytokines of pulmonary fibrosis: much learned, much more to learn. *Cytokine* 74, 88–100. doi: 10.1016/j.cyto.2014.11.008

Mannello, F., and Tonti, G. A. (2009). Concise review: no breakthroughs for human mesenchymal and embryonic stem cell culture: conditioned medium, feeder layer, or feeder-free; medium with fetal calf serum, human serum, or enriched plasma; serum-free, serum replacement nonconditioned medium, o. *Stem Cells* 25, 1603–1609. doi: 10.1634/stemcells.2007-0127

McElroy, M. C., and Kasper, M. (2004). The use of alveolar epithelial type I cell-selective markers to investigate lung injury and repair. *Eur. Respir. J.* 24, 664–673. doi: 10.1183/09031936.04.00096003

Miklavc, P., Frick, M., Wittekindt, O. H., Haller, T., and Dietl, P. (2010). Fusion-Activated Ca2+ entry: an "active zone" of elevated Ca2+ during the postfusion stage of lamellar body exocytosis in rat Type II Pneumocytes. *PLoS One* 5:e10982. doi: 10.1371/journal.pone.0010982

Moore, B. B., Lawson, W. E., Oury, T. D., Sisson, T. H., Raghavendran, K., and Hogaboam, C. M. (2013). Animal models of fibrotic lung disease. *Ame. J. Respir. Cell Mol. Biol.* 49, 167–179. doi: 10.1165/rcmb.2013-0094TR

Ntokou, A., Klein, F., Dontireddy, D., Becker, S., Bellusci, S., Richardson, W. D., et al. (2015). Characterization of the platelet-derived growth factor receptor-α-positive cell lineage during murine late lung development. *Am. J, Physiol. Lung Cell. Mol. Physiol.* 309, L942–L958. doi: 10.1152/ajplung.00272.2014

Oikonomou, N., Harokopos, V., Zalevsky, J., Valavanis, C., Kotaniduo, A., Szymkowski, D. E., et al. (2006). Soluble TNF mediates the transition from pulmonary inflammation to fibrosis. *PLoS One* 1:e108. doi: 10.1371/journal.pone.0000108

O'Reilly, S. (2013). Role of interleukin-13 in fibrosis, particularly systemic sclerosis. *BioFactors* 39, 593–596. doi: 10.1002/biof.1117

Palchesko, R. N., Zhang, L., Sun, Y., and Feinberg, A. W. (2012). Development of polydimethylsiloxane substrates with tunable elastic modulus to study cell mechanobiology in muscle and nerve. *PLoS One* 7:e0051499. doi: 10.1371/journal.pone.0051499

Pardo, A., and Selman, M. (2016). Lung fibroblasts, aging, and idiopathic pulmonary fibrosis. *Ann. Am. Thoracic Soc.* 13, S417–S421. doi: 10.1513/AnnalsATS.201605-341AW

Parker, M. W., Rossi, D., Peterson, M., Smith, K., Sikström, K., White, E. S., et al. (2014). Fibrotic extracellular matrix activates a profibrotic positive feedback loop. *J. Clin. Invest.* 124, 1622–1635. doi: 10.1172/JCI71386

Pfaffl, M. W. (2001). A new mathematical model for relative quantification in real-time RT-PCR. *Nucleic Acids Res.* 29:e45. doi: 10.1093/nar/29.9.e45

Pierce, E. M., Carpenter, K., Jakubzick, C., Kunkel, S. L., Evanoff, H., Flaherty, K. R., et al. (2007). Idiopathic pulmonary fibrosis fibroblasts migrate and proliferate to CC chemokine ligand 21. *Eur. Respir. J.* 29, 1082–1093. doi: 10.1183/09031936.00122806

Plantier, L., Crestani, B., Wert, S. E., Dehoux, M., Zweytick, B., Guenther, A., et al. (2011). Ectopic respiratory epithelial cell differentiation in bronchiolised distal airspaces in idiopathic pulmonary fibrosis. *Thorax* 66, 651–657. doi: 10.1136/thx.2010.151555

Quintanilla, M., Montero, L. M., Renart, J., and Villar, E. M. (2019). Podoplanin in inflammation and cancer. *Int. J. Mol. Sci.* 20:707. doi: 10.3390/ijms20030707

Raghu, G., Collard, H. R., Egan, J. J., Martinez, F. J., Behr, J., Brown, K. K., et al. (2011). An Official ATS/ERS/JRS/ALAT statement: idiopathic pulmonary fibrosis: evidence-based guidelines for diagnosis and management. *Am. J. Respir. Crit. Care Med.* 183, 788–824. doi: 10.1164/rccm.2009-040GL

Ran, F. A., Hsu, P. D., Wright, J., Agarwala, V., Scott, D. A., and Zhang, F. (2013). Genome engineering using the CRISPR-Cas9 system. *Nat. Protoc.* 8, 2281–2308. doi: 10.1038/nprot.2013.143

Reyfman, P. A., Walter, J. M., Joshi, N., Anekalla, K. R., McQuattie-Pimentel, A. C., Chiu, S., et al. (2019). Single-cell transcriptomic analysis of human lung provides insights into the pathobiology of pulmonary fibrosis. *Am. J. Respir. Crit. Care Med.* 199, 1517–1536. doi: 10.1164/rccm.201712-2410OC

Richeldi, L., Collard, H. R., and Jones, M. G. (2017). Idiopathic pulmonary fibrosis. *Lancet* 389, 1941–1952. doi: 10.1016/S0140-6736(17)30866-8

Ryu, J. H., Moua, T., Daniels, C. E., Hartman, T. E., Yi, E. S., Utz, J. P., et al. (2014). Idiopathic pulmonary fibrosis: evolving concepts. *Mayo Clin. Proc.* 89, 1130–1142. doi: 10.1016/j.mayocp.2014.03.016

Saito, A., Okazaki, H., Sugawara, I., Yamamoto, K., and Takizawa, H. (2003). Potential action of IL-4 and IL-13 as fibrogenic factors on lung fibroblasts in vitro. *Int. Arch. Allergy Immunol.* 132, 168–176. doi: 10.1159/000073718

Sayols, S., Scherzinger, D., and Klein, H. (2016). dupRadar: a bioconductor package for the assessment of PCR artifacts in RNA-Seq data. *BMC Bioinformatics* 17:428. doi: 10.1186/s12859-016-1276-2

Seibold, M. A., Wise, A. L., Speer, M. C., Steele, M. P., Brown, K. K., Loyd, J. E., et al. (2011). A common MUC5B promoter polymorphism and pulmonary fibrosis. *N. Engl. J. Med.* 364, 1503–1512. doi: 10.1056/NEJMoa1013660

Selman, M., and Pardo, A. (2001). Idiopathic pulmonary fibrosis: an epithelial/fibroblastic cross-talk disorder. *Respir. Res.* 3, 1–8. doi: 10.1186/rr175

Sgalla, G., Iovene, B., Calvello, M., Ori, M., Varone, F., and Richeldi, L. (2018). Idiopathic pulmonary fibrosis: pathogenesis and management. *Respir. Res.* 19:32. doi: 10.1186/s12931-018-0730-2

Shi, Y., Dong, Y., Duan, Y., Jiang, X., Chen, C., and Deng, L. (2013). Substrate stiffness influences TGF-β1-induced differentiation of bronchial fibroblasts into myofibroblasts in airway remodeling. *Mol. Med. Rep.* 7, 419–424. doi: 10.3892/mmr.2012.1213

Sime, P. J., Marr, R. A., Gauldie, D., Xing, Z., Hewlett, B. R., Graham, F. L., et al. (1998). Transfer of tumor necrosis factor-α to rat lung induces severe pulmonary inflammation and patchy interstitial fibrogenesis with induction of transforming growth factor-β1 and myofibroblasts. *Am. J. Pathol.* 153, 825–832. doi: 10.1016/S0002-9440(10)65624-6

Sime, P. J., Xing, Z., Graham, F. L., Csaky, K. G., and Gauldie, J. (1997). Adenovector-mediated gene transfer of active transforming growth factor- β1 induces prolonged severe fibrosis in rat lung. *J. Clin. Invest.* 100, 768–776. doi: 10.1172/JCI119590

Strunz, M., Simon, L. M., Ansari, M., Mattner, L. F., Angelidis, I., Mayr, C. H., et al. (2019). Longitudinal single cell transcriptomics reveals Krt8+ alveolar epithelial progenitors in lung regeneration. *bioRxiv* [preprint]. doi: 10.1101/705244

Stuart, B. D., Choi, J., Zaidi, S., Xing, C., Holohan, B., Chen, R., et al. (2015). Exome sequencing links mutations in PARN and RTEL1 with familial pulmonary fibrosis and telomere shortening. *Nat. Genet.* 47, 512–517. doi: 10.1038/ng.3278

Stucki, J. D., Hobi, N., Galimov, A., Stucki, A. O., Schneider-Daum, N., Lehr, C. M., et al. (2018). Medium throughput breathing human primary cell alveolus-on-chip model. *Sci. Rep.* 8:14359. doi: 10.1038/s41598-018-32523-x

Tahedl, D., Wirkes, A., Tschanz, S. A., Ochs, M., and Mühlfeld, C. (2014). How common is the lipid body-containing interstitial cell in the mammalian lung? *Am. J. Physiol. Lung Cell. Mol. Physiol.* 307, L386–L394. doi: 10.1152/ajplung.00131.2014

Thannickal, V. J., Lee, D. Y., White, E. S., Cui, Z., Larios, J. M., Chacon, R., et al. (2003). Myofibroblast differentiation by transforming growth factor-β1 is dependent on cell adhesion and integrin signaling via focal adhesion kinase. *J. Biol. Chem.* 278, 12384–12389. doi: 10.1074/jbc.M208544200

Trapnell, C., Hendrickson, D. G., Sauvageau, M., Goff, L., Rinn, J. L., and Pachter, L. (2013). Differential analysis of gene regulation at transcript resolution with RNA-seq. *Nat. Biotechnol.* 31, 46–53. doi: 10.1038/nbt.2450

Travaglini, K. J., Nabhan, A. N., Penland, L., Sinha, R., Gillich, A., Sit, R. V., et al. (2020). A molecular cell atlas of the human lung from single cell RNA sequencing. *bioRxiv* [Preprint]. doi: 10.1101/742320

Tschumperlin, D. J., Ligresti, G., Hilscher, M. B., and Shah, V. H. (2018). Mechanosensing and fibrosis. *J. Clin. Invest.* 128, 74–84. doi: 10.1172/JCI93561

Valenzi, E., Bulik, M., Tabib, T., Morse, C., Sembrat, J., Trejo Bittar, H., et al. (2019). Single-cell analysis reveals fibroblast heterogeneity and myofibroblasts in systemic sclerosis-associated interstitial lung disease. *Ann. Rheumat. Dis.* 78, 1379–1387. doi: 10.1136/annrheumdis-2018-214865

Wipff, P. J., Rifkin, D. B., Meister, J. J., and Hinz, B. (2007). Myofibroblast contraction activates latent TGF-β1 from the extracellular matrix. *J. Cell Biol.* 179, 1311–1323. doi: 10.1083/jcb.200704042

Wuyts, W. A., Agostini, C., Antoniou, K. M., Bouros, D., Chambers, R. C., Cottin, V., et al. (2013). The pathogenesis of pulmonary fibrosis: a moving target. *Eur. Respir. J.* 41, 1207–1218. doi: 10.1183/09031936.00073012

Xiao, M. W., Zhang, Y., Hong, P. K., Zhou, Z., Feghali-Bostwick, C. A., Liu, F., et al. (2006). Caveolin-1: a critical regulator of lung fibrosis in idiopathic pulmonary fibrosis. *J. Exp. Med.* 203, 2895–2906. doi: 10.1084/jem.20061536

Xie, T., Wang, Y., Deng, N., Huang, G., Taghavifar, F., Geng, Y., et al. (2018). Single-cell deconvolution of fibroblast heterogeneity in mouse pulmonary fibrosis. *Cell Rep.* 22, 3625–3640. doi: 10.1016/j.celrep.2018.03.010

Xu, Y., Mizuno, T., Sridharan, A., Du, Y., Guo, M., Tang, J., et al. (2016). Single-cell RNA sequencing identifies diverse roles of epithelial cells in idiopathic pulmonary fibrosis. *JCI Insight* 1:e90558. doi: 10.1172/jci.insight.90558

Yanaba, K., Yoshizaki, A., Asano, Y., Kadono, T., and Sato, S. (2011). Serum IL-33 levels are raised in patients with systemic sclerosis: association with extent of skin sclerosis and severity of pulmonary fibrosis. *Clin. Rheumatol.* 30, 825–830. doi: 10.1007/s10067-011-1686-5

Zepp, J., Zacharias, W., and Frank, D. (2017). Distinct mesenchymal lineages and niches promote epithelial self-renewal and myofibrogenesis in the lung. *Cell* 170, 1134–1148. doi: 10.1016/j.cell.2017.07.034

Zhu, Z., Homer, R. J., Wang, Z., Chen, Q., Geba, G. P., Wang, J., et al. (1999). Pulmonary expression of interleukin-13 causes inflammation, mucus hypersecretion, subepithelial fibrosis, physiologic abnormalities, and eotaxin production. *J. Clin. Invest.* 103, 779–788. doi: 10.1172/JCI5909

17

Tobacco Smoke and Inhaled Drugs Alter Expression and Activity of Multidrug Resistance-Associated Protein-1 (MRP1) in Human Distal Lung Epithelial Cells *in vitro*

Mohammed Ali Selo[1,2], Anne-Sophie Delmas[1], Lisa Springer[1], Viktoria Zoufal[1,3], Johannes A. Sake[1], Caoimhe G. Clerkin[1], Hanno Huwer[4], Nicole Schneider-Daum[5], Claus-Michael Lehr[5,6], Sabrina Nickel[1], Oliver Langer[3,7,8] and Carsten Ehrhardt[1*]*

[1] School of Pharmacy and Pharmaceutical Sciences and Trinity Biomedical Sciences Institute, Trinity College Dublin, Dublin, Ireland, [2] Faculty of Pharmacy, University of Kufa, Al-Najaf, Iraq, [3] Preclinical Molecular Imaging, AIT Austrian Institute of Technology GmbH, Seibersdorf, Austria, [4] Department of Cardiothoracic Surgery, Völklingen Heart Centre, Völklingen, Germany, [5] Helmholtz Institute for Pharmaceutical Research Saarland, Helmholtz Centre for Infection Research, Saarbrücken, Germany, [6] Department of Pharmacy, Saarland University, Saarbrücken, Germany, [7] Department of Clinical Pharmacology, Medical University of Vienna, Vienna, Austria, [8] Division of Nuclear Medicine, Department of Biomedical Imaging and Image-guided Therapy, Medical University of Vienna, Vienna, Austria

***Correspondence:**
Mohammed Ali Selo
mohammeda.mohsin@uokufa.edu.iq;
selom@tcd.ie
Carsten Ehrhardt
ehrhardc@tcd.ie

Multidrug resistance-associated protein-1 (MRP1/*ABCC1*) is highly expressed in human lung tissues. Recent studies suggest that it significantly affects the pulmonary disposition of its substrates, both after pulmonary and systemic administration. To better understand the molecular mechanisms involved, we studied the expression, subcellular localization and activity of MRP1 in freshly isolated human alveolar epithelial type 2 (AT2) and type 1-like (AT1-like) cells in primary culture, and in the NCI-H441 cell line. Moreover, the effect of cigarette smoke extract (CSE) and a series of inhaled drugs on MRP1 abundance and activity was investigated *in vitro*. MRP1 expression levels were measured by q-PCR and immunoblot in AT2 and AT1-like cells from different donors and in several passages of the NCI-H441 cell line. The subcellular localization of the transporter was studied by confocal laser scanning microscopy and cell surface protein biotinylation. MRP1 activity was assessed by bidirectional transport and efflux experiments using the MRP1 substrate, 5(6)-carboxyfluorescein [CF; formed intracellularly from 5(6)-carboxyfluorescein-diacetate (CFDA)] in AT1-like and NCI-H441 cell monolayers. Furthermore, the effect of CSE as well as several bronchodilators and inhaled corticosteroids on MRP1 abundance and CF efflux was investigated. MRP1 protein abundance increased upon differentiation from AT2 to AT1-like phenotype, however, *ABCC1* gene levels remained unchanged. MRP1 abundance in NCI-H441 cells were comparable to those found in AT1-like cells. The transporter was detected primarily in basolateral membranes of both cell types which was consistent with net basolateral efflux of CF. Likewise, bidirectional transport studies showed net apical-to-basolateral transport of CF which was sensitive to the MRP1 inhibitor MK-571. Budesonide, beclomethasone dipropionate, salbutamol sulfate, and CSE decreased

CF efflux in a concentration-dependent manner. Interestingly, CSE increased MRP1 abundance, whereas budesonide, beclomethasone dipropionate, salbutamol sulfate did not have such effect. CSE and inhaled drugs can reduce MRP1 activity *in vitro*, which implies the transporter being a potential drug target in the treatment of chronic obstructive pulmonary disease (COPD). Moreover, MRP1 expression level, localization and activity were comparable in human AT1-like and NCI-H441 cells. Therefore, the cell line can be a useful alternative *in vitro* model to study MRP1 in distal lung epithelium.

Keywords: COPD, ABC transporters, pulmonary drug disposition, inhalation biopharmaceutics, efflux transporters

INTRODUCTION

Multidrug resistance-associated protein-1 (MRP1, 190 kDa), a member of the ATP binding cassette (ABC) superfamily of transporters, is encoded by the *ABCC1* gene (Cole, 2014a). As an efflux transporter, MRP1 plays a pivotal role in physiological detoxification. Its substrates include glutathione, glucuronate, and sulfate conjugates of drugs and endogenous molecules (Cole, 2014a,b). The transporter is highly expressed in the human lung, including bronchial, bronchiolar and alveolar epithelial cells (Flens et al., 1996; Scheffer et al., 2002).

We have become interested in pulmonary MRP1 for two reasons, its impact on inhaled drugs disposition and its potential role as a target in the treatment of chronic obstructive pulmonary disease (COPD).

It has been hypothesized that MRP1 protects lung cells against toxic insults of xenobiotics and from damage induced by oxidative stress by maintaining intracellular glutathione-glutathione disulfide homeostasis (Cole and Deeley, 2006; Cole, 2014b; Nickel et al., 2016). Inhibition of MRP1 was observed to worsen cigarette smoke extract (CSE)-induced cytotoxicity *in vitro* (van der Deen et al., 2007) and pre-clinical and clinical data suggest that changes in abundance (van der Deen et al., 2006; Wu et al., 2019) or function (Budulac et al., 2010) of the transporter are associated with occurrence and severity of COPD. Moreover, recent *in vivo* data from our group showed that pulmonary distribution and clearance of the MRP1 substrate S-(6-(7-[^{11}C] methylpurinyl)) glutathione ([^{11}C]MPG), measured with positron emission tomography (PET), was significantly dependent on MRP1 abundance (Mairinger et al., 2020).

On a molecular level, the expression and activity of MRP1 in distal lung epithelium, however, remains poorly investigated. Thus, the aims of this study were to determine the expression, cellular localization and activity of MRP1 in freshly isolated human alveolar epithelial cells in primary culture and to compare these data to the human adenocarcinoma cell line NCI-H441, which present several features of human distal lung epithelium, such as an ability to form electrically tight monolayers of polarized cells. Further it has been previously proposed to be the most promising continuously growing *in vitro* surrogate of human distal lung epithelial cells (Salomon et al., 2014; Salomon et al., 2019). In addition, the influence of CSE and commonly prescribed inhaled drugs on the abundance and activity of MRP1 *in vitro* was studied.

MATERIALS AND METHODS

Cell Culture

NCI-H441 human distal lung epithelial cells (ATCC HTB-174) were purchased from LGC Standards (Teddington, United Kingdom). Human alveolar type 2 epithelial (AT2) cells were isolated from non-tumor lung tissue obtained from patients undergoing lung surgery according to a previously published protocol (Daum et al., 2012). The freshly isolated AT2 cells were either used directly for RNA and protein isolation or left for 2 days to attach on collagen/fibronectin coated surfaces. Alternatively, cells were cultured for 8–10 days to undergo transdifferentiation into an alveolar type 1-like (AT1-like) phenotype. Primary cell culture was performed using small airways growth medium (SAGM, Lonza, Verviers, Belgium) supplemented with penicillin (100 U/ml), streptomycin (100 µg/ml), and 1% fetal bovine serum (all purchased from Sigma-Aldrich, Dublin, Ireland). Where indicated, 10 ng/ml keratinocyte growth factor (KGF, ProSpec-Tany TechnoGene, Ltd., Rehovot, Israel) was added to the culture medium to inhibit differentiation of AT2 cells into an AT1-like phenotype. The use of human tissue specimens was approved by Saarland State Medical Board (Saarbrücken, Germany). All cell types were cultured in a humidified atmosphere at 37°C in 5% CO_2 as described in more detail by Nickel et al. (2017).

Preparation of CSE

The smoke of two University of Kentucky research cigarettes (3R4F) was bubbled into 20 ml of RPMI 1640 medium (Biosciences, Dublin, Ireland) using a vacuum pump to generate 100% CSE. The latter was sterile filtered to remove any particulate matter and further diluted with RPMI medium to prepare 5 and 10% CSE which was used for exposure studies. Human AT1-like and NCI-H441 cells were exposed to either freshly prepared or aged CSE, which was prepared and stored at room temperature for 14 days, to investigate their effect on MRP1 abundance and activity.

Isolation of RNA and Real-Time Polymerase Chain Reaction (q-PCR)

RNA was isolated from freshly isolated AT2 cells, which were cultured for 8–10 days to transdifferentiate into the AT1-like phenotype and NCI-H441 cells grown in six-well plates

(Greiner Bio-One GmbH, Frickenhausen, Germany) using Tri-Reagent (Sigma-Aldrich) according to the manufacturer's instructions and as described in a previously published protocol (Nickel et al., 2017). Semi-quantitative, one-step real time PCR (q-PCR) was carried out on a 7500 Real-Time PCR System (Applied Biosystems, Inc., Foster City, CA, United States) as described previously (Nickel et al., 2017) using KiCqStart predesigned primers [(Sigma-Aldrich) for *ACTB* (forward GACGACATGGAGAAAATCTG; reverse ATGATCTGGGTCATCTTCTC) and *ABCC1* (forward AGC AGAAAAATGTGTTAGGG; reverse TACCCACTGGTAATA CTTGG)].

Immunoblot

Western blotting was carried out to investigate MRP1 abundance in AT2, AT1-like and in NCI-H441 cells. It was also used to assess the influence of different cell culture conditions [i.e., whether growing cells under air-interfaced culture (AIC) or liquid-covered culture (LCC)] on MRP1 protein level in NCI-H441 cells. In addition, the analysis was used to determine the effect of CSE, budesonide and salbutamol sulfate on MRP1 abundance in NCI-H441 cells. Cells were grown in presence of 5 or 10 μM budesonide (Mundipharma Pharmaceuticals Limited, Dublin, Ireland) or 100 μM salbutamol sulfate (Sigma-Aldrich) for up to 6 days and compared with the negative control (medium alone) or incubated with the solvent [i.e., dimethyl sulfoxide (DMSO)] when appropriate.

Confluent cell monolayers were washed twice with ice cold phosphate buffered saline (PBS) and lysed with cell extraction buffer (Life Technologies, Eugene, OR, United States) supplemented with protease inhibitor cocktail (Roche, Mannheim, Germany). Subsequently, samples were sonicated and centrifuged at 12,000 × *g* for 15 min at 4°C. The total protein amount was determined by Pierce BCA protein assay kit (Thermo Fisher Scientific, Waltham, MA, United States) according to the manufacturer's instructions. Polyacrylamide gel electrophoresis was carried out as described previously (Nickel et al., 2017). Following transfer onto immunoblot polyvinylidine fluoride membranes, blots were blocked with washing buffer [PBS containing 0.05% Tween 20 (PBST)] supplemented with 3% (w/v) bovine serum albumin (BSA) for at least 1 h at room temperature before being incubated overnight at 4°C with rat monoclonal anti-MRP1 Ab (clone MRPr1, GTX13368, GeneTex, Inc., Irvine, CA, United States, 1:50) in PBST supplemented with 1% (w/v) BSA. The following day, membranes were washed three times and incubated with secondary anti-rat antibody (1:5000; Santa Cruz, Dallas, TX, United States) for 1 h at room temperature. Peroxidase activity was detected with Immobilon Western Chemiluminescent HRP substrate (Millipore, Carrigtwohill, Ireland). Signals were documented using a ChemiDoc system (Bio-Rad Laboratories, Hercules, CA, United States).

Biotinylation of Cell Surface Proteins

Cell surface protein biotinylation was carried out to determine whether MRP1 is localized at the apical or basolateral membranes of polarized AT1-like and NCI-H441 cells. The analysis was not carried out in freshly isolated AT2 cells due to their unpolarized phenotype. Apical or basolateral membrane proteins of confluent, Transwell-grown cell monolayers were labeled with sulpho-NHS-biotin (Thermo Fisher Scientific), isolated and analyzed as described in a previously published protocol (Schwagerus et al., 2015).

Immunohistochemistry and Confocal Laser Scanning Microscopy (CLSM)

NCI-H441, AT2, and AT1-like cells cultured in Lab-Tek chamber slides (Nunc A/S, Roskilde, Denmark) or on Transwell Clear inserts (either 12 mm or 6.5 mm in diameter, 0.4 μm pore size, Corning, Bedford, MA, United States) were used and processed for immunocytochemistry, as described previously (Nickel et al., 2017). Cells were fixed with 2% paraformaldehyde, incubated with 50 mM aqueous NH_4Cl and then permeabilized with 0.1% Triton X-100. Monolayers were blocked with 2% BSA in PBS and incubated overnight with rat monoclonal anti-MRP1 Ab (1:50 dilution). The following day, cell monolayers were washed twice and incubated with Alexa Fluor 488-conjugated goat anti-rat secondary antibody (ab150165, abcam, Cambridge, United Kingdom, 1:100) for 1 h at room temperature, followed by 5 min incubation with a Hoechst 33342 solution (1 μg/ml) to counterstain nuclei. Samples were visualized on a Leica SP8 confocal laser scanning microscope (Leica Microsystems, Wetzlar, Germany) with a 63× oil immersion objective, a 488 nm diode laser and 520 nm Alexa Fluor 488 detection filter (green antibody signal) and a 405 nm diode laser in combination with a Hoechst 33342 detection filter (blue nucleic signal).

Bidirectional 5(6)-Carboxyfluorescein Transport Studies

Multidrug resistance-associated protein-1 activity *in vitro* was determined by carrying out bidirectional transport studies of the MRP1 substrate 5(6)-carboxyfluorescein (CF) across polarized monolayers of AT1-like and NCI-H441 cells as described by Salomon et al. (2014). CF is formed intracellularly from the cleavage of its non-fluorescent diacetate conjugate (CFDA) which diffuses passively into the cells. Due to their unpolarized phenotype, transport studies could not be carried out in freshly isolated AT2 cells. Cells were grown in Transwell Clear inserts and studies were carried out only across monolayers with transepithelial electrical resistance (TEER) values exceeding 500 $\Omega \times cm^2$. Monolayers were washed twice with pre-warmed Krebs-Ringer buffer (KRB; 116.4 mM NaCl, 5.4 mM KCl, 0.78 mM NaH_2PO_4, 25 mM $NaHCO_3$, 5.55 mM glucose, 15 mM HEPES, 1.8 mM $CaCl_2$, and 0.81 mM $MgSO_4$; pH 7.4) and then pre-equilibrated with the buffer solution for 1 h in the presence or absence of the MRP1 inhibitor MK-571 (20 μM, Santa Cruz). Permeation studies were initiated by replacing the buffer solution in the donor chambers with 100 μM CFDA solution (Applied BioProbes, Rockville, MD, United States) with or without the inhibitor compound. Cells were maintained at 37°C and 200 μl samples were collected from the receptor chambers after 0, 15, 30, 45, 60, 75, and 90 min and replaced with the same volume of buffer solution. Fluorescence intensity was analyzed using an automated plate reader (FLUOstar Optima, BMG LABTECH, Offenburg, Germany) at excitation and emission wavelengths of 485 and 520 nm, respectively. TEER values were measured before and after the study to verify cell monolayer integrity. The apparent permeability coefficient (P_{app}) was calculated using the following equation:

$$P_{app} = \frac{\Delta Q/\Delta t}{A \times C_0} \quad (1)$$

where ΔQ is the change in the amount of CF over the designated period of time (Δt), A is the nominal surface area of the growth supports (i.e., 1.13 and 0.33 cm^2 in case of 3460 and 3470 Transwell inserts, respectively), and C_0 is the initial concentration of CFDA in the donor fluid.

CF Efflux Studies

Bidirectional CF efflux studies were carried out on polarized AT1-like and NCI-H441 cell monolayers grown in Transwell Clear inserts. Cell monolayers were washed twice and then incubated with KRB alone or supplemented with MK-571 (20 μM) for 1 h. Afterward, cells were loaded with 100 μM CFDA solutions (± MK-571) by adding 0.5 and 1.5 ml into the apical and basolateral chambers, respectively. Following 1 h incubation, monolayers were washed twice, and the donor solutions were replaced with the same volumes of fresh KRB alone or supplemented with the inhibitor compound. Afterward, 200 μl samples were collected from both apical and basolateral chambers every 15 min and up to 90 min and replaced with the same volumes of fresh KRB. At the end of experiments, TEER values were measured to confirm cell monolayers integrity.

Carboxyfluorescein efflux studies from AT-like and NCI-H441 cell monolayers grown in 24-well plates (Greiner Bio-One) were carried out to determine the effect of a series of inhaled drugs and CSE on MRP1 activity *in vitro*. As described above, cell monolayers were loaded with CFDA solution alone or containing either budesonide (5 or 10 μM), beclomethasone dipropionate (50 μM, Sigma-Aldrich), salbutamol sulfate (100 μM), salbutamol base (100 μM, Sigma-Aldrich), R-salbutamol HCl (100 μM, Sunovion Pharmaceuticals, Marlborough, MA, United States), S-salbutamol HCl, (100 μM, Sunovion Pharmaceuticals), terbutaline (100 μM, Sunovion Pharmaceuticals), formoterol fumarate (100 μM, Santa Cruz), L-sulforaphane (10 μM, Cayman Chemical, Ann Arbor, MI, United States), 5 or 10% CSE or the solvent [i.e., dimethyl sulfoxide (DMSO)] when appropriate. Following 1 h incubation, CFDA solutions were replaced with fresh KRB alone or supplemented with one of the above compounds and CF efflux was assessed by collecting 200 μl samples every 15 min. After 90 min, cell monolayers were washed twice with ice cold KRB and lysed in cell extraction buffer and fluorescence intensity was analyzed as described above. For standardization, the total protein concentration of whole cell lysate was determined by Pierce BCA assay (Thermo Fischer Scientific) according to the manufacturer's instructions and the amount of CF effluxed per μg of protein was calculated.

Data Analysis

Results are expressed as means ± SD. The significance of differences between mean values was determined either by unpaired, two-tailed Student's *t*-test or one-way ANOVA followed by Bonferroni's *post hoc* comparisons test. $P \leq 0.05$ was considered significant. All experiments were carried out at least in triplicate using cells from three different passages or donors.

RESULTS

Expression Analysis of MRP1/*ABCC1* in Human Alveolar Epithelial Cells

Semi-quantitative real-time PCR analysis revealed *ABCC1* mRNA expression at similar levels in freshly isolated AT2 cells and cells differentiated into an AT1-like phenotype (**Figure 1A**). Analysis of immunoblot data, however, revealed significantly ($P \leq 0.01$) lower MRP1 protein abundance in freshly isolated AT2 cells than in AT1-like cells from the same donors (**Figures 1B,C**). To exclude the probability that the lower protein levels observed in freshly isolated AT2 cells was an artifact due to cleavage of MRP1 protein by enzymes used for cell isolation, AT2 cells from the same donors were cultured in the presence or absence of 10 ng/ml KGF for at least 8 days. The growth factor has been shown to inhibit differentiation of AT2 cells into AT-like phenotype in primary culture (Demling et al., 2006). MRP1 abundance was, again, significantly ($P \leq 0.01$) lower in cells which retained their AT2 characteristics than in cells differentiated into an AT1-like phenotype (**Figures 1D,E**). CLSM analysis was inconclusive in terms of MRP1 localization in unpolarized AT2 cells (**Figure 1F**), but MRP1 signals were primarily localized to the basolateral cell membranes of AT1-like cells grown to monolayers for at least 8 days (**Figure 1G**). The localization of MRP1 in the basolateral membranes of AT1-like cells was further confirmed by cell surface protein biotinylation and subsequent analysis by Western blotting (**Figure 2A**).

Expression Analysis of MRP1/*ABCC1* in NCI-H441 Cells

Semi-quantitative real-time PCR and Western blot analyses showed stable MRP1/*ABCC1* expression across several passages of NCI-H441 cells. Neither passage number nor cell culture conditions (i.e., whether cells were grown in LCC or AIC conditions) had an influence on MRP1 abundance (**Figures 3A–C**). Protein levels of the transporter in the NCI-H441 cell line were comparable to AT1-like cells (**Figures 3D,E**). CLSM analysis of MRP1 in NCI-H441 cells grown under AIC (**Figure 3F**) and LCC (**Figure 3G**) conditions showed MRP1 signals mainly along the basolateral membranes. Cell surface protein biotinylation of Transwell-grown NCI-H441 monolayers further confirmed the basolateral localization of the protein (**Figure 2A**).

MRP1 Activity in Distal Lung Epithelial Cells

Multidrug resistance-associated protein-1 activity was studied *in vitro* by bidirectional transport and efflux studies of

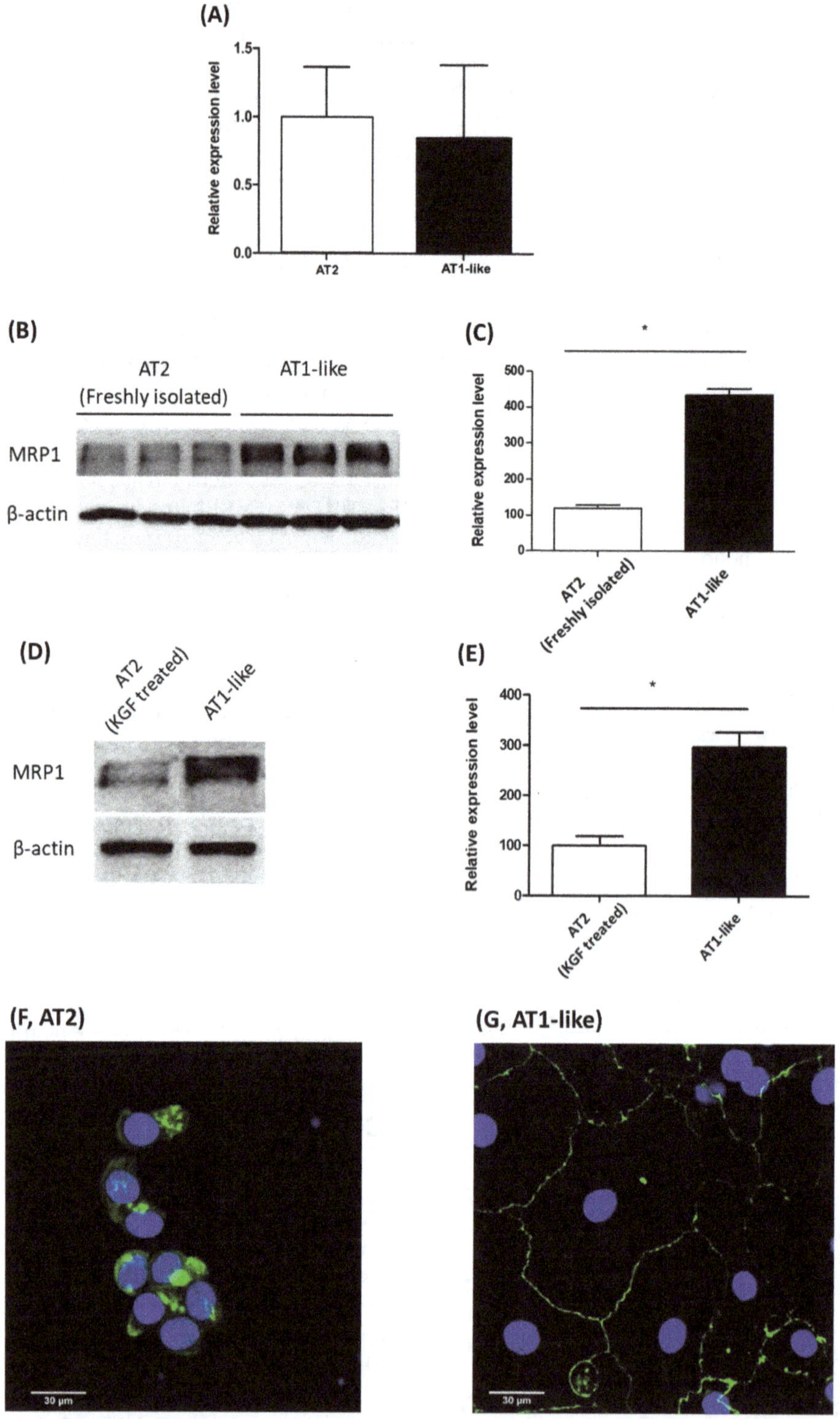

FIGURE 1 | Expression of multidrug resistance-associated protein-1 (MRP1)/*ABCC1* during transdifferentiation of human primary alveolar epithelial cells. **(A)** q-PCR analysis of *ABCC1* mRNA from three donors shows stable expression upon differentiation of alveolar type 2 epithelial (AT2) cells into an alveolar type 1-like (AT1-like) phenotype. **(B,C)** Representative Western blot and corresponding densitometric analyses of MRP1 protein in alveolar cells isolated from three donors show significantly lower levels in freshly isolated AT2 cells than cells differentiated into AT1-like phenotype. **(D,E)** show lower MRP1 abundance observed in cells cultured in the presence of KGF and thus retaining their AT2 properties than in cells differentiated into AT1-like cells in the absence of the growth factor. Data are represented as means + SD, $n \geq 3$, $^*P \leq 0.01$. Unpaired, two-tailed Student's *t*-test was used. Confocal laser scanning microscopic analysis of MRP1 (green signals) in AT2 cells cultured for 2 days **(F)** was inconclusive because of the non-polarized phenotype of the cells. **(G)** In AT1-like cells, the signals detected were mainly at the basolateral cell membranes. Cell nuclei were counterstained with Hoechst 33342 (blue signals).

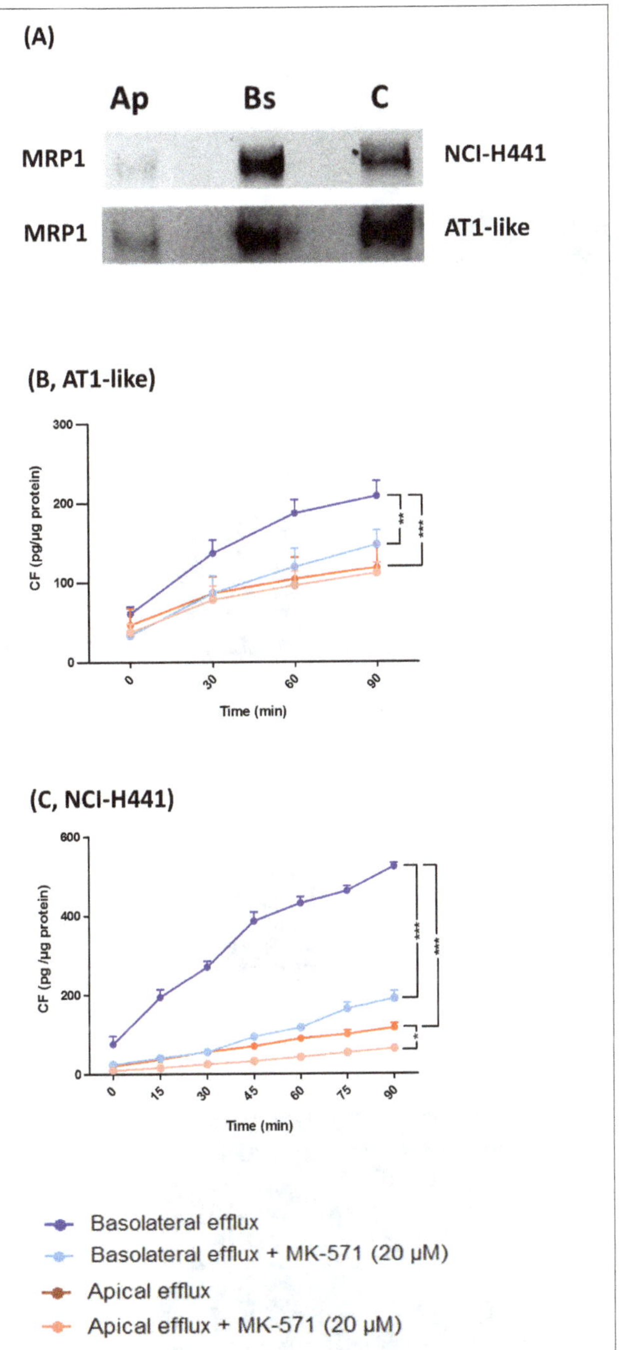

FIGURE 2 | Multidrug resistance-associated protein-1 is localized to the basolateral membranes of alveolar type 1-like (AT1-like) and NCI-H441 cells. **(A)** Apical or basolateral membranes proteins of polarized, Transwell-grown NCI-H441 **(upper)** and human AT1-like **(lower)** cell monolayers were biotinylated, isolated and detected by immunoblot. Immunoblots clearly show MRP1 localization in the basolateral membranes of both cell models. Ap and Bs, indicate apically and basolaterally sulfo-NHS-biotin treated cells, respectively, and C indicates whole cell lysate. **(B,C)** show bidirectional carboxyfluorescein (CF) efflux studies from AT1-like **(B)** and NCI-H441 **(C)** cell monolayers. Consistent with the basolateral localization of the transporter, MK-571 sensitive, net basolateral efflux of CF from both cell models was observed. Data are represented as means + SD, $n = 9$, *P (0.05, **P (0.01, ***P (0.001. One-way ANOVA followed by Bonferroni's post hocpost-hoc comparisons test was used.

CF in polarized, Transwell-grown AT1-like and NCI-H441 monolayers, respectively. Data obtained were consistent with a basolateral localization of the transporter. A significantly ($P = 0.001$) higher amount of CF was effluxed into the basolateral receiver chamber than the apical receiver chamber from human AT1-like (**Figure 2B**) as well as NCI-H441 (**Figure 2C**) monolayers. The CF efflux was sensitive to inhibition by MK-571. Likewise, bidirectional transport studies showed MK-571-sensitive, net apical-to-basolateral transport of CF across both cell types (**Figures 4A,B**).

Effect of Inhaled Drugs on MRP1 Activity and Abundance

Carboxyfluorescein efflux studies were carried out to assess the effect of a set of commonly prescribed inhaled drugs on MRP1 activity *in vitro*. Budesonide (5 or 10 μM) decreased CF efflux from AT1-like and NCI-H441 cell monolayers in a dose-dependent manner (**Figure 5A** and **Table 1**). Similarly, beclomethasone dipropionate (50 μM) and salbutamol sulfate (100 μM) resulted in a significant reduction of CF efflux from NCI-H441 cells. Other tested bronchodilator compounds had no such effect (**Table 1**).

Immunoblot analysis of NCI-H441 cells grown in the presence of either 5 or 10 μM budesonide or 100 μM salbutamol sulfate for up to 6 days showed no influence of the drugs on MRP1 abundance (**Figure 5B**).

Effect of CSE and Sulforaphane on MRP1 Activity and Abundance

Carboxyfluorescein efflux studies and immunoblot analysis were used to determine the influence of CSE on MRP1 activity and abundance in AT1-like and NCI-H441 cells. Twenty-four hours exposure to freshly prepared 10% CSE caused a significant ($P \leq 0.01$) reduction in CF efflux from AT1-like and NCI-H441 cell monolayers (**Figures 6A,B**). The effect of the freshly prepared CSE was dose-dependent and more pronounced than that of aged CSE in NCI-H441 cells (**Figure 6A**). Interestingly, CSE exposure resulted in a significant increase in MRP1 abundance in NCI-H441 cells (**Figures 6C,D**).

The nuclear factor erythroid 2 related factor 2 (Nrf2)-antioxidant response elements (ARE) pathway has been previously suggested to be involved in the regulation of MRP1 expression (Ji et al., 2013). CF efflux studies were, therefore, carried out in the presence of the Nrf2 activator, sulforaphane to determine if it can improve MRP1 activity. The compound increased CF efflux from AT1-like cell monolayers (**Figure 6B**) but it had no influence on MRP1 activity in NCI-H441 cells (data not shown).

DISCUSSION

Multidrug resistance-associated protein-1 has previously been found to be the most abundant ABC transporter in human lung tissue in a study using liquid chromatography-tandem mass spectrometry for protein quantification (Sakamoto et al., 2013). The protein has also been detected in bronchial and

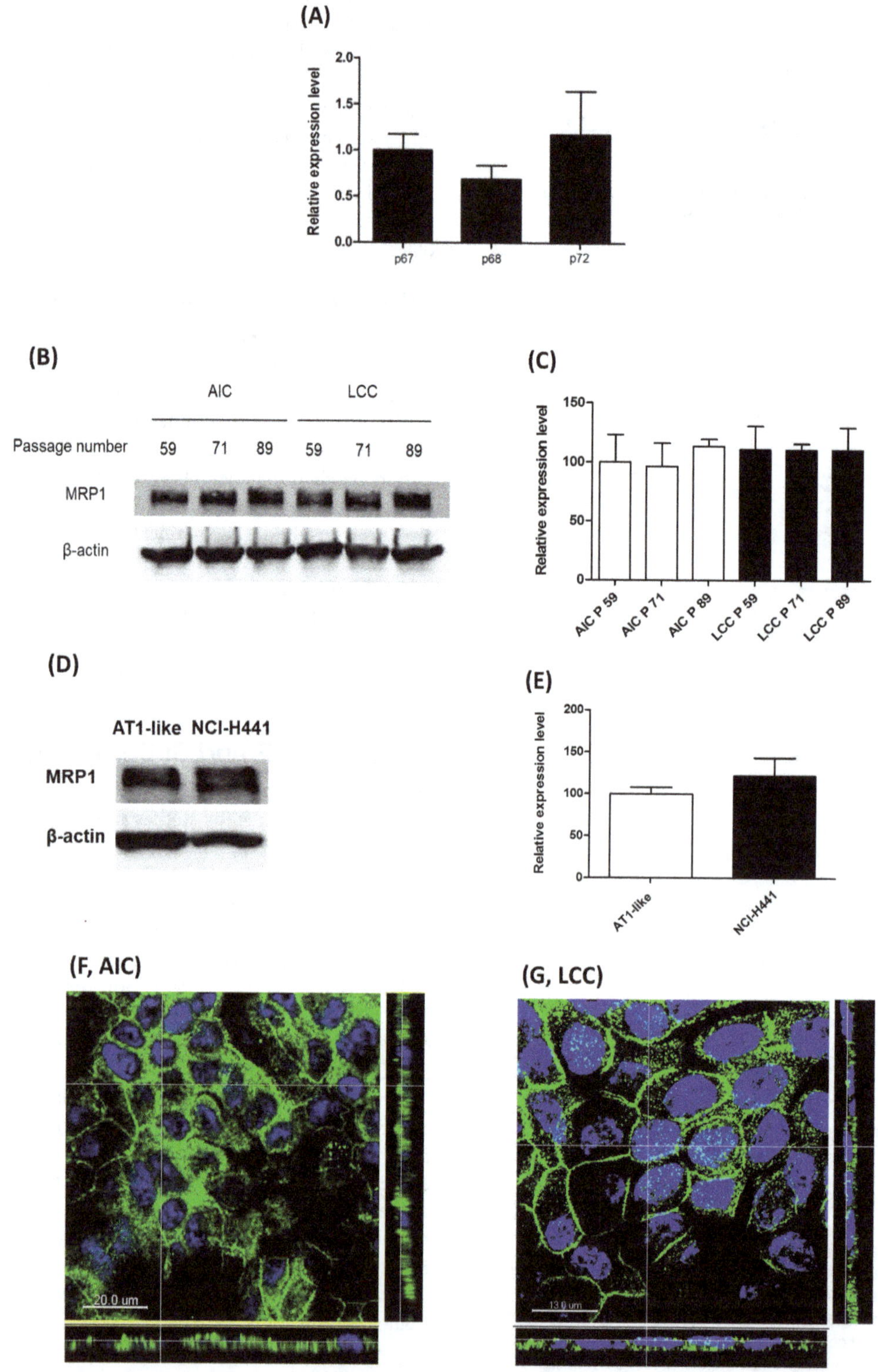

FIGURE 3 | Expression of multidrug resistance-associated protein-1 (MRP1)/*ABCC1* in NCI-H441 cells. **(A)** q-PCR analysis shows stable expression of *ABCC1* mRNA across several passages, p67, p68, and p72 indicate 67th, 68th, and 72th passage numbers, respectively. **(B,C)** Western blot and densitometric analyses of MRP1 in NCI-H441 cells grown either under air-interfaced culture (AIC) or liquid-covered culture (LCC) conditions for at least 7 days show similar abundance across different passage numbers and culture conditions. **(D,E)** Western blot and densitometric analysis showing similar protein levels of MRP1 in alveolar type 1-like (AT1-like) and NCI-H441 cells. Data are represented as means + SD, $n \geq 3$. Confocal laser scanning microscopy (CLSM) analysis of MRP1 (green signals) in NCI-H441 cells grown under AIC **(F)** and LCC **(G)** conditions show MRP1 signals primarily along the basolateral cell membranes. Cell nuclei were counterstained with Hoechst 33342 (blue signals).

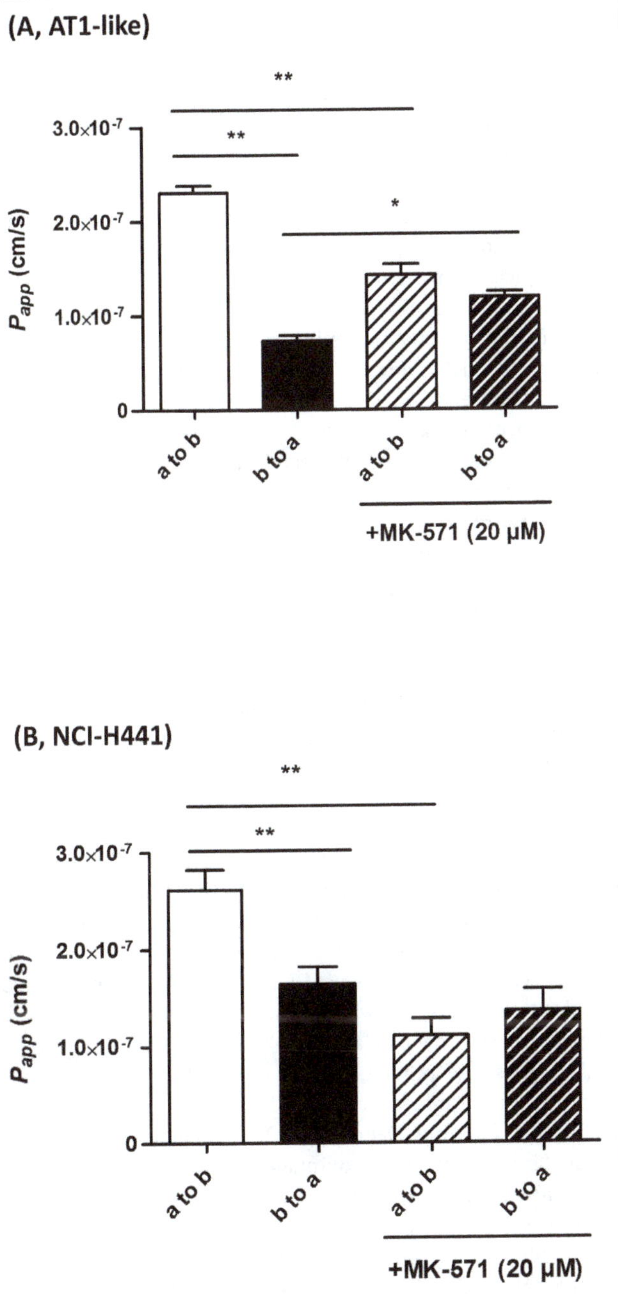

FIGURE 4 | Bidirectional transport studies of carboxyfluorescein (CF) across Transwell-grown confluent monolayers of human alveolar type 1-like (AT1-like) **(A)** and NCI-H441 **(B)** cells show significant net absorption of CF, consistent with the basolateral localization of multidrug resistance-associated protein-1 (MRP1). This net apical-to-basolateral transport can be attenuated by MK-571. Data represent means + SD, $n = 9$, $^{*}P \leq 0.05$, $^{**}P \leq 0.01$. One-way ANOVA followed by Bonferroni's *post hoc* comparisons test was used.

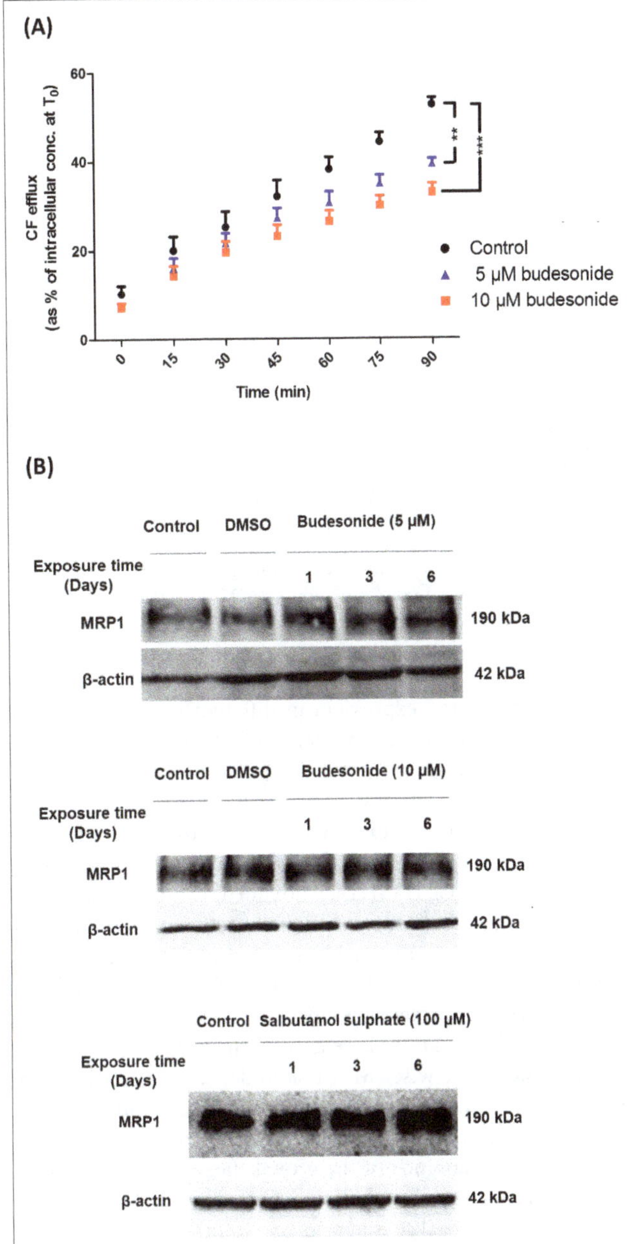

FIGURE 5 | Effect of several inhaled drugs on multidrug resistance-associated protein-1 (MRP1) activity and expression. **(A)** Efflux studies from alveolar type 1-like (AT1-like) cell monolayers show significant and dose-dependent reduction of carboxyfluorescein (CF) efflux in the presence of budesonide. **(B)** Immunoblot analysis shows that treatment of NCI-H441 cells with budesonide (5 or 10 μM) or salbutamol sulfate (100 μM) for up to 6 days has no effect on MRP1 abundance. Data are represented as means + SD, $n \geq 6$, $^{**}P \leq 0.01$, $^{***}P \leq 0.001$. One-way ANOVA followed by Bonferroni's *post hoc* comparisons test was used.

bronchiolar epithelial cells, alveolar macrophages, seromucinous glands and nasal epithelium (Flens et al., 1996; Bréchot et al., 1998; Wioland et al., 2000). The transporter has also been detected in normal human bronchial epithelial cells in primary culture with substantial variations in the expression levels in cells obtained from different donors (Lehmann et al., 2001). However, the expression, subcellular localization, and activity of the transporter are poorly investigated in distal lung epithelial cells. Previous reports have shown differences in mRNA and protein expression levels of several membrane transporters

TABLE 1 | Influence of Inhaled drugs on multidrug resistance-associated protein-1 (MRP1) activity in NCI-H441 cells.

Treatment	CF effluxed after 60 min (% of intracellular conc. at T_0)
KRB	45.4 ± 11.2
KRB + DMSO	47.2 ± 7.5
Budesonide 5 μM	36.5 ± 4.3
Budesonide 10 μM	34.2 ± 7.4*
Beclomethasone dipropionate 50 μM	20.4 ± 3.04***
Salbutamol sulfate 100 μM	35.1 ± 5.9*
Salbutamol base 100 μM	41.6 ± 2.3
R-Salbutamol HCl 100 μM	41.8 ± 2.5
S-Salbutamol HCl 100 μM	37.8 ± 6.2
Formoterol fumarate 100 μM	45.3 ± 3.6
Terbutaline 100 μM	43.7 ± 1.1

*Carboxyfluorescein (CF) efflux studies from NCI-H441 cells were carried out in presence of a set of beta-agonists and inhaled corticosteroids and compared with controls to assess their effect on MRP1 activity. Cells treated with transport buffer alone served as control. Data are represented as means ± SD, n ≥ 9. *P ≤ 0.05, ***P ≤ 0.001. One-way ANOVA followed by Bonferroni's post hoc comparisons test was used.*

both regarding spatial expression in different lung regions and regarding immortalized vs. primary cells (Endter et al., 2009; Salomon et al., 2012). To our knowledge, this is the first study in which the expression, subcellular localization, and activity of MRP1 is comprehensively investigated in human alveolar epithelial cells in primary culture and in the distal lung epithelial cell line NCI-H441. Data obtained revealed MRP1 to be expressed at high levels and functionally active in human distal lung epithelial cells. Immunoblots followed by densitometric analysis of samples from three donors showed a significant increase in MRP1 protein abundance upon differentiation of freshly isolated human AT2 cells into an AT1-like phenotype (**Figures 1B,C**). Likewise, MRP1 abundance was significantly lower in cells cultured in the presence of KGF and retaining their AT2 characteristics than in cells differentiated into AT1-like phenotype in the absence of the growth factor (**Figures 1D,E**). Similar results have previously been reported by Patel et al. (2008) in rat alveolar epithelial cells in primary culture. However, q-PCR analysis of *ABCC1* mRNA showed similar expression levels in AT2 cells and those differentiated into an AT1-like phenotype (**Figure 1A**). In fact, mRNA levels do not always strongly correlate with protein abundance due to distinct regulation controls at different stages and existence of numerous biological mechanisms that decouples gene level from protein level (Vogel and Marcotte, 2012; Fortelny et al., 2017).

Consistent with data previously reported in other lung epithelial cells (Bréchot et al., 1998; Hamilton et al., 2001), the subcellular localization experiments confirmed the transporter to be expressed primarily in the basolateral membranes of polarized AT1-like cells (**Figure 1G**, 2A lower panel). In NCI-H441 cells, MRP1/*ABCC1* expression was stable across several passage numbers. Moreover, the protein level and the subcellular localization of the transporter were comparable to human primary AT1-like cells (**Figures 3A–G**, 2A upper panel).

On a functional level, *in vitro* MRP1 activity data were also comparable between NCI-H441 cells and human AT1-like cells. Bidirectional CF efflux studies were consistent with a basolateral localization of the transporter in both cell types and the majority of substrate was effluxed into the basolateral receiver compartment. This efflux was sensitive to inhibition by MK-571 (**Figures 2B,C**). Small amounts of CF were also found in the apical compartment in both cell models, which may be due to paracellular transport of CF from the basolateral to the apical compartment. In addition, CF is a pan-MRP substrate and therefore a contribution of apically localized MRP2 and/or MRP4 to substrate efflux is conceivable as low *ABCC2* and *ABCC4* mRNA levels were reported previously in AT1-like cells (Endter et al., 2009). Bidirectional CF transport data were, again, comparable between human AT1-like and NCI-H441 cells. Consistent with basolateral localization of MRP1, MK-571 sensitive, net absorption of CF was observed in both cell models (**Figure 4**).

Multidrug resistance-associated protein-1, among other ABC transporters, plays a key role in the disposition of a wide variety of chemically unrelated drugs across various cellular and tissue barriers (Szakács et al., 2008). The transporter can, therefore, influence the pharmacokinetic profile and result in drug–drug interactions and modulation of pharmacologic activity of its drug substrates (Szakács et al., 2008; Marquez and Van Bambeke, 2011). The broad substrate spectrum together with the high abundance and functional activity of MRP1 observed at the alveolar epithelial barrier in our study suggest a potential role for the transporter in the pulmonary disposition of inhaled drug substrates. This is further supported by a recent *in vivo* study from our group in which profound differences in the pulmonary distribution and elimination kinetics of the MRP1 substrate [^{11}C]MPG were observed with PET imaging between wild type and $Abcc1^{(-/-)}$ rats following intratracheal aerosolisation of the radiotracer (Mairinger et al., 2020). In addition, a number of inhaled drugs have previously been reported to modulate MRP1 activity in the immortalized 16HBE14o- human bronchial cell line *in vitro* (van der Deen et al., 2008). Thus, we studied the potential interaction of a set of inhaled drugs with MRP1 in distal lung epithelial cells. Experiments carried out in human AT1-like and NCI-H441 monolayers showed a significant decrease of CF efflux in the presence of budesonide, beclomethasone dipropionate and salbutamol sulfate (**Table 1** and **Figure 5A**). Similar findings were reported with budesonide in previous studies performed on the 16HBE14o- (van der Deen et al., 2008) and the Calu-1 (Bandi and Kompella, 2002) epithelial cell lines. To determine whether the observed effect is attributed to a reduction of MRP1 protein levels, NCI-H441 cells were grown in the presence or absence of budesonide and salbutamol sulfate for up to 6 days. Immunoblot analysis showed no change in the transporter protein level suggesting that inhaled drugs above are either inhibitors or substrates of MRP1 (i.e., competing with CF). Due to complexity of lung anatomy, determination of clinically achievable concentrations of inhaled drugs in the lung fluid and epithelial cells is extremely challenging (van der Deen et al., 2008; Mukherjee et al., 2012). Thus, the concentrations applied in our study were mainly based on

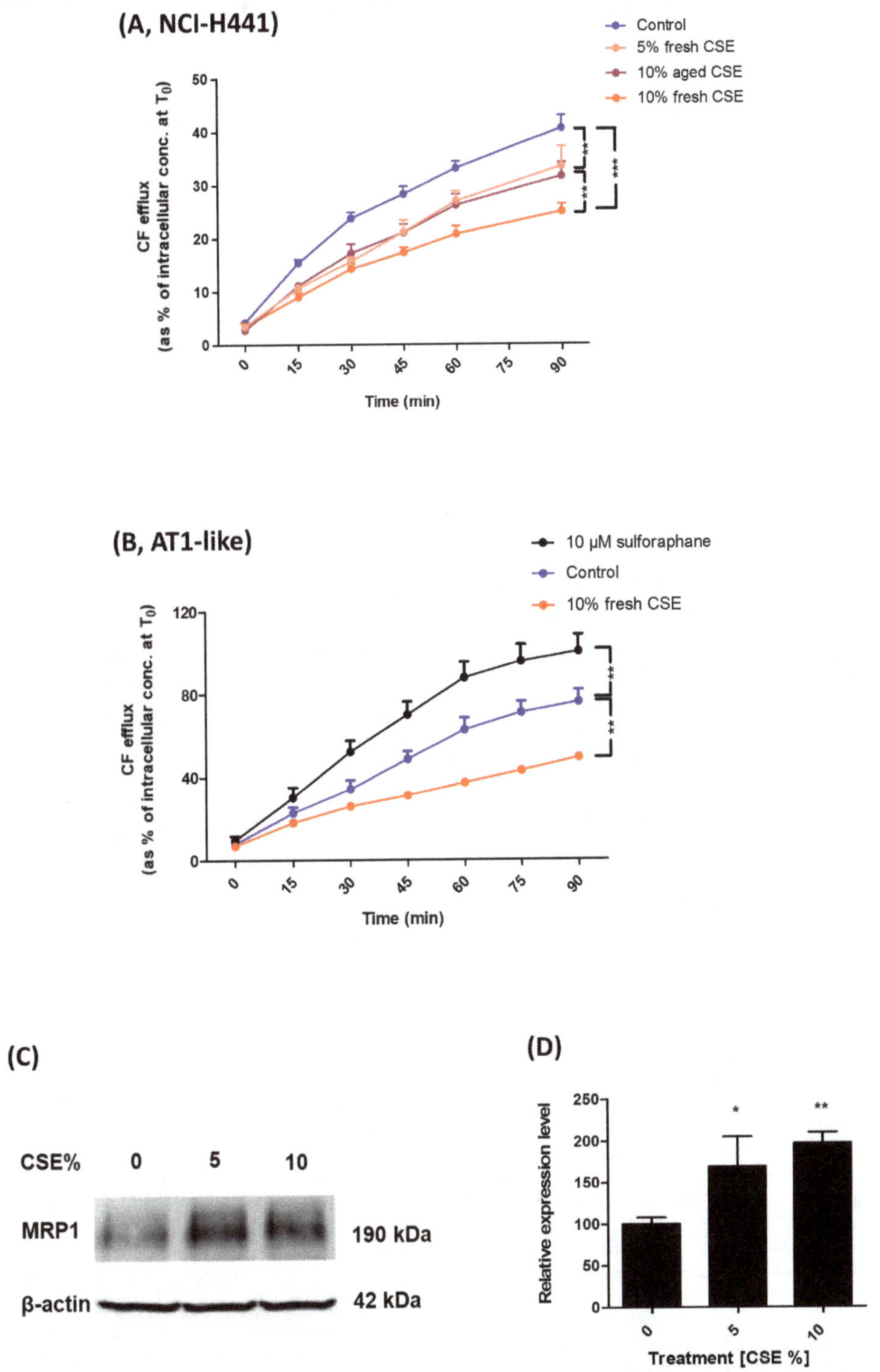

FIGURE 6 | Effect of cigarette smoke extract (CSE) and sulforaphane on multidrug resistance-associated protein-1 (MRP1) activity and abundance. Exposing NCI-H441 **(A)** and alveolar type 1-like (AT1-like) **(B)** cells to CSE for 24 h results in a significant and dose-dependent reduction of MRP1-mediated carboxyfluorescein (CF) efflux from both cell types. **(C,D)** Immunoblot analysis of NCI-H441 cells exposed to CSE show a dose-dependent increase in MRP1 abundance. Data are represented as means + SD, $n \geq 3$, $^{*}P \leq 0.05$, $^{**}P \leq 0.01$, $^{***}P \leq 0.001$. One-way ANOVA followed by Bonferroni's *post hoc* comparisons test was used.

previous *in vitro* studies (van der Deen et al., 2008; Mukherjee et al., 2012; Salomon et al., 2012). Reduced MRP1 activity observed with inhaled drug substrates may be a source of drug–drug interaction and variability in drug pharmacokinetics and could ultimately influence the safety and therapeutic efficacy of inhaled drugs.

Previous reports have suggested a potential role for MRP1 in smoking-related lung function loss and development of COPD. Reduced MRP1 protein levels were observed in lung tissue of COPD patients (van der Deen et al., 2006) and in an experimental rat model of COPD (Wu et al., 2019) using immunohistochemistry analysis. Moreover, the pulmonary clearance of inhaled [^{99m}Tc] methoxyisobutyl isonitrile ([^{99m}Tc] sestamibi), a radiolabeled MRP1 substrate, has been recorded to decrease in smokers and the decrement was attributed to modulation in MRP1 activity and expression profile (Mohan et al., 2019). The distal lung epithelium has been reported to be the initial site of development of tobacco smoke-induced diseases such as COPD (Baskoro et al., 2018). Thus, we investigated the potential impact of CSE on MRP1 activity and/or abundance in human AT1-like and NCI-H441 cells. Results showed a dose dependent reduction in CF efflux from monolayers of both cell types (**Figures 6A,B**). Immunoblot analysis, however, showed a dose dependent increase in MRP1 protein level upon exposure to CSE (**Figures 6C,D**). Given the protective role of MRP1 by extruding a variety of toxic xenobiotics out of lung epithelial cells, reduced MRP1 activity induced by CSE itself or inhaled drugs could further worsen the damage induced by tobacco smoke and may have a negative impact on the incidence and/or progression of COPD. The Nrf2-ARE pathway has been previously suggested to play a role in regulation of MRP1 expression (Ji et al., 2013). Therefore, we investigated whether the Nrf2 stimulator, sulforaphane, can improve MRP1 activity in distal lung epithelial cells. The compound had a positive impact on MRP1 activity in human AT1-like cells but not in NCI-H441 cells implying a possible beneficial effect in reversing the negative effect of CSE on MRP1 activity. The difference in response between both cell types could be, theoretically, attributed to differences in Nrf2-ARE pathway activity which requires further investigations.

CONCLUSION

Multidrug resistance-associated protein-1 is functionally expressed at high levels to the basolateral membranes of human alveolar AT1-like cells in primary culture. The expression and activity profile of the transporter in NCI-H441 cells and AT1-like cells are similar and thus the cell line can be used as an *in vitro* model to study MRP1 in the distal lung epithelial barrier. Furthermore, tobacco smoke, inhaled drugs and sulforaphane can modulate MRP1 activity and/or abundance in distal lung epithelial cells *in vitro*, implying the transporter could be a novel therapeutic target of COPD.

AUTHOR CONTRIBUTIONS

CE, MS, OL, and SN: conceptualization. MS, JS, SN, and CE: data analysis. OL, CE, CC, and MS: funding acquisition. MS, A-SD, LS, VZ, JS, CC, HH, NS-D, and SN: investigation. MS and CE: project administration. HH, NS-D, and C-ML: resources. MS, SN, and CE: supervision. MS and CE: original draft. MS, A-SD, LS, VZ, JS, CC, C-ML, SN, OL, and CE: manuscript review and editing. All authors contributed to the article and approved the submitted version.

ACKNOWLEDGMENTS

The authors would like to acknowledge the contribution of the COST Actions BM1201 and MP1404.

REFERENCES

Bandi, N., and Kompella, U. B. (2002). Budesonide reduces multidrug resistance-associated protein 1 expression in an airway epithelial cell line (Calu-1). *Eur. J. Pharmacol.* 437, 9–17. doi: 10.1016/s0014-2999(02)01267-0

Baskoro, H., Sato, T., Karasutani, K., Suzuki, Y., Mitsui, A., Arano, N., et al. (2018). Regional heterogeneity in response of airway epithelial cells to cigarette smoke. *BMC Pulm. Med.* 18:148. doi: 10.1186/s12890-018-0715-714

Bréchot, J. M., Hurbain, I., Fajac, A., Daty, N., and Bernaudin, J. F. (1998). Different pattern of MRP localization in ciliated and basal cells from human bronchial epithelium. *J. Histochem. Cytochem.* 46, 513–517. doi: 10.1177/002215549804600411

Budulac, S. E., Postma, D. S., Hiemstra, P. S., Kunz, L. I., Siedlinski, M., Smit, H. A., et al. (2010). Multidrug resistance-associated protein-1 (MRP1) genetic variants, MRP1 protein levels and severity of COPD. *Respir. Res.* 11:60. doi: 10.1186/1465-9921-11-60

Cole, S. P. (2014a). Multidrug resistance protein 1 (MRP1, ABCC1), a "multitasking". ATP-binding cassette (ABC) transporter. *J. Biol. Chem.* 289, 30880–30888. doi: 10.1074/jbc.R114.609248

Cole, S. P. (2014b). Targeting multidrug resistance protein 1 (MRP1, ABCC1): past, present, and future. *Annu. Rev. Pharmacol. Toxicol.* 54, 95–117. doi: 10.1146/annurev-pharmtox-011613-135959

Cole, S. P., and Deeley, R. G. (2006). Transport of glutathione and glutathione conjugates by MRP1. *Trends Pharmacol. Sci.* 27, 438–446. doi: 10.1016/j.tips.2006.06.008

Daum, N., Kuehn, A., Hein, S., Schaefer, U. F., Huwer, H., and Lehr, C. M. (2012). Isolation, cultivation, and application of human alveolar epithelial cells. *Methods Mol. Biol.* 806, 31–42. doi: 10.1007/978-1-61779-367-7_3

Demling, N., Ehrhardt, C., Kasper, M., Laue, M., Knels, L., and Rieber, E. P. (2006). Promotion of cell adherence and spreading: a novel function of RAGE, the highly selective differentiation marker of human alveolar epithelial type I cells. *Cell Tissue Res.* 323, 475–488. doi: 10.1007/s00441-005-0069-60

Endter, S., Francombe, D., Ehrhardt, C., and Gumbleton, M. (2009). RT-PCR analysis of ABC, SLC and SLCO drug transporters in human lung epithelial cell models. *J. Pharm. Pharmacol.* 61, 583–591. doi: 10.1211/jpp/61.05.0006

Flens, M. J., Zaman, G. J., van der Valk, P., Izquierdo, M. A., Schroeijers, A. B., Scheffer, G. L., et al. (1996). Tissue distribution of the multidrug resistance protein. *Am. J. Pathol.* 148, 1237–1247.

Fortelny, N., Overall, C. M., Pavlidis, P., and Freue, G. V. C. (2017). Can we predict protein from mRNA levels? *Nature* 547, E19–E20. doi: 10.1038/nature22293

Hamilton, K. O., Topp, E., Makagiansar, I., Siahaan, T., Yazdanian, M., and Audus, K. L. (2001). Multidrug resistance-associated protein-1 functional activity in Calu-3 cells. *J. Pharmacol. Exp. Ther.* 298, 1199–1205.

Ji, L., Li, H., Gao, P., Shang, G., Zhang, D. D., Zhang, N., et al. (2013). Nrf2 pathway regulates multidrug-resistance-associated protein 1 in small cell lung cancer. *PLoS One* 8:e63404. doi: 10.1371/journal.pone.0063404

Lehmann, T., Köhler, C., Weidauer, E., Taege, C., and Foth, H. (2001).). Expression of MRP1 and related transporters in human lung cells in culture. *Toxicology* 167, 59–72. doi: 10.1016/s0300-483x(01)00458-9

Mairinger, S., Sake, J. A., Hernandez Lozano, I., Filip, T., Sauberer, M., Stanek, J., et al. (2020). Assessing the activity of multidrug resistance-associated protein 1 at the lung epithelial barrier. *J. Nucl. Med.* (in press). doi: 10.2967/jnumed.120.244038

Marquez, B., and Van Bambeke, F. (2011). ABC multidrug transporters: target for modulation of drug pharmacokinetics and drug-drug interactions. *Curr. Drug Targets* 12, 600–620. doi: 10.2174/138945011795378504

Mohan, H. K., Livieratos, L., and Peters, A. M. (2019). Lung clearance of inhaled aerosol of Tc-99m-methoxyisobutyl isonitrile: relationships with cigarette smoking, age and gender. *Clin. Physiol. Funct. Imaging* 39, 236–239. doi: 10.1111/cpf.12562

Mukherjee, M., Pritchard, D. I., and Bosquillon, C. (2012). Evaluation of air-interfaced Calu-3 cell layers for investigation of inhaled drug interactions with organic cation transporters in vitro. *Int. J. Pharm.* 426, 7–14. doi: 10.1016/j.ijpharm.2011.12.036

Nickel, S., Clerkin, C. G., Selo, M. A., and Ehrhardt, C. (2016). Transport mechanisms at the pulmonary mucosa: implications for drug delivery. *Expert Opin. Drug Deliv.* 13, 667–690. doi: 10.1517/17425247.2016.1140144

Nickel, S., Selo, M. A., Fallack, J., Clerkin, C. G., Huwer, H., Schneider-Daum, N., et al. (2017). Expression and activity of breast cancer resistance protein (BCRP/ABCG2) in human distal lung epithelial cells in vitro. *Pharm. Res.* 34, 2477–2487. doi: 10.1007/s11095-017-2172-9

Patel, L. N., Uchiyama, T., Kim, K. J., Borok, Z., Crandall, E. D., Shen, W. C., et al. (2008). Molecular and functional expression of multidrug resistance-associated protein-1 in primary cultured rat alveolar epithelial cells. *J. Pharm. Sci.* 97, 2340–2349. doi: 10.1002/jps.21134

Sakamoto, A., Matsumaru, T., Yamamura, N., Uchida, Y., Tachikawa, M., Ohtsuki, S., et al. (2013). Quantitative expression of human drug transporter proteins in lung tissues: analysis of regional, gender, and interindividual differences by liquid chromatography-tandem mass spectrometry. *J. Pharm. Sci.* 102, 3395–3406. doi: 10.1002/jps.23606

Salomon, J. J., Endter, S., Tachon, G., Falson, F., Buckley, S. T., and Ehrhardt, C. (2012). Transport of the fluorescent organic cation 4-(4-(dimethylamino)styryl)-N-methylpyridinium iodide (ASP+) in human respiratory epithelial cells. *Eur. J. Pharm. Biopharm.* 81, 351–359. doi: 10.1016/j.ejpb.2012.03.001

Salomon, J. J., Gausterer, J. C., Selo, M. A., Hosoya, K. I., Huwer, H., Schneider-Daum, N., et al. (2019). OCTN2-mediated acetyl-l-carnitine transport in human pulmonary epithelial cells in vitro. *Pharmaceutics* 11:396. doi: 10.3390/pharmaceutics11080396

Salomon, J. J., Muchitsch, V. E., Gausterer, J. C., Schwagerus, E., Huwer, H., Daum, N., et al. (2014). The cell line NCl-H441 is a useful in vitro model for transport studies of human distal lung epithelial barrier. *Mol. Pharm.* 11, 995–1006. doi: 10.1021/mp4006535

Scheffer, G. L., Pijnenborg, A. C., Smit, E. F., Muller, M., Postma, D. S., Timens, W., et al. (2002). Multidrug resistance related molecules in human and murine lung. *J. Clin. Pathol.* 55, 332–339. doi: 10.1136/jcp.55.5.332

Schwagerus, E., Sladek, S., Buckley, S. T., Armas-Capote, N., Alvarez de la Rosa, D., Harvey, B. J., et al. (2015). Expression and function of the epithelial sodium channel delta-subunit in human respiratory epithelial cells in vitro. *Pflugers. Arch.* 467, 2257–2273. doi: 10.1007/s00424-015-1693-1695

Szakács, G., Váradi, A., Ozvegy-Laczka, C., and Sarkadi, B. (2008). The role of ABC transporters in drug absorption, distribution, metabolism, excretion and toxicity (ADME-Tox). *Drug Discov. Today* 13, 379–393. doi: 10.1016/j.drudis.2007.12.010

van der Deen, M., de Vries, E. G., Visserman, H., Zandbergen, W., Postma, D. S., Timens, W., et al. (2007). Cigarette smoke extract affects functional activity of MRP1 in bronchial epithelial cells. *J. Biochem. Mol. Toxicol.* 21, 243–251. doi: 10.1002/jbt.20187

van der Deen, M., Homan, S., Timmer-Bosscha, H., Scheper, R. J., Timens, W., Postma, D. S., et al. (2008). Effect of COPD treatments on MRP1-mediated transport in bronchial epithelial cells. *Int. J. Chron. Obstruct. Pulmon. Dis.* 3, 469–475. doi: 10.2147/copd.s2817

van der Deen, M., Marks, H., Willemse, B. W., Postma, D. S., Muller, M., Smit, E. F., et al. (2006). Diminished expression of multidrug resistance-associated protein 1 (MRP1) in bronchial epithelium of COPD patients. *Virchows Arch.* 449, 682–688. doi: 10.1007/s00428-006-0240-243

Vogel, C., and Marcotte, E. M. (2012). Insights into the regulation of protein abundance from proteomic and transcriptomic analyses. *Nat. Rev. Genet.* 13, 227–232. doi: 10.1038/nrg3185

Wioland, M. A., Fleury-Feith, J., Corlieu, P., Commo, F., Monceaux, G., Lacau-St-Guily, J., et al. (2000). CFTR, MDR1, and MRP1 immunolocalization in normal human nasal respiratory mucosa. *J. Histochem. Cytochem.* 48, 1215–1222. doi: 10.1177/002215540004800905

Wu, J., Wang, X., Yao, Z., Wu, Q., Fang, W., Li, Z., et al. (2019). Allyl isothiocyanate may reverse the expression of MRP1 in COPD rats via the Notch1 signaling pathway. *Arch. Pharm. Res* 42, 1000–1011. doi: 10.1007/s12272-019-01183-1184

18

The Fundamentals of Respiratory Physiology to Manage the COVID-19 Pandemic

*Edem Allado[1,2], Mathias Poussel[1,2], Simon Valentin[1,3], Antoine Kimmoun[4,5], Bruno Levy[4,5], Duc Trung Nguyen[6,7], Cécile Rumeau[1,6] and Bruno Chenuel[1,2]**

[1]EA 3450 DevAH-Développement, Adaptation et Handicap, Régulations cardio-respiratoires et de la motricité, Université de Lorraine, Nancy, France, [2]Explorations Fonctionnelles Respiratoires et de l'Aptitude à l'Exercice, Centre Universitaire de Médecine du Sport et Activité Physique Adaptée, CHRU-Nancy, Nancy, France, [3]Département de Pneumologie, CHRU-Nancy, Nancy, France, [4]Médecine Intensive et Réanimation Brabois, CHRU-Nancy, Nancy, France, [5]INSERM U1116, Université de Lorraine, Nancy, France, [6]ORL et Chirurgie Cervico-Faciale, CHRU-Nancy, Nancy, France, [7]INSERM U1254-IADI, Université de Lorraine, Nancy, France

***Correspondence:**
Bruno Chenuel
b.chenuel@chru-nancy.fr

The growing coronavirus disease (COVID-19) crisis has stressed worldwide healthcare systems probably as never before, requiring a tremendous increase of the capacity of intensive care units to handle the sharp rise of patients in critical situation. Since the dominant respiratory feature of COVID-19 is worsening arterial hypoxemia, eventually leading to acute respiratory distress syndrome (ARDS) promptly needing mechanical ventilation, a systematic recourse to intubation of every hypoxemic patient may be difficult to sustain in such peculiar context and may not be deemed appropriate for all patients. Then, it is essential that caregivers have a solid knowledge of physiological principles to properly interpret arterial oxygenation, to intubate at the satisfactory moment, to adequately manage mechanical ventilation, and, finally, to initiate ventilator weaning, as safely and as expeditiously as possible, in order to make it available for the next patient. Through the expected mechanisms of COVID-19-induced hypoxemia, as well as the notion of silent hypoxemia often evoked in COVID-19 lung injury and its potential parallelism with high altitude pulmonary edema, from the description of hemoglobin oxygen affinity in patients with severe COVID-19 to the interest of the prone positioning in order to treat severe ARDS patients, this review aims to help caregivers from any specialty to handle respiratory support following recent knowledge in the pathophysiology of respiratory SARS-CoV-2 infection.

Keywords: coronavirus disease-19, respiratory physiology, control of breathing, hypoxemia, respiratory failure

INTRODUCTION

The growing coronavirus disease (COVID-19) crisis has stressed worldwide healthcare systems probably as never before, requiring a tremendous increase of the capacity of intensive care units to handle the sudden increase of patients in critical status. In many countries, innovative solutions have been found to change the routine hospital organization and cope with limited resources, leading to massive task-shifting with suspension of elective medical and surgical procedures and reassignment of volunteers (Aziz et al., 2020; Meschi et al., 2020; Xie et al., 2020b). If lung infection resulting from severe acute respiratory syndrome coronavirus 2 (SARS-CoV-2) has been shown to encompass various clinical features, the most serious presentation is worsening arterial hypoxemia, eventually leading to acute respiratory distress syndrome (ARDS) promptly needing mechanical ventilation (Guan et al., 2020; Wu and McGoogan, 2020). The systematic recourse to intubation of every patient suffering from hypoxemia may be difficult to sustain and may not be deemed appropriate for all patients. Then, it is essential that caregivers have solid knowledge of physiological principles to properly interpret arterial oxygenation, to intubate at the satisfactory moment, to adequately manage mechanical ventilation, and, finally, to begin weaning from the ventilator, as safely and as expeditiously as possible, in order to make it available for the next patient.

COVID-19-RELATED HYPOXEMIA, INTERPRETATION OF BLOOD OXYGEN LEVELS, AND THE CONCEPT OF "SILENT HYPOXEMIA"

COVID-19-Related Hypoxemia and Suspected Physiopathological Mechanisms

Hypoxemia is a defining feature of COVID-19. Viral respiratory infection has been shown to cause interstitial pneumonia, leading to a reduction in lung capacity and evolving in some patients to ARDS and respiratory failure. The typical imaging characteristics of COVID-19 pneumonia are non-specific, including peripheral ground-glass opacities with or without consolidation (Bernheim et al., 2020; Lang et al., 2020). They reflect diffuse alveolar injury associated to interstitial thickening, greatly altering gas exchange. In that context, four basic mechanisms of hypoxemia can be discussed: hypoventilation, diffusion impairment, shunt (i.e., hypoventilated areas of the lung are hyperemic), and ventilation-perfusion inequality. However, the most important cause by far is ventilation-perfusion mismatch, resulting from blood perfusing lung regions that have either limited or no ventilation [i.e., regions with low ventilation-perfusion ratios $\dot{V}_A/\dot{Q}$ ratios) or intraparenchymal shunt, respectively], as Gattinoni et al. have reported in their cohort of COVID-19 patients with ARDS (Gattinoni et al., 2020c). They observed a shunt fraction around ~0.5 [i.e., venous to arterial shunt estimated by the shunted blood flow/total blood flow ratio ($\dot{Q}_s/\dot{Q}_T$ ratio) of 50%] and a large alveolar-to-arterial oxygen gradient (P_AO_2-P_aO_2 gradient), enhanced by impaired hypoxic vasoconstriction (Gattinoni et al., 2020c). In addition, COVID-19 is often associated to coagulopathy, providing microemboli which could divert lung perfusion to regions with low $\dot{V}_A/\dot{Q}$ ratios (Altemeier et al., 1998; Connors and Levy, 2020). Two major different phenotypes of COVID-19-associated ARDS have been described and probably involve different pathophysiological mechanisms: COVID-19 pneumonia type L depicted by high compliance (i.e., low elastance), low ventilation-to-perfusion ratio, and low recruitability, and COVID-19 pneumonia type H characterized by low compliance (i.e., high elastance), high right-to-left shunt (i.e., the hypoventilated areas of the lung are hyperemic), and high recruitability, analogous to what is experienced in common acute respiratory distress (Gattinoni et al., 2020a).

Therefore, in addition to the CT scan evaluation, the response to oxygen therapy can be helpful to distinguish the two phenotypes. The delivery of raised FIO_2 would increase PaO_2 and oxygen saturation in the L phenotype when ventilation-to-perfusion ratio mismatch drives hypoxia, avoiding or delaying the recourse to intubation and mechanical ventilation with satisfactory levels of arterial oxygenation by oxygen therapy. At the opposite, when hypoxia is mainly determined by a shunt, in H phenotype, a modest enhancement in oxygen saturation is expected by the delivery of high FIO_2, often requiring earlier invasive ventilator assistance (Gattinoni et al., 2020a).

The underlying physiopathology has not been fully elucidated but partly due to the SARS-CoV-2 infecting the host recognizing the angiotensin-converting enzyme 2 (ACE-2) receptor as a specific target (Hoffmann et al., 2020; Lu et al., 2020). It is a membrane-bound aminopeptidase expressed on many human cells (respiratory tract, lung, heart, arteries, veins, kidney, and intestines; Hamming et al., 2004). More particularly, the ACE-2 receptor is located in alveolar epithelial cells and vascular endothelium, and when SARS-CoV-2 binds to it, a reduction in intracellular ACE-2 protein activity is provided, resulting in a marked immune response with hyperinflammatory syndrome and widespread endothelial dysfunction (Connors and Levy, 2020; Mehta et al., 2020; Polidoro et al., 2020; Zhang et al., 2020). Physiologically, ACE-2 is a vasodepressor, at the opposite of the homologous enzyme ACE-1 acting as a vasoconstrictor, and both proteins form the oxygen-sensitive renin-angiotensin system (Hampl et al., 2015). Histopathologically, recent works have emphasized the development of alveolar and interstitial exudative inflammation characterized by macrophage and monocyte predominance and associated to focal respiratory epithelial desquamation, hemorrhage, and type 2 pneumocyte proliferation (Tian et al., 2020; Xu et al., 2020).

Hypoxemia has been shown to be an independent prognostic factor for the severe form of COVID-19 (Wei et al., 2020) and associated with in-hospital mortality (Xie et al., 2020a).

Interpretation of Blood Oxygenation From Pulse Oximetry, Caution, and Limits

The assessment of oxygen saturation in the arterial blood by pulse oximetry should be carefully interpreted. Indeed pulse oximetry provides an estimate of the arterial oxygen saturation (SpO_2) and is not a direct measurement, as CO-oximeters are able to do (SaO_2). By definition, oxygen saturation is the percentage of hemoglobin-binding sites occupied by oxygen, varying according to the arterial PO_2, as stipulated by the oxyhemoglobin dissociation curve. The difference between the two methods is not negligible, reaching as much as ±4% (Tobin, 1990).

The peculiar sigmoidal shape of the oxyhemoglobin dissociation curve involves several important features. In the higher range of partial pressures, the upper part of the curve is flat, impeding a significant decline in oxygen saturation when PO_2 starts to drop. In contrast, the steeper portion of the dissociation curve markedly enhances the carriage of oxygen in the lungs (on-loading) and oxygen delivery to the tissues (off-loading). As lung injury progresses, leading to further impairment of gas exchange, PO_2 may fall on the steep part of the dissociation curve (from 20 to 60 mmHg), allowing noticeable changes in the measured oxygen saturation with small changes in PO_2. In this context, the natural variability of ventilation due to physiological acts as talking, laughing, or breath holding may change the alveolar PO_2, thereby inducing similar variations in PaO_2. Then, oxygen saturation monitoring should be observed for at least several minutes. Moreover, the position of the dissociation curve itself can be modified by the patient's acid-base status. Acidemia shifts it rightward and alkalemia in the opposite way. In the early course of COVID-19 pneumonia, numerous patients begin to hyperventilate in order to compensate for their collapsing PaO_2. The hyperventilation consequently generates a respiratory alkalosis, shifting the dissociation curve to the left (increasing hemoglobin's oxygen affinity to facilitate oxygen loading) such that the predictable decrease in oxygen saturation with a falling PaO_2 will be dampened and, in some cases, prevented (Hamilton et al., 2004). In addition, with respect to the alveolar gas equation, the decreased alveolar CO_2 partial pressure ($PACO_2$) will lead to a comparable increase in alveolar oxygen partial pressure (PAO_2). These combined mechanisms are able to improve SaO_2 in hypocapnic hypoxic stimulation compared with an isocapnic or hypercapnic hypoxia. In contrast, a right shift in oxygen dissociation (decreasing hemoglobin's oxygen affinity to facilitate oxygen unloading) is expected with fever, an obvious clinical feature in COVID-19, leading to noticeable desaturation without any change in the chemosensitive drive of breathing.

Some important practical limits of pulse oximetry also need to be known. Movements of the digits (shivering patient, for example), avoiding to identify an adequate pulse signal, or bright artificial light as observed in an operating room can induce false low readings (Schnapp and Cohen, 1990; Sinex, 1999).

The pulse oximeter uses two different wavelengths to estimate oxygen saturation, generated by two light-emitting diodes, but both wavelengths of light are similarly absorbed by hemoglobin in arterial blood, capillary, venous blood, and other soft tissues. Then, it is necessary to distinguish the pulsatile signal of arterial blood flow in order to limit the signal-to-noise ratio and dispense a valid result (Sinex, 1999). Therefore, factors that are able to limit pulsatile blood flow in the digits, such as hypotension and use of vasoconstrictor agent as well as the presence of peripheral vascular disease or Raynaud's phenomenon, may worsen the signal-to-noise ratio, resulting in an inaccurate estimation of arterial oxygen saturation. Chilblains have been increasingly recognized in association with COVID-19 (Bouaziz et al., 2020; Gottlieb and Long, 2020; Tosti et al., 2020), and peripheral vascular disease has been found to be associated with the usual comorbidities in patients suffering from severe COVID-19, such as diabetes and coronary artery disease (Du et al., 2020; Wu and McGoogan, 2020). It is also important to know that pulse oximeters dispense misleading results in front of either carboxyhemoglobinemia or methemoglobinemia since they are not able to distinguish these dyshemoglobinemias from oxygenated and deoxygenated hemoglobin. If carboxyhemoglobinemia is involved in heavy smokers or individuals using grills or heaters in enclosed spaces, it has been demonstrated that methemoglobinemia can result from the use of some drugs, including chloroquine (Rizvi et al., 2012).

Other important sources of artifact need to be cited, such as nail polish and increased skin pigmentation, especially if the real oxygen saturation is diminished (Bickler et al., 2005; Sutcu Cicek et al., 2011).

Furthermore, it has been demonstrated that large SpO_2 to SaO_2 differences exist in patients in critical condition with mediocre reproducibility of SpO_2, specifically in shocked patients with low cardiac output or under high doses of vasopressor. In hemodynamically unstable patients, the detection limit of the sensor is most often exceeded (Van de Louw et al., 2001).

In addition to interpretation of blood oxygenation by pulse oximetry, to correctly assess the real efficacy of pulmonary gas exchange, it is required to know the fraction of inspired oxygen (FIO_2) in order to adequately calculate the P_AO_2-P_aO_2 gradient using the alveolar gas equation (cf. **Figure 1**). Then, if interpretation of blood oxygenation with supplemental oxygen is straightforward when a patient is breathing room air or is intubated, it is clearly problematic when a nasal cannula is used to deliver oxygen since the inspiratory fraction of oxygen is difficult to estimate. For example, depending on the effective patient's minute ventilation (more specifically tidal volume patient's demand), when a nasal cannula or a face mask is used to deliver pure oxygen flow rate at 2 l/min, FIO_2 can vary from 24 to 35% (Bazuaye et al., 1992). Therefore, the severity of hypoxemia cannot be assessed by the level of supplemental oxygen delivery. In practice, peculiar attention on the level of gas exchange impairment is recommended when high F_iO_2 is used to treat hypoxemia according to a simple target level on pulse oximetry, given the flatness of the upper portion of the dissociation curve (Bickler et al., 2017).

A synthesis is proposed in **Figure 2** in order to present a practical assessment of blood oxygenation using pulse oximetry and limitations.

Concept of "Silent Hypoxemia"

In one of the first largest studies on the clinical characteristics of coronavirus in China, shortness of breath has been reported in only 18.7% of 1,099 hospitalized patients with COVID-19 pneumonia, despite hypoxemia commonly requiring supplemental oxygen (41%) and abnormal results on CT scans (86.2%; Guan et al., 2020). Numerous reports worldwide have described a subset of patients with severe hypoxemia presenting no obvious respiratory difficulties or dyspnea, leading to abundant coverage in media with sensational headlines such as "happy hypoxia" or, more conventionally, "silent hypoxemia" (Couzin-Frankel, 2020; Levitan, 2020; Tobin et al., 2020b). However, in contrast to media's assertion, this questioning discrepancy is not really defying biology since fundamentals in respiratory physiology can account for most of it, with the specific effect of SARS-CoV-2 on control of breathing or chemoreceptors excepted.

Then, knowledge of the putative mechanisms involved in the genesis of dyspnea, basics of control of breathing, ventilatory response to hypoxia, and the role of PCO_2 is necessary to address the mystery.

Alveolar gas equation:

$$PA_{O_2} = PI_{O_2} - \frac{PA_{CO_2}}{R} + \left[PA_{CO_2} \cdot FI_{O_2} \cdot \frac{1 - R}{R} \right]$$

Where PA_{O2} = alveolar partial pressure of oxygen, PI_{O2} = Inspired partial pressure of oxygen, PA_{CO2}= alveolar partial pressure of CO_2, FI_{O2}= inspired fraction of oxygen and R = respiratory exchange ratio (from 0.7 to 1).
This is only valid if there is no CO_2 in inspired gas.

The term in square brackets is relatively small and an estimation of PA_{O2} can be provided by the following equation:

$$PA_{O_2} = PI_{O_2} - \frac{Pa_{CO_2}}{0.8}$$

With $PI_{O2}=FI_{O2}.(Patm-PH_2O)$; Patm= atmospheric pressure , PH_2O= water vapour pressure
On room air (FI_{O2} = 0.21, or 21%), at sea level (Patm = 760 mmHg) assuming 100% humidity in the alveoli (PH_2O = 47 mmHg at 37°C).

Alveolar–arterial gradient of oxygen partial pressure:

$$\text{A-a } (P_{O_2}) = PA_{O_2} - Pa_{O_2}$$

FIGURE 1 | Useful toolkit to interpret oxygenation in an appropriate way.

Patient Measurements in practice	Main Conditions limiting PO accuracy
Patient at rest with quiet breathing if possible	Poor perfusion (hypotension, hypovolemic or septic shock, cardiac failure...)
Use the index or middle finger (avoid the ear lobe or toe)	Dyshemoglobinemias (Carbon monoxide poisoning, methemoglobinemia, fetal hemoglobinemia)
Remove fingernail polish if needed	Dark pigmented skin (risk of overestimation of oxygen saturation with values < 80%)
Warm cold fingers	Sickle cell anemia (vasoocclusive crises)
Accept values only if the pulse signal is strong	Severe hyperbilirubinemia (> 30 mg/dL, due to increased heme metabolism (hemolysis) or decreased bilirubin metabolism (liver disease))
Use the most common value on readings for 1 to several minutes	Some drugs (affecting oxygen's affinity for hemoglobin)

FIGURE 2 | Blood oxygenation assessment with pulse oximetry (PO).

Dyspnea and Control of Breathing

Dyspnea is a highly multidimensional subjective experience needing careful assessment. It shows tremendous variability in regards to cultural and linguistic features and affective and cognitive factors (Anonymus, 1999; Parshall et al., 2012). The neurophysiologic mechanisms that give rise to the perception of dyspnea are incompletely understood, but the sensation of dyspnea probably results from a mismatch between efferent motor commands from the central nervous system (CNS) to the respiratory system and afferent sensory inputs (e.g., expected airflow, cage movements) from the respiratory system to the CNS (Adler and Janssens, 2019). It increases as inputs from receptors increase, and the central nervous system perceives that respiratory muscles cannot match the inputs and maintain adequate ventilation (Laviolette et al., 2014).

Chemoreceptors are certainly involved in the sensation of dyspnea, rising respiratory output and subsequently activating respiratory afferences, associated to corollary discharges and direct projections from chemoreceptors to forebrain structures (notably the limbic system, also underlying the genesis of pain sensation; Banzett et al., 2000; Evans et al., 2002; Buchanan and Richerson, 2009). The insular cortex appears to play a crucial role since it has been demonstrated that insular lesions are associated with a blunted perception of dyspnea (Schon et al., 2008).

With the lung injury due to SARS-CoV-2, numerous sources of stimulation of sensory receptors may gather information and feed it to the central controller, from inflammation of the respiratory tract and lungs to hypoxemia, leading to dyspnea (Tobin, 2020). However, the experience of the subjective sensation of breathlessness is not systematic, depending on the patient and circumstances and with great similarity to pain sensation (Lansing et al., 2009).

Ventilatory Response to Hypoxia and Dyspnea

In healthy humans, the ventilatory response to partial pressure of arterial oxygen (PaO_2) is hyperbolic (Rebuck and Campbell, 1974). Reducing the partial pressure of arterial oxygen (PaO_2) from its normal value to 60 mmHg has a marginal effect on pulmonary ventilation ($\dot{V}_E$) and $PaCO_2$ (Forster and Dempsey, 1981). Nevertheless, further reducing PaO_2, from about 60 to 30 mmHg, provides a progressive increase in $\dot{V}_E$ following an exponential pattern (hyperbolic curve) and a decrease in $PaCO_2$ (Forster and Dempsey, 1981). In contrast, the relationship between ventilation and arterial oxygen saturation (SaO_2) is linear (Rebuck and Campbell, 1974). Physiologically, in human subjects, the increase in ventilation occurs primarily because of a rise of tidal volume and only a small increase in the frequency of breathing (Reynolds and Milhorn, 1973; Bender et al., 1987). If tachypnea is one of the most important clinical indicators of respiratory distress, it could be without proportion to severe hypoxemia. Moreover, in COVID-19 patients, tachypnea would be more elicited by stimulation of lung receptors (pulmonary stretch, irritant, and J receptors) due to lung inflammation than by the hypoxic stimulus and therefore would not be the cornerstone of the intubation decision (Tobin, 2020).

It has been demonstrated that the level of hypoxia corresponding to the perception of air hunger in healthy subjects matches with the sharp increase of minute ventilation but far from all the subjects have complained as a strong increase in air hunger with a fall end-tidal oxygen partial pressure below 60 mmHg (Moosavi et al., 2003). Dyspnea often occurs when PaO_2 declines below 40 mmHg (Manning and Schwartzstein, 1995). Like the large variability of the resting respiratory drive, there is a great between-subject and within-subject variability of ventilatory response to hypoxia in healthy subjects (Sahn et al., 1977; Tobin et al., 1988; Matsuzawa et al., 1989). It has been demonstrated that the ventilatory response to hypoxia is decreased by half in elderly healthy people (Kronenberg and Drage, 1973; Peterson et al., 1981). The decrease is even more pronounced in patients suffering from diabetes (Nishimura et al., 1989; Weisbrod et al., 2005), who not only presented an impaired perception of sensory input from organs but also demonstrated an increased threshold for the perception of respiratory sensations has been (O'Donnell et al., 1988). Since diabetes is among the most frequently reported comorbidities and the median age is easily over 60 years in patients infected with COVID-19, it is not so surprising to observe numerous cases of "silent hypoxemia" (Grasselli et al., 2020; Huang et al., 2020; Richardson et al., 2020).

Furthermore, hypoxia is also well known to depress ventilation at the central nervous system level, possibly masking unpleasant sensations (Berry et al., 1989).

Modulation of the Hypoxic Ventilatory Response by CO_2

In the absence of isocapnia, the ventilatory response to hypoxia is severely attenuated by hypocapnia associated with hyperventilation. This attenuation is due to an effect on the peripheral chemoreceptors (carotid body essentially) as well as to reduced drive from the central chemoreceptors (Lahiri and DeLaney, 1975; Fitzgerald and Dehghani, 1982; Moore et al., 1984). It has been demonstrated that moderate hypocapnia, corresponding to $PaCO_2$ values from 5 to 10 mmHg below eucapnia, flattened the hypoxic response, suggesting that a minimum level of CO_2 is required to generate the hypoxic ventilatory response (Jounieaux et al., 2002; Corne et al., 2003; Wilson and Teppema, 2016). In order to elicit a valuable rise in ventilation, severe hypoxia must be associated to baseline $PaCO_2$ that exceeds 39 mmHg (Moosavi et al., 2003). Since hypoventilation is uncommon with COVID-19, hypoxemia accompanied by a normal alveolar-to-arterial oxygen gradient and increase in $PaCO_2$ is highly unlikely, especially in the early phase of lung injury. In the great majority of severe cases, hypoxemia is accompanied by an increased alveolar-to-arterial oxygen gradient reflecting either ventilation-perfusion mismatch or intrapulmonary shunting and the compensatory ventilatory response to hypoxemia, leading to noticeable hypocapnia (Tobin, 2020).

Consequently, knowledge of the accompanying $PaCO_2$ is imperative to assess the severity of the respiratory failure associated to hypoxemia, another reason to claim that isolated monitoring of SaO_2 is insufficient to guide clinical decisions.

Taken together, it would not be so astonishing that many COVID-19 patients face hypoxemia and rapid respiratory failure without evidence of dyspnea.

LESSONS FROM HIGH ALTITUDE AND AVIATION PHYSIOLOGY: ARE THE SIMILARITIES BETWEEN COVID-19 ARDS AND HIGH-ALTITUDE PULMONARY EDEMA RELEVANT?

The common clinical pattern of COVID-19 lung injury is based upon a noticeable imbalance between relatively well-preserved lung compliance and a severely impaired pulmonary gas exchange, resulting in hypoxemia without corresponding signs of dyspnea or respiratory distress. Since the physiological characteristics of the hypocapnic ventilatory response to hypoxia have been extensively investigated in high altitude physiology and aviation medicine, learnings from them could be helpful in order to better manage the COVID-19 pandemic.

Beyond the apparent similarity between the COVID-19 silent hypoxemia and the non-lethal high altitude-induced hypoxemia associated to respiratory alkalosis, even allowing climbers to exercise in ascent despite very low levels of PaO_2, some authors have advocated parallelism between COVID-19 acute respiratory distress syndrome and high-altitude pulmonary edema (HAPE), with great amplification *via* social media (Solaimanzadeh, 2020).

With the first descriptions of the clinical features of severe COVID-19 pneumonia, a debate has emerged on the development of typical ARDS or not, allowing specific and important clinical implications (Gattinoni et al., 2020b,c). Most of the patients with severe COVID-19 pneumonia meet the criteria that define internationally the ARDS [ARDS Berlin definition: acute onset of hypoxemia assessed by the PaO_2/FIO_2 ratio ≤ 300 mmHg in a ventilated patient with a positive end-expiratory pressure (PEEP) of at least 5 cmH_2O and bilateral lung infiltrates not fully explained by heart failure or volume overload (Force et al., 2012)], but unusual presentations exist (Gattinoni et al., 2020b,c). The main difference is relatively well-preserved lung mechanics with maintenance of a relatively high respiratory system compliance (close to the normal value of 50 ml/cm H_2O), in contrast to typical severe ARDS (Gattinoni et al., 2020b,c). For some authors, the hypothesis for such hypoxemia associated to compliant lungs could be a hypoxic vasoconstriction (Gattinoni et al., 2020c). HAPE and ARDS are a non-cardiogenic form of pulmonary edema characterized by diffuse bilateral opacities on chest imaging caused by an imbalance in Starling forces, thus inducing fluid accumulation in the interstitial and alveolar spaces. However, the pathogenesis of such pulmonary edema is radically different between the two entities. HAPE is related to an excessive hypoxia-mediated increase in pulmonary vascular resistance or hypoxic pulmonary vasoconstriction increasing microvascular pressure and leading to a substantial increase in pulmonary artery pressure with overperfusion of some regions of the lung, elevated pulmonary capillary hydrostatic pressure, and leakage of fluid into the alveolar space (Swenson and Bartsch, 2012). Consequently, HAPE is a life-threatening condition that is favorably influenced (often reversed) by oxygen therapy, exposure to hyperbaric environment (using portable hyperbaric chambers), or descent/evacuation to lower altitude and, finally, very unusually needs intensive care (Swenson and Bartsch, 2012; Strapazzon et al., 2020). Since hypoxic vasoconstriction is the fundamental pathogenesis mechanism in HAPE, increasing the alveolar PO_2 decreases pulmonary artery pressure, allowing the resolution of alveolar and interstitial edema and full recovery within hours to a few days of exposure. Distinctly, the underlying pathophysiological mechanisms in ARDS due to COVID-19 involve multi-organ viral-mediated inflammatory responses leading in the lung to genesis of alveolar epithelial inflammation and dysfunction of surfactant and alveolar fluid clearance, finally leading to alveolar collapse and/or filling and marked ventilation-perfusion mismatch (Gattinoni et al., 2020a). Therefore, in marked contrast to HAPE, the delivery of supplemental oxygen in COVID-19 pneumonia may increase oxygen availability but will not be able to counteract the underlying inflammation or lung injury (Luks and Swenson, 2020; Strapazzon et al., 2020). This major distinction has crucial clinical implications since drugs well known to inhibit hypoxic pulmonary vasoconstriction—acetazolamide, systemic vasodilators like calcium channel blockers, or phosphodiesterase-5 inhibitors—are not only inappropriate but also expected to worsen ventilation/perfusion mismatch by raising prefusion blood flow to poorly and/or nonventilated lung regions, exacerbating hypoxemia and provoking hypotension in COVID-19 patients (Archer et al., 2020; Brugger et al., 2020; Luks and Swenson, 2020; Strapazzon et al., 2020).

ON THE INTEREST OF PRONE POSITIONING IN COVID-19 PNEUMONIA, NOT ONLY TO IMPROVE GAS EXCHANGE BUT ALSO AS A STRATEGY TO DELAY OR AVOID MECHANICAL VENTILATION

Prone positioning, i.e., when a patient is repositioned from supine position to lie on their front, has been used for more than 45 years to improve oxygenation in patients with acute respiratory failure and more specifically with ARDS (Guerin, 2014). Historically, in the 1970s, Mellins observed that children suffering from advanced cystic fibrosis spontaneously position themselves on their hands and knees to improve their ventilation, while Bryan hypothesized that, in acute respiratory failure with consequent impairment of functional residual capacity and enhancement of dependent airway closure, the prone position might recruit and stabilize the dependent lung (Bryan, 1974; Mellins, 1974). Since then, numerous randomized controlled trials and meta-analyses have demonstrated a conclusive and important mortality reduction using prone positioning early and for a prolonged time in subjects with severe ARDS (Abroug et al., 2008; Alsaghir and Martin, 2008; Guerin et al., 2013; Beitler et al., 2014; Hu et al., 2014; Lee et al., 2014; Bloomfield et al., 2015; Munshi et al., 2017). Nowadays, prone positioning is used not only as an efficient treatment in case of life-threatening hypoxemia but also in the prevention of ventilatory-induced lung injury (VILI; Chiumello and Brioni, 2016; Guerin, 2017; Mitchell and Seckel, 2018).

The main underlying physiologic mechanism for the ensuing improvement in patients' oxygenation with prone position is the decrease in intrapulmonary shunting, but an improvement of ventilatory mechanics is also involved (Gattinoni et al., 2013; Guerin et al., 2014). Prone positioning provides reduction in intrapulmonary shunt ($\dot{Q}_s/\dot{Q}_T$), variation in lung ventilation ($\dot{V}_A$), and lung perfusion ($\dot{Q}$) distribution with improved $\dot{V}_A/\dot{Q}$ matching. By recruiting dorsal regions which have a larger number of alveolar units and by obtaining an increase in chest wall elastance, better ventilation to the perfused lung is provided, improving the ventilation/perfusion ratio and allowing a more homogeneous distribution of ventilation. This leads to a decrease in lung strain and, consecutively, reduction of VILI, reducing the risk of right heart failure (Gattinoni et al., 2013; Guerin et al., 2014; Ruste et al., 2018). The improvement of oxygenation in ARDS patients during a prone session is observed in ~75% of the cases and sometimes intense (Guerin, 2014). The positive oxygenation response is commonly defined as an improvement in PaO_2 by 20% or an increase in the PaO_2/FIO_2 ratio by 20 mmHg (Guerin, 2014). It has been demonstrated that prone positioning reduced relative shunt fraction by about 30% and improved PaO_2/FIO_2 ratio by 34–62%, with a variable temporal response (from an immediate response to a continued response for up to 24 h; Kallet, 2015; Scholten et al., 2017).

Additional data are also important to note concerning the drainage of secretions which improves when prone, with material in the dorsal lung traveling more easily to open airways. Nevertheless, no significant reduction in the incidence of ventilator-associated pneumonia has been observed in a recent prospective study cohort of patients with severe ARDS (Ayzac et al., 2016). Major improvements in thoraco-abdominal compliance were particularly observed in patients with higher body mass index (Kallet, 2015).

During the COVID-19 pandemic, the use of prone positioning was proposed not only in ARDS patients requiring mechanical ventilation, as it is internationally recommended (Alhazzani et al., 2020; Wilson et al., 2020), but also in order to avoid or delay the recourse to intubation in the dramatic context of limited resources and capacity of intensive care units (Chad and Sampson, 2020; Elharrar et al., 2020; Sartini et al., 2020; Villarreal-Fernandez et al., 2020).

Innovative solutions have been found worldwide to cope with limited resources and to include the prone positioning in the management of patients requiring mechanical ventilation, even at the surge of the outbreak, resulting in the emergence of prone teams (Doussot et al., 2020; Kimmoun et al., 2020; Settembre et al., 2020).

In COVID-19 patients, the Surviving Sepsis campaign recommends a trial of prone positioning in mechanically ventilated patients who meet the moderate-to-severe ARDS definition (Alhazzani et al., 2020). Periods of 12–16 h are suggested, based upon evidence for non-COVID ARDS (Alhazzani et al., 2020).

In conscious non-ventilated COVID-19 patients, it is expected that the underlying mechanism leading to an improvement in oxygenation is analogous, but only few studies evaluated the benefits of the prone position and no clear recommendations have emerged (Elharrar et al., 2020; Sartini et al., 2020). Short-term improvements of oxygenation are observed in such patients, but further studies are needed to clarify the real benefit, particularly on mortality.

PHYSIOLOGICAL BASIS FOR VENTILATORY SUPPORT

If the initial message from the Chinese medical teams at the surge of the outbreak was to intubate early, the current ventilatory approach is to delay intubation if it clinically appears safe and feasible (Alhazzani et al., 2020). Currently, any therapy that could prevent intubation and mechanical ventilation (MV) or enhance MV weaning without further deterioration is welcome. Regrettably, "safe" lung-protective ventilation does not really exist; thus, ventilatory support needs to be individualized as the best compromise among respiratory mechanics, recruitability, gas exchange, and hemodynamics to minimize VILI and to ensure adequate oxygenation when arterial hypoxemia is refractory to oxygen therapy.

The spectrum of therapies and the different lung support which have been proposed to the management of ARDS with critical hypoxemia (i.e., severe ARDS, with PaO_2/FIO_2 <100 mmHg) encompass the delivery of oxygen therapy by high-flow nasal cannula (HFNC) system and non-invasive positive pressure ventilation (NIPPV). In severe COVID-19 patients, these therapies should only be used in selected patients with hypoxemic respiratory failure and who are closely observed for early detection of further deterioration (Pfeifer et al., 2020).

With oxygen flow rates that can reach 60–80 L per minute, HFNC systems can more accordingly ensure the ventilatory demands of patients with respiratory distress and respiratory failure compared to the standard nasal cannula (Suffredini and Allison, 2020). They are able to reduce dead space, raise the end-expiratory lung volume, improve compliance, and reduce the work of breathing, resulting in improvement of pulmonary gas exchange (Suffredini and Allison, 2020). There is limited data to promote or refute the use of HFNC in SARS-CoV-2 and in ARDS patients; the failure rate has been found to be relatively high (Messika et al., 2015). However, it has been proposed to be combined with prone positioning (Colla et al., 2020; Suffredini and Allison, 2020; Villarreal-Fernandez et al., 2020). Decisions to continue HFNC treatment might depend on the results of periodic clinical assessments and repeated biological measurements corroborating clinical stability or improvement (Suffredini and Allison, 2020).

The use of NIPPV with a pressure support tailored to ensure a tidal volume between 7 and 10 ml/kg and a PEEP set between 2 and 10 cm H_2O could also lessen the intrapulmonary shunt and diminish the work of breathing, but just as the HFNC, NIPPV is associated with a high risk of failure and associated risks of a delayed start of invasive mechanical ventilation (Evans, 2001). The clinical result of the use of NIPPV needs to be carefully assessed, and if, following the first few hours, no significant improvement in pulmonary gas exchange is observed, it should be ceased and invasive mechanical ventilation should be initiated (Evans, 2001). More specifically, the magnitude of oxygenation disturbance is a predictor of NIPPV failure, and a PaO_2/FIO_2 ratio <150 mmHg is described as the decisive threshold for increased mortality (Bellani et al., 2017). However, some very recent works have emphasized the interest on non-invasive strategies in COVID-19, especially in order to avoid intubation (Brusasco et al., 2020; Oranger et al., 2020; Tobin et al., 2020a).

Invasive Mechanical Ventilation

The decision to intubate mainly relies on the clinical judgment of the critical care physician but is also based upon combined features such as level of hypoxemia, respiratory distress, increased work of breathing, fatigue, and gas exchange (Tobin, 2020). In the peculiar context of the COVID-19 pandemic, the most appropriate timing for the intubation of hypoxic patients with severe lung injury is not well known and also depends on the local capacity for mechanical ventilation.

The main objective of mechanical ventilation is to lessen work and the oxygen cost of breathing, allowing oxygen stores to be redirected to vulnerable tissue beds (Tobin et al., 2012). In patients in acute respiratory distress, it has been demonstrated that the oxygen cost of breathing is enhanced to as much as 50% of total oxygen consumption (Field et al., 1984).

The basic principles of the assist-control ventilation are based upon the delivery of a breath under positive pressure provided by the ventilator, either triggered by the inspiratory effort achieved by the patient (pressure or flow triggered) or, independently, if such an effort is not performed within a preselected time period.

The main challenge for the physician then is to cycle the rhythm of the ventilator in synchrony with the patient's central respiratory rhythm while improving gas exchange. Three critical points have been identified: triggering (cycling on), post-trigger inflation, and inspiration-expiration switchover (cycling off; Tobin et al., 2012; Tobin, 2018).

The two most common modes used for mechanical ventilation are pressure-controlled ventilation (PCV), using a predetermined inflation pressure applied for a predetermined inflation time, and volume-controlled ventilation (VCV), using a predetermined volume.

With PCV, the delivered volume varies according to the properties of the respiratory system and also to the patient's effort and the inspiratory flow displays a decelerating shape; in VCV, the delivered volume is maintained constant, independently of the patient's effort, while the airway pressure is non-uniform and the inspiratory flow has a fixed shape.

It is important to note that the amount of active work performed by a patient in volume-cycled assist-control crucially relies on the sensitivity of the trigger and inspiratory flow settings. Despite optimal selected settings, it has been established that patients actively perform about a third of the work carried out by the ventilator during passive conditions (Marini et al., 1985). Pressure support can efficiently decrease the work of inspiration, but the level of inspiratory muscle unloading appears highly labile, with a coefficient of variation reaching up to 96% among patients (Jubran et al., 1995).

If mechanical ventilation is a valid life-saving intervention, it can also enhance lung injury and, through VILI, contribute to multi-organ failure in patients with ARDS (Slutsky and Ranieri, 2013). The major determinant of VILI is the genesis of non-physiologic stress (tension) and strain (deformation), which relies not only on the size of the delivered tidal volume but also on the amount of lung resting volume (Gattinoni et al., 2012).

Therefore, the most common strategy to minimize VILI is low tidal volume (V_T) ventilation. A V_T from 4 to 8 ml/kg of predicted body weight is recommended in mechanically ventilated adults with COVID-19 and ARDS (Alhazzani et al., 2020). Along with low V_T ventilation, lower airway pressure use [i.e., plateau pressure (P_{plat}) $\leq$30 cmH$_2$O] is a lung-protective strategy (Petrucci and De Feo, 2013).

Ventilator Weaning

Considering the side effects of mechanical ventilation and, additionally, the limitation of the intensive care resources during the COVID-19 pandemic, it is critical to get patients off the ventilator at the earliest possible time.

Since a delayed initiation of the weaning process has recurrently been observed, weaning predictor tests have been developed (Yang and Tobin, 1991; Tobin and Jubran, 2006). Among the physiological measurements that can alert a physician at initiating the weaning process, the level of rapid shallow breathing, quantified by frequency of breathing-to-V_T ratio (fb/V_T), has been shown to be the best predictor of weaning outcome (Yang and Tobin, 1991; Tobin and Jubran, 2006). Synchronized mandatory ventilation is not recommended (Brochard et al., 1994).

Several approaches are used to manage weaning: from the use of a T-tube circuit allowing bouts of spontaneous breathing trials to the gradual reduction in the level of ventilator assistance (Tobin et al., 2012). Almost invariably, weaning failure arises within the first hour of attempted spontaneous breathing (Tobin, 2018).

CONCLUSION

In COVID-19 lung injury, as observed in many other respiratory diseases, control of breathing is the cornerstone of the clinical presentation, from dyspnea to respiratory failure, not only explaining symptoms but also allowing appropriate levels of physiological compensations in order to maintain efficient spontaneous ventilation. However, when overwhelmed, a patient critically requires ventilator assistance, which also greatly involves the key elements of the control of breathing.

A clear view of COVID-19-related hypoxemia needs an appropriate interpretation of blood oxygenation from pulse oximetry, keeping in mind cautions and limits of accuracy. The role of the position of the dissociation curve associated to changes of the patient's acid-base status or hyperventilation-related hypocapnia, as well as the calculation of the P_AO_2-P_aO_2 gradient using the alveolar gas equation, is crucial to assess the real efficacy of pulmonary gas exchange. The participation of ventilatory response to hypoxia in the genesis of dyspnea and its modulation by CO_2 can help to explain that many COVID-19 patients face hypoxemia and rapid respiratory failure without evidence of dyspnea.

When mechanical ventilation is decided in critical COVID-19 patients, the usual strategies to tailor it are involved, based upon the basis of respiratory physiology to lessen work and the oxygen cost of breathing. The safe discontinuation of mechanical ventilation needs a careful assessment of physiological parameters (level of rapid shallow breathing) in order to warn a physician that a ventilated patient might be able to come off the ventilator in order to make it available for the next patient in such a peculiar context of the COVID-19 pandemic.

AUTHOR CONTRIBUTIONS

EA, MP, AK, CR, and BC contributed to conception of this work: literature search, drafting, writing, and critical review of the text. SV, DN, and BL contributed to literature search, writing, and critical review of the final document. All authors contributed to the article and approved the submitted version.

REFERENCES

Abroug, F., Ouanes-Besbes, L., Elatrous, S., and Brochard, L. (2008). The effect of prone positioning in acute respiratory distress syndrome or acute lung injury: a meta-analysis. Areas of uncertainty and recommendations for research. *Intensive Care Med.* 34, 1002–1011. doi: 10.1007/s00134-008-1062-3

Adler, D., and Janssens, J. P. (2019). The pathophysiology of respiratory failure: control of breathing, respiratory load, and muscle capacity. *Respiration* 97, 93–104. doi: 10.1159/000494063

Alhazzani, W., Moller, M. H., Arabi, Y. M., Loeb, M., Gong, M. N., Fan, E., et al. (2020). Surviving sepsis campaign: guidelines on the management of critically ill adults with coronavirus disease 2019 (COVID-19). *Intensive Care Med.* 46, 854–887. doi: 10.1007/s00134-020-06022-5

Alsaghir, A. H., and Martin, C. M. (2008). Effect of prone positioning in patients with acute respiratory distress syndrome: a meta-analysis. *Crit. Care Med.* 36, 603–609. doi: 10.1097/01.CCM.0000299739.98236.05

Altemeier, W. A., Robertson, H. T., Mckinney, S., and Glenny, R. W. (1998). Pulmonary embolization causes hypoxemia by redistributing regional blood flow without changing ventilation. *J. Appl. Physiol.* 85, 2337–2343. doi: 10.1152/jappl.1998.85.6.2337

Anonymus (1999). Dyspnea. Mechanisms, assessment, and management: a consensus statement. American Thoracic Society. *Am. J. Respir. Crit. Care Med.* 159, 321–340. doi: 10.1164/ajrccm.159.1.ats898

Archer, S. L., Sharp, W. W., and Weir, E. K. (2020). Differentiating COVID-19 pneumonia from acute respiratory distress syndrome and high altitude pulmonary edema: therapeutic implications. *Circulation* 142, 101–104. doi: 10.1161/CIRCULATIONAHA.120.047915

Ayzac, L., Girard, R., Baboi, L., Beuret, P., Rabilloud, M., Richard, J. C., et al. (2016). Ventilator-associated pneumonia in ARDS patients: the impact of prone positioning. A secondary analysis of the PROSEVA trial. *Intensive Care Med.* 42, 871–878. doi: 10.1007/s00134-015-4167-5

Aziz, S., Arabi, Y. M., Alhazzani, W., Evans, L., Citerio, G., Fischkoff, K., et al. (2020). Managing ICU surge during the COVID-19 crisis: rapid guidelines. *Intensive Care Med.* 46, 1303–1325. doi: 10.1007/s00134-020-06092-5

Banzett, R. B., Mulnier, H. E., Murphy, K., Rosen, S. D., Wise, R. J., and Adams, L. (2000). Breathlessness in humans activates insular cortex. *Neuroreport* 11, 2117–2120. doi: 10.1097/00001756-200007140-00012

Bazuaye, E. A., Stone, T. N., Corris, P. A., and Gibson, G. J. (1992). Variability of inspired oxygen concentration with nasal cannulas. *Thorax* 47, 609–611. doi: 10.1136/thx.47.8.609

Beitler, J. R., Shaefi, S., Montesi, S. B., Devlin, A., Loring, S. H., Talmor, D., et al. (2014). Prone positioning reduces mortality from acute respiratory distress syndrome in the low tidal volume era: a meta-analysis. *Intensive Care Med.* 40, 332–341. doi: 10.1007/s00134-013-3194-3

Bellani, G., Laffey, J. G., Pham, T., Madotto, F., Fan, E., Brochard, L., et al. (2017). Noninvasive ventilation of patients with acute respiratory distress syndrome. Insights from the LUNG SAFE study. *Am. J. Respir. Crit. Care Med.* 195, 67–77. doi: 10.1164/rccm.201606-1306OC

Bender, P. R., Weil, J. V., Reeves, J. T., and Moore, L. G. (1987). Breathing pattern in hypoxic exposures of varying duration. *J. Appl. Physiol.* 62, 640–645. doi: 10.1152/jappl.1987.62.2.640

Bernheim, A., Mei, X., Huang, M., Yang, Y., Fayad, Z. A., Zhang, N., et al. (2020). Chest CT findings in coronavirus disease-19 (COVID-19): relationship to duration of infection. *Radiology* 295:200463. doi: 10.1148/radiol.2020200463

Berry, D. T., Mcconnell, J. W., Phillips, B. A., Carswell, C. M., Lamb, D. G., and Prine, B. C. (1989). Isocapnic hypoxemia and neuropsychological functioning. *J. Clin. Exp. Neuropsychol.* 11, 241–251.

Bickler, P. E., Feiner, J. R., Lipnick, M. S., Batchelder, P., Macleod, D. B., and Severinghaus, J. W. (2017). Effects of acute, profound hypoxia on healthy humans: implications for safety of tests evaluating pulse oximetry or tissue oximetry performance. *Anesth. Analg.* 124, 146–153. doi: 10.1213/ANE.0000000000001421

Bickler, P. E., Feiner, J. R., and Severinghaus, J. W. (2005). Effects of skin pigmentation on pulse oximeter accuracy at low saturation. *Anesthesiology* 102, 715–719. doi: 10.1097/00000542-200504000-00004

Bloomfield, R., Noble, D. W., and Sudlow, A. (2015). Prone position for acute respiratory failure in adults. *Cochrane Database Syst. Rev.* 2015:CD008095. doi: 10.1002/14651858.CD008095.pub2

Bouaziz, J. D., Duong, T., Jachiet, M., Velter, C., Lestang, P., Cassius, C., et al. (2020). Vascular skin symptoms in COVID-19: a french observational study. *J Eur Acad Dermatol. Venereol.* 34, e451–e452. doi: 10.1111/jdv.16544

Brochard, L., Rauss, A., Benito, S., Conti, G., Mancebo, J., Rekik, N., et al. (1994). Comparison of three methods of gradual withdrawal from ventilatory support during weaning from mechanical ventilation. *Am. J. Respir. Crit. Care Med.* 150, 896–903. doi: 10.1164/ajrccm.150.4.7921460

Brugger, H., Basnyat, B., Ellerton, J., Hefti, U., Strapazzon, G., and Zafren, K. (2020). Letter to the editor: COVID-19 lung injury is different from high altitude pulmonary edema. *High Alt. Med. Biol.* 21, 204–205. doi: 10.1089/ham.2020.0061

Brusasco, C., Corradi, F., Di Domenico, A., Raggi, F., Timossi, G., Santori, G., et al. (2020). Continuous positive airway pressure in Covid-19 patients with moderate-to-severe respiratory failure. *Eur. Respir. J.* 8:2002524. doi: 10.1183/13993003.02524-2020

Bryan, A. C. (1974). Conference on the scientific basis of respiratory therapy. Pulmonary physiotherapy in the pediatric age group. Comments of a devil's advocate. *Am. Rev. Respir. Dis.* 110, 143–144. doi: 10.1164/arrd.1974.110.6P2.143

Buchanan, G. F., and Richerson, G. B. (2009). Role of chemoreceptors in mediating dyspnea. *Respir. Physiol. Neurobiol.* 167, 9–19. doi: 10.1016/j.resp.2008.12.002

Chad, T., and Sampson, C. (2020). Prone positioning in conscious patients on medical wards: a review of the evidence and its relevance to patients with COVID-19 infection. *Clin. Med.* 20, e97–e103. doi: 10.7861/clinmed.2020-0179

Chiumello, D., and Brioni, M. (2016). Severe hypoxemia: which strategy to choose. *Crit. Care* 20:132. doi: 10.1186/s13054-016-1304-7

Colla, J., Rodos, A., Seyller, H., and Weingart, S. (2020). Fighting COVID-19 hypoxia with one hand tied behind our back: blanket prohibition of high-flow oxygen and noninvasive positive end-expiratory pressure in US hospitals. *Ann. Emerg. Med.* 75, 791–792. doi: 10.1016/j.annemergmed.2020.04.015

Connors, J. M., and Levy, J. H. (2020). COVID-19 and its implications for thrombosis and anticoagulation. *Blood* 135, 2033–2040. doi: 10.1182/blood.2020006000

Corne, S., Webster, K., and Younes, M. (2003). Hypoxic respiratory response during acute stable hypocapnia. *Am. J. Respir. Crit. Care Med.* 167, 1193–1199. doi: 10.1164/rccm.2203019

Couzin-Frankel, J. (2020). The mystery of the pandemic's 'happy hypoxia. *Science* 368, 455–456. doi: 10.1126/science.368.6490.455

Doussot, A., Ciceron, F., Cerutti, E., Salomon Du Mont, L., Thines, L., Capellier, G., et al. (2020). Prone positioning for severe acute respiratory distress syndrome in COVID-19 patients by a dedicated team: a safe and pragmatic reallocation of medical and surgical work force in response to the outbreak. *Ann. Surg.* 272, e311–e315. doi: 10.1097/SLA.0000000000004265

Du, Y., Tu, L., Zhu, P., Mu, M., Wang, R., Yang, P., et al. (2020). Clinical features of 85 fatal cases of COVID-19 from Wuhan. A retrospective observational study. *Am. J. Respir. Crit. Care Med.* 201, 1372–1379. doi: 10.1164/rccm.202003-0543OC

Elharrar, X., Trigui, Y., Dols, A. M., Touchon, F., Martinez, S., Prud'homme, E., et al. (2020). Use of prone positioning in nonintubated patients with COVID-19 and hypoxemic acute respiratory failure. *JAMA* 323, 2336–2338. doi: 10.1001/jama.2020.8255

Evans, T. W. (2001). International consensus conferences in intensive care medicine: non-invasive positive pressure ventilation in acute respiratory failure. Organised jointly by the American Thoracic Society, the European Respiratory Society, the European Society of Intensive Care Medicine, and the Societe de reanimation de langue Francaise, and approved by the ATS Board of Directors, December 2000. *Intensive Care Med.* 27, 166–178. doi: 10.1007/s001340000721

Evans, K. C., Banzett, R. B., Adams, L., Mckay, L., Frackowiak, R. S., and Corfield, D. R. (2002). BOLD fMRI identifies limbic, paralimbic, and cerebellar activation during air hunger. *J. Neurophysiol.* 88, 1500–1511. doi: 10.1152/jn.2002.88.3.1500

Field, S., Sanci, S., and Grassino, A. (1984). Respiratory muscle oxygen consumption estimated by the diaphragm pressure-time index. *J. Appl. Physiol. Respir. Environ. Exerc. Physiol.* 57, 44–51. doi: 10.1152/jappl.1984.57.1.44

Fitzgerald, R. S., and Dehghani, G. A. (1982). Neural responses of the cat carotid and aortic bodies to hypercapnia and hypoxia. *J. Appl. Physiol. Respir. Environ. Exerc. Physiol.* 52, 596–601. doi: 10.1152/jappl.1982.52.3.596

Force, A. D. T., Ranieri, V. M., Rubenfeld, G. D., Thompson, B. T., Ferguson, N. D., Caldwell, E., et al. (2012). Acute respiratory distress syndrome: the Berlin definition. *JAMA* 307, 2526–2533. doi: 10.1001/jama.2012.5669

Forster, H. V., and Dempsey, J. A. (1981). "Ventilatory adaptations" in *Lung biology in health and disease. Regulation of breathing*. ed. T. Hornbein (New York: Dekker M), 845–904.

Gattinoni, L., Carlesso, E., and Caironi, P. (2012). Stress and strain within the lung. *Curr. Opin. Crit. Care* 18, 42–47. doi: 10.1097/MCC.0b013e32834f17d9

Gattinoni, L., Chiumello, D., Caironi, P., Busana, M., Romitti, F., Brazzi, L., et al. (2020a). COVID-19 pneumonia: different respiratory treatments for different phenotypes? *Intensive Care Med.* 46, 1099–1102. doi: 10.1007/s00134-020-06033-2

Gattinoni, L., Chiumello, D., and Rossi, S. (2020b). COVID-19 pneumonia: ARDS or not? *Crit. Care* 24:154. doi: 10.1186/s13054-020-02880-z

Gattinoni, L., Coppola, S., Cressoni, M., Busana, M., Rossi, S., and Chiumello, D. (2020c). COVID-19 does not Lead to a "typical" acute respiratory distress syndrome. *Am. J. Respir. Crit. Care Med.* 201, 1299–1300. doi: 10.1164/rccm.202003-0817LE

Gattinoni, L., Taccone, P., Carlesso, E., and Marini, J. J. (2013). Prone position in acute respiratory distress syndrome. Rationale, indications, and limits. *Am. J. Respir. Crit. Care Med.* 188, 1286–1293. doi: 10.1164/rccm.201308-1532CI

Gottlieb, M., and Long, B. (2020). Dermatologic manifestations and complications of COVID-19. *Am. J. Emerg. Med.* 38, 1715–1721. doi: 10.1016/j.ajem.2020.06.011

Grasselli, G., Zangrillo, A., Zanella, A., Antonelli, M., Cabrini, L., Castelli, A., et al. (2020). Baseline characteristics and outcomes of 1591 patients infected with SARS-CoV-2 admitted to ICUs of the lombardy region, Italy. *JAMA* 323, 1574–1581. doi: 10.1001/jama.2020.5394

Guan, W. J., Ni, Z. Y., Hu, Y., Liang, W. H., Ou, C. Q., He, J. X., et al. (2020). Clinical Characteristics of Coronavirus Disease 2019 in China. *N. Engl. J. Med.* 382, 1708–1720. doi: 10.1056/NEJMoa2002032

Guerin, C. (2014). Prone ventilation in acute respiratory distress syndrome. *Eur. Respir. Rev.* 23, 249–257. doi: 10.1183/09059180.00001114

Guerin, C. (2017). Prone positioning acute respiratory distress syndrome patients. *Ann Transl Med* 5:289. doi: 10.21037/atm.2017.06.63

Guerin, C., Baboi, L., and Richard, J. C. (2014). Mechanisms of the effects of prone positioning in acute respiratory distress syndrome. *Intensive Care Med.* 40, 1634–1642. doi: 10.1007/s00134-014-3500-8

Guerin, C., Reignier, J., Richard, J. C., Beuret, P., Gacouin, A., Boulain, T., et al. (2013). Prone positioning in severe acute respiratory distress syndrome. *N. Engl. J. Med.* 368, 2159–2168. doi: 10.1056/NEJMoa1214103

Hamilton, C., Steinlechner, B., Gruber, E., Simon, P., and Wollenek, G. (2004). The oxygen dissociation curve: quantifying the shift. *Perfusion* 19, 141–144. doi: 10.1191/0267659104pf734oa

Hamming, I., Timens, W., Bulthuis, M. L., Lely, A. T., Navis, G., and Van Goor, H. (2004). Tissue distribution of ACE2 protein, the functional receptor for SARS coronavirus. A first step in understanding SARS pathogenesis. *J. Pathol.* 203, 631–637. doi: 10.1002/path.1570

Hampl, V., Herget, J., Bibova, J., Banasova, A., Huskova, Z., Vanourkova, Z., et al. (2015). Intrapulmonary activation of the angiotensin-converting enzyme type 2/angiotensin 1-7/G-protein-coupled mas receptor axis attenuates pulmonary hypertension in Ren-2 transgenic rats exposed to chronic hypoxia. *Physiol. Res.* 64, 25–38. doi: 10.33549/physiolres.932861

Hoffmann, M., Kleine-Weber, H., Schroeder, S., Kruger, N., Herrler, T., Erichsen, S., et al. (2020). SARS-CoV-2 cell entry depends on ACE2 and TMPRSS2 and is blocked by a clinically proven protease inhibitor. *Cell* 181, 271.e8–280.e8. doi: 10.1016/j.cell.2020.02.052

Hu, S. L., He, H. L., Pan, C., Liu, A. R., Liu, S. Q., Liu, L., et al. (2014). The effect of prone positioning on mortality in patients with acute respiratory distress syndrome: a meta-analysis of randomized controlled trials. *Crit. Care* 18:R109. doi: 10.1186/cc13896

Huang, C., Wang, Y., Li, X., Ren, L., Zhao, J., Hu, Y., et al. (2020). Clinical features of patients infected with 2019 novel coronavirus in Wuhan, China. *Lancet* 395, 497–506. doi: 10.1016/S0140-6736(20)30183-5

Jounieaux, V., Parreira, V. F., Aubert, G., Dury, M., Delguste, P., and Rodenstein, D. O. (2002). Effects of hypocapnic hyperventilation on the response to hypoxia in normal subjects receiving intermittent positive-pressure ventilation. *Chest* 121, 1141–1148. doi: 10.1378/chest.121.4.1141

Jubran, A., Van De Graaff, W. B., and Tobin, M. J. (1995). Variability of patient-ventilator interaction with pressure support ventilation in patients with chronic obstructive pulmonary disease. *Am. J. Respir. Crit. Care Med.* 152, 129–136. doi: 10.1164/ajrccm.152.1.7599811

Kallet, R. H. (2015). A comprehensive review of prone position in ARDS. *Respir. Care* 60, 1660–1687. doi: 10.4187/respcare.04271

Kimmoun, A., Levy, B., and Chenuel, B. (2020). Usefulness and safety of a dedicated team to prone patients with severe ARDS due to COVID-19. *Crit. Care* 24:509. doi: 10.1186/s13054-020-03128-6

Kronenberg, R. S., and Drage, C. W. (1973). Attenuation of the ventilatory and heart rate responses to hypoxia and hypercapnia with aging in normal men. *J. Clin. Invest.* 52, 1812–1819.

Lahiri, S., and Delaney, R. G. (1975). Stimulus interaction in the responses of carotid body chemoreceptor single afferent fibers. *Respir. Physiol.* 24, 249–266. doi: 10.1016/0034-5687(75)90017-1

Lang, M., Som, A., Mendoza, D. P., Flores, E. J., Reid, N., Carey, D., et al. (2020). Hypoxaemia related to COVID-19: vascular and perfusion abnormalities on dual-energy CT. *Lancet Infect. Dis.* 20, 1365–1366. doi: 10.1016/S1473-3099(20)30367-4

Lansing, R. W., Gracely, R. H., and Banzett, R. B. (2009). The multiple dimensions of dyspnea: review and hypotheses. *Respir. Physiol. Neurobiol.* 167, 53–60. doi: 10.1016/j.resp.2008.07.012

Laviolette, L., Laveneziana, P., and Faculty, E. R. S. R. S. (2014). Dyspnoea: a multidimensional and multidisciplinary approach. *Eur. Respir. J.* 43, 1750–1762. doi: 10.1183/09031936.00092613

Lee, J. M., Bae, W., Lee, Y. J., and Cho, Y. J. (2014). The efficacy and safety of prone positional ventilation in acute respiratory distress syndrome: updated study-level meta-analysis of 11 randomized controlled trials. *Crit. Care Med.* 42, 1252–1262. doi: 10.1097/CCM.0000000000000122

Levitan, R. (2020). The infection that's silently killing coronavirus patients. The New York Times, April 20.

Lu, R., Zhao, X., Li, J., Niu, P., Yang, B., Wu, H., et al. (2020). Genomic characterisation and epidemiology of 2019 novel coronavirus: implications for virus origins and receptor binding. *Lancet* 395, 565–574. doi: 10.1016/S0140-6736(20)30251-8

Luks, A. M., and Swenson, E. R. (2020). COVID-19 lung injury and high-altitude pulmonary edema. A false equation with dangerous implications. *Ann. Am. Thorac. Soc.* 17, 918–921. doi: 10.1513/AnnalsATS.202004-327FR

Manning, H. L., and Schwartzstein, R. M. (1995). Pathophysiology of dyspnea. *N. Engl. J. Med.* 333, 1547–1553. doi: 10.1056/NEJM199512073332307

Marini, J. J., Capps, J. S., and Culver, B. H. (1985). The inspiratory work of breathing during assisted mechanical ventilation. *Chest* 87, 612–618. doi: 10.1378/chest.87.5.612

Matsuzawa, Y., Fujimoto, K., Kobayashi, T., Namushi, N. R., Harada, K., Kohno, H., et al. (1989). Blunted hypoxic ventilatory drive in subjects susceptible to high-altitude pulmonary edema. *J. Appl. Physiol.* 66, 1152–1157. doi: 10.1152/jappl.1989.66.3.1152

Mehta, P., Mcauley, D. F., Brown, M., Sanchez, E., Tattersall, R. S., Manson, J. J., et al. (2020). COVID-19: consider cytokine storm syndromes and immunosuppression. *Lancet* 395, 1033–1034. doi: 10.1016/S0140-6736(20)30628-0

Mellins, R. B. (1974). Pulmonary physiotherapy in the pediatric age group. *Am. Rev. Respir. Dis.* 110, 137–142. doi: 10.1164/arrd.1974.110.6P2.137

Meschi, T., Rossi, S., Volpi, A., Ferrari, C., Sverzellati, N., Brianti, E., et al. (2020). Reorganization of a large academic hospital to face COVID-19 outbreak: the model of Parma, Emilia-Romagna region, Italy. *Eur. J. Clin. Investig.* 50:e13250. doi: 10.1111/eci.13250

Messika, J., Ben Ahmed, K., Gaudry, S., Miguel-Montanes, R., Rafat, C., Sztrymf, B., et al. (2015). Use of high-flow nasal cannula oxygen therapy in subjects with ARDS: a 1-year observational study. *Respir. Care* 60, 162–169. doi: 10.4187/respcare.03423

Mitchell, D. A., and Seckel, M. A. (2018). Acute respiratory distress syndrome and prone positioning. *AACN Adv. Crit. Care* 29, 415–425. doi: 10.4037/aacnacc2018161

Moore, L. G., Huang, S. Y., Mccullough, R. E., Sampson, J. B., Maher, J. T., Weil, J. V., et al. (1984). Variable inhibition by falling CO2 of hypoxic ventilatory response in humans. *J. Appl. Physiol. Respir. Environ. Exerc. Physiol.* 56, 207–210. doi: 10.1152/jappl.1984.56.1.207

Moosavi, S. H., Golestanian, E., Binks, A. P., Lansing, R. W., Brown, R., and Banzett, R. B. (2003). Hypoxic and hypercapnic drives to breathe generate equivalent levels of air hunger in humans. *J. Appl. Physiol.* 94, 141–154. doi: 10.1152/japplphysiol.00594.2002

Munshi, L., Del Sorbo, L., Adhikari, N. K. J., Hodgson, C. L., Wunsch, H., Meade, M. O., et al. (2017). Prone position for acute respiratory distress syndrome. A systematic review and meta-analysis. *Ann. Am. Thorac. Soc.* 14, S280–S288. doi: 10.1513/AnnalsATS.201704-343OT

Nishimura, M., Miyamoto, K., Suzuki, A., Yamamoto, H., Tsuji, M., Kishi, F., et al. (1989). Ventilatory and heart rate responses to hypoxia and hypercapnia in patients with diabetes mellitus. *Thorax* 44, 251–257. doi: 10.1136/thx.44.4.251

O'Donnell, C. R., Friedman, L. S., Russomanno, J. H., and Rose, R. M. (1988). Diminished perception of inspiratory-resistive loads in insulin-dependent diabetics. *N. Engl. J. Med.* 319, 1369–1373. doi: 10.1056/NEJM198811243192102

Oranger, M., Gonzalez-Bermejo, J., Dacosta-Noble, P., Llontop, C., Guerder, A., Trosini-Desert, V., et al. (2020). Continuous positive airway pressure to avoid intubation in SARS-CoV-2 pneumonia: a two-period retrospective case-control study. *Eur. Respir. J.* 56:2001692. doi: 10.1183/13993003.01692-2020

Parshall, M. B., Schwartzstein, R. M., Adams, L., Banzett, R. B., Manning, H. L., Bourbeau, J., et al. (2012). An official American Thoracic Society statement: update on the mechanisms, assessment, and management of dyspnea. *Am. J. Respir. Crit. Care Med.* 185, 435–452. doi: 10.1164/rccm.201111-2042ST

Peterson, D. D., Pack, A. I., Silage, D. A., and Fishman, A. P. (1981). Effects of aging on ventilatory and occlusion pressure responses to hypoxia and hypercapnia. *Am. Rev. Respir. Dis.* 124, 387–391. doi: 10.1164/arrd.1981.124.4.387

Petrucci, N., and De Feo, C. (2013). Lung protective ventilation strategy for the acute respiratory distress syndrome. *Cochrane Database Syst. Rev.* 2013: CD003844. doi: 10.1002/14651858.CD003844.pub4

Pfeifer, M., Ewig, S., Voshaar, T., Randerath, W. J., Bauer, T., Geiseler, J., et al. (2020). Position paper for the state-of-the-art application of respiratory support in patients with COVID-19. *Respiration* 99, 521–542. doi: 10.1159/000509104

Polidoro, R. B., Hagan, R. S., De Santis Santiago, R., and Schmidt, N. W. (2020). Overview: systemic inflammatory response derived from lung injury caused by SARS-CoV-2 infection explains severe outcomes in COVID-19. *Front. Immunol.* 11:1626. doi: 10.3389/fimmu.2020.01626

Rebuck, A. S., and Campbell, E. J. (1974). A clinical method for assessing the ventilatory response to hypoxia. *Am. Rev. Respir. Dis.* 109, 345–350. doi: 10.1164/arrd.1974.109.3.345

Reynolds, W. J., and Milhorn, H. T. Jr. (1973). Transient ventilatory response to hypoxia with and without controlled alveolar PCO2. *J. Appl. Physiol.* 35, 187–196. doi: 10.1152/jappl.1973.35.2.187

Richardson, S., Hirsch, J. S., Narasimhan, M., Crawford, J. M., Mcginn, T., Davidson, K. W., et al. (2020). Presenting characteristics, comorbidities, and outcomes among 5700 patients hospitalized with COVID-19 in the new York City area. *JAMA* 323, 2052–2059. doi: 10.1001/jama.2020.6775

Rizvi, I., Zaman, S., Zaidi, N., Asif, M. S., and Abdali, N. (2012). Acute life-threatening methaemoglobinaemia following ingestion of chloroquine. *BMJ Case Rep.* 2012:bcr1220115383. doi: 10.1136/bcr.12.2011.5383

Ruste, M., Bitker, L., Yonis, H., Riad, Z., Louf-Durier, A., Lissonde, F., et al. (2018). Hemodynamic effects of extended prone position sessions in ARDS. *Ann. Intensive Care* 8:120. doi: 10.1186/s13613-018-0464-9

Sahn, S. A., Zwillich, C. W., Dick, N., Mccullough, R. E., Lakshminarayan, S., and Weil, J. V. (1977). Variability of ventilatory responses to hypoxia and hypercapnia. *J. Appl. Physiol. Respir. Environ. Exerc. Physiol.* 43, 1019–1025. doi: 10.1152/jappl.1977.43.6.1019

Sartini, C., Tresoldi, M., Scarpellini, P., Tettamanti, A., Carcò, F., Landoni, G., et al. (2020). Respiratory parameters in patients with COVID-19 after using noninvasive ventilation in the prone position outside the intensive care unit. *JAMA* 323, 2338–2340. doi: 10.1001/jama.2020.7861

Schnapp, L. M., and Cohen, N. H. (1990). Pulse oximetry. Uses and abuses. *Chest* 98, 1244–1250.

Scholten, E. L., Beitler, J. R., Prisk, G. K., and Malhotra, A. (2017). Treatment of ARDS with prone positioning. *Chest* 151, 215–224. doi: 10.1016/j.chest.2016.06.032

Schon, D., Rosenkranz, M., Regelsberger, J., Dahme, B., Buchel, C., and Von Leupoldt, A. (2008). Reduced perception of dyspnea and pain after right insular cortex lesions. *Am. J. Respir. Crit. Care Med.* 178, 1173–1179. doi: 10.1164/rccm.200805-731OC

Settembre, N., Maurice, P., Paysant, J., Theurel, J., Claudon, L., Kimmoun, A., et al. (2020). The use of exoskeletons to help with prone positioning in the intensive care unit during COVID-19. *Ann. Phys. Rehabil. Med.* 63, 379–382. doi: 10.1016/j.rehab.2020.05.004

Sinex, J. E. (1999). Pulse oximetry: principles and limitations. *Am. J. Emerg. Med.* 17, 59–67. doi: 10.1016/S0735-6757(99)90019-0

Slutsky, A. S., and Ranieri, V. M. (2013). Ventilator-induced lung injury. *N. Engl. J. Med.* 369, 2126–2136. doi: 10.1056/NEJMra1208707

Solaimanzadeh, I. (2020). Acetazolamide, Nifedipine Phosphodiesterase inhibitors: rationale for their utilization as adjunctive countermeasures in the treatment of coronavirus disease 2019 (COVID-19). *Cureus* 12:e7343. doi: 10.7759/cureus.7343

Strapazzon, G., Hilty, M. P., Bouzat, P., Pratali, L., Brugger, H., and Rauch, S. (2020). To compare the incomparable: COVID-19 pneumonia and high-altitude disease. *Eur. Respir. J.* 55:2001362. doi: 10.1183/13993003.01362-2020

Suffredini, D. A., and Allison, M. G. (2020). A rationale for use of high flow nasal cannula for select patients with suspected or confirmed severe acute respiratory syndrome Coronavirus-2 infection. *J. Intensive Care Med.* 36, 9–17. doi: 10.1177/0885066620956630

Sutcu Cicek, H., Gumus, S., Deniz, O., Yildiz, S., Acikel, C. H., Cakir, E., et al. (2011). Effect of nail polish and henna on oxygen saturation determined by pulse oximetry in healthy young adult females. *Emerg. Med. J.* 28, 783–785. doi: 10.1136/emj.2010.096073

Swenson, E. R., and Bartsch, P. (2012). High-altitude pulmonary edema. *Compr. Physiol.* 2, 2753–2773. doi: 10.1002/cphy.c100029

Tian, S., Hu, W., Niu, L., Liu, H., Xu, H., and Xiao, S. Y. (2020). Pulmonary pathology of early-phase 2019 novel coronavirus (COVID-19) pneumonia in two patients with lung cancer. *J. Thorac. Oncol.* 15, 700–704. doi: 10.1016/j.jtho.2020.02.010

Tobin, M. J. (1990). Respiratory monitoring. *JAMA* 264, 244–251. doi: 10.1001/jama.1990.03450020096034

Tobin, M. J. (2018). Physiologic basis of mechanical ventilation. *Ann. Am. Thorac. Soc.* 15, S49–S52. doi: 10.1513/AnnalsATS.201705-417KV

Tobin, M. J. (2020). Basing respiratory management of COVID-19 on physiological principles. *Am. J. Respir. Crit. Care Med.* 201, 1319–1320. doi: 10.1164/rccm.202004-1076ED

Tobin, M. J., and Jubran, A. (2006). Variable performance of weaning-predictor tests: role of Bayes' theorem and spectrum and test-referral bias. *Intensive Care Med.* 32, 2002–2012. doi: 10.1007/s00134-006-0439-4

Tobin, M. J., Jubran, A., and Laghi, F. (2020a). Noninvasive strategies in COVID-19: epistemology, randomised trials, guidelines, physiology. *Eur. Respir. J.* doi: 10.1183/13993003.04247-2020 [Epub ahead of print]

Tobin, M. J., Laghi, F., and Jubran, A. (2012). Ventilatory failure, ventilator support, and ventilator weaning. *Compr. Physiol.* 2, 2871–2921. doi: 10.1002/cphy.c110030

Tobin, M. J., Laghi, F., and Jubran, A. (2020b). Why COVID-19 silent hypoxemia is baffling to physicians. *Am. J. Respir. Crit. Care Med.* 202, 356–360. doi: 10.1164/rccm.202006-2157CP

Tobin, M. J., Mador, M. J., Guenther, S. M., Lodato, R. F., and Sackner, M. A. (1988). Variability of resting respiratory drive and timing in healthy subjects. *J. Appl. Physiol.* 65, 309–317. doi: 10.1152/jappl.1988.65.1.309

Tosti, G., Barisani, A., Queirolo, P., Pennacchioli, E., Villa, L., Lodeserto, A. M., et al. (2020). Skin signs resembling vascular acrosyndromes during the COVID-19 outbreak in Italy. *Clin. Exp. Dermatol.* 45, 757–758. doi: 10.1111/ced.14267

Van De Louw, A., Cracco, C., Cerf, C., Harf, A., Duvaldestin, P., Lemaire, F., et al. (2001). Accuracy of pulse oximetry in the intensive care unit. *Intensive Care Med.* 27, 1606–1613. doi: 10.1007/s001340101064

Villarreal-Fernandez, E., Patel, R., Golamari, R., Khalid, M., Dewaters, A., and Haouzi, P. (2020). A plea for avoiding systematic intubation in severely hypoxemic patients with COVID-19-associated respiratory failure. *Crit. Care* 24:337. doi: 10.1186/s13054-020-03063-6

Wei, Y. Y., Wang, R. R., Zhang, D. W., Tu, Y. H., Chen, C. S., Ji, S., et al. (2020). Risk factors for severe COVID-19: evidence from 167 hospitalized patients in Anhui, China. *J. Infect.* 81, e89–e92. doi: 10.1016/j.jinf.2020.04.010

Weisbrod, C. J., Eastwood, P. R., O'driscoll, G., and Green, D. J. (2005). Abnormal ventilatory responses to hypoxia in type 2 diabetes. *Diabet. Med.* 22, 563–568. doi: 10.1111/j.1464-5491.2005.01458.x

Wilson, K. C., Chotirmall, S. H., Bai, C., and Rello, J. (2020). COVID-19: Interim Guidance on Management Pending Empirical Evidence. From an American Thoracic Society-led International Task Force: A.T. Society; on behalf of the International Task Force on COVID-19. Available at: https://www.thoracic.org/covid/covid-19-guidance.pdf (Accessed May 9, 2020).

Wilson, R. J., and Teppema, L. J. (2016). Integration of central and peripheral respiratory Chemoreflexes. *Compr. Physiol.* 6, 1005–1041. doi: 10.1002/cphy.c140040

Wu, Z., and Mcgoogan, J. M. (2020). Characteristics of and important Lessons from the coronavirus disease 2019 (COVID-19) outbreak in China: summary of a report of 72314 cases from the Chinese Center for Disease Control and Prevention. *JAMA* 323, 1239–1242. doi: 10.1001/jama.2020.2648

Xie, J., Covassin, N., Fan, Z., Singh, P., Gao, W., Li, G., et al. (2020a). Association between hypoxemia and mortality in patients with COVID-19. *Mayo Clin. Proc.* 95, 1138–1147. doi: 10.1016/j.mayocp.2020.04.006

Xie, J., Tong, Z., Guan, X., Du, B., Qiu, H., and Slutsky, A. S. (2020b). Critical care crisis and some recommendations during the COVID-19 epidemic in China. *Intensive Care Med.* 46, 837–840. doi: 10.1007/s00134-020-05979-7

Xu, Z., Shi, L., Wang, Y., Zhang, J., Huang, L., Zhang, C., et al. (2020). Pathological findings of COVID-19 associated with acute respiratory distress syndrome. *Lancet Respir. Med.* 8, 420–422. doi: 10.1056/NEJM199105233242101

Yang, K. L., and Tobin, M. J. (1991). A prospective study of indexes predicting the outcome of trials of weaning from mechanical ventilation. *N. Engl. J. Med.* 324, 1445–1450. doi: 10.1056/NEJM199105233242101

Zhang, H., Penninger, J. M., Li, Y., Zhong, N., and Slutsky, A. S. (2020). Angiotensin-converting enzyme 2 (ACE2) as a SARS-CoV-2 receptor: molecular mechanisms and potential therapeutic target. *Intensive Care Med.* 46, 586–590. doi: 10.1007/s00134-020-05985-9

19

Methods and Applications in Respiratory Physiology: Respiratory Mechanics, Drive and Muscle Function in Neuromuscular and Chest Wall Disorders

*Nina Patel, Kelvin Chong and Ahmet Baydur**

[1]Dornsife College of Letters, Arts and Sciences, Division of Pulmonary, Critical Care and Sleep Medicine, Keck School of Medicine and University of Southern California, Los Angeles, CA, United States

***Correspondence:**
Ahmet Baydur
baydur@usc.edu

Individuals with neuromuscular and chest wall disorders experience respiratory muscle weakness, reduced lung volume and increases in respiratory elastance and resistance which lead to increase in work of breathing, impaired gas exchange and respiratory pump failure. Recently developed methods to assess respiratory muscle weakness, mechanics and movement supplement traditionally employed spirometry and methods to evaluate gas exchange. These include recording postural change in vital capacity, respiratory pressures (mouth and sniff), electromyography and ultrasound evaluation of diaphragmatic thickness and excursions. In this review, we highlight key aspects of the pathophysiology of these conditions as they impact the patient and describe measures to evaluate respiratory dysfunction. We discuss potential areas of physiologic investigation in the evaluation of respiratory aspects of these disorders.

Keywords: neuromuscular disease, respiratory mechanics, dyspnea, control of ventilation, expiratory flow limitation, diaphragmatic fatigue, gas exchange, respiratory pressures

INTRODUCTION

Neuromuscular and chest wall disorders impact breathing in a manner different from injury to the lungs. Respiratory muscle weakness, reduced lung volume and increases in respiratory elastance and resistance lead to increase in work of breathing, respiratory pump failure and impaired gas exchange (Campbell, 1965). The main objective of this review is to highlight key aspects of the pathophysiology of these conditions as they impact the patient and describe recently developed measures to evaluate respiratory dysfunction. We describe key aspects of normal respiratory muscle structure and function, how they are affected in neuromuscular disorders (NMDs), current methods of functional evaluation, and recent advances in their assessment. We finish with suggestions for potential applications of newer techniques that may be considered for their evaluation. We focus primarily on the pathophysiology of NMDs as they impact adults but will refer to changes in children where relevant.

PATHOPHYSIOLOGY

Normal Respiratory Muscle Function

The respiratory system functions to secure gas exchange between ambient air and blood to maintain arterial blood gas pressures within certain acceptable values. It consists of the lungs, chest wall

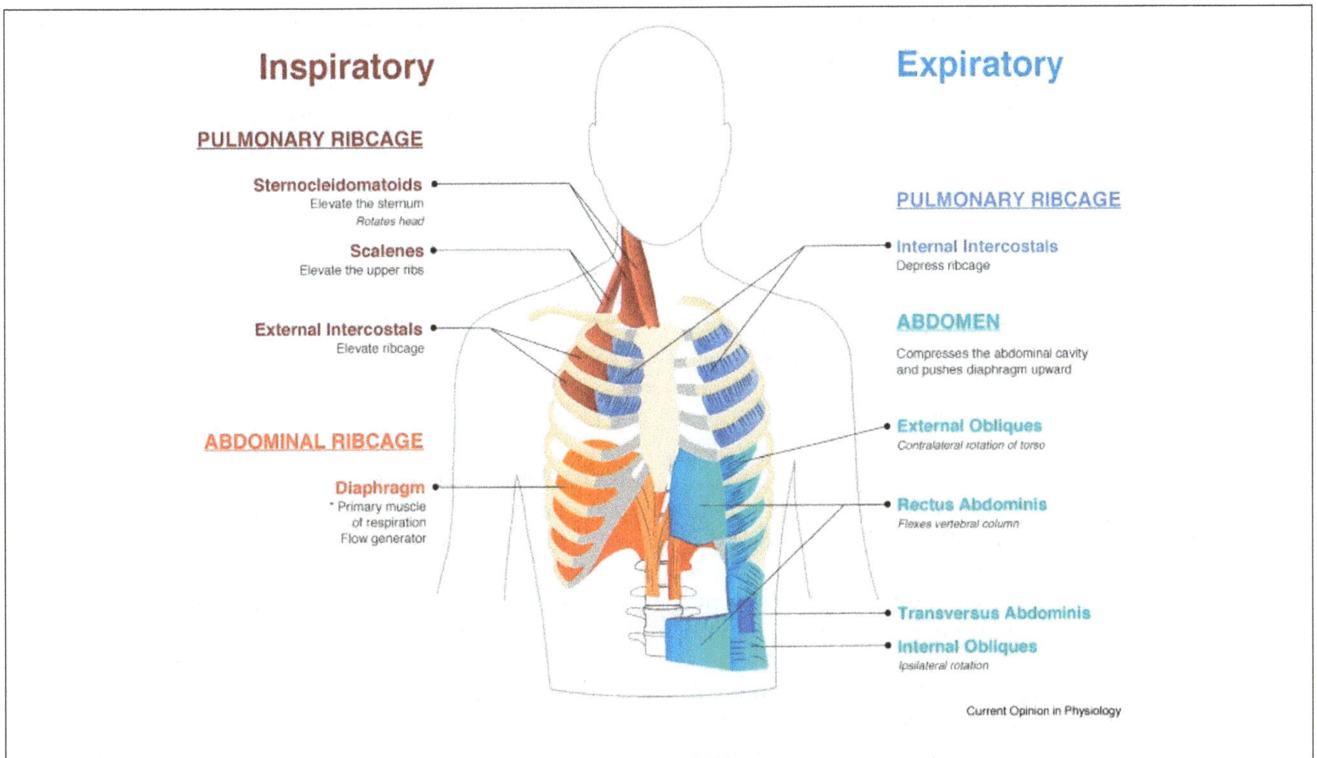

FIGURE 1 | Muscles involved in normal inspiration and expiration. From Welch et al., 2019.

(including respiratory muscles), controllers of breathing, and spinal cord and peripheral nerves that communicate with the respiratory system. Neuromuscular and chest wall disorders affect these structures in varied ways, depending on the age of onset, distribution of neuro/myopathic involvement and rate of progression of the disorder.

Respiratory muscles are classified into those with inspiratory and expiratory function (**Figure 1**) (Campbell, 1965; Benditt, 2019; Welch et al., 2019). In healthy individuals during quiet breathing, the diaphragm is the only active inspiratory muscle; expiration is achieved by passive relaxation of the lungs. During increased demand such as exercise, other muscles become selectively active depending on the relative increase in inspiratory or expiratory requirements, or both. Upper airway dilator muscles maintain patency of the pharynx and larynx, preventing upper airway occlusion, an event occuring frequently with bulbar dysfunction and exacerbated during sleep-disordered breathing.

Diaphragm

The diaphragm is a thin sheet of muscle acting as a piston, decreasing intrathoracic pressure and drawing air into the lungs. It enables the ribs to move up and outwards ("bucket handle" action), increasing their transverse span (Benditt, 2019). It is configured like an elliptical cylindroid with a dome cap. The cylindrical portion of the diaphragm shortens during inspiration while the dome changes little. Two components counterbalance the

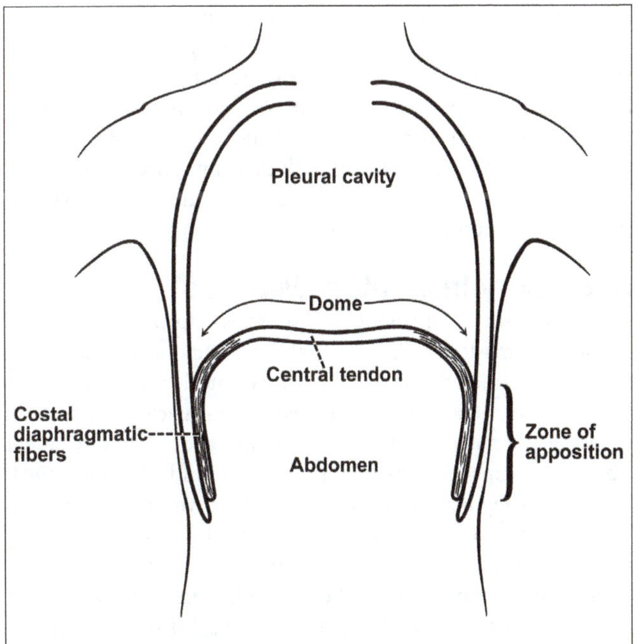

FIGURE 2 | Zone of apposition of the diaphragm. The muscle fibers of the diaphragm originate from the circumference of the thoracic outlet, in particular the lower ribs, and converge to insert into a central tendon). From their origins on the lower ribs the fibers run mainly cranially and are directly parallel (apposed) to the inner aspect of the lower rib cage, constituting the "zone of apposition." From (Troyer and Wilson, 2016).

inspiratory action: the appositional and insertional components. The zone of apposition is represented by the muscular portion inserted into and parallel to posterolateral aspect of the abdominal wall (**Figure 2**). The increase in abdominal pressure on the lower rib cage constitutes the appositional portion while the action of the diaphragm in relation to the rib cage constitutes the insertion portion (Mead, 1979; Loring and Mead, 1982; Troyer and Wilson, 2016). During tidal breathing in upright position the diaphragm and intercostal muscles contribute to 70% and 30% of the Vt, respectively (Druz and Sharp, 1981). In supine posture the contribution of diaphragm increases to 90% (Mognoni et al., 1969; Druz and Sharp, 1981), predisposing to orthopnea. The diaphragm generates only 10–20% of its maximum force generation during quiet breathing (Benditt, 2019; Welch et al., 2019).

Intercostal muscles

Intercostal muscles span the intercostal space as two thin layers. The inner intercostal fibers run in the caudal-dorsal direction from the sternocostal junction to near the tubercles of the ribs (De Troyer and Estenne, 1984). Fibers of the external intercostals run caudal-ventrally, extending from the tubercles of the ribs to the costochondral junction.

The functions of intercostal muscles have been controversial, particularly because they cannot be activated individually and are inaccessible. De Troyer et al. (De Troyer and Estenne, 1984) found that external intercostal muscles possess a substantial inspiratory mechanical advantage that decreases in the caudal and ventral directions until it is reversed into an expiratory mechanical advantage. The internal intercostals primarily exhibit an expiratory mechanical advantage (Benditt, 2019) while the intertriginous portion of the internal (parasternal) intercostals also possess an inspiratory advantage (De Troyer and Estenne, 1984; Benditt, 2019). External intercostal muscles additionally stabilize (stiffen) the rib cage, minimizing its inward collapse during inspiration while maintaining ventilation-perfusion relationships (Roussos).

Accessory Inspiratory Muscles

The accessory inspiratory muscles consist of the sternocleidomastoids (SCM), scalenes, pectoralis major and minor, and inferior fibers of serratus anterior and latissimus dorsi. The sternocleidomastoids elevate the clavicles and first rib, reducing pleural pressure and cause the abdomen and lateral ribcage to expand outward (De Troyer and Estenne, 1984; Roussos). They become active at high tidal volume generation, such as during exercise (Roussos). Sternocleidomastoid activity increases during respiratory distress from any cause, but has been mainly documented in patients with chronic obstructive pulmonary disease (COPD) (Sarkar et al., 2019): more than a 5 mm upward movement of the clavicle is associated with severe airflow limitation, reflected by an FEV_1 of 0.6 L or less (Sarkar et al., 2019). The scalenes arise from the transverse processes of the lower cervical vertebra and insert into the first 2 ribs. They contract under increased stress and metabolic demand, expanding the upper rib cage to augment tidal breathing.

Bastir et al. (Bastir et al., 2017) showed that expansion and contraction (kinematics) of the pulmonary and diaphragmatic parts of the thorax differed in their modes of shape change during breathing while the degree of shape change was similar in both compartments. The diaphragmatic part exhibited expansion more than the pulmonary part, therefore the upper thorax has to undergo greater deformation to expand to the same degree as the lower thorax. This has important implications with regard to respiratory muscles weakened at different times. For example, in ascending paralysis, the lower rib cage is likely to exhibit inward retraction and collapse as the intercostals weaken, while the diaphragm and accessory neck muscles assume increasing inspiratory activity. Thus, variability in regional lung expansion, ventilation-perfusion matching and gas exchange ensue depending on which thoracic muscles are impaired and the time over which these changes evolve (Roussos).

Abdominal Muscles

Four primary abdominal muscles augment expiratory force—the rectus abdominus, transverse abdominus, internal abdominal oblique and external abdominal oblique (Welch et al., 2019; Roussos). They increase intraabdominal pressure by pulling the abdominal wall inwards and displacing the diaphragm up into the thoracic cavity. In addition they lower the ribs, pulling them medially thereby deflating the ribcage, key during forced expiration such as coughing.

Abdominal muscles indirectly aid with inspiration. They compress the lungs to below their normal end-expiratory volume, storing elastic energy in the chest wall during expiration, facilitating passive inspiration. This action increases the curvature of the diaphragm and its force generation (based on Laplace's Law) (Roussos).

Upper Airway Dilator Muscles

Dilator muscles of the pharynx and larynx facilitate air flow by minimizing upper airway resistance during inspiration, an important function compromised in patients with bulbar dysfunction, and more so in individuals with obstructive sleep apnea (Oliven et al., 2018). Airway patency is maintained by coordinated co-activation of inspiratory and upper airway muscles, including the genioglossus, and preventing collapse of pharyngeal soft tissues (Van de Graaff et al., 1984; Kobayashi et al., 1996; Malhotra et al., 2000; Eckert et al., 2007; Fauroux and Khirani, 2014; Oliven et al., 2018). Posterior movement of the hyoid during inspiration can increase airway resistance and limit airflow, especially during sleep, an action opposed by contraction of the sternothyroid, thyrohyoid, sternohyoid, and geniohyoid muscles to preserve upper airway patency (Van de Graaff et al., 1984).

REDUCTIONS IN RESPIRATORY SYSTEM COMPLIANCE AND VOLUMES

Patients with NMD exhibit reduced vital capacity (Fauroux and Khirani, 2014; Lo Mauro and Aliverti, 2016) and respiratory (lung + chest wall) compliance (increase in respiratory elastance) (**Figure 3**), in part due to alveolar collapse and, when present, scoliosis. Recurrent aspiration contributes to further reduction in

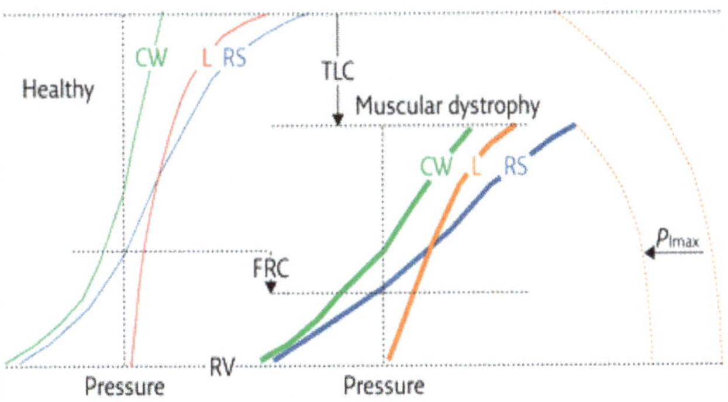

FIGURE 3 | Respiratory mechanics in individual with muscular dystrophy compared to that of a healthy individual. Shown are the presumed pressure–volume curves of the respiratory system (RS, blue curves) and its two components, the chest wall (CW, green curves) and lung (L, red curves), for healthy subjects (thin curves on the left panel) and patients with muscular dystrophy (thick curves on the right panel). The maximal inspiratory pressure (Plmax) is also shown (dashed curves). Key features include 1) decreased total lung capacity (TLC); 2) decreased compliance of chest wall (CCW), lungs (CL) and respiratory system, a consequence of reduced thoracic volume (slopes of the corresponding pressure–volume curves); 3) reduced Plmax; 4) decreased inspiratory capacity (IC = TLC–FRC); and 5) reduced expiratory reserve volume (ERV = FRC–RV). Functional residual capacity (FRC) may be reduced or even normal. Residual volume (RV) is usually preserved. Plmax represents the force of inspiratory muscles, while the volume variations are the resulting action of their contraction. The compliance of the respiratory system is decreased because of **(A)** lung atelectasis and fibrosis, the former a consequence of hypoventilation, and the latter from recurrent aspirations; and **(B)** scoliosis, induced by assymmetric involvement of trunk muscles. Figure caption modified from (Lo Mauro and Aliverti, 2016).

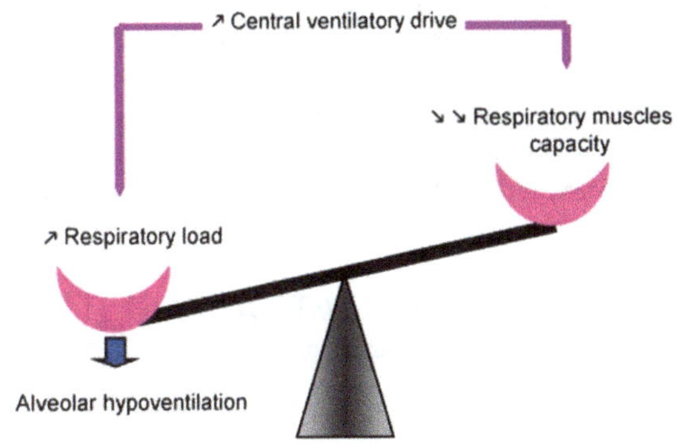

FIGURE 4 | Maintenance of spontaneous ventilation depends on balance between function of the respiratory muscles on one side and the respiratory load, determined by respiratory mechanics, on the other. Central respiratory drive is regulated such that work of breathing is minimized by adjusting tidal volume and respiratory rate to compensate for the load. Alveolar hypoventilation ensues when the respiratory load exceeds the ability of the central drive and respiratory muscles to maintain adequate gas exchange, often associated with respiratory muscle fatigue. From (Fauroux and Khirani, 2014).

lung compliance with loss of aerated alveolar volume, as seen with acute respiratory distress syndrome, and a serious complication of aspiration (Zaloga, 2002). Upper airway collapse from bulbar dysfunction further increases resistance to breathing (Benditt, 2019). Such changes in compliance contribute to increase in work of breathing. Work of breathing is kept at the lowest level by adjusting tidal volume and respiratory rate to compensate for the load. Alveolar hypoventilation results from the respiratory load exceeding the ability of the central drive and respiratory muscles to maintain adequate gas exchange (**Figure 4**).

In supine posture gravitational pressure from abdominal contents impairs tidal excursions of the diaphragm. In most NMDs a decrease in VC upon assuming supine posture (by 25% or more) is a sensitive index of diaphragmatic weakness (Fromageot et al., 2001; Lechtzin et al., 2002; Prigent et al., 2012; Chen et al., 2013). In this connection, in the upright position, application of an abdominal wrap below the lower rib margin displaces the diaphragm cephalad, lengthening its fibers, increasing its force generation and reducing dyspnea, a technique widely adopted by poliomyelitis patients during the epidemic of the 1940s and 1950s to improve activities of daily living and quality of life (Bach, 2017). Individuals with high cervical cord injury and others with weak abdominal musculature also find abdominal wraps to be helpful with breathing (Goldman et al., 1986; McCool et al., 1986; Scott et al., 1993; Berlowitz et al., 2016). Their VC increases as diaphragmatic fibers lengthen with increase in force generation and reversal of platypnea (Fugl-Meyer and Grimby, 1984; Baydur et al., 2001; Terson de Paleville et al., 2014). This finding is in line with studies in able-bodied individuals in which maximal force generation of the transdiaphragmatic pressure (Pdi) decreases as lung volume increases (Beck et al., 1998) and would explain the increase in diaphragmatic strength in the supine spinal cord-injured patient.

EFFECTS OF OBESITY

Similar to able-bodied people, individuals with NMD are at risk for developing chronic diseases resulting from obesity and a sedentary lifestyle. Aitkens et al. (Aitkens et al., 2005) found that 55% of their NMD patients met criteria for metabolic syndrome. Bauman et al. (Bauman et al., 1992) determined that cardiovascular disease was the leading cause of death in individuals with spinal cord injury and occurred at a younger age than in able-bodied persons.

Changes in respiratory mechanics occurring in NMD are augmented with obesity. Oxygen cost and work of breathing are increased to overcome respiratory resistance or inertance (Dempsey et al., 1966; Sharp et al., 1986; Kress et al., 1999). Despite the increase in gravitational load of the chest wall in the supine position, functional residual capacity (FRC) does not fall below seated values in obese subjects with reduced FRC when seated. In supine position inspiratory muscle activity maintains dynamic hyperinflation above relaxation volume presumably because of greater muscle length and force generation (Yap et al., 1995).

In a retrospective study of 34 patients with Duchenne muscular dystrophy (DMD, mean age 13.7 years) Chew et al. (Chew et al., 2016) found that BMI was positively related to FVC, contrary to what one might expect in obese individuals (Sharp et al., 1964; Thomas et al., 1989; Salome et al., 2010). The observed association may have been the result of corticosteroid therapy resulting in greater muscle mass and strength, although the study did not take into account changes in muscle and fat mass, edema or growth, also known to occur in DMD (Durnin and Rahaman, 1967; Stanbury and Graham, 1998; Pessolano et al., 2003).

CONTROL OF VENTILATION AND ITS RELATION TO RESPIRATORY LOAD COMPENSATION

The link between the nervous system and respiratory muscles are the motor neurons located in the brain stem. The ventral medulla regulates exhalation while the dorsal medulla is responsible for inhalation. Communication between the two parts of the medulla is through integration of input from peripheral and central respiratory muscles to generate a cyclical respiratory rhythm. The pontine group allows for regulation of the medullary signals to ensure smooth inspiration and expiration transition. Central chemoreceptors located within the medulla and retrotrapezoid nucleus to sense pH changes related to carbon dioxide concentrations in the cerebrospinal fluid (Panitch, 2009). Peripheral chemoreceptors (carotid and aortic bodies) respond primarily to changes in arterial oxygen tension.

As early as the poliomyelitis epidemic (Whittenberger and Sarnoff, 1950; Plum and Swanson, 1958), changes in central control of ventilation have been described in various NMDs (Kilburn et al., 1959; Carroll et al., 1976; Rosenow and Engel, 1978a; Borel et al., 1993; Rialp et al., 2013). A blunting of the ventilatory response to hypercapnia implies a decrease in chemoreceptor sensitivity; however, in the presence of diffuse muscle weakness and abnormal respiratory mechanics, determining the exact contribution of the medullary motoneurons to a decrease in ventilatory response can be a challenge (Borel et al., 1993; Rialp et al., 2013). Measurement of occlusion pressure ($P_{0.1}$) provides a more reliable assessment of central drive as it is not influenced by change in lung volume and flow resistance (Whitelaw et al., 1975). Indeed, some studies have demonstrated normal or increased $P_{0.1}$ (McCool et al., 1988; Baydur, 1991), indicating that central drive is intact. In many cases, sleep-disordered breathing contributes to nocturnal hypoventilation even as the patient is able to maintain normal daytime gas exchange (Aboussouan, 2015; Fermin et al., 2016). An inspiratory vital capacity of less than 60% predicts sleep disordered breathing in children and adolescents with NMD [59 Fermin]. Overnight polysomnography confirms presence of sleep-disordered breathing. Sleep abnormalities of central origin can be seen in myotonic dystrophy, which may be separate from the muscular deficit. We refer the reader to excellent reviews on sleep-disordered breathing for in-depth discussions of their diagnosis and management (Aboussouan, 2015; Fermin et al., 2016).

Axen (Axen, 1982) described variable changes in ventilatory control (tidal volume and inspiratory duration) in cervical cord-injured men in response to elastic and resistive loads, assuming identical respiratory muscle pressure (Pmus) wave forms in the unloaded and loaded states. Afferent pathways from the mouth, lung, and/or diaphragm modulated the phrenic discharge during the first loaded breath. In chest wall disorders such as kyphoscoliosis (KS), respiratory elastance and resistance are increased, and breathing pattern is rapid and shallow, resulting in defense of tidal volume (Vt) in the face of inspiratory resistive loading. Baydur and Carlson (Baydur and Carlson, 1996) computed passive elastance (Ers) and active elastance and resistance (E′rs and R′rs, respectively) in anesthetized patients according to previously described techniques (Behrakis et al., 1983; Baydur et al., 1989). The difference between passive and active respiratory elastance represents changes in thoracic mechanical properties (stiffening) related to chest wall distortion during added loads. With resistive loading, driving pressure and inspiratory time were prolonged compared to healthy subjects, while percent reduction in Vt and minute ventilation was less in KS. Increased intrinsic impedance, Pmus, and differences in changes in neural timing in anesthetized kyphoscoliotics contributed to modestly greater Vt defense, compared to that of anesthetized subjects free of cardiorespiratory disease.

Elastic Load Compensation

If someone were to hold a 20-lb weight with arm outstretched and had a 1-lb weight added to the load, they are not likely to feel the added weight as afferent sensory receptors adapt to the high muscle tension; by contrast, they are more likely to feel the addition of a 10-lb weight which noticeably adds to the tension. A similar analogy can be applied in individuals with increased elastic respiratory loads. To evaluate the effects of abnormal respiratory mechanics and neuromuscular drive on the various components of elastic load compensation, Baydur et al. (Baydur et al., 1989) studied anesthetized patients with KS whose mean passive and active respiratory elastance, active respiratory resistance, and peak inspiratory occlusion pressure were, respectively, 89%, 84%, 100%, and 37% greater, and inspiratory duration (Ti) 13% less than corresponding values in anesthetized control subjects. The increased intrinsic elastance and resistance and decreased Ti contributed to Vt defense in KS in the absence of vagal modulation. Characteristics of elastic load compensation in anesthetized KS patients are nevertheless similar to those of anesthetized normal subjects.

Post-Inspiratory Diaphragmatic Braking Activity

The diaphragm has been shown to exhibit post-inspiratory activity during passive expiration (pliometric activity) (Muller et al., 1979; Muller et al., 1980; Zin et al., 1983; Baydur, 1992; Easton et al., 1999) resulting in preservation of lung volume. Such activity may be of benefit in patients with chest wall disorders in preventing airway collapse (Muller et al., 1980; Baydur, 1992). Absence of pliometric activity may result in reduction in lung volume and atelectasis.

DYSPNEA IN PATIENTS WITH NEUROMUSCULAR DISEASE: CONCEPT OF AIR HUNGER VS. PERCEPTION OF RESPIRATORY WORK AND EFFORT

The sensation of an urge to breathe is referred to as "air hunger", for example, when it develops during a long breath hold (Banzett et al., 2021) it occurs when urgent homeostatic needs to maintain gas exchange are not met. Stimuli that increase air hunger include hypercapnia, hypoxia, exercise, and acidosis; tidal expansion of the lungs (spontaneous or assisted) reduces air hunger. As such, it is not affected by respiratory muscle activity and is thought to be regulated by central chemoreceptors in the brain stem (Banzett et al., 1990). By contrast, when respiratory muscle fatigue or an increase in breathing load (such as occurs with pneumonia) calls for increase in muscle contraction, a sensation of increased work or effort is described; it likely arises from respiratory muscle afferents or from the brainstem or cerebral cortex.

A striking example of these events is that of a chronically over-ventilated muscular dystrophy patient whose $PaCO_2$ has gradually decreased to the 20–30 mm Hg range (a common issue as patients feels better with sensation of increase in chest wall expansion with increase in Vt. Patients receiving nocturnal ventilation often maintain a lower PCO_2 during the following day. Possible explanations include: 1) Reducing daytime work of breathing by resting respiratory muscles at night, and 2) CO_2 elimination at night promotes bicarbonate excretion with a lower set point for ventilatory control as metabolic alkalosis is corrected. Allowing the PCO_2 to increase by intermittently reducing the delivered Vt (even by 30–50 ml at a time) or respiratory rate become uncomfortable for the patient, increasing demand that ventilator settings be restored to their original state (personal observation). These symptoms suggest a re-set of the threshold for CO_2 sensitivity such that even a slight rise in PCO_2 induces air hunger despite (or because of) the chronic hypocapnia. Coughing induced by airway irritation can aggravate the sensation of air hunger and might be vagally mediated but central mechanisms cannot be ruled out (Nishino et al., 2008).

By contrast, individuals will describe a sensation of feeling "hard to breathe" when experiencing a respiratory infection because of alterations in respiratory compliance and resistance (with little or no change in blood gases). Changing ventilator settings by increasing the Vt or respiratory rate relieves their symptoms, but at the cost of inducing a chronic respiratory alkalosis. The resulting reduction in plasma bicarbonate stores increases vulnerability to metabolic acidosis resulting from sepsis, shock and other causes.

RESPIRATORY MUSCLE FATIGUE

Respiratory muscle fatigue is defined by loss in capacity for developing force against a constant load (Roussos and Koutsoukou, 2003). The higher the diaphragmatic force generation is as a function of maximal pressure the diaphragm can sustain, the greater the chance the diaphragm is likely to fatigue. Multiple factors contribute depending on how the NMD affects the central nervous system, transmission of signals between the CNS and muscle (central fatigue) or even the muscle itself (peripheral fatigue). Central muscle fatigue results from a deficit in the capacity to recruit all muscle units, while peripheral fatigue is due to a failure of muscle fibers to respond maximally during full activation (Edwards, 1979). Weakening of respiratory muscles produces paradoxical breathing (asynchronous movement) between abdomen and ribcage (Troyer and Wilson, 2016). As the diaphragm fatigues, inspiratory action assumed by the accessory muscles of the neck results in inward retraction of the ribcage and outward displacement of the abdominal wall (Benditt, 2019).

Measurement of transdiaphragmatic pressure (Pdi) (using esophageal and gastric balloons) is a more precise means of recording diaphragmatic force generation (Pdi) and endurance (Roussos et al., 1979a; Bellemare and Grassino, 1982). It is, however, invasive and requires coaching for naïve individuals, and therefore primarily used in research. The individual is asked to breathe through a series of inspiratory flow resistors to achieve a target pressure on an oscilloscope or computer screen. From these measurements, the tension-time index [TTdi = (Pdi/Pdimax) (Ti/Ttot), where Ti is the inspiratory time and Ttot is the duration of respiratory cycle] can be computed. TTdi values of >0.18 are associated with respiratory muscle fatigue and reduced endurance (Roussos et al., 1979a; Bellemare and Grassino, 1982). The technique is capable of producing inspiratory pressures generated by rib cage muscles in the absence of diaphragmatic contribution. A potential clinical application of Pdi in individuals with NMD is to determine which inspiratory muscles contribute to respiratory insufficiency and cough impairment (as a result of loss of lung volume and elastic recoil): Alternating amplitude of Pdi and gastric pressure (Pga) indicates recruitment and derecruitment of different groups of inspiratory muscles (Roussos et al., 1979a).

A non-invasive alternative is to measure the tension-time index of the inspiratory muscles as a whole (TTlim) during mouth breathing without the use of esophageal and gastric balloons (Ramonatxo et al., 1995). An increase in mean inspiratory pressure in relation to the maximal inspiratory pressure produces an increase in TTlim. Another noninvasive tool analogous to the TTdi is the breathing intolerance index (BIT), used to assess the ability of patients with NMD and other conditions to wean off ventilation (Koga et al., 2206). It makes use of the relation of breathing pattern to vital capacity (VC) [(Vt/VC) (Ti/Ttot)]. In this analysis, lung volumes replace respiratory muscle pressures so that the ratios comprising BIT can be affected by lung and chest wall mechanics in addition to respiratory muscle strength. Later, Baydur and Chen (Baydur and Chen, 2013) found BIT in patients with obesity (a chest wall disorder) tended to be higher than in healthy controls in contrast to patients with chronic obstructive pulmonary disease.

Sarmento and colleagues (Sarmento et al., 2021) found that *1)* inspiratory rib cage muscles (sternocleidomastoids, scalenes and parasternals) differed in their responses to fatigue and recovery, as reflected by changes in spectral surface EMG variables, *2)* loss of mechanical power in rib cage muscles resulted from reduced shortening velocity, and *3)* relaxation properties recovered better from fatigue than do contractile characteristics. Recovery of fatigue varied, with median frequency returning to pre-fatigue values faster than the high/low (H/L) frequency spectrum suggesting that mechanisms of fatigue differed depending on the specific inspiratory muscle. Furthermore, changes in relaxation rates were strongly associated with the H/L frequency spectrum and predicted inspiratory ribcage muscle recovery. Again, the rate of progression of respiratory impairment (or stabilization) will vary depending on which groups of muscles are involved and their characteristics of fatigability. In addition to twitch characteristics assessed by EMG (Bellemare and Roussos, 1995), muscle fatigue characteristics may be presaged by periodic analysis of their H/L frequency spectrum.

PHYSIOLOGY OF COUGH: NEUROMECHANICAL COUPLING

Patients with NMD experience difficulty clearing airway secretions due to ineffective cough (Perrin et al., 2204; Yang and Finkel, 2010; Sahni and Wolfe, 2018; Allen, 2010). For an effective cough, one needs to take a deep breath, while the glottis closes to increase intrathoracic pressure, followed by its opening explosively in conjunction with abdominal contraction to expel air. Peak cough flows below 160 L/min are considered ineffective (Bach, 2017). Glottic and bulbar dysfunction lead to accumulation of saliva in the valleculae and pyriform sinuses (Silbergleit et al., 1991; Sonies and Dalakas, 1991). As a result, ineffective airway clearance predispose to recurrent pneumonia a major cause of mortality and morbidity (Chatwin et al., 2018).

The cough reflex is chiefly mediated by vagal afferent nerve fibers innervating the larynx, large airways and parenchyma; its components comprise both myelinated (rapidly and slowly adapting receptors) and unmyelinated rapidly adapting and noniceptive pulmonary fiber (C-fiber) receptors (Widdicombe, 1954; Paintal et al., 1986). The latter fibers assume a major role in cough and related reflexes. Deep inspiration stimulates airway irritant receptors, therefore an impaired inspiratory effort will diminish triggers to cough as well as the effort. Other neural pathways regulating the cough reflex include the glossopharyngeal and phrenic nerves which have many sensory as well as motor fibers. Efferent pathways include (again) the *1)* vagus (motor nerve for the muscles of the pharynx and larynx); *2)* the spinal motor nerves of which the thoracic supply the intercostal muscles and the lumbar nerves the abdominal muscles; and *3)* the trigeminal, facial, hypoglossal and accessory nerves innervating the upper airway and accessory muscles, called into play during cough (Bouros and Green, 1971).

Patients with spinal cord injury exhibit respiratory muscle dysfunction to the extent reflected by the level of cord injury (Ledsome and Sharp, 1981; Fugl-Meyer and Grimby, 1984; Baydur et al., 2001). High cord injuries leave intact residual action by the diaphragm and accessory muscles with cough generation dependent on high lung elastic recoil. Even with such injuries, however, active expiration in quadriplegic individuals can be augmented by contraction of the clavicular portion of the pectoralis major (innervated by the 5th through 7th cervical segments) which displaces the manubrium and upper ribs downward, contracting the upper rib cage (De Troyer et al., 1986), an important consideration for cough generation. By contrast, the lower rib cage expanded, at least in early inspiration, as a result of increase in abdominal pressure. Estenne et al. (Estenne et al., 1994) later showed that despite weak expiratory muscles, quadriplegic individuals were able to enhance their cough ability as a result of dynamic compression of tracheal and large airways enabling marked increase in expiratory flow, even though peak pleural pressures were 74–92% less than in normal subjects.

RESPIRATORY FAILURE

Respiratory failure develops from impairment of ventilation and gas exchange due to lung or chest wall dysfunction. Increases in respiratory elastance and resistance due to lung volume reduction and thoracic cage distortion lead to increase in work of breathing and respiratory muscle fatigue. Typically, arterial oxygen tensions lower than 8.0 kPa and arterial carbon dioxide tensions above 6.0 kPa define respiratory failure. These values should serve as guides to identifying respiratory failure, not as rigid cut-offs (Roussos and Koutsoukou, 2003; Welch et al., 2019).

There are two types of respiratory failure—hypoxemia with and without hypercapnia (Roussos and Koutsoukou, 2003). The former is a result of inadequate ventilation due to reduced neural drive and muscular power as occurs with progressive NMDs. Hypercapnic failure reflects increase in physiological dead space, manifested during rapid, shallowing breathing due to abnormal chest wall mechanics (Welch et al., 2019). Hypoxemia without hypercapnia results from impaired oxygen transfer, a consequence of atelectasis and chest wall distortion (Campbell, 1965; Welch et al., 2019). Microatelectasis results in an increase in the alveolar-arterial oxygen difference (AaDO2), reflected by a normal PaO_2, sometimes in conjunction with a reduced $PaCO_2$ while breathing room air. In individuals with sleep apnea, loss of upper airway muscle tone and collapse coupled with weakening thoracic cage muscles lead to impaired gas exchange, exaggerated during REM sleep (Benditt, 2019). As sleep disordered breathing worsens, hypercapnia persists throughout day and night.

Acute decompensation may result from aspiration due to bulbar dysfunction-induced dysphagia or gastroesophageal reflux (Allen, 2010; Wijdicks, 2017; Welch et al., 2019), requiring assisted ventilation. In this connection, long-term ventilatory support can result in further weakening of the diaphragm due to muscle atrophy (Roussos et al., 1979b; Jaber et al., 2011) and passive increase in end-expiratory volume by application of positive end-expiratory pressure (PEEP) (Jansen et al., 2021).

EVALUATION OF RESPIRATORY MUSCLE FUNCTION AND PHYSIOLOGIC CHANGES IN NMD

Electrophysiologic Techniques

Relating the electrical activity of the diaphragm to its force generation during quiet breathing or maximal respiratory efforts is used to assess diaphragmatic weakness and its propensity to fatigue under conditions of increased load (Bellemare and Grassino, 1982; Bellemare and Roussos, 1995; Sarmento et al., 2021). Assessing the ratio of diaphragm compound muscle action potential (CMAP) amplitude to transdiaphragmatic twitch pressure is also used to distinguish between defects in neuromuscular transmission defects (when both quantities decrease) and defects in muscle contractility (when twitch pressure is decreased in presence of a normal CMAP) (Aldrich et al., 1986).

Respiratory Pressures

Traditionally, respiratory muscle strength has been measured with maximal inspiratory and expiratory mouth pressures (Black and Hyatt, 1971; Leech et al., 1983; Vincken et al., 1987). Padkao and Boonla (Padkao and Boonla, 2020) showed that Pimax and Pemax were significantly related to middle and lower thoracic wall expansion, suggesting that respiratory muscle strength was more closely associated with chest wall expansion and diaphragmatic descent than with expiratory muscle strength. If thoracic cage muscles are weakened by disease, rib cage expansion is impaired and the rib cage fails to expand, these maneuvers are, however, difficult to perform by patients with weak muscles, as they require cooperation and coordination, Pimax (MIP) and Pemax (MEP) are ideally generated at residual volume and total capacity, respectively, and need to be maintained for 4 s, a challenge even for able-bodied individuals (Aldrich and Spiro, 1995).

As alluded to earlier, respiratory impairment depends on the pattern of muscle and/or nerve involvement and on the rate of progression of disease. Respiratory muscles are often involved in patients with proximal limb weakness, as in certain myopathies (Rosenow and Engel, 1978b; Braun et al., 1983; Mellies et al., 2005; Bi et al., 2021). Braun et al. (Braun et al., 1983) studied 53 patients with proximal myopathy (16 with lung disease). Hypercapnia was inversely related to VC (which, however, could be as high as 55% predicted), as well as to respiratory muscle strength (RMS, average of Pimax and Pemax). The latter relationship (an occlusive maneuver devoid of airflow and with negligible change in lung volume) reflected respiratory muscle weakness more than a decrease in VC which is affected by lung disease. Carbon dioxide retention did not occur until RMS was less than 50% predicted (Braun et al., 1983).

More recently, measurement of sniff nasal inspiratory pressures (SNIP) have been found to be better tolerated and reproducible (Ti and Fit Ting, 1999; Sarmento et al., 2021). Nasal pressure is measured in an occluded nostril as the patient sniffs through the opposite nasal passage and is closely associated with and easier to perform than Pimax (Laroche et al., 1988; Ti and Fit Ting, 1999) and FVC (Nicot et al., 2006) measurements. In a study of 61 patients with NMD and COPD, recording of esophageal pressure during a maximal sniff was found to be useful in assessing inspiratory muscle strength and easier to perform than the MIP (Sarmento et al., 2021). Many patients had normal sniff Pes despite low MIPs, suggesting that performing MIP was challenging because of dyspnea and weakness of facial muscles with difficulty in maintaining static pressures.

Transdiaphragmatic pressure (Pdi) can be recorded while breathing spontaneously or during maximal inspiratory maneuvers, such as a sniff (Perrin et al., 2204; Yang and Finkel, 2010). It can also be measured during magnetic stimulation of the phrenic nerve and has the advantage of greater accuracy for measuring diaphragm strength, especially in individuals with airflow limitation in whom airway opening pressure or SNIP would not accurately reflect esophageal pressure because of reduced lung elastic recoil and gas decompression. Measurement of Pdi and its role in the evaluation of diaphragmatic fatigue is described in detail in **section 7**.

Spirometry and Lung Volumes

Spirometry is essential in the diagnosis and management of pulmonary diseases and can be performed in children as young as 6 years old (**Table 1**) (Steier et al., 2007; Sharma, 2009; Caruso et al., 2015; Chiang et al., 2018). It facilitates assessment of functional capacity, following the course of illness, and response to management.

The forced expiratory volume in one second (FEV_1) and FVC will show different rates of decline, depending on the course of illness. However, the ratio FEV1/FVC remains within normal range (80–100%). Using FEV1, respiratory health can be graded from mild to very severe: mild >70% predicted; moderate 60–69%; moderately severe 50–59%; severe ranging 35–49%; and very severe <35% (Sahni and Wolfe, 2018; Allen, 2010). **Table 1** lists tests useful for evaluating respiratory function in patients with NMD and chest wall disorders. In a study of 60 patients with Duchenne muscular dystrophy, FVC and peak expiratory flow (PEF or Pemax) decreased linearly by 5 percent per year (Mayer et al., 2015). An FVC of <40% predicted was associated with a $PaCO_2$ ≥45 mm Hg and a base excess of >4 mmol/L. Some have reported the value of determining the plateau VC which correlates with severity of Duchenne dystrophy (DMD) and risk of developing severe scoliosis (Welch et al., 2019). Following the VC plateau may indicate the best point to initiate air stacking to maximum lung insufflations (Benditt, 2019). Inspiratory muscle weakness is detected by a 20% or more reduction in VC upon assuming supine posture (Fromageot et al., 2001; Lechtzin et al., 2002; Prigent et al., 2012; Chen et al., 2013) and indicates need for assisted ventilation (Chen et al., 2013) (**Figure 5**). The reduction in lung volume also results in a decrease in maximal transdiaphragmatic sniff pressure (Pdimax sniff) (**Figure 6**). In general, assisted ventilation is indicated for patients whose VC has decreased below 1 L or 30% predicted (Steier et al., 2007; Sharma, 2009; Mayer et al., 2015; Chiang et al., 2018). Decline in FVC can be variable in patients with amyotrophic lateral sclerosis (ALS) (Ackrivo et al., 2019a), indicating phenotypes with differing prognostic implications (Elamin et al., 2015; Ackrivo et al., 2019b) (**Figure 7**).

Lung volume subdivisions can be measured using body plethysmography, gas dilution, or washout techniques (**Table 1**). If airflow limitation is suspected, plethysmography is the preferred method to avoid underestimating volume of trapped gas (Sharma, 2009; Mayer et al., 2015; Chiang et al., 2018). The method distinguishes air trapping from effects of obesity; both conditions result in reduction of expiratory reserve volume, while inspiratory capacity is reduced with air trapping but is increased with obesity. In advanced stages, preferential weakening of abdominal muscles with decrease in maximal

TABLE 1 | Respiratory function tests commonly used to evaluate individuals with neuromuscular disorders.

Lung Volumes
Total lung capacity (TLC)
Residual volume (RV)
Spirometry
Peak flow rate (PFR)
Cough peak flow (CPF)
Forced vital capacity (FVC) (preferably in seated and supine positions)
Forced expiratory volume in 1 s (FEV_1)
Maximum insufflation capacity (MIC)
Respiratory muscle strength
Maximal expiratory pressure (MEP) (preferably in seated and supine positions)
Maximal inspiratory pressure (MIP) (preferably in seated and supine positions)
Sniff test (SNIP)
Gas exchange
Oxyhemoglobin saturation by pulse oximetry
Capnography: end-tidal CO_2 (PetCO2) measurement
Arterial or venous blood gas profile

Modified from (Sharma, 2009).

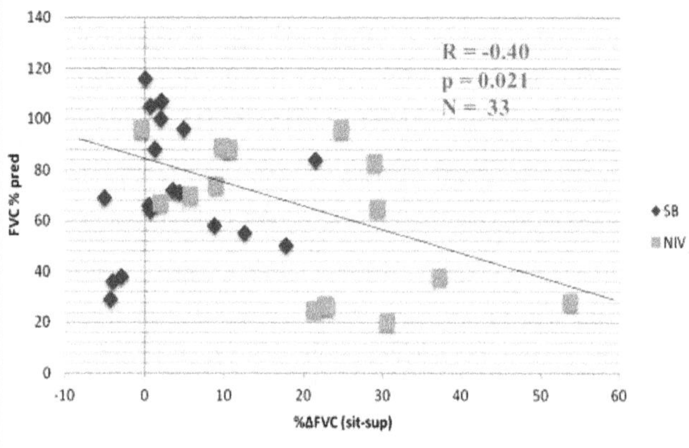

FIGURE 5 | Relationship between % change in forced vital capacity (FVC) from seated (sit) to supine (sup) posture and baseline FVC in seated position in patients with neuromuscular disease (FVCsit, % predicted). Black diamonds, spontaneous breathing (SB); grey squares, noninvasive ventilation (NIV). Patients with greater than 20% decrease in FVC when supine required NIV. From (Chen et al., 2013).

expiratory pressure (Pemax) may explain the preservation or increase in residual volume. Spasticity of rib cage muscles prevents outward recoil of the chest wall from being reduced further helping to maintain FRC and preserve residual volume (RV). Patients may experience difficulty in performing panting maneuvers in the body box because of bulbar weakness. Excessive upper airway and cheek compliance may also result in underestimation of FRC and RV (Jaeger, 1982).

Measurement of Flow Limitation and Airway Resistance--Old and New Techniques

The presence of intrathoracic airflow limitation has been determined using the negative expiratory pressure (NEP) technique (**Figure 8**) in patients with NMDs (Baydur, 2013). It avoids technical challenges posed by spirometry such as lung history and inhomogeneity, forced expiratory maneuvers, and the speed of forced expiration, all influenced by viscoelastic properties of the lung and chest wall. NEP consists of comparing the tidal expiratory flow during application of gentle negative pressure (about −5 cm H_2O) at the onset of expiration to the immediately preceding tidal expiratory flow. Expiratory flow should increase in healthy individuals while it changes little or not all in airflow limitation. Obese individuals or those with weakened bulbar musculature may exhibit transient decreases in tidal expiratory flow as upper airway soft tissues appose each other during application of NEP (**Figure 8C**). Such patients may be at risk for obstructive apneas during sleep as the upper airway may collapse during inspiratory efforts.

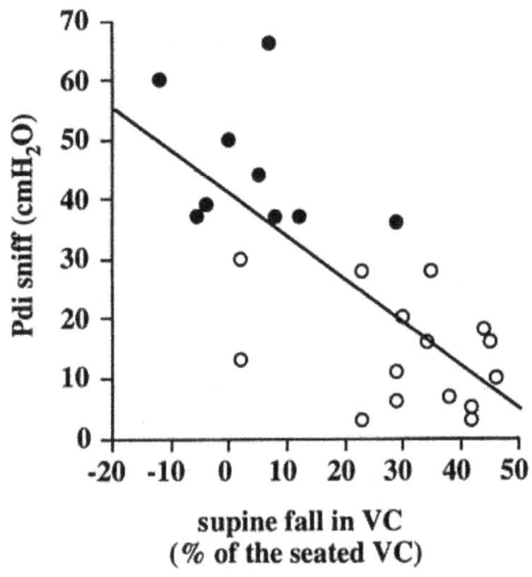

FIGURE 6 | Relation between transdiaphragmatic sniff pressure (Pdi sniff) and supine fall in VC. Open symbols indicate patients with paradoxical diaphragmatic motion and closed symbols indicate patients without paradoxical diaphragmatic motion. From (Fromageot et al., 2001).

The forced oscillation technique (FOT) or impulse oscillometry (IOS) until recently was employed in infants and young children as a useful alternative to spirometry to assess airway mechanics. More recently, it has been increasingly used to assess respiratory resistance and impedance in older individuals with obstructive and restrictive disorders (Lappas et al., 2016). Even fewer studies have evaluated respiratory mechanics in individuals with neuromuscular disorders. Impedance measurements can be easily obtained as they require little cooperation and no forced respiratory maneuvers. In one study normal respiratory impedance (Xrs) characteristics were found, while respiratory resistance (Rrs) was somewhat higher than those found in normal subjects (Wesseling et al., 1992). Van Noord et al. (Van Noord et al., 1991) found that patients with kyphoscoliosis (TLC 41% based on arm span) exhibited an increase in total respiratory resistance and elastance.

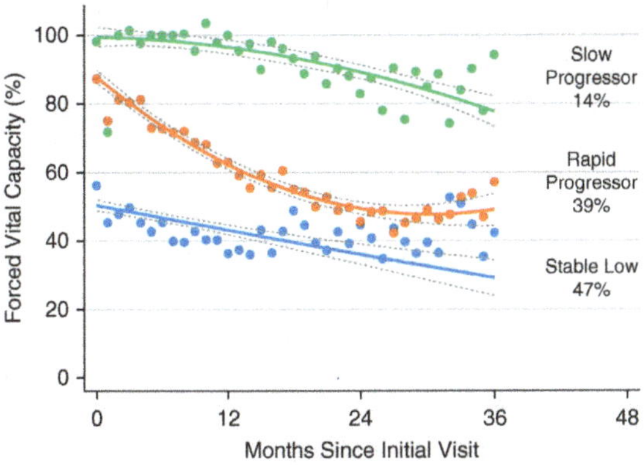

FIGURE 7 | The Penn Comprehensive ALS Center cohort trajectories of forced vital capacity (FVC) percent predicted with 95% confidence intervals. Three groups of patients with amyotrophic lateral sclerosis (ALS) are indicated by slow progressors (green), rapid progressors (red), and stable low (blue). Percentages represent proportion of the cohort with the corresponding group number as the highest predicted posterior probability. From (Ackrivo et al., 2019a).

Assessment of Control of Ventilation

The measurement of ventilatory drive by occlusion pressure recorded 100 msec after the onset of inspiratory effort ($P_{0.1}$) is a noninvasive method that assesses central drive and has been measured in NMD(Whitelaw et al., 1975; Baydur, 1991). Several factors, however, can alter the relation between P0. 1 and central drive, including presence of dynamic hyperinflation, expiratory muscle activity, chest wall distortion, respiratory muscle weakness, neuromuscular junction blockade, and the shape of the inspiratory pressure waveform (Whitelaw and Derenne, 1993). Central respiratory drive is blunted in patients with hypercapnic respiratory failure associated with NMD. In one study, NMD patients exhibited a hypercapnic drive response of only 30% that of normal subjects (García Río et al., 1994). The difference could be attributed to the reduced sensitivity of the chemoreceptors to chemical CO_2.

Peak Expiratory and Cough Flows

Peak expiratory flow and cough flow (PEF and PCF, respectively) are used to assess ability to cough and clear airway secretions. Values of PEF less than 160 L/min are associated with increased risk for retained secretions, atelectasis and pneumonia (Bach and Saporito, 1996; Bach et al., 1997; Bach, 2017). Suarez and colleagues (Suárez et al., 2002) found differences between PEF and PCF to be 46%, 43% and 11% in normal subjects, patients with DMD and those with ALS, respectively, the last finding because of poor glottic closure. Determination of PEF and PCF can be applied to estimate respiratory muscle strength if maximal static mouth pressures cannot be performed (Suárez et al., 2002). Patients with PCF below 160 L/min benefit from mechanical in-exsufflation (Bach and Saporito, 1996; Bach et al., 1997; Polkey and Moxham, 2001; Suárez et al., 2002; Miller and Mayer, 2021).

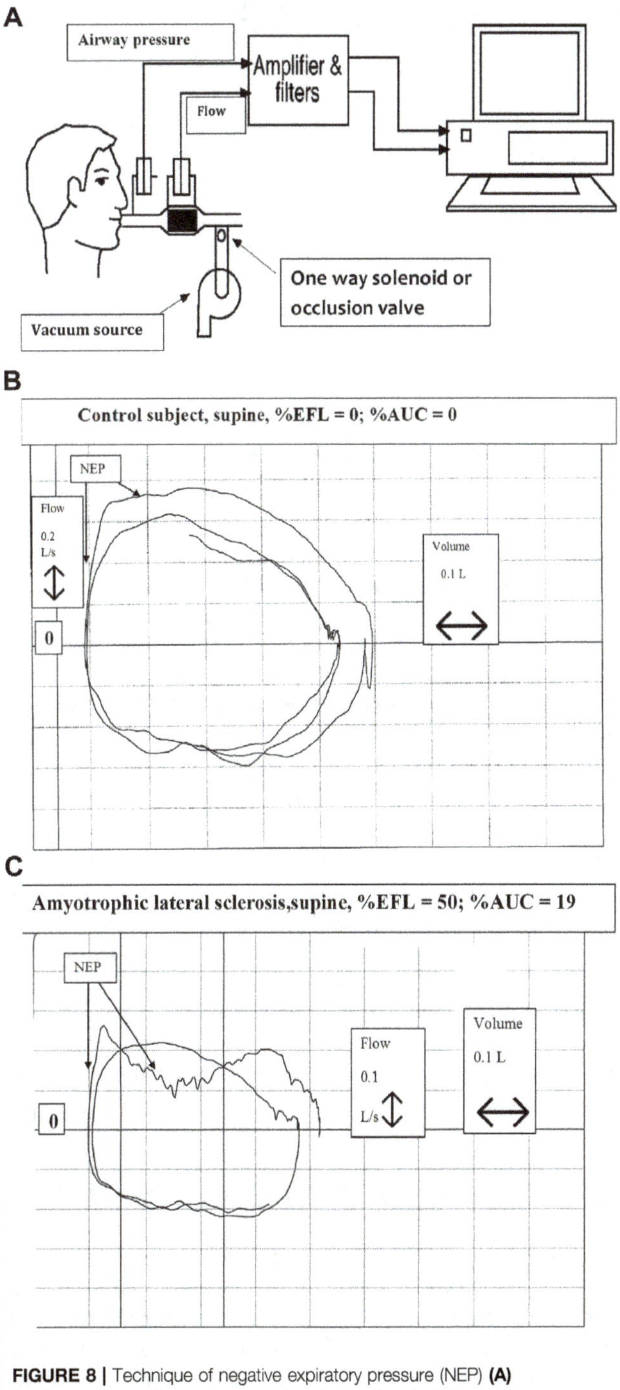

FIGURE 8 | Technique of negative expiratory pressure (NEP) **(A)** Equipment setup for assessment of expiratory flow limitation during spontaneous breathing. NEP is applied at beginning of tidal expirartion **(B)** Tracings of airway pressure, volume and flow during quiet breathing in a healthy supine individual. Application of negative expiratory pressure at the onset of expiration is indicated by NEP **(C)** Tracings of airway pressure, volume and flow during quiet breathing in a supine individual with amyotrophic lateral sclerosis. Application of negative expiratory pressure at the onset of expiration is indicated by NEP. In C, the "dip" in expiratory flow during NEP indicates upper airway narrowing, suggestive of bulbar impairment. From (Baydur, 2013).

Dyspnea and Sleep Quality

The reporting of dyspnea in patients with NMD may be related to sleep deprivation. Rault et al. (Rault et al., 2020) recently reported that a single night of sleep deprivation in a cohort of 20 healthy subjects reduced respiratory endurance during an inspiratory loading trial, accompanied by an increased sensation of dyspnea. More recently, using a questionnaire survey, the same group showed that the same individuals described a sensation of smothering more often than in a non-sleep-deprived control group (Rault et al., 2021). Thus, sleep deprivation modifies the sensation of dyspnea. While similar studies have yet to be done in individuals with NMD, increased respiratory elastance, and resistance, sleep deprivation should result in an increased sensation of breathlessness.

Oximetry and Capnography

Oximetry and capnography are useful to monitor gas exchange during studies of sleep disordered breathing. In patients with OSA (a chest wall disorder), oximetry may exhibit a sawtooth pattern during oxygen desaturation (Won et al., 2016) which represents cyclical variation in chemoreceptor response to fluctuations in ventilation or cardiac output (slow circulation time). Oximetry is more reliable when used in junction with capnography. While not as reliable as arterial blood gas analysis (because of changes in pH and CO_2), the latter is invasive and increases work for the technologist and/or nursing. Capnography records CO_2 tensions continuously using an end-tidal sensor or transcutaneous sensor. Disadvantages include expense, need for repeated calibration and susceptibility to external influences. A study simultaneously recording end-tidal and transcutaneous CO_2 found that transcutaneous capnometry registered higher values of CO_2 than the end-tidal method (Won et al., 2016). Using only end-tidal capnometry, the patient would not have been considered hypercapnic and thereby not offered assisted ventilation. Differences in recorded values should be considered when deciding to give a patient end-tidal or transcutaneous capnometry.

RECENT AND FUTURE DEVELOPMENTS

A number of recent molecular and physiologic approaches have demonstrated potential roles in further evaluation of respiratory function and treatment in NMD. Their continued role in clinical evaluation and management of neuromuscular-respiratory issues remains to be determined with more extended trials and clinical experience.

Gene Therapy

Recent developments in gene therapy have markedly improved care for NMDs (Markham et al., 2015; Harada et al., 2020; Oechsel and Cartwright, 2021; Paul et al., 2021). For instance, a new therapy called Poloxamer 188 NF improved respiratory function and measurements in dystrophic mice by targeting cardiomyocytes and improving intracellular calcium concentrations (Vincken et al., 1987). Plethysmographic measurements of dystrophic mice were similar to wild-type mice showing that the effects of muscular dystrophy could be minimized with the Poloxamer. Nusinersen, and onasemnogene aveparvovec (AVCS-101), a gene replacement therapy, have resulted in promising improvements in respiratory function and quality of life (Harada et al., 2020; Oechsel and Cartwright, 2021; Paul et al., 2021).

Electrical Stimulation of Muscles

In ALS reinnervation of denervated muscle fibers is crucial for preserving motor function as a means of compensating for motor neuron degeneration in long-term survivors. Diaphragm pacing has been advocated as a means of preserving respiratory muscle function, or at least, slowing its deterioration, but remains controversial (DiPALS, writing committee, DiPALS, Study Group Collaborators, 2015; Bermejo et al., 2016). Its mechanism was originally thought to be related to an increase in muscle fiber tone, thereby increasing its contractile properties.

Electrical stimulation of motor nerves leads to a reverse recruitment of motor units, in which larger fibers with less input resistance are activated before the smaller fibers. Recent studies in ALS have shown the opposite effect with an accelerated deterioration in respiratory function and increase in mortality (Bermejo et al., 2016). The RespistimALS group (Bermejo et al., 2016) reported that pacing in individuals with ALS failed to exhibit, over time, a significant increase in maximal amplitude of motor unit potentials (MUPs). These patients eventually required noninvasive ventilation and experienced decreased survival. By contrast, those who did not receive muscle stimulation showed a progressive increase in MUPs over time. Because efficient reinnervation leads to motor unit enlargement with an increase in muscle fiber content of surviving units, the authors concluded that the absence of increase in MUP amplitude over time in the active stimulation group supported the concept of a pacing-induced defective reinnervation.

In contrast to directly stimulating the muscle, the phrenic nerve can also be stimulated in cases of muscle deterioration to strengthen the diaphragm. However, the efficacy of this technique is disputed by some. In a study assessing the effects of phrenic nerve stimulation in 13 patients with myasthenia gravis, Mier et al. (Mier et al., 1992) demonstrated absence of change in diaphragmatic action potentials and even a reduction in 5 of the patients' action potentials. A study testing phrenic nerve stimulation in humans with ALS was terminated early because of an excessive mortality rate and complications such as pneumothorax and acute respiratory failure occurring in the test group (Gonzalez-Bermejo et al., 2016).

Magnetic Stimulation of Respiratory Muscles

Contrary to electrical stimulation, magnetic stimulation is more of a diagnostic tool. Through different positions and placements of electrodes, the phrenic nerve can be stimulated by cervical, anterior pre-sternal and unilateral/bilateral anterolateral magnetic stimulation, and CMAP can be recorded (Man et al., 2004). These assessments indicate which parts of the diaphragm would benefit from rehabilitation and prognosticate the muscle's recovery.

Imaging of Respiratory Muscles

Ultrasound imaging of the diaphragm is a non-invasive means of measuring diaphragm thickness and inspiratory thickening because an increase in diaphragm thickness leads to inspiratory strength (Roussos et al., 1979b; Boussuges et al., 2021). When applied by experienced users it provides reproducible results, with good inter- and intra-observer reliability (Cohn et al., 1997; Schepens et al., 2015). The thickness of the diaphragm can be determined in more than 85% of measurements, with a low coefficient of variation (0.09–0.14). Goligher et al. (Roussos et al., 1979b) assessed the validity of ultrasound in assessing diaphragm thickness and function in patients on mechanical ventilation. They found that only the right hemidiaphragm thickness is able to be measured, not the left, to help track the patient's status while on mechanical ventilation unless the patent had a unilateral injury. Thickness of the right hemidiaphragm is also related to the degree of contractile activation of muscle during ventilation, so this technique can be used to assess diaphragm atrophy (Roussos et al., 1979b). The technique has the potential to be applied in NMD to assess changes in diaphragm thickness and motion over time, but requires skill and experience. It would be best applied in individuals who have not received assisted ventilation in order to monitor any progressive muscle loss from the NMD itself.

More recently kinematic analysis of the diaphragm from three-dimensional magnetic resonance images has been able to assess diaphragm mechanics (Mogalle et al., 2016) and is more sensitive than lung function testing in detecting weakness of the muscle; individuals with Pompé disease compensate for impaired diaphragm function with increase in chest wall movement.

Evaluation of Respiratory Mechanics During Mechanical Ventilation in NMD and Chest Wall Disorders

An interesting concept to consider is the phenomenon of airway opening pressure (AOP) during inspiration from FRC to total lung capacity (TLC) in individuals with restrictive respiratory disorders such as NMD and chest wall deformities receiving mechanical ventilation. As noted above, such patients may exhibit expiratory flow limitation (EFL) (Baydur, 2013). In such situations, it is possible to record the pressure-volume relationships to assess respiratory compliance and the AOP to facilitate adjustment of tidal volume and positive end-expiratory pressure (PEEP) and optimize gas exchange.

The question arises as to the relation of AOP to expiratory flow limitation (EFL): do they correspond? An analogy of this feature can be made with acute respiratory distress syndrome (ARDS). Using the airway occlusion technique, Guerin et al. (Guérin et al., 2020) showed that in semi-recumbent ARDS patients at PEEP 5 cm H_2O, EFL and AOP did not occur simultaneously. While most patients with EFL exhibited an AOP, nearly half of patients with AOP did not have EFL. The additional tissue resistance measured at the end of inspiration was higher in patients with EFL than in those without EFL but did not differ amongst patients with and without AOP. Meanwhile, the interrupter resistance (of the conducting airways) did not differ between EFL and non-EFL patients, suggesting that EFL occurred in small airways. Thus, applying increasing levels of PEEP results in higher AOP without abolishing EFL. In addition, lung dynamic elastance was higher in FL than in non-FL patients and had a good accuracy for detecting EFL.

While the histopathologic features of ARDS are different from that of the microatelectatic changes seen with thoracic cage disorders, the lung mechanical properties of the latter conditions should be similar to that of ARDS with increases in respiratory resistance and elastance. If the curve depicting the lung transpulmonary pressure-volume relationship in a ventilated neuromuscular or scoliotic patient shown in **Figure 3** were recorded at lower lung volumes, a discreet inflection point and its relationship to the presence or absence of EFL could be detected. Thus, application of PEEP would be expected to shift AOP towards higher airway pressures. In turn, determination of the location of AOP would optimize ventilator settings to improve gas exchange while avoiding volutrauma. It is not known how differences in lung mechanics between ARDS and NMD/chest wall disorder patients would influence the relation between EFL and AOP. This aspect of respiratory mechanics is a suggested opportunity for further study.

OPPORTUNITIES FOR FUTURE RESEARCH

Serum Biomarkers for Inflammation

COPD causes inflammation resulting in skeletal muscle dysfunction. COPD increases inflammatory factors such as IL-6, TNF-α, IL-8, and C-reactive protein, as well as an increase in the generation of reactive oxygen species (ROS) (Kim et al., 2008). The combination of inflammatory factors and ROS may be the cause of muscle wasting in COPD. Muscle atrophy from COPD can also severely affect inspiratory muscles, limiting their function. These events are similar in patients with NMDs depending on the etiologic origin of muscle weakness, so in both diseases, serum biomarkers can be used to noninvasively evaluate muscle breakdown and effects on the inspiratory muscles. Therefore, future research could evaluate the association between respiratory impairment and these biomarkers.

The neurodegenerative changes associated with NMD are, in some ways, similar to the myriad changes documented with COPD and aging (Kim et al., 2008; Dobrowolny et al., 2021). Neuromuscular junctions (NMJ) undergo functional, morphological, and molecular alterations during aging, resulting in a progressive decrease in skeletal muscle mass and strength (sarcopenia), changes common in NMD. In addition to the intrinsic myoneural changes inherent of NMDs, ROS homeostasis can contribute to changes in the neuromuscular junction morphology and stability, leading to reduction in fiber number and innervation. For example, Puig-Vilanova et al. (Puig-Vilanova et al., 2014) found that in the diaphragm of COPD patients, compared to control subjects, muscle-specific microRNA expression was downregulated, while histone acetyltransferases (HATs) and deacetylases and myocyte enhancer factor 2C protein levels were higher; by contrast, DNA methylation levels, muscle fiber types and sizes did not differ between patients and controls. The authors concluded that these epigenetic events act as adaptive mechanisms used to overcome the continuous inspiratory loads of the respiratory system in COPD. As respiratory muscles in NMDs are subject to mechanical and oxidative stresses similar to those observed in COPD, epigenetic events may also regulate respiratory muscle dysfunction and are a potential fertile area of investigation in this group of disorders.

Changes in Respiratory Pressures Influenced by Inspiratory Maneuvers

The updated guidelines by the ERS in 2019 (Laveneziana et al., 2019) do not provide much detail about performance of the SNIP test, limiting the instructions to: "the test is performed at FRC and the subject is instructed to sniff quickly and deeply". Although considered a more physiological maneuver, an individual can perform a sniff test suboptimally when not appropriately instructed. In the evaluation of respiratory muscle strength, the diaphragmatic control performed during the SNIP test influences the inspiratory pressure and contractile properties of inspiratory muscles This occurs due to changes in the pattern of muscle recruitment, which change the force velocity characteristics of muscles. Benicio et al. instructed patients to perform a maximal effort starting from relaxed FRC according to ATS/ERS guidelines (Laveneziana et al., 2019). Participants were initially trained to breathe with a slow diaphragmatic breathing pattern, allowing bulging of the anterior abdominal wall (also known as ballistic contraction, diaphC). They were then instructed to inhale deeply through the nose, while simultaneously moving the abdominal wall outward (ballistic inspiratory maneuver). The main findings of this study showed that the maneuver with diaphC compared to without diaphC 1) significantly reduced the SNIP value, 2) reduced contraction times and electrical activity of accessory inspiratory muscles, and 3) decreased absolute values of maximum relaxation rate ($p < 0.01$), maximum rate of pressure development (MRPD). These findings confirmed that SNIP values diminish when a ballistic contraction of the diaphragm muscle is performed during a sniff maneuver. Thus, instructions on diaphC are recommended for specifically targeting diaphragm activity and better performance of the SNIP test.

Power Spectrum of EMG

Analysis of the power spectrum of EMG is a relatively old technique to assess muscle fatigue in patients during and after exercise with and without COPD and has not been employed in NMDs. Casabona et al. (Casabona et al., 2021) studied the possibility of using the power spectrum of EMG with non-fatigueable exercises to estimate muscle fiber composition in patients with COPD due to the different spectral content of the sEMG signal, which depends on the fiber type composition. The conclusion was that the power spectrum of COPD patients was at higher frequencies, which aligned with the severity of the disease. Even though this experiment was done on leg muscles, the same principle may be applied to the diaphragm and other inspiratory muscles by using surface electrodes, or better, esophageal electrodes situated at the cardia. Profiles of electromyographic power spectrum can be generated during repetitive maximal diaphragmatic contractions during deep breathing maneuvers. Future research could focus on this potential for detecting respiratory muscle fatigue before it affects VC, Pimax or Pdi.

Muscle Fiber Type

Changes in fiber type composition occur in NMDs (Glaser et al., 2018). New investigational approaches may elucidate how muscle fiber type specification occurs during disease conditions. For example, skeletal muscle cell culture from human pluripotent cell resources can provide a new instrument to study differentiation of human skeletal myocytes into myotubes with specific fiber types in culture (Hosoyama et al., 2014; Jiwlawat et al., 2017). Such studies could elucidate mechanisms involved in changes of fiber composition and ratio in the skeletal muscle of certain NMDs, and how they influence respiratory muscle kinematics and pathology. Such work carries the potential to create an *in vitro* model of contractile sarcomeric myofibrils for disease modeling and drug screening to study neuromuscular diseases.

CONCLUSION

Thoracic cage disorders are characterized by reduced lung volumes and respiratory compliance. Both upper and lower airway changes contribute to increase in airway resistance. While respiratory muscle weakness is a key feature that contributes to respiratory failure, central drive may be increased as characterized by increase in P0.1. Changes in respiratory mechanics contribute to elastic and resistive load compensation. Diaphragmatic braking action during expiration helps prevent further reduction in lung volume and atelectasis. Diagnostic studies focus on the evaluation of lung volumes and flows, respiratory muscle strength, ventilatory drive and recording of electromechanical dissociation of respiratory muscles. Ultrasound evaluation of diaphragmatic thickness and motion may prove useful in predicting respiratory muscle fatigue and failure. Mechanical ventilation affords an opportunity for further assessment of diaphragmatic function and airway properties such as expiratory flow limitation and airway opening pressure, which may provide guidance in applying appropriate ventilator settings. Finally, utilizing biochemical, genetic modeling and cell culture techniques have the potential to elucidate mechanisms of neuromuscular degeneration and the potential for discovering therapeutic approaches to halting or even stabilizing the loss of skeletal muscle, including respiratory muscles.

AUTHOR CONTRIBUTIONS

AB searched and selected the literature, conceived of the structure of the paper, guided the students who wrote the major portion of the paper, contributed to and revised the text and figures. NP searched and selected the literature, wrote most of the text, selected some of the figures. KC searched and selected appropriate literature, contributed to the text and created the table.

REFERENCES

Aboussouan, L. S. (2015). Sleep-disordered Breathing in Neuromuscular Disease. Am. J. Respir. Crit. Care *Med.* 191, 979–989. doi:10.1164/rccm.201412-2224ci

Ackrivo, J., Hansen-Flaschen, J., Jones, B. L., Wileyto, E. P., Schwab, R. J., Elman, L., et al. (2019). Classifying Patients with Amyotrophic Lateral Sclerosis by Changes in FVC. A Group-Based Trajectory Analysis. *Am. J. Respir. Crit. Care. Med.* 200 (2), 1513–1521. doi:10.1164/rccm.201902-0344OC

Ackrivo, J., Hansen-Flaschen, J., Wileyto, E. P., Schwab, R. J., Elman, L., and Kawut, S. M. (2019). Development of a Prognostic Model of Respiratory Insufficiency or Death in Amyotrophic Lateral Sclerosis. *Eur. Respir. J.* 53, 1802237. doi:10.1183/13993003.02237-2018

Aitkens, S., Kilmer, D. D., Wright, N. C., and McCrory, M. A. (2005). Metabolic Syndrome in Neuromuscular Disease. *Archives Phys. Med. Rehabilitation* 86 (5), 1030–1036. doi:10.1016/j.apmr.2004.09.012

Aldrich, T. K., Shander, A., Chaudhry, I., and Nagashima, H. (1986). Fatigue of Isolated Rat Diaphragm: Role of Impaired Neuromuscular Transmission. *J. Appl. Physiology* 61 (3), 1077–1083. doi:10.1152/jappl.1986.61.3.1077

Aldrich, T. K., and Spiro, P. (1995). Maximal Inspiratory Pressure: Does Reproducibility Indicate Full Effort? *Thorax* 50 (1), 40–43. doi:10.1136/thx.50.1.40

Allen, J. (2010). Pulmonary Complications of Neuromuscular Disease: A Respiratory Mechanics Perspective. *Paediatr. Respir. Rev.* 11 (1), 18–23. doi:10.1016/j.prrv.2009.10.002

Axen, K. (1982). Ventilatory Responses to Mechanical Loads in Cervical Cord-Injured Humans. *J. Appl. Physiology* 52 (3), 748–756. doi:10.1152/jappl.1982.52.3.748.48

Bach, J. R., Ishikawa, Y., and Kim, H. (1997). Prevention of Pulmonary Morbidity for Patients with Duchenne Muscular Dystrophy. *Chest* 112 (4), 1024–1028. doi:10.1378/chest.112.4.1024

Bach, J. R. (2017). Noninvasive Respiratory Management of Patients with Neuromuscular Disease. *Ann. Rehabil. Med.* 41 (4), 519–538. doi:10.5535/arm.2017.41.4.519

Bach, J. R., and Saporito, L. R. (1996). Criteria for Extubation and Tracheostomy Tube Removal for Patients with Ventilatory Failure. *Chest* 110 (6), 1566–1571. doi:10.1378/chest.110.6.1566

Banzett, R. B., Lansing, R. W., and Binks, A. P. (2021). Air Hunger: A Primal Sensation and a Primary Element of Dyspnea. *Compr. Physiol.* 11 (2), 1449–1483. doi:10.1002/cphy.c200001

Banzett, R. B., Lansing, R. W., Brown, R., Topulos, G. P., Yager, D., Steele, S. M., et al. (1990). 'Air Hunger' from Increased PCO2 Persists after Complete Neuromuscular Block in Humans. *Respir. Physiol.* 81, 1–17. doi:10.1016/0034-5687(90)90065-7

Bastir, M., García-Martínez, D., Torres-Tamayo, N., Sanchis-Gimeno, J. A., O'Higgins, P., Utrilla, C., et al. (2017). *In Vivo* 3D Analysis of Thoracic Kinematics: Changes in Size and Shape during Breathing and Their Implications for Respiratory Function in Recent Humans and Fossil Hominins. *Anat. Rec.* 300 (2), 255–264. doi:10.1002/ar.23503

Bauman, W. A., Spungen, A. M., Raza, M., Rothstein, J., Zhang, R. L., Zhong, Y. G., et al. (1992). Coronary Artery Disease: Metabolic Risk Factors and Latent Disease in Individuals with Paraplegia. *Mt. Sinai J. Med.* 59, 163–168.

Baydur, A., and Carlson, M. (1996). Immediate Response to Inspiratory Resistive Loading in Anesthetized Patients with Kyphoscoliosis: Spirometric and Neural Effects. *Lung* 174, 99–118. doi:10.1007/BF00177704

Baydur, A., Adkins, R. H., and Milic-Emili, J. (2001). Lung Mechanics in Individuals with Spinal Cord Injury: Effects of Injury Level and Posture. *J. Appl. Physiology* 90 (2), 405–411. doi:10.1152/jappl.2001.90.2.405

Baydur, A., and Chen, Z. (2013). Breathing Intolerance Index in COPD and Obesity: A Comparative Observational Study. *Ojrd* 03, 119–127. doi:10.4236/ojrd.2013.33019

Baydur, A. (1992). Decay of Inspiratory Muscle Pressure during Expiration in Anesthetized Kyphoscoliosis Patients. *J. Appl. Physiology* 72 (2), 712–720. doi:10.1152/jappl.1992.72.2.712

Baydur, A. (2013). Expiratory Flow Limitation in Intra and Extrathoracic Respiratory Disorders: Use of the Negative Expiratory Pressure Technique - Review and Recent Developments. *InTechOpen*. doi:10.5772/53270

Baydur, A. (1991). Respiratory Muscle Strength and Control of Ventilation in Patients with Neuromuscular Disease. *Chest* 99 (2), 330–338. doi:10.1378/chest.99.2.330

Baydur, A., Swank, S. M., Stiles, C. M., and Sassoon, C. S. (1989). Respiratory Elastic Load Compensation in Anesthetized Patients with Kyphoscoliosis. *J. Appl. Physiology* 67, 1024–1031. doi:10.1152/jappl.1989.67.3.1024

Beck, J., Sinderby, C., Lindström, L., and Grassino, A. (1998). Effects of Lung Volume on Diaphragm EMG Signal Strength during Voluntary Contractions. *J. Appl. Physiology* 85 (3), 1123–1134. doi:10.1152/jappl.1998.85.3.1123

Behrakis, P. K., Higgs, B. D., Baydur, A., Zin, W. A., and Milic-Emili, J. (1983). Active Inspiratory Impedance in Halothane-Anesthetized Humans. *J. Appl. Physiology* 54, 1477–1481. doi:10.1152/jappl.1983.54.6.1477

Bellemare, F., and Grassino, A. (1982). Effect of Pressure and Timing of Contraction on Human Diaphragm Fatigue. *J. Appl. Physiology* 53, 1190–1195. doi:10.1152/jappl.1982.53.5.1190

Bellemare, F. (1995). "Strength of the Respiratory Muscles," in *The ThoraxLung Biology Biology in Health and Disease*. Editor Ch. Roussos, 85, 1161–1197. part B, ch. 40.

Benditt, J. O. (2019). Respiratory Care of Patients with Neuromuscular Disease. *Respir. Care* 64 (6), 679–688. doi:10.4187/respcare.06827

Berlowitz, D. J., Wadsworth, B., and Ross, J. (2016). Respiratory Problems and Management in People with Spinal Cord Injury. *Breathe* 12, 328–340. doi:10.1183/20734735.012616

Bermejo, J. G., Morélot-Panzini, C., Tanguy, M. L., Meininger, V., Pradat, P. F., Lenglet, T., et al. (2016). Early Diaphragm Pacing to Delay Non-invasive Ventilation in Patients with Amyotrophic Lateral Sclerosis (RespiStimALS): A Multicenter, Triple-Blind, Randomized Controlled Trial. *Eur. Respir. J.* 48, OA270. doi:10.1183/13993003.congress-2016.oa270

Bi, T., Zhang, J., Strohl, K. P., and Han, F. (2021). Hypercapnia and Hypoxemia in a Young Woman. *Ann. ATS* 18 (3), 527–533. doi:10.1513/annalsats.202006-699cc

Black, L. F., and Hyatt, R. E. (1971). Maximal Static Respiratory Pressures in Generalized Neuromuscular Disease. *Am. Rev. Respir. Dis.* 103 (5), 641–650. doi:10.1164/arrd.1971.103.5.641

Borel, C. O., Teitelbaum, J. S., and Hanley, D. F. (1993). Ventilatory Drive and Carbon Dioxide Response in Ventilatory Failure Due to Myasthenia Gravis and Guillain-Barré Syndrome. *Crit. Care Med.* 21 (11), 1717–1726. doi:10.1097/00003246-199311000-00022

Bouros, D., and Green, M. (1971). "Cough. "Physiological and Pathophysiological Considerations," in *The Thorax, Part B: Applied Physiology*. Editor Ch. Roussos (New York: Lung Biology in Health and Disease, Marcel Dekker, Inc.), 85, 1335–1354.

Boussuges, A., Rives, S., Finance, J., Chaumet, G., Vallée, N., Risso, J.-J., et al. (2021). Ultrasound Assessment of Diaphragm Thickness and Thickening: Reference Values and Limits of Normality when in a Seated Position. *Front. Med.* 8, 742703. doi:10.3389/fmed.2021.742703

Braun, N. M., Arora, N. S., and Rochester, D. F. (1983). Respiratory Muscle and Pulmonary Function in Polymyositis and Other Proximal Myopathies. *Thorax* 38, 616–623. doi:10.1136/thx.38.8.616

Campbell, E. J. M. (1965). Respiratory Failure. *Bmj* 1 (5448), 1451–1460. doi:10.1136/bmj.1.5448.1451

Carroll, J. E., Zwillich, C., Weil, J. V., and Brooke, M. H. (1976). Depressed Ventilatory Response in Oculocraniosomatic Neuromuscular Disease. *Neurology* 26, 140. doi:10.1212/wnl.26.2.140

Caruso, P., Albuquerque, A. L. P. d., Santana, P. V., Cardenas, L. Z., Ferreira, J. G., Prina, E., et al. (2015). Diagnostic Methods to Assess Inspiratory and Expiratory Muscle Strength. *J. Bras. Pneumol.* 41 (2), 110–123. doi:10.1590/s1806-37132015000004474

Casabona, A., Valle, M. S., Laudani, L., Crimi, C., Russo, C., Malaguarnera, L., et al. (2021). Is the Power Spectrum of Electromyography Signal a Feasible Tool to Estimate Muscle Fiber Composition in Patients with COPD? *Jcm* 10 (17), 3815. doi:10.3390/jcm10173815

Chatwin, M., Toussaint, M., Gonçalves, M. R., Sheers, N., Mellies, U., Gonzales-Bermejo, J., et al. (2018). Airway Clearance Techniques in Neuromuscular Disorders: A State of the Art Review. *Respir. Med.* 136, 98–110. doi:10.1016/j.rmed.2018.01.012

Chen, J., Nguyen, N., and Soong, M. (2013). Postural Change of FVC in Patients with Neuromuscular Disease: Relation to Initiating Non-invasive Ventilation. *J. Pulmon Resp. Med.* 3, 2. doi:10.4172/2161-105X.1000147

Chew, K., carey, K., Ho, G., Mallitt, K.-A., Widger, J., and Farrar, M. (2016). The Relationship of Body Habitus and Respiratory Function in Duchenne Muscular Dystrophy. *Respir. Med.* 119, 35–40. doi:10.1016/j.rmed.2016.08.018

Chiang, J., Mehta, K., and Amin, R. (2018). Respiratory Diagnostic Tools in Neuromuscular Disease. *Children* 5 (6), 78. doi:10.3390/children5060078

Cohn, D., Benditt, J. O., Eveloff, S., and McCool, F. D. (1997). Diaphragm Thickening during Inspiration. *J. Appl. Physiology* 83, 291–296. doi:10.1152/jappl.1997.83.1.291

De Troyer, A., and Estenne, M. (1984). Coordination between Rib Cage Muscles and Diaphragm during Quiet Breathing in Humans. *J. Appl. Physiology* 57 (3), 899–906. doi:10.1152/jappl.1984.57.3.899

De Troyer, A., Estenne, M., and Heilporn, A. (1986). Mechanism of Active Expiration in Tetraplegic Subjects. *N. Engl. J. Med.* 314, 740–744. doi:10.1056/nejm198603203141203

Dempsey, J. A., Reddan, W., Balke, B., and Rankin, J. (1966). Work Capacity Determinants and Physiologic Cost of Weight-Supported Work in Obesity. *J. Appl. Physiology* 21, 1815–1820. doi:10.1152/jappl.1966.21.6.1815

DiPALS, writing committee, DiPALS, Study Group Collaborators (2015). Safety and Efficacy of Diaphragm Pacing in Patients with Respiratory Insufficiency Due to Amyotrophic Lateral Sclerosis (DiPALS): a Multicentre, Open-Label, Randomised Controlled Trial. *Lancet Neurol.* 14, 883–892. doi:10.1016/S1474-4422(15)00152-0

Dobrowolny, G., Barbiera, A., Sica, G., and Scicchitano, B. M. (2021). Age-related Alterations at Neuromuscular Junction: Role of Oxidative Stress and Epigenetic Modifications. *Cells* 10 (6), 1307. doi:10.3390/cells10061307

Druz, W. S., and Sharp, J. T. (1981). Activity of Respiratory Muscles in Upright and Recumbent Humans. *J. Appl. Physiology* 51 (6), 1552–1561. doi:10.1152/jappl.1981.51.6.1552

Durnin, J. V. G. A., and Rahaman, M. M. (1967). The Assessment of the Amount of Fat in the Human Body from Measurements of Skinfold Thickness. *Br. J. Nutr.* 21, 681–689. doi:10.1079/bjn19670070

Easton, P. A., Katagiri, M., Kieser, T. M., and Platt, R. S. (1999). Postinspiratory Activity of Costal and Crural Diaphragm. *J. Appl. Physiology* 87, 582–589. doi:10.1152/jappl.1999.87.2.582

Eckert, D. J., McEvoy, R. D., George, K. E., Thomson, K. J., and Catcheside, P. G. (2007). Genioglossus Reflex Inhibition to Upper-Airway Negative-Pressure Stimuli during Wakefulness and Sleep in Healthy Males. *J. Physiol.* 581 (Pt 3), 1193–1205. doi:10.1113/jphysiol.2007.132332

Edwards, R. H. (1979). The Diaphragm as a Muscle. Mechanisms Underlying Fatigue. *Am. Rev. Respir. Dis.* 119, 81–84. doi:10.1164/arrd.1979.119.2P2.81

Elamin, M., Bede, P., Montuschi, A., Pender, N., Chio, A., and Hardiman, O. (2015). Predicting Prognosis in Amyotrophic Lateral Sclerosis: a Simple Algorithm. *J. Neurol.* 262, 1447–1454. doi:10.1007/s00415-015-7731-6

Estenne, M., Van Muylem, A., Gorini, M., Kinnear, W., Heilporn, A., and De Troyer, A. (1994). Evidence of Dynamic Airway Compression during Cough in Tetraplegic Patients. *Am. J. Respir. Crit. Care Med.* 150 (4), 1081–1085. doi:10.1164/ajrccm.150.4.7921440

Fauroux, B., and Khirani, S. (2014). Neuromuscular Disease and Respiratory Physiology in Children: Putting Lung Function into Perspective. *Respirology* 19 (6), 782–791. doi:10.1111/resp.12330

Fermin, A. M., Afzal, U., and Culebras, A. (2016). Sleep in Neuromuscular Diseases. *Sleep. Med. Clin.* 11 (1), 53–64. doi:10.1016/j.jsmc.2015.10.005

Fromageot, C., Lofaso, F., Annane, D., Falaize, L., Lejaille, M., Clair, B., et al. (2001). Supine Fall in Lung Volumes in the Assessment of Diaphragmatic Weakness in Neuromuscular Disorders. *Archives Phys. Med. Rehabilitation* 82 (1), 123–128. doi:10.1053/apmr.2001.18053

Fugl-Meyer, A. R., and Grimby, G. (1984). Respiration in Tetraplegia and in Hemiplegia: a Review. *Int. Rehabil. Med.* 6 (4), 186–190. doi:10.3109/03790798409165962

García Río, F., Prados, C., Diez Tejedor, E., Diaz Lobato, S., Alvarez-Sala, R., Villamor, J., et al. (1994). Breathing Pattern and Central Ventilatory Drive in Mild and Moderate Generalised Myasthenia Gravis. *Thorax* 49 (7), 703–706. doi:10.1136/thx.49.7.703

Glaser, J., and Suzuki, M. (2018). "Skeletal Muscle Fiber Types in Neuromuscular Diseases." In *Muscle Cell and Tissue*. Ed by K. Sakuma. In London, United Kingdom: In Tech. doi:10.5772/intechopen.79474

Goldman, J. M., Rose, L. S., Williams, S. J., Silver, J. R., and Denison, D. M. (1986). Effect of Abdominal Binders on Breathing in Tetraplegic Patients. *Thorax* 41, 940–945. doi:10.1136/thx.41.12.940

Gonzalez-Bermejo, J., Morélot-Panzini, C., Tanguy, M.-L., Meininger, V., Pradat, P.-F., Lenglet, T., et al. (2016). Early Diaphragm Pacing in Patients with Amyotrophic Lateral Sclerosis (RespiStimALS): a Randomised Controlled Triple-Blind Trial. *Lancet Neurology* 15 (12), 1217–1227. doi:10.1016/s1474-4422(16)30233-2

Guérin, C., Terzi, N., Galerneau, L.-M., Mezidi, M., Yonis, H., Baboi, L., et al. (2020). Lung and Chest Wall Mechanics in Patients with Acute Respiratory Distress Syndrome, Expiratory Flow Limitation, and Airway Closure. *J. Appl. Physiology* 128, 1594–1603. doi:10.1152/japplphysiol.00059.2020

Harada, Y., Rao, V. K., Arya, K., Kuntz, N. L., DiDonato, C. J., Napchan-Pomerantz, G., et al. (2020). Combination Molecular Therapies for Type 1 Spinal Muscular Atrophy. *Muscle Nerve* 62 (4), 550–554. doi:10.1002/mus.27034

Hosoyama, T., McGivern, J. V., Van Dyke, J. M., Ebert, A. D., and Suzuki, M. (2014). Derivation of Myogenic Progenitors Directly from Human Pluripotent Stem Cells Using a Sphere-Based Culture. *Stem Cells Transl. Med.* 3, 564–574. doi:10.5966/sctm.2013-0143

Jaber, S., Petrof, B. J., Jung, B., Chanques, G., Berthet, J.-P., Rabuel, C., et al. (2011). Rapidly Progressive Diaphragmatic Weakness and Injury during Mechanical Ventilation in Humans. *Am. J. Respir. Crit. Care Med.* 183, 364–371. doi:10.1164/rccm.201004-0670oc

Jaeger, M. J. (1982). Effect of the Cheeks and the Compliance of Alveolar Gas on the Measurement of Respiratory Variables. *Respir. Physiol.* 47 (3), 325–340. doi:10.1016/0034-5687(82)90061-5

Jansen, D., Jonkman, A. H., Vries, H. J. d., Wennen, M., Elshof, J., Hoofs, M. A., et al. (2021). Positive End-Expiratory Pressure Affects Geometry and Function of the Human Diaphragm. *J. Appl. Physiology* 131, 1328–1339. doi:10.1152/japplphysiol.00184.2021

Jiwlawat, S., Lynch, E., Glaser, J., Smit-Oistad, I., Jeffrey, J., Van Dyke, J. M., et al. (2017). Differentiation and Sarcomere Formation in Skeletal Myocytes Directly Prepared from Human Induced Pluripotent Stem Cells Using a Sphere-Based Culture. *Differentiation* 96, 70–81. doi:10.1016/j.diff.2017.07.004

Benício, K. (2021). Effects of Diaphragmatic Control on Multiparametric Analysis of the Sniff Nasal Inspiratory Pressure Test and Inspiratory Muscle Activity in Healthy Subjects. *PLoS One* 16 (7), e0253132. doi:10.1371/journal.pone.0253132

Kilburn, K. H., Eagan, J. T., Sieker, H. O., and Heyman, A. (1959). Cardiopulmonary Insufficiency in Myotonic and Progressive Muscular Dystrophy. *N. Engl. J. Med.* 261, 1089–1096. doi:10.1056/nejm195911262612201

Kim, H. C., Mofarrahi, M., and Hussain, S. N. (2008). Skeletal Muscle Dysfunction in Patients with Chronic Obstructive Pulmonary Disease. *Int. J. Chron. Obstruct Pulmon Dis.* 3 (4), 637–658. doi:10.2147/copd.s4480

Kobayashi, I., Perry, A., Rhymer, J., Wuyam, B., Hughes, P., Murphy, K., et al. (1996). Inspiratory Coactivation of the Genioglossus Enlarges Retroglossal Space in Laryngectomized Humans. *J. Appl. Physiology* 80, 1595–1604. doi:10.1152/jappl.1996.80.5.1595

Koga, T., Watanabe, K., Sano, M., Ishikawa, Y., and Bach, J. R. (2206). Breathing Intolerance Index: A New Indicator for Ventilator Use. *Am. J. Phys. Med. Rehabil.* 85 (1), 24–30. doi:10.1097/01.phm.0000184237.62628.e1

Kress, J. P., Pohlman, A. S., Alverdy, J., and Hall, J. B. (1999). The Impact of Morbid Obesity on Oxygen Cost of Breathing (Vo2RESP) at Rest. *Am. J. Respir. Crit. Care Med.* 160, 883–886. doi:10.1164/ajrccm.160.3.9902058

Lappas, A. S., Tzortzi, A. S., and Behrakis, P. K. (2016). Forced Oscillations in Applied Respiratory Physiology: Clinical Applications. *Clin. Res. Pulmonol.* 2 (2), 1016.

Laroche, C. M., Mier, A. K., Moxham, J., and Green, M. (1988). The Value of Sniff Esophageal Pressures in the Assessment of Global Inspiratory Muscle Strength. *Am. Rev. Respir. Dis.* 138, 598–603. doi:10.1164/ajrccm/138.3.598

Laveneziana, P., Albuquerque, A., Aliverti, A., Babb, T., Barreiro, E., Dres, M., et al. (2019). ERS Statement on Respiratory Muscle Testing at Rest and during Exercise. *Eur. Respir. J.* 53 (6), 1801214. doi:10.1183/13993003.01214-2018

Lechtzin, N., Wiener, C. M., Shade, D. M., Clawson, L., and Diette, G. B. (2002). Spirometry in the Supine Position Improves the Detection of Diaphragmatic Weakness in Patients with Amyotrophic Lateral Sclerosis. *Chest* 121 (2), 436–442. doi:10.1378/chest.121.2.436

Ledsome, J. R., and Sharp, J. M. (1981). Pulmonary Function in Acute Cervical Cord Injury. *Am. Rev. Respir. Dis.* 124, 41–44. doi:10.1164/arrd.1981.124.1.41

Leech, J. A., Ghezzo, H., Stevens, D., and Becklake, M. R. (1983). Respiratory Pressures and Function in Young Adults1-4. *Am. Rev. Respir. Dis.* 128 (1), 17–23. doi:10.1164/arrd.1983.128.1.17

Lo Mauro, A., and Aliverti, A. (2016). Physiology of Respiratory Disturbances in Muscular Dystrophies. *Breathe* 12 (4), 318–327. doi:10.1183/20734735.012716

Loring, S. H., and Mead, J. (1982). Action of the Diaphragm on the Rib Cage Inferred from a Force-Balance Analysis. *J. Appl. Physiology* 53 (3), 756–760. doi:10.1152/jappl.1982.53.3.756

Malhotra, A., Fogel, R. B., Edwards, J. K., Shea, S. A., and White, D. P. (2000). Local Mechanisms Drive Genioglossus Activation in Obstructive Sleep Apnea. *Am. J. Respir. Crit. Care Med.* 161, 1746–1749. doi:10.1164/ajrccm.161.5.9907109

Man, W. D.-C., Moxham, J., and Polkey, M. I. (2004). Magnetic Stimulation for the Measurement of Respiratory and Skeletal Muscle Function. *Eur. Respir. J.* 24 (5), 846–860. doi:10.1183/09031936.04.00029004

Markham, B. E., Kernodle, S., Nemzek, J., Wilkinson, J. E., and Sigler, R. (2015). Chronic Dosing with Membrane Sealant Poloxamer 188 NF Improves Respiratory Dysfunction in Dystrophic *Mdx And Mdx/Utrophin-/-* Mice. *PLoS ONE* 10 (8), e0134832. doi:10.1371/journal.pone.0134832

Mayer, O. H., Finkel, R. S., Rummey, C., Benton, M. J., Glanzman, A. M., Flickinger, J., et al. (2015). Characterization of Pulmonary Function in Duchenne Muscular Dystrophy. *Pediatr. Pulmonol.* 50 (5), 487–494. doi:10.1002/ppul.23172

McCool, F. D., Brown, R., Mayewski, R. J., and Hyde, R. W. (1988). Effects of Posture on Stimulated Ventilation in Quadriplegia. *Am. Rev. Respir. Dis.* 138 (1), 101–105. doi:10.1164/ajrccm/138.1.101

McCool, F. D., Pichurko, B. M., Slutsky, A. S., Sarkarati, M., Rossier, A., and Brown, R. (1986). Changes in Lung Volume and Rib Cage Configuration with Abdominal Binding in Quadriplegia. *J. Appl. Physiology* 60, 1198–1202. doi:10.1152/jappl.1986.60.4.1198

Mead, J. (1979). Functional Significance of the Area of Apposition of Diaphragm to Rib Cage [proceedings]. *Am. Rev. Respir. Dis.* 119 (2), 31–32. doi:10.1164/arrd.1979.119.2P2.31

Mellies, U., Dohna-Schwake, C., and Voit, T. (2005). Respiratory Function Assessment and Intervention in Neuromuscular Disorders. *Curr. Opin. Neurol.* 18, 543–547. doi:10.1097/01.wco.0000180662.03544.5f

Mier, A., Brophy, C., Moxham, J., and Green, M. (1992). Repetitive Stimulation of Phrenic Nerves in Myasthenia Gravis. *Thorax* 47 (8), 640–644. doi:10.1136/thx.47.8.640

Miller, K., and Mayer, O. H. (2021). Pulmonary Function Testing in Patients with Neuromuscular Disease. *Pediatr. Pulmonol.* 56 (4), 693–699. doi:10.1002/ppul.25182

Mogalle, K., Perez-Rovira, A., Ciet, P., Wens, S. C. A., van Doorn, P. A., Tiddens, H. A. W. M., et al. (2016). Quantification of Diaphragm Mechanics in Pompe Disease Using Dynamic 3D MRI. *PloS ONE* 11 (7), e0158912. doi:10.1371/journal.pone.0158912

Mognoni, P., Saibene, F., and Sant'Ambrogio, G. (1969). Contribution of the Diaphragm and the Other Inspiratory Muscles to Different Levels of Tidal Volume and Static Inspiratory Effort in the Rabbit. *J. Physiol.* 202, 517–534. doi:10.1113/jphysiol.1969.sp008825

Muller, N., Bryan, A. C., and Zamel, N. (1980). Tonic Inspiratory Muscle Activity as a Cause of Hyperinflation in Histamine-Induced Asthma. *J. Appl. Physiology* 49, 869–874. doi:10.1152/jappl.1980.49.5.869

Muller, N., Volgyesi, G., Becker, L., Bryan, M. H., and Bryan, A. C. (1979). Diaphragmatic Muscle Tone. *J. Appl. Physiology* 47, 279–284. doi:10.1152/jappl.1979.47.2.279

Nicot, F., Hart, N., Forin, V., Boulé, M., Clément, A., Polkey, M. I., et al. (2006). Respiratory Muscle Testing. *Am. J. Respir. Crit. Care Med.* 174 (1), 67–74. doi:10.1164/rccm.200512-1841oc

Nishino, T., Isono, S., Shinozuka, N., and Ishikawa, T. (2008). Coughing Induced by Airway Irritation Modulates the Sensation of Air Hunger. *J. Physiol.* 586 (2), 649–658. doi:10.1113/jphysiol.2007.145276

Oechsel, K. F., and Cartwright, M. S. (2021). Combination Therapy with Onasemnogene and Risdiplam in Spinal Muscular Atrophy Type 1. *Muscle Nerve* 64 (4), 487–490. doi:10.1002/mus10.1002/mus.27375

Oliven, R., Cohen, G., Dotan, Y., Somri, M., Schwartz, A. R., and Oliven, A. (2018). Alteration in Upper Airway Dilator Muscle Coactivation during Sleep: Comparison of Patients with Obstructive Sleep Apnea and Healthy Subjects. *J. Appl. Physiology* 124, 421–429. doi:10.1152.japplphysiol.01067.201610.1152/japplphysiol.01067.2016

Padkao, T., and Boonla, O. (2020). Relationships between Respiratory Muscle Strength, Chest Wall Expansion, and Functional Capacity in Healthy Nonsmokers. *J. Exerc Rehabil.* 16 (2), 189–196. doi:10.12965/jer.2040080.040

Paintal, A. S. (1986). "Chapter 1 the Visceral Sensations - Some Basic Mechanisms," in *Progress in Brain Research*. Editors F. Gervero and J. F. B. Morrison (Amsterdam: Elsevier Scientific Publishers), 3–19. doi:10.1016/s0079-6123(08)62752-1

Panitch, H. B. (2009). Diurnal Hypercapnia in Patients with Neuromuscular Disease. *Paediatr. Respir. Rev.* 11 (1), 3–8. doi:10.1016/j.prrv.2009.10.0010.1016/j.prrv.2009.10.005

Paul, G. R., Gushue, C., Kotha, K., and Shell, R. (2021). The Respiratory Impact of Novel Therapies for Spinal Muscular Atrophy. *Pediatr. Pulmonol.* 56 (4), 721–728. doi:10.1002/ppul.25135

Perrin, C., Unterborn, J. N., Ambrosio, C. D., and Hill, N. S. (2204). Pulmonary Complications of Chronic Neuromuscular Diseases and Their Management. *Muscle Nerve* 29 (1), 5–27. doi:10.1002/mus.10487

Pessolano, F., Suarez, A., Monteiro, S., Mesa, L., Dubrovsky, A., Roncoroni, A., et al. (2003). Nutritional Assessment of Patients with Neuromuscular Diseases. *Am. J. Phys. Med. Rehabil.* 82, 182–185. doi:10.1097/00002060-200303000-00005

Plum, F., and Swanson, A. G. (1958). Abnormalities in Central Regulation of Respiration in Acute and Convalescent Poliomyelitis. *Arch. NeurPsych* 80, 267–285. doi:10.1001/archneurpsyc.1958.02340090003001

Polkey, M. I., and Moxham, J. (2001). Clinical Aspects of Respiratory Muscle Dysfunction in the Critically Ill. *Chest* 119 (3), 926–939. doi:10.1378/chest.119.3.926

Prigent, H., Orlikowski, D., Laforêt, P., Letilly, N., Falaize, L., Pellegrini, N., et al. (2012). Supine Volume Drop and Diaphragmatic Function in Adults with Pompe Disease: Table 1-. *Eur. Respir. J.* 39, 1545–1546. doi:10.1183/09031936.00169011

Puig-Vilanova, E., Aguiló, R., Rodríguez-Fuster, A., Martínez-Llorens, J., Gea, J., and Barreiro, E. (2014). Epigenetic Mechanisms in Respiratory Muscle Dysfunction of Patients with Chronic Obstructive Pulmonary Disease. *PLoS One* 9 (11), e111514. doi:10.1371/journal.pone.0111514

Ramonatxo, M., Boulard, P., and Prefaut, C. (1995). Validation of a Noninvasive Tension-Time Index of Inspiratory Muscles. *J. Appl. Physiology* 78 (2), 646–653. doi:10.1152/jappl.1995.78.2.646

Rault, C., Heraud, Q., Ragot, S., Robert, R., and Drouot, X. (2021). Sleep Deprivation Increases Air Hunger rather Than Breathing Effort. *Am. J. Respir. Crit. Care Med.* 203 (5), 642–645. doi:10.1164/rccm.202004-1478le

Rault, C., Sangaré, A., Diaz, V., Ragot, S., Frat, J.-P., Raux, M., et al. (2020). Impact of Sleep Deprivation on Respiratory Motor Output and Endurance. A Physiological Study. *Am. J. Respir. Crit. Care Med.* 201, 976–983. doi:10.1164/rccm.201904-0819oc

Rialp, G., Raurich, J. M., Llompart-Pou, J. A., Ayestaran, I., and Ibanez, J. (2013). Central Respiratory Drive in Patients with Neuromuscular Diseases. *Respir. Care* 58 (3), 450–457. doi:10.4187/respcare.01873

Rosenow, E. C., and Engel, A. G. (1978). Acid Maltase Deficiency in Adults Presenting as Respiratory Failure. *Am. J. Med.* 64, 485–491. doi:10.1016/0002-9343(78)90235-8

Rosenow, E. C., and Engel, A. G. (1978). Acid Maltase Deficiency in Adults Presenting as Respiratory Failure. *Am. J. Med.* 64 (3), 485–491. doi:10.1016/0002-9343(78)90235-8

Roussos, C. (1978). Function and Fatigue of Respiratory Muscles. *Chest* 88 (2), 124S–132S. doi:10.1378/chest.88.2.124s

Roussos, C., Fixley, M., Gross, D., and Macklem, P. T. (1979). Fatigue of Inspiratory Muscles and Their Synergic Behavior. *J. Appl. Physiology* 46 (5), 897–904. doi:10.1152/jappl.1979.46.5.897

Roussos, C., Fixley, M., Gross, D., and Macklem, P. T. (1979). Fatigue of Inspiratory Muscles and Their Synergic Behavior. *J. Appl. Physiology* 46 (5), 897–904. doi:10.1152/jappl.1979.46.5.897

Roussos, C., and Koutsoukou, A. (2003). Respiratory Failure. *Eur. Respir. J.* 22 (Suppl. 47), 3s–14s. doi:10.1183/09031936.03.00038503

Sahni, A. S., and Wolfe, L. (2018). Respiratory Care in Neuromuscular Diseases. *Respir. Care* 63 (5), 601–608. doi:10.4187/respcare.06210

Salome, C. M., King, G. G., and Berend, N. (2010). Physiology of Obesity and Effects on Lung Function. *J. Appl. Physiology* 108, 206–211. doi:10.1152/japplphysiol.00694.2009

Sarkar, M., Bhardwaz, R., and Madabhavi, I. (2019). Physical Signs in Patients with Chronic Obstructive Pulmonary Disease. *Lung India* 36 (1), 38–47. doi:10.4103/lungindia.lungindia_145_1810.1378/chest.88.2_supplement.124s

Sarmento, A., Fregonezi, G., Lira, M., Marques, L., Pennati, F., Resqueti, V., et al. (2021). Changes in Electromyographic Activity, Mechanical Power, and Relaxation Rates Following Inspiratory Ribcage Muscle Fatigue. *Sci. Rep.* 11, 12475. doi:10.1038/s41598-021-92060-y

Schepens, T., Verbrugghe, W., Dams, K., Corthouts, B., Parizel, P. M., and Jorens, P. G. (2015). The Course of Diaphragm Atrophy in Ventilated Patients Assessed with Ultrasound: a Longitudinal Cohort Study. *Crit. Care.* 19, 422–430. doi:10.1186/s13054-015-1141-0

Scott, M., Frost, F., and Supinski, G. (1993). The Effect of Body Position and Abdominal Binders in Chronic Tetraplegic Subjects More Than 15 Years Post-injury. *J. Am. Paraplegia Soc.* 16, 117.

Sharma, G. D. (2009). Pulmonary Function Testing in Neuromuscular Disorders. *Pediatrics* 123, S219–S221. doi:10.1542/peds.2008-2952d

Sharp, J. T., Druz, W. S., and Kondragunta, V. R. (1986). Diaphragmatic Responses to Body Position Changes in Obese Patients with Obstructive Sleep Apnea1-3. *Am. Rev. Respir. Dis.* 133 (1), 32–37. doi:10.1164/arrd.1986.133.1.32

Sharp, J. T., Henry, J. P., Sweany, S. K., Meadows, W. R., and Pietras, R. J. (1964). The Total Work of Breathing in Normal and Obese Men*. *J. Clin. Investig.* 43 (4), 728–739. doi:10.1172/JCI104957

Silbergleit, A. K., Waring, W. P., Sullivan, M. J., and Maynard, F. M. (1991). Evaluation, Treatment, and Follow-Up Results of Post Polio Patients with Dysphagia. *Otolaryngol. Head. Neck Surg.* 104, 333–338. doi:10.1177/019459989110400308

Sonies, B. C., and Dalakas, M. C. (1991). Dysphagia in Patients with the Post-Polio Syndrome. *N. Engl. J. Med.* 324, 1162–1167. doi:10.1056/nejm199104253241703

Stanbury, R. M., and Graham, E. M. (1998). Systemic Corticosteroid Therapy---side effects and their management. *Br. J. Ophthalmol.* 82, 704–708. doi:10.1136/bjo.82.6.704

Steier, J., Kaul, S., Seymour, J., Jolley, C., Rafferty, G., Man, W., et al. (2007). The value of multiple tests of respiratory muscle strength. *Thorax* 62 (11), 975–980. doi:10.1136/thx.2006.072884

Suárez, A. A., Pessolano, F. A., Monteiro, S. G., Ferreyra, G., Capria, M. E., Mesa, L., et al. (2002). Peak flow and peak cough flow in the evaluation of expiratory muscle weakness and bulbar impairment in patients with neuromuscular disease. *Am. J. Phys. Med. Rehabilitation* 81 (7), 506–511. doi:10.1097/00002060-200207000-00007

Terson de Paleville, D. G. L., Sayenko, D. G., Aslan, S. C., Folz, R. J., McKay, W. B., and Ovechkin, A. V. (2014). Respiratory motor function in seated and supine positions in individuals with chronic spinal cord injury. *Respir. Physiology Neurobiol.* 203, 9–14. doi:10.1016/j.resp.2014.08.013

Thomas, P. S., Cowen, E. R., Hulands, G., and Milledge, J. S. (1989). Respiratory function in the morbidly obese before and after weight loss. *Thorax* 44, 382–386. doi:10.1136/thx.44.5.382

Ti, D. S., and Fit Ting, J.-W. (1999). Sniff Nasal Inspiratory Pressure. *Am. J. Respir. Crit. Care Med.* 159 (1), 107–111. doi:10.1164/ajrccm.159.1.9804052

Troyer, A. D., and Wilson, T. A. (2016). Action of the diaphragm on the rib cage. *J. Appl. Physiology* 121 (2), 391–400. doi:10.1152/japplphysiol.00268.2016

Van de Graaff, W. B., Gottfried, S. B., Mitra, J., van Lunteren, E., Cherniack, N. S., and Strohl, K. P. (1984). Respiratory function of hyoid muscles and hyoid arch. *J. Appl. Physiology* 57, 197–204. doi:10.1152/jappl.1984.57.1.197

Van Noord, J. A., Cauberghs, M., Van De Woestijne, K. P., and Demedts, M. (1991). Total respiratory resistance and reactance in ankylosing spondylitis and kyphoscoliosis. *Eur. Respir. J.* 4 (8), 945–951.

Vincken, W., Ghezzo, H., and Cosio, M. G. (1987). Maximal static respiratory pressures in adults: normal values and their relationship to determinants of respiratory function. *Bull. Eur. Physiopathol. Respir.* 23 (5), 435–439.

Welch, J. F., Kipp, S., and Sheel, A. W. (2019). Respiratory muscles during exercise: mechanics, energetics, and fatigue. *Curr. Opin. Physiology* 10, 102–109. doi:10.1016/j.cophys.2019.04.023

Wesseling, G., Quaedvlieg, F. C. M., and Wouters, E. F. M. (1992). Oscillatory mechanics of the respiratory system in neuromuscular disease. *Chest* 102, 1752–1757. doi:10.1378/chest.102.6.1752

Whitelaw, W. A., Derenne, J.-P., and Milic-Emili, J. (1975). Occlusion pressure as a measure of respiratory center output cm conscious man. *Respir. Physiol.* 23 (2), 181–199. doi:10.1016/0034-5687(75)90059-6

Whitelaw, W. A., and Derenne, J. P. (1993). Airway occlusion pressure. *J. Appl. Physiology* 74, 1475–1483. doi:10.1152/jappl.1993.74.4.1475

Whittenberger, J. L., and Sarnoff, S. J. (1950). Physiologic principles in the treatment of respiratory failure. *Med. Clin. N. Am.* 34, 1335–1362. doi:10.1016/s0025-7125(16)35367-6

Widdicombe, J. G. (1954). Receptors in the trachea and bronchi of the cat. *J. Physiol. Lond.* 123, 71–104. doi:10.1113/jphysiol.1954.sp005034

Wijdicks, E. F. M. (2017). The neurology of acutely failing respiratory mechanics. *Ann. Neurol.* 81 (4), 485–494. doi:10.1002/ana.24908

Won, Y. H., Choi, W. A., Lee, J. W., Bach, J. R., Park, J., and Kang, S.-W. (2016). Sleep transcutaneous vs. end-tidal CO2 monitoring for patients with neuromuscular disease. *Am. J. Phys. Med. Rehabil.* 95 (2), 91–95. doi:10.1097/phm.0000000000000345

Yang, M. L., and Finkel, R. S. (2010). Overview of paediatric neuromuscular disorders and related pulmonary issues: diagnostic and therapeutic considerations. *Paediatr. Respir. Rev.* 11 (1), 9–17. doi:10.1016/j.prrv.2009.10.009

Yap, J. C., Watson, R. A., Gilbey, S., and Pride, N. B. (1995). Effects of posture on respiratory mechanics in obesity. *J. Appl. Physiology* 79, 1199–1205. doi:10.1152/jappl.1995.79.4.1199

Zaloga, G. P. (2002). Aspiration-related illnesses: Definitions and diagnosis. *JPEN J. Parenter. Enter. Nutr.* 26, S2–S8. doi:10.1177/014860710202600602

Zin, W. A., Pengelly, L. D., and Milic-Emili, J. (1983). Decay of inspiratory muscle pressure during expiration in anesthetized cats. *J. Appl. Physiology* 54 (2), 408–413. doi:10.1152/jappl.1983.54.2.408

Permissions

All chapters in this book were first published by Frontiers; hereby published with permission under the Creative Commons Attribution License or equivalent. Every chapter published in this book has been scrutinized by our experts. Their significance has been extensively debated. The topics covered herein carry significant findings which will fuel the growth of the discipline. They may even be implemented as practical applications or may be referred to as a beginning point for another development.

The contributors of this book come from diverse backgrounds, making this book a truly international effort. This book will bring forth new frontiers with its revolutionizing research information and detailed analysis of the nascent developments around the world.

We would like to thank all the contributing authors for lending their expertise to make the book truly unique. They have played a crucial role in the development of this book. Without their invaluable contributions this book wouldn't have been possible. They have made vital efforts to compile up to date information on the varied aspects of this subject to make this book a valuable addition to the collection of many professionals and students.

This book was conceptualized with the vision of imparting up-to-date information and advanced data in this field. To ensure the same, a matchless editorial board was set up. Every individual on the board went through rigorous rounds of assessment to prove their worth. After which they invested a large part of their time researching and compiling the most relevant data for our readers.

The editorial board has been involved in producing this book since its inception. They have spent rigorous hours researching and exploring the diverse topics which have resulted in the successful publishing of this book. They have passed on their knowledge of decades through this book. To expedite this challenging task, the publisher supported the team at every step. A small team of assistant editors was also appointed to further simplify the editing procedure and attain best results for the readers.

Apart from the editorial board, the designing team has also invested a significant amount of their time in understanding the subject and creating the most relevant covers. They scrutinized every image to scout for the most suitable representation of the subject and create an appropriate cover for the book.

The publishing team has been an ardent support to the editorial, designing and production team. Their endless efforts to recruit the best for this project, has resulted in the accomplishment of this book. They are a veteran in the field of academics and their pool of knowledge is as vast as their experience in printing. Their expertise and guidance has proved useful at every step. Their uncompromising quality standards have made this book an exceptional effort. Their encouragement from time to time has been an inspiration for everyone.

The publisher and the editorial board hope that this book will prove to be a valuable piece of knowledge for researchers, students, practitioners and scholars across the globe.

List of Contributors

Rocio J. Jimenez-Valdes, Uryan I. Can and Brian F. Niemeyer
Division of Pulmonary Sciences and Critical Care Medicine, Department of Medicine, University of Colorado Anschutz Medical Campus, Aurora, CO, United States

Kambez H. Benam
Division of Pulmonary Sciences and Critical Care Medicine, Department of Medicine, University of Colorado Anschutz Medical Campus, Aurora, CO, United States
Department of Bioengineering, University of Colorado Denver, Aurora, CO, United States
Linda Crnic Institute for Down Syndrome, University of Colorado Anschutz Medical Campus, Aurora, CO, United States

Arun Lingampally, Matthew R. Jones, Shirisha Bagari, Stefano Rivetti and Saverio Bellusci
Key Laboratory of Interventional Pulmonology of Zhejiang Province, Department of Pulmonary and Critical Care Medicine, First Affiliated Hospital of Wenzhou Medical University, Wenzhou, China
Department of Pulmonary and Critical Care Medicine and Infectious Diseases, Universities of Giessen and Marburg Lung Center (UGMLC), Member of the German Center for Lung Research (DZL), Cardio-Pulmonary Institute, Justus-Liebig University Giessen, Giessen, Germany

Chengshui Chen
Key Laboratory of Interventional Pulmonology of Zhejiang Province, Department of Pulmonary and Critical Care Medicine, First Affiliated Hospital of Wenzhou Medical University, Wenzhou, China

Aylin Cidem
Respiratory Technology, Woolcock Institute of Medical Research, Sydney, NSW

Peta Bradbury, Daniela Traini and Hui Xin Ong
Respiratory Technology, Woolcock Institute of Medical Research, Sydney, NSW, Australia
Faculty of Medicine and Health, University of Sydney, Sydney, NSW, Australia

Cristina García-Mouton, Alberto Hidalgo, Raquel Arroyo, Mercedes Echaide, Antonio Cruz and Jesús Pérez-Gil
Department of Biochemistry and Molecular Biology, Faculty of Biology, Research Institute "Hospital 12 de Octubre (imas12)," Complutense University, Madrid, Spain

Justus C. Horstmann, Patrick Carius and Claus-Michael Lehr
Helmholtz Institute for Pharmaceutical Research Saarland (HIPS), Saarbrücken, Germany
Department of Pharmacy, Saarland University, Saarbrücken, Germany

Chelsea R. Thorn
Clinical and Health Science, University of South Australia, Adelaide, SA, Australia

Florian Graef, Xabier Murgia and Cristiane de Souza Carvalho-Wodarz
Helmholtz Institute for Pharmaceutical Research Saarland (HIPS), Saarbrücken, Germany

Jia-Wei Yang, Ko-Chih Lin, Sheng-Jen Cheng, Shiue-Luen Chen, Chong-You Chen and Shien-Fong Lin
Department of Electrical and Computer Engineering, College of Electrical and Computer Engineering National Chiao Tung University, Hsinchu, Taiwan
Institute of Biomedical Engineering, College of Electrical and Computer Engineering, National Chiao Tung University, Hsinchu, Taiwan

Yu-Chih Shen
Institute of Biomedical Engineering, College of Electrical and Computer Engineering, National Chiao Tung University, Hsinchu, Taiwan
Ph.D. Degree Program of Biomedical Science and Engineering, National Chiao Tung University, Hsinchu, Taiwan

Priyank V. Kumar
School of Chemical Engineering, University of New South Wales, Sydney, NSW, Australia

Huai-En Lu
Bioresource Collection and Research Center, Food Industry Research and Development Institute, Hsinchu, Taiwan

Guan-Yu Chen
Department of Electrical and Computer Engineering, College of Electrical and Computer Engineering National Chiao Tung University, Hsinchu, Taiwan
Institute of Biomedical Engineering, College of Electrical and Computer Engineering, National Chiao Tung University, Hsinchu, Taiwan
Department of Biological Science and Technology, National Chiao Tung University, Hsinchu, Taiwan

Cameron Yamanishi, Eric Parigoris and Shuichi Takayama
Wallace H. Coulter Department of Biomedical Engineering, Georgia Institute of Technology, Atlanta, GA, United States
The Parker H. Petit Institute of Bioengineering and Bioscience, Georgia Institute of Technology, Atlanta, GA, United States

Raphael Brandt and Elena Lopez-Rodriguez
Institute of Functional Anatomy, Charité - Universitätsmedizin Berlin, Berlin, Germany

Sara Timm
Core Facility Electron Microscopy, Charité - Universitätsmedizin Berlin, Berlin, Germany

Jacob L. Gorenflos López and Christian P. R. Hackenberger
Department Chemical Biology, Leibniz-Forschungsinstitut für Molekulare Pharmakologie (FMP), Berlin, Germany
Department of Chemistry, Humboldt Universität zu Berlin, Berlin, Germany

Jubilant Kwame Abledu
Institute of Physiology, Charité-Universitätsmedizin Berlin, Berlin, Germany

Wolfgang M. Kuebler
Institute of Physiology, Charité-Universitätsmedizin Berlin, Berlin, Germany
German Center for Lung Research (DZL), Berlin, Germany

Matthias Ochs
Institute of Functional Anatomy, Charité - Universitätsmedizin Berlin, Berlin, Germany
Core Facility Electron Microscopy, Charité - Universitätsmedizin Berlin, Berlin, Germany
German Center for Lung Research (DZL), Berlin, Germany

Shani Elias-Kirma, Arbel Artzy-Schnirman, Prashant Das, Metar Heller-Algazi, Netanel Korin and Josué Sznitman
Department of Biomedical Engineering, Technion - Israel Institute of Technology, Haifa, Israel

Sandrine Le Guellec
INSERM, Research Center for Respiratory Diseases, U1100, Tours, France
DTF Aerodrug, Tours, France
Université de Tours, Tours, France

Laurine Allimonnier, Nathalie Heuzé-Vourc'h and Maria Cabrera
INSERM, Research Center for Respiratory Diseases, U1100, Tours, France
Université de Tours, Tours, France

Frédéric Ossant
Inserm U1253, Imagerie et Cerveau, Tours, France

Jérémie Pourchez
Mines Saint-Etienne, Univ. Lyon, Univ. Jean Monnet, INSERM, U1059 Sainbiose, Centre CIS, Saint-Etienne, France

Laurent Plantier
INSERM, Research Center for Respiratory Diseases, U1100, Tours, France
Université de Tours, Tours, France
CHRU de Tours, Service de Pneumologie et Explorations Fonctionnelles Respiratoires, Tours, France

Caroline Majoral, Alain Le Pape and Laurent Vecellio
INSERM, Research Center for Respiratory Diseases, Tours, France
Université de Tours, Tours, France

Allan L. Coates
Hospital for Sick Children, Toronto, ON, Canada

Moira L. Aitken, Ranjani Somayaji and Maricela Pier
Department of Medicine, School of Medicine, University of Washington, Seattle, WA, United States

Thomas R. Hinds
Department of Pharmacy, School of Medicine, University of Washington, Seattle, WA, United States

Karla Droguett, Mariana Rios and Manuel Villalon
Department of Physiology, Faculty of Biological Sciences, Pontificia Universidad Católica de Chile, Santiago, Chile

Shawn J. Skerrett
Department of Medicine, School of Medicine, University of Washington, Seattle, WA, United States
Department of Physiology, Faculty of Biological Sciences, Pontificia Universidad Católica de Chile, Santiago, Chile

Barbara Drasler, Bedia Begum Karakocak, Esma Bahar Tankus, Hana Barosova, Mauro Sousa de Almeida and Barbara Rothen-Rutishauser
Institut Adolphe Merkle, Faculté des Sciences et de Médecine, Université de Fribourg, Fribourg, Switzerland

Jun Abe
Department of Oncology, Microbiology and Immunology, Faculty of Science and Medicine, University of Fribourg, Fribourg, Switzerland

Alke Petri-Fink
Institut Adolphe Merkle, Faculté des Sciences et de Médecine, Université de Fribourg, Fribourg, Switzerland
Département de Chimie, Faculté des Sciences et de Médecine, Université de Fribourg, Fribourg, Switzerland

Jarred R. Mondoñedo
Department of Biomedical Engineering, College of Engineering, Boston University, Boston, MA, United States
Boston University School of Medicine, Boston, MA, United States
Elizabeth Bartolák-Suki, Samer Bou Jawde, Kara Nelson, Kun Cao, Walter Patrick Obrochta, Jasmin Imsirovic and Béla Suki
Department of Biomedical Engineering, College of Engineering, Boston University, Boston, MA, United States

Adam Sonnenberg
Department of Systems Engineering, College of Engineering, Boston University, Boston, MA, United States

Sumati Ram-Mohan and Ramaswamy Krishnan
Department of Emergency Medicine, Beth Israel Deaconess Medical Center, Harvard Medical School, Boston, MA, United States

Ali Doryab, Andreas Schröppel, Sezer Orak, Carola Voss, Markus Rehberg, Tobias Stöger and Otmar Schmid
Comprehensive Pneumology Center Munich, Member of the German Center for Lung Research, Munich, Germany
Helmholtz Zentrum München—German Research Center for Environmental Health, Institute of Lung Biology and Disease, Munich, Germany

Mehmet Berat Taskin, Philipp Stahlhut and Jürgen Groll
Department of Functional Materials in Medicine and Dentistry, Bavarian Polymer Institute, University of Würzburg, Würzburg, Germany

Arti Ahluwalia
Research Center "E. Piaggio", University of Pisa, Pisa, Italy
Department of Information Engineering, University of Pisa, Pisa, Italy

Anne Hilgendorff
Comprehensive Pneumology Center Munich, Member of the German Center for Lung Research, Munich, Germany
Helmholtz Zentrum München—German Research Center for Environmental Health, Institute of Lung Biology and Disease, Munich, Germany
Center for Comprehensive Developmental Care (CDeCLMU), Dr. von Haunersches Children's Hospital University, Hospital of the Ludwig-Maximilians University, Munich, Germany

Julia Nemeth, Annika Schundner, Veronika E. Winkelmann and Manfred Frick
Institute of General Physiology, Ulm University, Ulm, Germany

Karsten Quast
Boehringer Ingelheim Pharma GmbH & Co. KG, Biberach, Germany

Mohammed Ali Selo
School of Pharmacy and Pharmaceutical Sciences and Trinity Biomedical Sciences Institute, Trinity College Dublin, Dublin, Ireland
Faculty of Pharmacy, University of Kufa, Al-Najaf, Iraq

Anne-Sophie Delmas, Lisa Springer, Johannes A. Sake, Caoimhe G. Clerkin, Sabrina Nickel and Carsten Ehrhardt
School of Pharmacy and Pharmaceutical Sciences and Trinity Biomedical Sciences Institute, Trinity College Dublin, Dublin, Ireland

Viktoria Zoufal
School of Pharmacy and Pharmaceutical Sciences and Trinity Biomedical Sciences Institute, Trinity College Dublin, Dublin, Ireland
Preclinical Molecular Imaging, AIT Austrian Institute of Technology GmbH, Seibersdorf, Austria

Hanno Huwer
Department of Cardiothoracic Surgery, Völklingen Heart Centre, Völklingen, Germany

Nicole Schneider-Daum
Helmholtz Institute for Pharmaceutical Research Saarland, Helmholtz Centre for Infection Research, Saarbrücken, Germany

Claus-Michael Lehr
Helmholtz Institute for Pharmaceutical Research Saarland, Helmholtz Centre for Infection Research, Saarbrücken, Germany
Department of Pharmacy, Saarland University, Saarbrücken, Germany

Oliver Langer
Preclinical Molecular Imaging, AIT Austrian Institute of Technology GmbH, Seibersdorf, Austria
Department of Clinical Pharmacology, Medical University of Vienna, Vienna, Austria
Division of Nuclear Medicine, Department of Biomedical Imaging and Image-guided Therapy, Medical University of Vienna, Vienna, Austria

Edem Allado, Mathias Poussel and Bruno Chenuel
EA 3450 DevAH-Développement, Adaptation et Handicap, Régulations cardio-respiratoires et de la motricité, Université de Lorraine, Nancy, France
Explorations Fonctionnelles Respiratoires et de l'Aptitude à l'Exercice, Centre Universitaire de Médecine du Sport et Activité Physique Adaptée, CHRU-Nancy, Nancy, France

Simon Valentin
EA 3450 DevAH-Développement, Adaptation et Handicap, Régulations cardio-respiratoires et de la motricité, Université de Lorraine, Nancy, France
Département de Pneumologie, CHRU-Nancy, Nancy, France

Antoine Kimmoun and Bruno Levy
Médecine Intensive et Réanimation Brabois, CHRU-Nancy, Nancy, France
INSERM U1116, Université de Lorraine, Nancy, France

Duc Trung Nguyen
ORL et Chirurgie Cervico-Faciale, CHRU-Nancy, Nancy, France
INSERM U1254-IADI, Université de Lorraine, Nancy, France

Cécile Rumeau
EA 3450 DevAH-Développement, Adaptation et Handicap, Régulations cardio-respiratoires et de la motricité, Université de Lorraine, Nancy, France
ORL et Chirurgie Cervico-Faciale, CHRU-Nancy, Nancy, France

Nina Patel, Kelvin Chong and Ahmet Baydur
Dornsife College of Letters, Arts and Sciences, Division of Pulmonary, Critical Care and Sleep Medicine, Keck School of Medicine and University of Southern California, Los Angeles, CA, United States

Index

www.ingramcontent.com/pod-product-compliance
Lightning Source LLC
LaVergne TN
LVHW082126200926
848484LV00008B/2014